Improving Functional Outcomes in Physical Rehabilitation,

Second Edition

Improving Functional Outcomes in Physical Rehabilitation,

Second Edition

SUSAN B. O'SULLIVAN, PT, EdD
Professor Emerita
Department of Physical Therapy
College of Health Sciences
University of Massachusetts Lowell
Lowell, Massachusetts

THOMAS J. SCHMITZ, PT, PhD
Professor Emeritus
Department of Physical Therapy
School of Health Professions
Long Island University
Brooklyn Campus
Brooklyn, New York

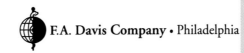

F.A. Davis Company • Philadelphia

F. A. Davis Company
1915 Arch Street
Philadelphia, PA 19103
www.fadavis.com

Printed in the United States of America

Last digit indicates print number: 10 9 8 7 6 5 4 3 2 1

Senior Acquisitions Editor: Melissa Duffield
Developmental Editor: Molly Ward
Director of Content Development: George Lang
Art and Design Manager: Carolyn O'Brien

As new scientific information becomes available through basic and clinical research, recommended treatments and drug therapies undergo changes. The author(s) and publisher have done everything possible to make this book accurate, up to date, and in accord with accepted standards at the time of publication. The author(s), editors, and publisher are not responsible for errors or omissions or for consequences from application of the book, and make no warranty, expressed or implied, in regard to the contents of the book. Any practice described in this book should be applied by the reader in accordance with professional standards of care used in regard to the unique circumstances that may apply in each situation. The reader is advised always to check product information (package inserts) for changes and new information regarding dose and contraindications before administering any drug. Caution is especially urged when using new or infrequently ordered drugs.

Library of Congress Cataloging-in-Publication Data

Names: O'Sullivan, Susan B., author. | Schmitz, Thomas J., author.
Title: Improving functional outcomes in physical rehabilitation / Susan B.
  O'Sullivan, Thomas J. Schmitz.
Description: Second edition. | Philadelphia : F.A. Davis Company, [2016] |
  Includes bibliographical references and index.
Identifiers: LCCN 2015049619 | ISBN 9780803646124
Subjects: | MESH: Physical Therapy Modalities | Treatment Outcome | Case
  Reports
Classification: LCC RM700 | NLM WB 460 | DDC 615.8/2—dc23 LC record available at http://lccn.loc.gov/2015049619

PREFACE

Our goal is to present an integrated model of therapeutic intervention applicable to a wide spectrum of adult patients engaged in physical rehabilitation. Part I, Promoting Function, first addresses the foundations of clinical decision-making and provides a conceptual framework for improving functional outcomes. The organization of content provides the student a logical learning progression of interventions used to improve motor function, with an emphasis on task-specific, motor learning, and neuromotor strategies (Chapters 1 and 2). Chapter 3 presents an overview of Proprioceptive Neuromuscular Facilitation. Chapters 4 through 13 then present strategies and interventions within the context of functional skills critical to independent function and optimal rehabilitation outcomes. Each chapter includes descriptions of suggested interventions accompanied by a discussion of lead-up skills and progressions. Also provided are descriptions of patient outcomes consistent with the American Physical Therapy Association's *Guide to Physical Therapist Practice,* together with clinical applications and patient examples. The interventions presented address many types of impairments and activity limitations that patients may exhibit across practice patterns. They should not be considered as practice pattern-specific but rather specific to the physical therapy *diagnosis* and *plan of care.* Our goal is to provide useful, practical examples of interventions that can be used to enhance functional performance.

Part II presents 15 case studies in narrative form. In addition, each case study includes an accompanying video addressing selected elements of the physical therapy plan of care available online at Davis*Plus* (www.fadavis.com). An outstanding group of clinicians from across the country have provided examples of patient management strategies based on effective clinical decision-making for patients with a variety of diagnoses, among them are traumatic brain injury, stroke, Parkinson's disease, cerebellar glioblastoma, Guillain Barré syndrome, peripheral vestibular dysfunction, spinal cord injury, and transfemoral amputation. The guiding questions included with each case study are designed to enhance clinical decision-making and to challenge the student to address the unique needs of the individual patients presented. The video captures each patient at three critical points within the episode of care: (1) at the initial examination, (2) during a treatment session, and (3) at discharge from physical therapy intervention. Our hope is that the case studies will facilitate meaningful dialogue between and among physical therapy students and faculty.

The text utilizes several pedagogical applications. Important information is emphasized using boxes and tables for easy reference. Key terms appear in *boldface italic* font in blue ink and are defined in the text. The *Red Flag* feature alerts the student to precautions or preventative safety measures. The *Clinical Note* feature provides additional insights based on clinical observations. Chapters in Part I include group Student Practice Activities to enhance learning. These activities provide an opportunity to share knowledge and skills with student peers and to confirm or clarify the student's understanding of the interventions. Each student in a group is encouraged to contribute his or her understanding of, or questions about, the technique or treatment activity being discussed and demonstrated. Dialogue should continue until a consensus of understanding is reached.

The case studies in Part II conclude with guiding questions designed to enhance students' critical thinking skills. Answers to the guiding questions for Case Studies 1 through 10 are provided to students (and instructors) online at Davis*Plus* (www.fadavis.com). Answers to the guiding questions for Case Studies 11 through 15 are provided only to instructors online at Davis*Plus* (www.fadavis.com). The intention of selected answer availability for Case Studies 11 through 15 is to provide faculty greater options for incorporating case materials into course assignments, laboratory activities, and group discussions. Student feedback to the guiding questions based on the answers developed by the case study contributors can be obtained from the course instructor(s).

The text recognizes the continuing growth of the profession and the importance of basic and applied clinical research in guiding and informing evidence-based practice. It also integrates terminology and interventions presented in the *Guide to Physical Therapist Practice.*

Our greatest hope is that this text enhances students' understanding of strategies to improve functional outcomes that lead to independence and ultimately an improved quality of life for our patients.

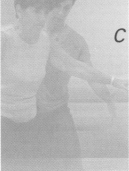

CONTRIBUTING AUTHORS

Edward William Bezkor, PT, DPT, OCS, MTC
Faculty, Doctor of Physical Therapy Program
San Diego State University School of Exercise &
    Nutritional Sciences, San Diego, California
Physical Therapist
University of California, San Diego Health System,
    Perlman Clinic, Rehabilitation Services, La Jolla,
    California
Faculty, Professional Doctorate Program
Pacific College of Oriental Medicine, Mission Valley,
    California

Cristiana K. Collins, PT, PhD, CFMT, NCS
Assistant Professor
Physical Therapy Department, Long Island University,
    Brooklyn, New York

George D. Fulk, PT, PhD
Chair and Associate Professor
Department of Physical Therapy, Clarkson University,
    Center for Health Sciences, Potsdam, New York

Sharon A. Gutman, PhD, OTR
Associate Professor
Programs in Occupational Therapy, Columbia University,
    New York, New York

Jennifer Hastings, PT, PhD, NCS
Professor and Director
School of Physical Therapy, University of Puget Sound,
    Tacoma, Washington

JoAnn Moriarty-Baron, PT, DPT
Instructor
Department of Physical Therapy, University of
    Massachusetts Lowell, Lowell, Massachusetts

David M. Morris, PT, PhD
Associate Professor
Department of Physical Therapy, University of Alabama at
    Birmingham, Birmingham, Alabama

Marianne H. Mortera, PhD, OTR
Assistant Professor of Clinical Occupational Therapy
Programs in Occupational Therapy, Columbia University,
    New York, New York

Coby Nirider, PT, DPT
Area Director of Therapy Services
Touchstone Neurorecovery Center, Conroe, Texas

Susan B. O'Sullivan, PT, EdD
Professor Emerita
Department of Physical Therapy, School of Health and
    Environment, University of Massachusetts Lowell,
    Lowell, Massachusetts

Vicky Saliba Johnson, PT, FFFMT, FAAOMPT
President
Institute of Physical Art, Inc.
Director
Functional Manual Therapy Foundation
Director
FMTF Orthopedic Residency
Steamboat Springs, Colorado

Thomas J. Schmitz, PT, PhD
Professor Emeritus
Department of Physical Therapy, School of Health
    Professions, Long Island University, Brooklyn,
    New York

Edward Taub, PhD
University Professor
Director CI Therapy Research Group and Taub Training
    Clinic, Department of Psychology, University of
    Alabama at Birmingham, Birmingham, Alabama

CASE STUDY CONTRIBUTORS

CASE STUDY 1. Patient With Traumatic Brain Injury

Temple T. Cowden, PT, MPT
Adult Brain Injury Service
Rancho Los Amigos National Rehabilitation Center,
Downey, California

CASE STUDY 2. Patient With Traumatic Brain Injury: Balance and Locomotor Training

Heidi Roth, PT, MSPT, NCS
Research and Clinical Physical Therapist
Rehabilitation Institute of Chicago, Chicago, Illinois

Jason Barbas, PT, MPT, NCS
Outpatient Rehabilitation
Rehabilitation Institute of Chicago, Chicago, Illinois

CASE STUDY 3. Patient With Incomplete Spinal Cord Injury, T4: Locomotor Training

Elizabeth Ardolino, PT, MS
Magee Rehabilitation Center
Philadelphia, Pennsylvania

Elizabeth Watson, PT, DPT, NCS
Magee Rehabilitation Center
Philadelphia, Pennsylvania

Andrea L. Behrman, PT, PhD
Associate Professor
College of Public Health and Health Professions
University of Florida
Department of Physical Therapy
Gainesville, Florida

Susan Harkema, PhD
Associate Professor
Department of Neurological Surgery
University of Louisville
Louisville, Kentucky
Owsley B. Frazier Chair in Neurological Rehabilitation
Rehabilitation Research Director
Kentucky Spinal Cord Injury Research Center
Louisville, Kentucky
Research Director
Frazier Rehab Institute
Louisville, Kentucky
Director of the NeuroRecovery Network
Louisville, Kentucky

Mary Schmidt-Read, PT, DPT, MS
Magee Rehabilitation Center
Philadelphia, Pennsylvania

CASE STUDY 4. Patient With Stroke: Home Care Rehabilitation

Lynn Wong, PT, DPT, MS, GCS
Caritas Home Care, Methuen, Massachusetts

CASE STUDY 5. Patient With Stroke: Constraint-Induced Movement Therapy

David M. Morris, PT, PhD
Professor, Department of Physical Therapy
University of Alabama at Birmingham, Birmingham,
Alabama

Sonya L. Pearson, PT, DPT
University of Alabama at Birmingham, Birmingham,
Alabama

Edward Taub, PhD
University Professor
Director CI Therapy Research Group and Taub Training
    Clinic
Department of Psychology, University of Alabama at
    Birmingham
Birmingham, Alabama

CASE STUDY 6. Patient With Parkinson's Disease

Edward William Bezkor, PT, DPT, OCS, MTC
Faculty, Doctor of Physical Therapy Program
San Diego State University
School of Exercise & Nutritional Sciences
San Diego, California
Physical Therapist
University of California, San Diego Health System
Perlman Clinic, Rehabilitation Services
La Jolla, California
Faculty, Professional Doctorate Program
Pacific College of Oriental Medicine
Mission Valley, California
Filmed at Rusk Institute of Rehabilitation Medicine
New York, New York

CASE STUDY 7. Patient With Complete Spinal Cord Injury, T9

Paula Ackerman, MS, OTR/L
Shepherd Center, Inc.
Atlanta, Georgia

Myrtice Atrice, BS, PT
Shepherd Center, Inc.
Atlanta, Georgia

Teresa Foy, BS, OTR/L
Shepherd Center, Inc.
Atlanta, Georgia

Sarah Morrison, BS, PT
SCI Program Director
Shepherd Center, Inc.
Atlanta, Georgia

Polly Hopkins, MOTR/L
Shepherd Center, Inc.
Atlanta, Georgia

Shari McDowell, BS, PT
Shepherd Center, Inc.
Atlanta, Georgia

CASE STUDY 8. Patient With Incomplete Spinal Cord Injury, C7

Maria Stelmach, PT, DPT, NCS
Clinical Specialist/Physical Therapist
NYU Langone Medical Center
Rusk Institute for Rehabilitation
New York, New York

Sophie Benoist, PT, DPT
NYU Langone Medical Center
Rusk Institute for Rehabilitation
New York, New York

CASE STUDY 9. Patient With Peripheral Vestibular Dysfunction

JoAnn Moriarty-Baron, PT, DPT
Instructor
Department of Physical Therapy
University of Massachusetts Lowell
Lowell, Massachusetts
Filmed at Southern New Hampshire Rehabilitation Center
Nashua, New Hampshire

CASE STUDY 10. Patient With Complete Spinal Cord Injury, T10

Darrell Musick, PT
Director of Physical Therapy
Craig Hospital
Englewood, Colorado

Laura S. Wehrli, PT, DPT, ATP
Craig Hospital
Englewood, Colorado

CASE STUDY 11. Patient With Cerebellar Glioblastoma

Catherine Printz, PT, DPT, NCS
Physical Therapist
University of California San Diego Medical Center
Thornton Hospital
San Diego, California

Melissa S. Doyle, PT, DPT, NCS
Physical Therapist
University of California San Diego Medical Center
Thornton Hospital
San Diego, California

Carter McElroy, PT, MPT
Physical Therapist
University of California San Diego Medical Center
Thornton Hospital
San Diego, California

CASE STUDY 12. Patient With Guillain Barré Syndrome and Tetraplegia

Kate Rough, PT, DPT, NCS
University of Washington Medical Center
Seattle, Washington

Victoria Stevens PT, NCS
Neuroclinical Specialist
University of Washington Medical Center
Seattle, Washington

Stacia Lee, PT, NCS
Physical Therapy Manager
University of Washington Medical Center
Seattle, Washington

Katie R. Sweet, PT, DPT
Physical Therapist
University of Washington Medical Center

CASE STUDY 13. Patient With Stroke

Lauren Snowdon, PT, DPT
Clinical Manager, Inpatient Physical Therapy
Kessler Institute for Rehabilitation, West Orange, New Jersey

CASE STUDY 14. Patient With Motor Incomplete Spinal Cord Injury, C4

Sally M. Taylor, PT, DPT, NCS
Allied Health Manager/Physical Therapist
Rehabilitation Institute of Chicago
Chicago, Illinois

CASE STUDY 15. Patient With Transfemoral Amputation

Kyla L. Dunlavey, PT, MPT, OCS
Walter Reed National Military Medical Center
Bethesda, Maryland

Barri L. Schnall, PT, MPT
Biomechanics Lab Clinical Research Specialist
Walter Reed National Military Medical Center
Bethesda, Maryland

ACKNOWLEDGMENTS

Improving Functional Outcomes in Physical Rehabilitation is a product of our combined years of experience in both clinical practice and teaching physical therapy students. From the outset, it has been a collaborative venture, bringing together a talented group of contributing authors from both academic and clinical practice settings. Without question, the text has benefited enormously from their participation. Their willingness to share their expertise as well as their interest in the professional development of physical therapy students was continually evident throughout project development. We are honored by their participation in the project. The breadth and scope of their professional knowledge and expertise are well reflected in their contributions. We extend heartfelt gratitude to the outstanding authors who contributed to the chapters and the expert clinicians and educators who contributed case studies.

We convey our gratitude to the following individuals who contributed their exceptional skills to create the numerous figures used throughout the text: Mitchell Shuldman, EdD, Librarian and Director of Media Services, University of Massachusetts Lowell, Lowell, Massachusetts; Paul Coppens, former Director of Media Services, University of Massachusetts Lowell, Lowell, Massachusetts; Christopher F. Lenney, University Photographer, Clarkson University, Potsdam, New York; Jason Torres, N.Y. Vintage Cameraworks, Ltd., Poughkeepsie, New York; Mark Lozier, Mark Lozier Photography, Cherry Hill, New Jersey; Lauray MacElhern, MBA, Center for Integrative Medicine, University of California San Diego; Kerry A. McCullough, PT, DPT, University of California San Diego Health System, San Diego, California; and Sara Beck-Pancer, Pacific College of Oriental Medicine, San Diego, California.

We are indebted to the generous models who cordially posed for photographs. For their gracious time commitment, belief in the importance of the project, and unfailing patience, we recognize Carole A. Remsay, Leonore Gordon, Joseph Lerner, Emmanuel R. Torrijos, Cynthia Gilbertson, Eric Bell, Stacie Caldwell, Natasha Chevalier-Richards, Paul Colbert, Aaron Hastings, Sally Healy, Emma Larson, Joel Lindstrom, Laura MacElhern, Philomena (Mini) G. Mungiole, Whitney Odle, Natalie Pieczynski, Robert Margeson, Sr., Celso Marquez, Khushbu Shah, J. Anthony Tomaszewski, Catherine Wright, and Mitchell Young. We also thank those who assisted in locating photography subjects and equipment: Cristiana K. Collins, PT, PhD, CFMT, NCS, Long Island University; Stephen Carp, PT, PhD, GCS, Temple University; Robin Dole, PT, EdD, PCS, Widener University; and Tom Weis, Long Island University.

For her patience and competent attention to detail, we extend our gratitude to Molly Mullen Ward, Developmental Editor. Our thanks also go to those who contributed to the production and editing of the case study videos that accompany the text: Mitchell Shuldman, EdD, Librarian and Head, Division of Media Services, University of Massachusetts Lowell, Lowell, Massachusetts; and Rob Kates at Kates Media.

We extend our appreciation to the dedicated professionals at F. A. Davis Company, Philadelphia, Pennsylvania: Margaret M. Biblis, Publisher; Melissa A. Duffield, Senior Acquisitions Editor; George W. Lang, Director of Content Development; Kirk Pedrick, Manager of Electronic Product Development; Carolyn O'Brien, Art and Design Manager; and Nichole Liccio, Editorial Assistant Health Professions and Medicine. Their continued support, encouragement, and unwavering commitment to excellence have contributed significantly to the development of this text as well as to the expansion of the physical therapy literature. Our appreciation is considerable.

Last, although hardly least, we wish to thank our students and patients who continually challenge us to improve our teaching and clinical skills. It is our sincere hope that this text proves to be a valuable resource in the development of clinical decision-making and practice skills of aspiring professionals.

Susan B. O'Sullivan
Thomas J. Schmitz

TABLE OF CONTENTS

Promoting Function

Part 1, Promoting Function, introduces the reader to foundational elements of patient care in terms of clinical decision-making and developing an appropriate, effective plan of care, then expands on those elements with chapters that specifically address key motor functions.

Chapter 1, Framework for Clinical Decision-Making and Client Management, provides the foundational context for clinical decision-making. It addresses the International Classification of Functioning, Disability, and Health model as the basis for planning. Chapter 1 presents a brief overview of motor control and motor learning and considers strategies to examine motor function. The chapter is organized around the characteristics of three critical elements for planning: the task, the individual, and the environment. The major focus of Chapter 2, Interventions to Improve Motor Function, is to help the learner acquire a conceptual framework for developing a comprehensive plan of care to improve functional outcomes. It directs attention to the components of task analysis and progresses to a discussion of task-oriented, activity-based strategies as the foundation of intervention. Motor learning strategies are organized and discussed according to stages of motor learning.

Chapters 3 through 13 present strategies and interventions to promote enhanced motor function and independence in key functional skills. The interventions presented in these chapters include descriptions of the general characteristics of each activity (e.g., base of support provided, location of center of mass, impact of gravity and body weight) and descriptions of required lead-up skills, appropriate interventions, and progressions. The chapters describe patient outcomes consistent with the *Guide to Physical Therapist Practice,*[1] clinical applications, and patient examples. The student practice activities included here enhance student learning.

The chapters are organized around a broad range of postures and activities required for normal human function (e.g., functional mobility skills, basic and instrumental activities of daily living). Postures and activities such as rolling and side-lying are presented first, with progression through upright

(text continues on page 2)

PART

I

standing and locomotion. Although the content is presented as a sequence from dependent to independent postures and activities, it should not be viewed as a "lock-step" progression. This means there are no absolute requirements for how the activities are sequenced or integrated into an individual plan of care. The sequencing presented has several implications for clinical practice:

- It will be the exception, rather than the norm, for an individual patient to require or benefit from the entire sequence of interventions presented.
- Evaluation of examination data will guide selection and sequencing of interventions for an individual patient.
- Interventions may be organized in a different sequence, used concurrently, expanded, or eliminated (i.e., deemed inappropriate) when developing a plan of care.
- The content should be viewed and used as a source of treatment ideas based on the desired functional outcome and not as a prescribed sequence. For example, if a patient requires improved core (trunk) strength or increased ankle range of motion, consideration is given to those strategies and interventions designed to address the specific impairments.
- The interventions include suggested therapist *positioning* and *hand placements*. These suggestions reflect effective strategies for applying assistance or resistance and maintaining appropriate and safe body mechanics. Again, these are not intended to be prescriptive; multiple factors influence selection of hand placements and therapist positioning. Although not an inclusive list of factors, several examples include: specific movement components at which the intervention is directed, height and size of the treatment surface, desired outcomes, type and severity of impairments and activity limitations, characteristics of the patient (e.g., height, weight, and size of individual body segments), and the physical therapist's body size and type.

Finally, the interventions address many types of impairments and activity limitations across practice patterns. They should not be considered practice pattern specific but rather specific to the physical therapy *diagnosis* and *plan of care.*

[1]American Physical Therapy Association. *Guide to Physical Therapist Practice*, Version 3.0. Alexandria, VA, APA, 2014. Retrieved September 9, 2014, from http://guidetoptpractice.apta.org.

Framework for Clinical Decision-Making and Patient Management

SUSAN B. O'SULLIVAN, PT, EdD

Optimal functional recovery is the primary goal of all rehabilitation. Although people have traditionally been identified or categorized by their disease or medical condition (e.g., spinal cord injury [SCI]), the World Health Organization's *International Classification of Functioning, Disability, and Health* (ICF) model[1] provides an important framework for examining and treating the patient by clearly defining health condition, impairment, activity limitation, and participation restriction. The American Physical Therapy Association in its *Guide to Physical Therapist Practice, Version 3.0*, has adopted this framework.[2] Thus the patient with SCI presents with paralysis; sensory loss; autonomic dysfunction (impairments); loss of independent function in bed mobility, dressing, bathing, and locomotion (activity limitations); and an inability to work or go to school (participation restrictions). Physical therapist practice intervenes primarily at the level of impairments, activity limitations, and participation restrictions. Effective clinical decision-making is based on an understanding of the ICF model and related contextual factors (environmental and personal factors) to arrive at effective choices for intervention. In addition, clinicians must understand factors that improve quality of life, prevention, wellness, and fitness. An effective plan of care (POC) clarifies risk factors and seeks to fully involve the patient in determining meaningful functional goals. This text focuses on improving motor function (motor control and motor learning) and muscle performance (strength, power, and endurance) through activities and exercises that optimize functional outcomes. Definitions of terminology of functioning, disability, and health are presented in Box 1.1.

An effective POC is based on the concept that normal motor function emerges from the practice of activity-based tasks. A successful POC uses a logical, sequential progression in terms of increasing difficulty. In general, the patient learns to control increasingly larger segments of the body simultaneously with gradual increases in the effects of gravity and body weight. Thus, during the progression of activities, the base of support (BOS) is gradually narrowed while the center of mass (COM) is elevated, increasing the demands on postural control and balance. Activity-based training helps the patient develop motor skills using synergistic patterns of muscles with movements that occur in multiple axes and planes of movement. Different types and combinations of muscle contractions (concentric, eccentric, isometric) are utilized. The types and variations of contractions used more closely represent the work muscles typically do during the execution of daily activities as compared to those trained using other methods, such as progressive resistance exercise. Somatosensory, vestibular, and visual inputs from the body assist in movement control and balance. Owing to the inherent use of body weight and gravity, enhanced demands for postural control are placed on the trunk and limb segments during performance. Activity-based training activities are complex movements in which the primary focus is coordinated action, not isolated muscle or joint control.

The key to successful intervention is a thorough understanding of the patient through processes of examination, evaluation, diagnosis, and prognosis to develop the POC.[2] Foundational concepts discussed in this chapter include understanding the task, the patient's performance capabilities, and the environment (Fig. 1.1).

Foundational Concepts

Motor Control

The foundational underlying theories on which motor function is based include *motor control* and *motor learning theory*. *Systems theory* describes motor function as the result of a series of interacting systems that contribute to different aspects of control. For example, the musculoskeletal system, the sensory system, and the neural control systems (synergistic control, coordination, and balance) all contribute to the movements produced. *Motor programming theory* is based on the concept of a *motor program*, which is defined as an abstract code that, when initiated, produces a coordinated movement sequence. Thus movement patterns are stored and can be initiated using preprogrammed instructions without peripheral inputs or feedback information (termed an *open-loop system*). Movement patterns can also be initiated and modified using sensory inputs and feedback information (termed a *closed-loop system*). In a closed-loop system, feedback is used to detect errors and to modify the movement responses, as seen when learning a new skill.

BOX 1.1 Terminology: Functioning, Disability, and Health

From World Health Organization's *International Classification of Functioning, Disability, and Health*[1]
Health condition is an umbrella term for disease, disorder, injury, or trauma and may also include other circumstances, such as aging, stress, congenital anomaly, or genetic predisposition. It may also include information about pathogeneses and/or etiology.
Body functions are physiological functions of body systems (including psychological functions).
Body structures are anatomical parts of the body such as organs, limbs, and their components.
Impairments are the problems in body function or structure such as a significant deviation or loss.
Activity is the execution of a task or action by an individual.
Participation is involvement in a life situation.
Activity limitations are difficulties an individual may have in executing activities.
Participation restrictions are problems an individual may experience in involvement in life situations.
Contextual factors represent the entire background of an individual's life and living situation.

- **Environmental factors** make up the physical, social, and attitudinal environment in which people live and conduct their lives, including social attitudes, architectural characteristics, and legal and social structures.
- **Personal factors** are the particular background of an individual's life, including gender, age, coping styles, social background, education, profession, past and current experience, overall behavior pattern,

character, and other factors that influence how disability is experienced by an individual.
Performance describes what an individual does in his or her current environment.
Capacity describes an individual's ability to execute a task or an action (highest probable level of functioning in a given domain at a given moment).

From *Guide to Physical Therapist Practice, 3.0*[2]
Pathology/pathophysiology (disease, disorder, condition) describes an abnormality characterized by a particular cluster of signs and symptoms and recognized by either the patient/client or the practitioner as abnormal. It is primarily identified at the cellular level.
Impairment is the loss or abnormality of anatomical, physiological, mental, or psychological structure or function.
Functional limitation is the restriction of the ability to perform, at the level of the whole person, a physical action, task, or activity in an efficient, typically expected, or competent manner.
Disability is the inability to perform or a limitation in the performance of actions, tasks, and activities usually expected in specific social roles that are customary for the individual or expected for the person's status or role in a specific sociocultural context and physical environment. Categories are self-care, home management, work (job/school/play), and community/leisure.
Health status describes the state or status of the conditions that constitute good health.

TASK ⇔	**INDIVIDUAL** ⇔	**ENVIRONMENT**
Functions: BADL, IADL	Arousal, Attention	Physical Environment
Attributes:	Cognition, Motivation	Variability
Mobility	Sensory-Perceptual Integrity	Regulatory Features
Stability	Muscle Strength, Motor Function	Psychosocial Factors
Controlled Mobility	Posture, ROM, Flexibility	
Skill	Gait, Locomotion, Balance	
Characteristics:	Aerobic Capacity/Endurance	
Velocity	Comorbidities, Complications	
Amplitude	Activity Limitations	
	Disability	
	Overall Health Status	

MOTOR FUNCTION

FIGURE 1.1 Motor function emerges from interactions among the task, the person, and the environment.
BADL, basic activities of daily living; IADL, instrumental activities of daily living; ROM, range of motion.

Motor learning theory is based on concepts of feedback and practice that are used to influence the type and degree of learning and lead to relatively permanent changes in performance capabilities. Use of appropriate motor learning strategies (discussed under Motor Learning Strategies in Chapter 2) enhances motor skill acquisition. Organized practice schedules and appropriate feedback delivery are essential elements. Motor control terminology is presented in Box 1.2. For a thorough review of these concepts, the reader is referred to the excellent works of Schmidt and Lee[3] and Shumway-Cook and Woollacott.[4]

The acquisition of motor skills in infants and children that are critical to independent function (such as rolling over, sitting up, sitting, crawling, kneeling, standing up, standing, walking, and eye-hand coordination) is a function of neuromuscular maturation and practice. These activities, sometimes termed *developmental skills* or *developmental sequence skills,* form the basis of a set of skills needed for lifelong independent function. Motor milestones that emerge at somewhat predictable ages mark motor control development in the infant and child. Development generally progresses from head to foot (cephalo-caudal) and proximal to distal. In infants and children, motor function development is viewed as a spiral progression with considerable variability, not as a strict linear progression. Primitive and static attitudinal reflexes become integrated as the central nervous system (CNS)

matures and higher-level postural reactions (e.g., righting and equilibrium reactions) and postural synergies emerge. Emerging motor behaviors depend on practice and the maturation and function of different system components during critical stages in development.

In the adult, the motor skills acquired early in life are maintained, adapted, and remain relatively stable across the life span. Skills such as rolling over and sitting up are used every day as a normal part of life. However, these movement patterns are responsive to change and can be modified by a number of different factors. Primary factors include overall health and activity levels. Changes are also associated with aging causing a decline in overall function of the CNS, including sensory decline in visual, somatosensory, and vestibular functions; changes in synergistic control of movement and timing; and a decline in balance. Secondary and potentially modifiable factors include changing body dimensions (changes in body weight, body shape and topography, and posture), level of physical activity (changes in muscle strength, flexibility, and range of motion [ROM] associated with inactivity), nutrition, and environmental factors. The physically frail older adult and the physically dependent person will likely demonstrate the greatest changes in basic motor skills. The CNS's ability for ongoing reorganization of motor skills is lifelong. As in infants and children, no one predictable pattern of movement to accomplish functional goals characterizes all adults or older adults.[5,6]

> **BOX 1.2** Terminology: Motor Control

Degrees of freedom: the number of separate independent dimensions of movement in a system that must be controlled[4(p463)]

Motor control: the underlying substrates of neural, physical, and behavioral aspects of movement

- **Reactive motor control:** Movements are adapted in response to ongoing feedback (e.g., muscle stretch causes an increase in muscle contraction in response to a forward weight shift).
- **Proactive (anticipatory) motor control:** Movements are adapted in advance of ongoing movements via feedforward mechanisms (e.g., the postural adjustments made in preparation for catching a heavy, large ball).

Motor plan: an idea or plan for purposeful movement that is made up of component motor programs

Motor program: an abstract representation that, when initiated, results in the production of a coordinated movement sequence[3(p497)]

Motor learning: a set of internal processes associated with feedback or practice leading to relatively permanent changes in the capability for motor skill[3(p497)]

Motor recovery: the reacquisition of movement skills lost through injury

Schema: a set of rules, concepts, or relationships formed on the basis of experience[3(p499)]; schema serve to provide a basis for movement decisions and are stored in memory for the reproduction of movement

- **Recall schema:** the relationship among past parameters, past initial conditions, and the movement outcomes produced by these combinations
- **Recognition schema:** the relationship among past initial conditions, past movement outcomes, and the sensory consequences produced by these combinations

Task analysis: a process of determining the underlying abilities and structure of a task or occupation[3(p500)]

Task organization: how the components of a task are interrelated or interdependent

- **Low organization:** Task components are relatively independent.
- **High organization:** Task components are highly interrelated.

Motor Recovery

In the adult patient with activity limitations and participation restrictions, motor skills are modified in the presence of musculoskeletal, neuromuscular, cardiorespiratory, integumentary, and/or cognitive impairments. *Motor recovery,* the reacquisition of movement skills lost through injury, is highly variable and individualized. Complete recovery, in which the performance of reacquired skills is identical in every way to preinjury performance, may not be possible. Rather, it is likely that the preinjury skills are modified in some way. For example, the patient with stroke regains walking ability but now walks with a slowed gait and increased hip and knee flexion on the more affected side. *Motor compensation* is defined as performance of an old movement in a new manner. This can be achieved through adaptive compensation (using alternative motor patterns to accomplish a task) or behavioral substitution (using alternate body segments or effectors to accomplish a task). For example, the patient with stroke learns to dress independently using the less affected upper extremity (UE). Or the patient with a complete T1 SCI learns to roll using both UEs and momentum. *Spontaneous recovery* refers to the restoration of function in neural tissues initially lost after injury, resulting from naturally occurring repair processes within the CNS. For example, the patient with stroke regains some motor function approximately 2 to 3 weeks after insult as cerebral edema resolves. *Function-induced recovery* (use-dependent cortical reorganization) refers to the nervous system's ability to modify itself in response to changes in activity and the environment.[7] Stimulation early after injury is important to prevent *learned nonuse.*[8] This behavioral learned response to paresis associated with preferential use of less affected limbs can interfere with recovery from neurological insult.[6] For example, the patient with stroke who undergoes limited rehabilitation learns to use the less affected extremities to achieve functional goals and fails to use the more affected extremities. For later rehabilitation to be successful, these faulty patterns must be unlearned while patterns that incorporate the more involved side are recruited. Early exposure to training can prevent learned nonuse and the development of faulty or poor motor patterns. There is ample evidence that training is also effective for patients with chronic disability. For example, patients with stroke for more than 1 year respond positively to functional task-oriented training using constraint-induced (CI) movement therapy (see Chapter 12: Constraint-Induced Movement Therapy and Case Study 5). Locomotor training using partial body weight support, a treadmill, and early assisted limb movements has also been shown to promote function-induced recovery (see Chapter 10: Interventions to Improve Locomotor Skills and Case Study 3). The elements essential for success with these interventions are that (1) practice is task specific and (2) practice is intense, with steady increases in duration and frequency. For example, in CI therapy, the patient with stroke practices grasping and manipulating objects during daily tasks using the more affected UE 4 to 6 hours per day, every day. The less-affected UE may be constrained with a mitt, thereby preventing all attempts at compensatory movements. Box 1.3 presents terminology related to motor recovery and neuroplasticity.

Motor Learning

Motor learning is a complex process that requires spatial, temporal, and hierarchical organization within the CNS that allows for acquisition and modification of movement. As mentioned earlier, changes in the CNS are not directly observable but rather are inferred from improvement

---

BOX 1.3 Terminology: Motor Recovery and Neuroplasticity[5]

Function-induced recovery: the restoration of the ability to perform a movement in the same or similar manner as it was performed before the injury; use-dependent cortical reorganization occurring in response to changes in activity and the environment

Learned nonuse: a behavioral learned response to paresis associated with preferential use of unaffected limbs; can interfere with recovery from neurological insult

Motor compensation: performance of an old movement in a new manner[a]

- **Adaptive compensation:** appearance of alternative motor patterns during the accomplishment of a task[b]

- **Substitutive compensation:** successful task accomplishment using alternative body segments or motor elements[b]

Motor recovery: restoration of the ability to perform a movement in the same manner as it was performed before injury[a]; successful task accomplishment using limbs or end effectors typically used by nondisabled people[b]

Neuroplasticity: the brain's ability to change and repair itself

Spontaneous recovery: restoration of function in neural tissue initially lost after injury, resulting from naturally occurring repair processes within the CNS

[a]Level of human functioning as classified by the ICF model: Body Functions/Structure (performance)[1]

[b]Level of human functioning as classified by the ICF model: activity (functional)[1]

in performance as a result of practice or experience. Individual differences in learning are expected and influence both the rate and degree of learning possible. Motor learning abilities vary across three main foundational categories: cognitive ability, perceptual speed ability, and psychomotor ability. Differences occur as a result of both genetics and experience. The therapist should be sensitive to such factors as alertness, anxiety, memory, speed of processing information, speed and accuracy of movements, uniqueness of the setting, and environment. In addition, recovering patients may vary in their learning potential according to the pathology present, the number and type of impairments, recovery potential, general health status, and comorbidities. Although most skills can be learned through practice or experience, the therapist should be sensitive to the patient's underlying capabilities (abilities) that support certain skills. For example, some patients with SCI may not be able to learn to manage curbs using "wheelies" because of the difficulty of the task, their residual abilities, and general health status.

Stages of Motor Learning

Fitts and Posner[9] described three main stages in learning a motor skill. Their model provides a useful framework for examining and developing strategies to improve motor learning and is used here in this work (see Chapter 2, Table 2.2, Characteristics of Stages of Motor Learning and Training Strategies).

Cognitive Stage

In the early *cognitive stage,* the learner develops an understanding of the task. During practice, *cognitive mapping* allows the learner to assess abilities and task demands, identify relevant and important stimuli, and develop an initial movement strategy (motor program) based on explicit memory of prior movement experiences. The learner performs initial practice of the task and retains some strategies while discarding others to develop an initial movement strategy. During successive practice trials, the learner modifies and refines the movements. During this stage, there is considerable cognitive activity, and each movement requires a high degree of conscious attention and thought. The learner is highly dependent on visual feedback. Performance is initially inconsistent with large gains occurring as the patient progresses to the next stage. The basic "What to do" decision is made.

Associative Stage

The second and middle stage is the *associative stage* of motor learning. During this stage, the learner practices and refines the motor patterns, making subtle adjustments. Spatial and temporal organization increases, while errors and extraneous movements decrease. Performance becomes more consistent, and cognitive activity decreases. The learner is less dependent on visual feedback, and the use of

proprioceptive feedback increases. Thus the learner begins to learn the "feel" of the movement. This stage can persist for a long time, depending upon the learner and the level of practice. The "How to do" decision is made.

Autonomous Stage

The third and final stage is the *autonomous stage* of motor learning. The learner continues to practice and refine motor patterns. The spatial and temporal components of movement become highly organized. Performance is at a very high level (e.g., skilled walking at all speeds and in all environments). At this stage of learning, movements are largely error-free and automatic with only a minimal level of cognitive monitoring and attention. The "How to succeed" decision is made.

Clinical Note: Many patients undergoing active rehabilitation are discharged before achieving this final stage of learning. For these patients, refinement of skills comes only after continued practice in home and community environments. The patient with traumatic brain injury (TBI) and significant cognitive impairment may never achieve this level of independent function, continuing to need structure and assistance for the rest of his or her life.

Understanding the Task

Tasks are commonly grouped into functional categories. *Activities of daily living (ADL)* refer to those daily living skills necessary for an adult to manage life. *Basic ADL (BADL)* include grooming skills (oral hygiene, showering or bathing, dressing), toilet hygiene, feeding, and use of personal devices (see Chapter 11: Interventions to Improve Upper Extremity Skills). *Instrumental ADL (IADL)* include money management, functional communication and socialization, functional and community mobility, and health maintenance.

Functional mobility skills (FMS) refer to those skills involved in:

- Bed mobility: rolling, bridging, and scooting in bed, moving from supine-to-sit and sit-to-supine
- Sitting: scooting
- Transfers: moving from sit-to-stand and stand-to-sit, transfers from one surface to another (e.g., bed-to-wheelchair and back, on and off a toilet, to and from a car seat), and moving from floor-to-stand
- Standing: stepping
- Walking and stair climbing.

Control can also be examined in other postures, including prone-on-elbows, quadruped (hands and knees), kneeling, and half-kneeling. It is important to remember that there is considerable variability in motor performance of

FMS across the life span. Thus, the activities of rolling over and sitting up may vary considerably between two adults of different size, age, or health.

Categories of Motor Skills

Movements can also be grouped according to the actions and type of motor control (neuromotor processes) required during performance of the task. These include (1) transitional mobility, (2) stability (static postural control), (3) controlled mobility (dynamic postural control), and (4) skill. Difficulty varies according to the degree of postural and movement control required. Thus those tasks with increased degrees of freedom and attentional demands, such as standing and walking, are more difficult than prone or supine tasks with limited body segments to control.[10]

Transitional Mobility

Transitional mobility is the ability to move from one position to another (e.g., rolling, supine-to-sit, sit-to-stand, transfers) independently and safely. Common characteristics of normal mobility include the ability to initiate movement, control movement, and terminate movement while maintaining postural control. Deficits in mobility range from failure to initiate or sustain movements to poorly controlled movement to failure to successfully terminate the movement. At the very lowest level, the impaired patient is only able to roll partially over to side-lying and exhibits poor ability to sustain movements. At a higher level, the patient is asked to sit up from supine and stand up from sitting. An impaired patient may exhibit difficulty standing up (may require several attempts) but once up is able to stand independently. Key elements the therapist should observe and document include (1) the ability to initiate movements, (2) strategies utilized and overall control of movement, (3) the ability to terminate movement, (4) the level and type of assistance required (manual cues, verbal cues, guided movements), and (5) environmental constraints that influenced performance.

Stability

Stability (static postural control) is the ability to maintain postural stability and orientation with the COM over the BOS and the body at rest. For example, the patient demonstrates stability in sitting or standing if he or she is able to maintain the posture with minimum sway, no loss of balance, and no handhold. Key elements the therapist should observe and document include (1) the BOS, (2) the position and stability of the COM within the BOS, (3) the degree of postural sway, (4) the degree of stabilization from upper extremities (UEs) or lower extremities (LEs) (e.g., handhold in sitting or standing, legs hooked around support in sitting), (5) number of episodes and direction of loss of balance (LOB) and fall safety risk, (6) the level and type of assistance required (manual cues, verbal cues,

guided movements), and (7) environmental constraints that influenced performance.

Dynamic Postural Control

Dynamic postural control (dynamic balance or *controlled mobility)* is the ability to maintain postural stability (a stable, nonmoving BOS, COM within the BOS) while parts of the body are in motion. Thus a person can shift his or her weight or rock back and forth or side to side in a posture (e.g., sitting or standing) without losing control. Being able to adjust postural control while performing a secondary task with a limb freed from weight-bearing is also evidence of dynamic postural control (sometimes called *static-dynamic control*). The initial weight shift and redistributed weight-bearing places increased demands for stability on the support segments while the dynamic limb challenges control. For example, a patient with TBI is positioned in quadruped and demonstrates difficulty when asked to lift either an upper or lower limb or to lift the opposite upper and lower limbs together. In sitting, the patient with stroke is unable to reach forward and toward the affected side with the less affected limb without losing balance and falling over. In standing, the patient with cerebellar ataxia is unable to step forward, backward, or out to the side without losing balance. Key elements the therapist should observe and document include (1) the degree of postural stability maintained by the weight-bearing segments, (2) the range and degree of control of the dynamically moving segments, (3) the level and type of assistance required (e.g., verbal cues, manual cues, guided movements), and (4) environmental constraints that influenced performance.

Skill

Skill is the ability to consistently perform coordinated movement sequences for the purposes of attaining an action goal. Skilled behaviors allow for purposeful investigation and interaction with the physical and social environment (e.g., manipulation or transport). Skills require voluntary control, so reflexes or involuntary movements are not considered skilled movements. Skills are learned and are the direct result of practice and experience with actions organized in advance of movement using a motor plan. Skilled movements can be variable and not constrained by one set movement pattern, but rather are organized by the action goal and the environment. Thus a skilled person is able to adapt movements easily to changes in task demands and the environments in which they occur. For example, control of walking is evident in the clinic as well as in home and community environments. Skills can be performed using a stationary or variable base (e.g., bouncing a ball while in standing position or walking). Conditions that influence performance can vary from a stationary closed environment (e.g., a quiet room within the clinic) to motion in an open environment (e.g., a busy community gym).[11]

Motor skills can be further categorized. Kicking a ball is an example of a *discrete skill,* with a recognizable beginning and end. Walking is a *continuous skill* that has no recognizable beginning and end. Playing a piano represents a *serial skill,* a series of discrete actions strung together. A movement skill performed in a stable, nonchanging environment is called a *closed motor skill,* whereas a movement skill performed in a variable, changing environment is called an *open motor skill.*[3] A skilled person is also able to perform a simultaneous secondary task while moving *(dual-task control).* For example, the patient with stroke is able to stand or walk while holding or manipulating an object (e.g., holding a tray with a full glass of water on it), talking, or performing a cognitive task (counting backward by 3s from 100). The terms may serve as anchor points along a continuum (e.g., open skill versus closed skill). It is important to remember that skills can fall anywhere along that continuum, not just at either end. Box 1.4 presents terminology related to motor skills.

The term *skill* also designates performance quality. Thus skilled movements are characterized by consistency, steadiness, speed, precise timing, and economy of effort in achieving the target goal (e.g., how well the person accomplishes the action). Skills require coordinated actions of trunk and limb segments. For example, the trunk and proximal segments stabilize while the hands complete a skilled action, say, eating with a knife and fork or getting dressed. Motor skill performance also has been defined by the timing of movement. *Reaction time (RT)* is the interval of time between the onset of the initial stimulus to move and the initiation of a movement response. *Movement time (MT)* is the interval of time between the initiation of movement and the completion of movement. The sum of both is called *response time,* which can be expected to improve as skill learning progresses as evidenced by a decrease in overall time. *Speed-accuracy trade-off* is a principle of motor skill performance that defines the influence of the speed of performance by movement accuracy demands. The trade-off is that increasing speed decreases accuracy, whereas decreasing speed improves accuracy. Speed-accuracy demands are task specific. In tasks with high accuracy requirements such as aiming tasks (e.g., throwing a football), speed must be kept within reasonable limits to permit accuracy. Speed-accuracy trade-off typically affects older adults. For example, with declining postural and balance abilities, movements such as walking are slowed in order to permit accurate and safe progression. When the older adult tries to walk fast, the result may be a loss of control and a fall.[10] Table 1.1 presents a classification of motor skills according to movement function.

Lead-Up Skills

Learning a motor skill is a difficult process. For patients with motor dysfunction, whole-task training may not be possible initially. For example, the patient with poor head and trunk control after TBI cannot relearn head control first in unsupported standing. There are simply too many body segments to control to be successful. This scenario is known as a *degrees of freedom problem.* In these situations, the therapist is challenged to make critical decisions

BOX 1.4 Terminology: Motor Skills

Ability: a genetically predetermined characteristic or trait of a person that underlies performance of certain motor skills
Adaptation: alteration of a skill or the environment to achieve a task goal
Coordinative structures (synergies): functionally linked muscles that are constrained by the CNS to act cooperatively to produce an intended movement
Motor skill: an action or task that has a goal to achieve; acquisition of skill is dependent on practice and experience and is not genetically defined. *Alternative definition:* an indicator of the quality of performance

- **Gross motor skills:** motor skills that involve large musculature and a goal where precision of movement is not important to the successful execution of the skill (e.g., running or jumping)
- **Fine motor skills:** motor skills that require control of small muscles of the body to achieve the goal of skill; this type of task (e.g., writing, typing, or buttoning a shirt) typically requires a high level of eye-hand coordination.
- **Closed motor skill:** a skill performed in a stable or predictable environment (e.g., walking in a quiet hall)

- **Open motor skill:** a skill performed in a variable or unpredictable environment (e.g., walking across a busy gym)
- **Discrete motor skills:** skills that have distinct beginning and end points defined by the task itself (e.g., locking the brake on a wheelchair)
- **Serial motor skills:** skills that are discrete or individual skills put together in a series (e.g., the highly individual steps required to transfer from a bed to a wheelchair).
- **Continuous motor skills:** skills that have arbitrary beginning and end points defined by the performer or some external agents (e.g., swimming, running)
- **Simple motor skills:** movements that involve a single motor program that produces an individual movement response (e.g., kicking a ball while sitting in a chair)
- **Complex motor skills:** movements that involve multiple actions and motor programs combined to produce a coordinated movement response (e.g., running and kicking a soccer ball during a game)
- **Dual-task skills:** movements that involve simultaneous actions (motor programs) performed together (e.g., walking and carrying a tray, walking and talking)

TABLE 1.1 Classification of Motor Skills According to Movement Function[a]

Category	Postural and Movement Characteristics	Postural and Movement Examples	Indicators of Impaired Function
Transitional mobility	Ability to move from one posture to another; BOS and/or COM are changing	Rolling; supine-to-sit; sit-to-stand; transfers	Failure to initiate or sustain movements through the range; poorly controlled movements
Stability (static postural control)	Ability to maintain postural stability and orientation with the COM over the BOS with the body not in motion; BOS is fixed	Holding in antigravity postures: prone-on-elbows, quadruped, sitting, kneeling, half-kneeling, plantigrade, or standing	Failure to maintain a steady posture; excessive postural sway; wide BOS; high guard arm position or UE handhold; loss of balance; COM exceeds BOS
Dynamic postural control (controlled mobility)	Ability to maintain postural stability and orientation with the COM over the BOS while parts of the body are in motion; BOS is fixed	Weight shifting; limb movements (UE reaching, LE stepping in plantigrade or standing)	Failure to maintain or control posture during weight shifting or dynamic trunk or extremity movements; loss of balance
Skill	Ability to consistently perform coordinated movement sequences for the purposes of investigation and interaction with the physical and social environment; during locomotion COM is in motion and BOS is changing	UE skills: grasp and manipulation; bipedal locomotion	Poorly coordinated movements (dyssynergia, dysmetria, dysdiadochokinesia); lack of precision, control, consistency, and economy of effort; inability to achieve a task goal

COM, center of mass; BOS, base of support; UE, upper extremity; LE, lower extremity.

[a]From O'Sullivan, S and Schmitz T. *Categories of Motor Skills*, ed 6. F.A. Davis, Philadelphia, 2014, Table 5.11 (with permission).

about how to break the task down into its component parts (*lead-up skills* or simple motor skills) within a functionally relevant context. Each lead-up skill represents a component of a larger functional task, referred to as the *criterion skill.* A single lead-up skill may involve a number of criterion skills. For example, lower trunk rotation is an important lead-up skill to upright stepping as well as rolling and scooting. *Parts-to-whole training* addresses mastery of individual component skills, with progression to a criterion skill. It also has the positive benefit of reducing fear and desensitizing patients who might be afraid to perform higher level or complex movements. For example, bridging activities can be used to prepare patients for sit-to-stand transfers. Hip extensor control is enhanced while the degrees of freedom problem and fear of falling during upright activity are reduced. Skills with highly independent parts (e.g., bed-to-wheelchair transfer) can usually be successfully trained using this strategy. Parts-to-whole transfer is generally less successful with skills that have highly integrated parts, such as walking. In this situation, it is generally better to implement practice of the criterion skill (whole-task training) as soon as possible. The successes therapists have had with locomotor training using body weight support and a motorized treadmill (see

Chapter 10: Interventions to Improve Locomotor Skills and Case Study 3) illustrate this point.

Clinical Note: Prolonged practice of lead-up skills without accompanying practice of the criterion skill can lead to limited motor transfer. Thus the patient is able to perform lead-up skills but cannot demonstrate the required criterion skill. Some patients are unable to make the transfer due to CNS dysfunction. For example, the patient with severe stroke and perceptual-motor impairments may develop *splinter skills.* These are skills that are acquired in a manner inconsistent with, or incapable of being integrated with, those already present.[12] Thus they cannot be easily modified to other skills or to other environments.

Understanding the Individual Patient

The first step in the treatment planning process is an accurate examination of the patient. This includes taking a history, performing systems review, and conducting definitive tests and measures as indicated. Evaluating the data permits the therapist to identify impairments and activity limitations upon which the POC is based.[2] For example, impairments in muscle strength and motor function, joint flexibility and ROM, sensory and perceptual integrity, cognition and attention, and endurance will all influence the selection of interventions and activities. Some of these impairments will need to be resolved before progressing to advanced skills such as walking. For example, the patient will be unable to practice sit-to-stand activities if hip joint ROM is limited and hip flexion contractures are present. Some impairments can be successfully addressed during activity-based training. For example, hip extensor weakness can be strengthened using bridging activities before standing.

The POC focuses on increasing overall levels of activity, reducing activity limitations and participation restrictions, and improving quality of life. The therapist must accurately complete a functional examination of BADL and FMS skills.[13] For example, many rehabilitation facilities use the Functional Independence Measure (FIM).[14] The therapist must also identify those activities that are meaningful for the patient and that the patient is capable of achieving. The skilled clinician is also able to recognize *environmental risk factors* defined as the behaviors, attributes, or environmental influences that increase the chances of developing impairments, functional limitations, or disability. The development of an *asset list* is also an important part of the clinical decision-making process. Assets include the patient's strengths, abilities, and positive behaviors or helping strategies that can be reinforced and emphasized during therapy. Using the asset list gives the therapist an opportunity to provide positive reinforcement and allows the patient to experience success. For example, the therapist always begins and ends a therapy session by having the patient perform a skill that has been mastered (or almost mastered) and can be performed with relative ease. This allows the patient to experience success, thereby improving motivation and participation in subsequent rehabilitation.

Measures of Motor Learning

Performance changes result from practice or experience and are a frequently used measure of learning. For example, with practice, a person can develop appropriate sequencing

of movement components with improved timing and reduced effort and concentration. Performance, however, is not always an accurate reflection of learning. It is possible to practice enough to temporarily improve performance but not retain the learning. Conversely, factors such as fatigue, anxiety, poor motivation, and medications may cause performance to deteriorate, although learning may still occur. Because performance can be affected by a number of factors, it may reflect a temporary change in motor behavior seen during practice sessions.

Retention is an important measure of learning. It is the ability of the learner to demonstrate the skill over time and after a period of no practice *(retention interval)*. A *retention test* looks at performance after a retention interval and compares it with the performance observed during the original learning trial. Performance can be expected to decrease slightly, but it should return to original levels after relatively few practice trials (termed *warm-up decrement*). For example, riding a bike is a well-learned skill that is generally retained even though a person may not have ridden for years.

The ability to apply a learned skill to the learning of other, similar tasks is termed *adaptability* or *generalizability* and is another important measure of learning. A *transfer test* looks at the person's ability to perform variations of the original skill (e.g., performing step-ups applied to climbing stairs and curbs). The time and effort required to organize and perform these new skill variations efficiently are reduced if learning the original skill was adequate. Finally, *resistance to contextual change* is another important measure of learning. This is the adaptability required to perform a motor task in altered environmental situations. Thus a person who has learned a skill (e.g., walking with a cane on indoor level surfaces) should be able to apply that learning to new and variable situations (e.g., walking outdoors or walking on a busy sidewalk). Box 1.5 provides definitions of measures of motor learning.[3]

The patient who is able to engage in introspection, self-evaluation of performance, and problem solving demonstrates an important outcome of successful rehabilitation. In an era of fiscal responsibility and limitations on the number of physical therapy sessions allowed, many patients are able to learn only the very basic skills while in active rehabilitation. Much of the necessary learning

BOX 1.5 Terminology: Measures of Motor Learning

Performance test: an examination of observable improvements with attention to the quality of movements and the success of movement outcomes after a period of skill practice
Retention: the ability of the learner to demonstrate a learned skill over time and after a period of no practice (termed a *retention interval*)
Retention test: an examination of a learned skill administered after a period of no practice *(retention interval)*

Generalizability (adaptability of skills): the ability to apply a learned skill to the performance of other similar or related skills
Resistance to contextual change (adaptability of context): the ability to perform a learned skill in altered environmental situations
Transfer test: an examination of performance of similar or related skills compared to a previously learned skill

of functional skills occurs after discharge and during out-patient episodes of care. The therapist cannot possibly structure practice sessions to meet all of the functional challenges the patient may face. The patient's acquiring independent problem-solving/decision-making skills ensures that the final goal of rehabilitation—independent function—can be achieved.

Some therapists may overemphasize guided movements and errorless practice. Although this may be important for safety reasons, lack of exposure to performance errors may preclude the patient from developing capabilities for self-evaluation and active problem solving. The therapist needs to observe, document, and promote this very important function.

Patients need to be encouraged to solve their own problems as movement challenges are presented. They also need to be challenged to critique their own movements with questions like *"How did you do that time?"* and *"How can you improve your next attempt?"* The success of successive movement attempts needs to be monitored and discussed with the patient.

Learning Style

People vary in their *learning style,* defined as their characteristic mode of acquiring, processing, and storing knowledge. Learning styles differ according to a number of factors, including personality characteristics, reasoning styles (inductive or deductive), initiative (active or passive), and so forth. Some people utilize an *analytical/objective* learning style. They process information in a step-by-step order and learn best with factual information and structure. Others are more *intuitive/global* learners. They tend to process information all at once, and learn best when information is personalized and presented within the context of practical, real-life examples. They may have difficulty in ordering steps and comprehending details. Some people rely heavily on visual processing and demonstration to learn a task. Others depend more on auditory processing, talking themselves through a task. Individual characteristics and preferences are best determined by talking with the patient and family, using careful listening and observation skills. The medical record may also provide information concerning relevant premorbid history (e.g., educational level, occupation, interests). A thorough understanding of each of these factors allows the therapist to appropriately structure the learning environment and therapist-patient interactions.

Psychosocial Factors

A number of psychosocial factors can influence a person's ability to successfully participate in rehabilitation, including motivation, personality factors, emotional state, spirituality, life roles, and educational level. Preexisting psychiatric and psychosocial conditions can have a marked impact on rehabilitation training and outcomes. Psychosocial adaptation to disability and chronic illness is an ongoing and evolving process. At any point in an episode of care, patients can exhibit grief, mourning, anxiety, denial, depression, anger, acknowledgment, or adjustment. Coping style is also an important variable. Patients with effective coping strategies are better able to participate in rehabilitation, seeking the information they need and demonstrating effective problem-solving skills. They are also better able to utilize social supports and are likely to have more positive outcomes. Patients with maladaptive coping skills are likely to fix blame and are less able to participate effectively in rehabilitation. Avoidance and escape along with substance abuse are examples of maladaptive behaviors.[15]

Understanding the Environment

Environmental factors influence motor function and functional recovery and include the physical and social environments in which the patient functions and lives. They can have a positive effect on rehabilitation, enabling successful motor learning and performance. Or, they can have a negative effect, limiting motor learning and performance. They can also significantly affect disability and overall quality of life.

Physical Environment

An accurate examination of the patient's ability to perform within the clinic, home, and community environments is essential in developing a POC that successfully restores function and returns the patient to his or her habitual environment. (See Schmitz[16] for a thorough discussion of this topic.)

The environment in which people normally function varies and changes; it is not static. Examination of *complex activities* in which the patient performs in changing and real-world environments is therefore critical to developing the POC and ensuring independent function. The therapist must also understand the needs of the patient and the speed in which transitioning environments can occur. For example, the patient may begin by practicing walking in a quiet clinic hallway with few interruptions. Progression is then to walking in a hallway with increased activity to finally a busy hospital lobby or outside on sidewalks and grass.

The environment in which people normally function also includes varying levels of regulatory features. *Anticipation timing* (time-to-contact) refers to the ability to time movements to a target or an event (e.g., doorway threshold) in the environment, requiring precise control of movements. It is a function of dynamic processing of visual information. Moving through a stationary target—for example, a doorway—is easier than intercepting a moving target. For example, walking through a revolving door or onto a moving walkway requires that the person match the speed of movements to the speed of the objects to safely progress. The term *visual proprioception* refers to the ability to perceive movements and positions of the body in space and in the environment during movement. Thus vision is critical in interpreting environmental cues and adapting our actions.[1] Box 1.6

BOX 1.6 Terminology: Motor Function and the Environment

Skill movements are shaped to the specific environments in which they occur.

Anticipation timing (time-to-contact): the ability to time movements to a target or an event (e.g., an obstacle) in the environment, requiring precise control of movements (e.g., running to kick a soccer ball)

Regulatory conditions: those features of the environment to which movement must be molded to be successful (e.g., stepping on a moving walkway or into a revolving door)

- **Closed skills:** movements performed in a stable or fixed environment (e.g., activities practiced in a quiet room)

- **Open skills:** movements performed in a changing or variable environment (e.g., activities practiced in a busy gym)
- **Self-paced skills:** movements that are initiated at will and whose timing is controlled or modified by the person (e.g., walking)
- **Externally paced skills:** movements that are initiated and paced by dictates of the external environment (e.g., walking in time with a metronome)

Visual proprioception: visual information as a strong basis for perception of the movements and positions of the body in space

---

provides definitions of terms related to motor function and the environment.

Social Environment

Adequate family involvement and social support are critical in helping patients achieve favorable outcomes. Spouses, family, and significant others can offer considerable help in the form of emotional support, financial support, and physical assistance. Rehabilitation outcomes and quality of life are dramatically improved in patients who have strong social support over those who have no one able to provide assistance. Social isolation is a frequent outcome of lack of social support.[16] The therapist must accurately identify and understand the impact of these factors on the patient undergoing rehabilitation.

Empowering patients to participate in collaborative planning and evaluation of outcomes *(patient-centered approach)* is a critical factor in determining successful outcomes. The patient is viewed as an active participant and partner who is fully involved in goal setting, makes informed choices regarding the POC, and assumes responsibility for his or her own health care. Therapists need to place strong emphasis on communicating effectively; educating patients, families, and caregivers; and teaching self-management skills to maximize motivation, adherence, and positive rehabilitation outcomes. The overall goal of a successful rehabilitation program must be to have patients learn to manage their lives in the context of ongoing disability and to promote overall health and wellness.[17,18]

SUMMARY

This chapter has presented an overview of a framework for clinical decision-making and client management. Successful intervention is based on a thorough understanding of motor function and motor learning. The therapist must carefully examine the patient and consider three basic elements in developing the POC: the nature and requirements of the task, the patient's performance capabilities, and the environment in which the task must be performed.

REFERENCES

1. The World Health Organization. International Classification of Functioning, Disability, and Health Resources (ICF). Geneva, Switzerland, World Health Organization, 2002.
2. American Physical Therapy Association. Guide to Physical Therapist Practice, Version 3.0. Alexandria, VA, 2014. Retrieved September 9, 2014, from http://guidetoptpractice.apta.org.
3. Schmidt, R, and Lee, T. Motor Control and Learning—A Behavioral Emphasis, ed 5. Champaign, IL, Human Kinetics, 2011.
4. Shumway-Cook, A, and Woollacott, M. Motor Control—Translating Research into Clinical Practice, ed 4. Philadelphia, Lippincott Williams & Wilkins, 2012.
5. VanSant, A. Life span development in functional tasks. Phys Ther, 1990; 70:788.
6. Green, L, and Williams, K. Differences in developmental movement patterns used by active vs sedentary middle-aged adults coming from a supine position to erect stance. Phys Ther, 1992; 72:560.
7. Levin, M, Kleim, J, and Wolf, S. What do motor "recovery" and "compensation" mean in patients following stroke? Neurorehabil Neural Repair, 2009; 23:3134.
8. Taub, E, et al. Technique to improve chronic motor deficit after stroke. Arch Phys Med Rehabil, 1993; 74:347.
9. Fitts, P, and Posner, M. Human Performance. Belmont, CA, Brooks/Cole, 1969.
10. O'Sullivan, SB. Examination of motor function: motor control and motor learning. In O'Sullivan, SB, and Schmitz, TJ. Physical Rehabilitation, ed 6. Philadelphia, FA Davis, 2014, 161.
11. Gentile, A. Skill acquisition: Action, movement, and neuromotor processes. In Carr, JH, et al (eds). Movement Science: Foundations for Physical Therapy in Rehabilitation, ed 2. Gaithersburg, MD, Aspen, 2000, 111.
12. Unsworth, C. Cognitive and perceptual dysfunction. In O'Sullivan, SB, and Schmitz, TJ. Physical Rehabilitation, ed 6. Philadelphia, FA Davis, 2014, 1222.
13. Scalzitti, D. Examination of function. In O'Sullivan, SB, and Schmitz, TJ. Physical Rehabilitation, ed 6. Philadelphia, FA Davis, 2014, 308.
14. UB Foundation Activities, Inc. *Guide for the Uniform Data Set for Medical Rehabilitation* (Adult FIM, Version 4.0). *Uniform Data System for Medical Rehabilitation*, Buffalo, NY, UB Foundation Activities, Inc, 1993.
15. Precin, P. Psychosocial disorders. In O'Sullivan, SB, and Schmitz, TJ. Physical Rehabilitation, ed 6. Philadelphia, FA Davis, 2014, 1175.
16. Schmitz, T. Examination of the environment. In O'Sullivan, SB, and Schmitz, TJ. Physical Rehabilitation, ed 6. Philadelphia, FA Davis, 2014, 338.
17. Ozer, M, Payton, O, and Nelson, C. Treatment Planning for Rehabilitation—A Patient-Centered Approach. New York, McGraw-Hill, 2000.
18. Drench, M, et al. Psychosocial Aspects of Health Care, ed 2. Upper Saddle River NJ, Pearson Education Inc, 2007.

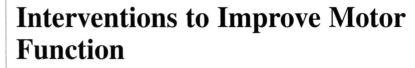

Careful examination and evaluation of impairments, activity limitations, and participation restrictions enable the therapist to identify movement deficiencies to target during rehabilitation. *Restorative interventions* focus on targeted movement deficiencies and utilize activity-based interventions and motor learning strategies. To be most effective, restorative interventions include three basic elements: (1) repetitive and intense practice of task-oriented, functional activities, (2) strategies that enhance active motor learning and adherence-enhancing behaviors, and (3) strategies that encourage use of more-impaired body segments while limiting use of less-impaired segments. During early recovery, patients with limited motor function who are unable to perform voluntary movements or have limited control (e.g., patients with stroke or traumatic brain injury [TBI]) may benefit from *augmented intervention strategies*. This is a more hands-on approach to training and includes guided, assisted, or facilitated movements. Neuromotor approaches such as *Proprioceptive Neuromuscular Facilitation (PNF)* and *Neurodevelopmental Treatment (NDT)* incorporate a number of strategies and techniques to promote movement. Patients with severe movement deficiencies, limited recovery potential, and multiple comorbidities and impairments (e.g., the patient with severe stroke and severe cardiac and respiratory compromise) benefit from *compensatory intervention strategies* designed to promote early resumption of function. Interventions include using altered movement strategies, focusing on using less-involved body segments for function, assistive devices, and environmental adaptation.

Interventions organized around a behavioral goal meaningful to the patient are the best way to promote functional recovery and retention. *Impairment-specific interventions* that target specific impairments (e.g., spasticity, contracture, weakness) may be necessary during the course of treatment but should not be the primary focus of treatment. The intended outcome of any rehabilitation plan of care (POC) is functional independence. Remediation of specific impairments can be built into a functional training activity. For example, in hooklying position, lower trunk rotation in which the knees move from side to side (knee rocks) can increase the strength of hip extensors and abductors while reducing lower extremity (LE) extensor tone. Functionally it promotes independent bed mobility.

The diversity of problems experienced by the patient with disordered motor function negates the idea that any one approach or intervention strategy can be successful for all patients. As patients recover, their needs and functional abilities change. The successful therapist understands the full continuum of intervention strategies available to aid patients with impaired motor function and uses them effectively during rehabilitation (Box 2.1).

Task Analysis

Task analysis is the process of breaking an activity down into its component parts to understand and evaluate the demands of the task. It begins with an understanding of normal movements and normal kinesiology associated with the task. The therapist examines and evaluates the patient's performance and analyzes the differences compared with "typical" or expected performance. Early in the treatment process, the therapist needs to identify what activities are important to the patient as determined by the patient's own interests, roles, and living environments. The patient's interest in the activity and motivation to complete the activity successfully can influence the level of performance observed.

Critical skills in this process include the ability to observe accurately, recognize and interpret movement deficiencies, ascertain how underlying impairments relate to the movements, and determine how the environment affects the movements observed. The therapist evaluates what needs to be altered and determines how to modify it by examining the blocks or obstacles to moving in the correct pattern and seeing how can they be changed. For example, the patient who is unable to transfer from bed to wheelchair may lack postural stability, adequate LE extensor control (strength), and coordinated movement control of the trunk and LEs. In addition, the patient with TBI may be highly distractible and have severely limited attention. The busy clinic environment in which the activity is performed renders this patient incapable of listening to instructions or concentrating on the activity. Sociocultural influences must also be considered to understand the patient's performance. For example, in some cultures, close hands-on assistance may be viewed as a violation of the patient's personal space or inappropriate if the therapist is of the opposite gender.

BOX 2.1 Interventions to Improve Motor Function.[1]

Restorative Interventions

Activity-Based Intervention
Task-specific training:
- Functional mobility skills
- Activities of daily living
Environmental context
Behavioral shaping
Safety awareness training

Motor Learning Strategies
Strategy development
Feedback
Practice
Transfer of learning
Active decision-making

Impairment-Specific and Augmented Interventions

Impairment Interventions
Strength, power, endurance
Flexibility
Coordination and agility
Postural control and balance
Gait and locomotion
Aerobic capacity/endurance
Relaxation

Augmented Interventions
Neuromuscular facilitation
Proprioceptive Neuromuscular Facilitation
Neurodevelopmental Treatment
Sensory stimulation
Biofeedback
Neuromuscular electrical stimulation
Sensory stimulation techniques

Compensatory Interventions

Substitution training:
- Alternate movement strategies
- Less-involved body segments
Assistive/supportive devices
Environmental modification

Categories of tasks include *basic activities of daily living (BADL)* or *BADL* (self-care tasks such as dressing, feeding, and bathing) and *instrumental activities of daily living (IADL)* or *IADL* (home management tasks such as cooking, cleaning, shopping, and managing a checkbook). *Functional mobility skills (FMS)* are those skills involved in moving by changing body position or location. Examples of FMS include rolling, supine-to-sit, sit-to-stand, transfers, stepping, walking, and running. The term *activity demands* refers to the requirements imbedded in each step of the activity. The term *environmental demands* refers to the physical characteristics of the environment required for successful performance. Questions posed in Box 2.2 can be used as a guide for qualitative task analysis.

Video recording of patients' performance is a useful tool for examining patients with marked movement disturbances (e.g., the patient with pronounced ataxia or dyskinesias). The therapist can review the performance repeatedly on the video without unnecessarily tiring the patient. Video-recorded motor performance can also serve as a useful training tool to aid patients in understanding their movement deficiencies.

Activity-Based Intervention

Function-Induced Recovery

Function-induced recovery *(use-dependent cortical reorganization)* refers to the ability of the nervous system to

modify itself in response to changes in activity and the environment. Repetitive learning behaviors have been shown to prevent degradation and atrophy, enable neuron growth, strengthen synaptic connections, alter cortical field representations, and expand topographical areas of motor activity. In addition, receptive fields are altered, processing time is improved, and evoked responses demonstrate increased strength and consistency with improved synchronicity. Improvements in functional outcomes are correlated with observed changes in neural adaptation. For example, these can include improved fine and gross motor coordination, sensory discrimination, postural control and balance, procedural memory, and adaptability.[2–7] In rehabilitation, constraint-induced movement (CIM) therapy and locomotor training using partial body-weight support (BWS) and a treadmill (TM) are examples of targeted interventions to promote function-induced recovery. For example, intervention for the patient with stroke and upper extremity (UE) involvement focuses on use of the more involved UE during daily tasks, whereas use of the less-involved extremities is minimized (e.g., CIM therapy).[8–16] Initial tasks are selected to ensure patient success and motivation (e.g., reach, grasp and manipulation of objects in the hand, feeding and dressing activities). (See Chapter 12: Constraint-Induced Movement Therapy.) Using partial BWS and a motorized TM provides a means of early and intense locomotor training for patients with stroke or incomplete spinal cord injury (SCI).[17–24] (See Chapter 10: Interventions to Improve

BOX 2.2 Guiding Questions for Task Analysis[a]

A. What are the normal requirements of the functional activity being observed?

1. What is the overall movement sequence (motor plan)?
2. What are the normal kinesiological requirements of the movement being attempted?
3. What are the initial conditions required? Starting position and initial alignment?
4. How and where is the movement initiated?
5. How is the movement performed?
6. What are the musculoskeletal and biomechanical components required for successful completion of the task?
7. What are the cognitive and sensory/perceptual components required for successful completion of the task?
8. What are the motor control requirements of the activity: *mobility, stability, dynamic stability,* or *skill?*
9. What are the requirements for timing, force, and direction of movements?
10. What are the requirements for postural control and balance?
11. How is the movement terminated?

B. How successful is the patient's overall movement in terms of outcome?

1. Was the overall movement sequence completed (successful outcome)?
2. What components of the patient's movements are normal in terms of kinesiological efficiency? Almost normal?
3. What components of the patient's movements are abnormal?
4. What components of the patient's movements are missing? Delayed?
5. If abnormal, are the movements compensatory and functional or are they noncompensatory and nonfunctional?

6. What are the underlying impairments that constrain or impair the movements?
7. Do the movement errors increase over time? Is fatigue a constraining factor?
8. Is this a mobility level activity? Are the requirements met?
9. Is this a stability level activity? Are the requirements met?
10. Is this a dynamic stability level activity? Are the requirements met?
11. Is this a skill level activity? Are the requirements met?
12. Are the requirements for postural control and balance met? Is patient safety maintained throughout the activity?
13. Can the patient effectively analyze his or her own movements?
14. Can the patient successfully adapt to changing activity or task demands?
15. What difficulties do you expect this patient will have with other functional activities?
16. What compensatory strategies are evident?
17. What adaptive equipment is required? What is the level of success in using the adaptive equipment?

C. What environmental factors must be considered?

1. What environmental factors constrain or impair the movements?
2. Can the patient adapt to changing environmental demands?
3. What difficulties do you expect this patient will have in other environments?
4. Are there any sociocultural factors that influence performance?

[a]Adapted from American Physical Therapy Association. A Compendium for Teaching Professional Level Neurologic Content. Neurology Section, Alexandria, VA, 2000.

Locomotor Skills.) Changes occur at the level of body function (i.e., the patient moves the limb in a more efficient pattern) and at the activity level (the patient reaches or walks with a more efficient movement pattern). The therapist's overall goal is to challenge the patient with the appropriate level of task difficulty at the appropriate time to promote optimal recovery.

Activity-Based, Task-Oriented Intervention

Activity or task selection is guided by evaluation of functional status and activity performance data. The therapist selects activities to be practiced based on the patient's abilities/strengths, impairments, activity limitations, interests and experience, and health status. Practice parameters are determined. Generally the level of practice is intense (e.g., daily practice, for extended time periods). Activities are continually modified to increase the level of difficulty. Motor learning strategies are utilized, including *behavioral shaping techniques* that use reinforcement and reward to promote skill development. The environment is structured to enhance concentration and reduce distractors. The patient is encouraged to actively problem-solve to reach solutions to movement challenges.[25] This approach represents a shift away from the traditional neuromotor approaches that utilize an extensive hands-on approach (e.g., guided or facilitated movements). Although initial movements can be guided, active movements are the overall goal in this approach. The therapist's role is one of coach, structuring the practice and providing appropriate feedback while encouraging the patient. Box 2.3 presents a summary of activity-based, task-oriented intervention guidelines to promote function-induced recovery.

BOX 2.3 Functional, Task-Oriented Training Strategies[1]

Emphasize Early Training
- To promote use-dependent cortical plasticity and overcome learned nonuse.

Define the Goal of Task Practice
- Involve the patient in goal setting and decision-making, thereby enhancing motivation and promoting active commitment to recovery.

Determine the Activities to Be Practiced
- Consider the patient's history, health status, age, interests, and experience.
- Consider the patient's abilities and strengths, recovery level, learning style, impairments, and activity limitations.
- Determine a set of activities to be practiced for each training goal.
- Select activities that are interesting, stimulating, and important to the patient.
- Choose activities with the greatest potential for patient success and intersperse more difficult tasks with easier tasks.
- Target active movements involving the more involved extremities.
- Limit use of less-involved extremities; set parameters, impose time limits for use of constraints.
- Prevent or limit compensatory strategies.

Determine the Parameters of Practice
- Manage fatigue; determine rest and practice times.
- Model ideal performance; establish a *reference of correctness.*
- Establish requirements for intensity, minimal number of repetitions.
- Establish practice schedule of tasks (blocked or variable); shift to variable practice as soon as possible to enhance retention.
- Determine the practice order of tasks (constant, serial, random); shift to random order as soon as possible to enhance retention.
- Control use of instructions and augmented feedback to promote learning.
- Control use of assisted or guided movements to promote initial learning; ensure the patient successfully transitions to active movements as soon as possible.

Utilize Behavioral Shaping Techniques
- Gradually modify the task to increase the challenge and make it progressively more difficult as patient performance improves.
- Provide immediate and explicit feedback; recognize and acknowledge small improvements in task performance.
- Emphasize positive aspects of performance.
- Avoid excessive effort and fatigue; they degrade performance and dampen motivation.

Promote Problem-Solving
- Have the patient evaluate performance, identify obstacles, generate potential solutions.
- Have the patient practice the chosen movement (solution) and evaluate outcome.
- Relate successes to overall goals.

Structure the Environment
- Promote initial practice in a supportive environment, free of distractors (closed environment for highly distractible patients).
- Progress to variable practice in real-world environments (open environments).

Establish Parameters for Practice Outside of Therapy
- Identify specific goals and strategies for unsupervised practice; maximize opportunities.
- Utilize a written behavioral contract; have the patient agree to targeted behaviors to be carried out during the day.
- Have patient document unsupervised practice using an activity log or home exercise diary.

Maintain Focus on Active Learning
- Minimize hands-on therapy
- Maximize therapist's role as *training coach.*

Monitor Recovery Closely and Document Progress
- Use sensitive, valid, and reliable functional outcome measures.

Be cautious about timetables and predictions: recovery is highly individualized and may take longer than expected.

Clinical Note: Activity-based, task-oriented training effectively counteracts the effects of immobility and the development of indirect impairments such as muscle weakness and loss of flexibility. It prevents *learned nonuse* of the more involved segments while stimulating recovery of the central nervous system (CNS).[8]

The selection and use of activities depend on the movement potential, degree of recovery, and severity of motor deficits the patient exhibits. Patients who are not able to participate in intense activity-based training include those who lack initial voluntary control or have limited cognitive function. The patient with TBI who is in the early recovery stages has limited potential to participate in training that involves complex activities. Similarly, patients with stroke who experience profound UE paralysis would not be eligible for activity training emphasizing the more involved UE. One of the consistent exclusion criteria for CIM therapy has been the inability to perform voluntary wrist and finger extension of the involved hand; thus, *threshold abilities* to perform the basic components of the task need to be identified. The therapist needs to answer this question: *What is the patient's potential to perform the intended movement?* For example, during locomotor training using BWS and a motorized TM, limited stepping and pelvic motions can be guided initially into an efficient motor pattern. However, absence of basic head and trunk stability during upright positioning would preclude patients from being candidates for this training.

Clinical Note: Improvements in function and recovery have been noted in patients who undergo intensive task-specific training years after an initial insult (e.g., the patient with chronic stroke defined as 1 year or more after insult). The therapist should not underestimate the potential of the nervous system to adapt and change to achieve motor skill acquisition.

Functional Postures

The therapist must determine what functional postures and activities to include in the POC. As postures progress in difficulty by elevating the center of mass (COM) and decreasing the base of support (BOS), more and more body segments must be coordinated. This scenario has been referred to as the *degrees of freedom problem* (the difficulty of controlling multiple, independently moving body parts[26]). Patients are likely to demonstrate increasing problems in synergistic control, posture, and balance. Thus the patient with TBI and significant movement deficiencies (e.g., pronounced ataxia) may need to begin activity training in more stable four-limb postures such as quadruped or modified plantigrade. With recovery, training can then progress to more challenging upright postures such as sitting, kneeling, and standing. Table 2.1 identifies the primary focus, potential treatment benefits, and activities that can be practiced in each posture.

Interventions to Remediate Impairments

Identifying and correcting impairments (e.g., limited range of motion [ROM], decreased strength) are essential

TABLE 2.1 Postures: Primary Focus, Potential Treatment Benefits, and Activities[a]	
Posture/Description	**Primary Focus/Benefits/Activities**
Prone on Elbows	
Prone, weightbearing on elbows Stable posture Wide BOS Low COM	• Focus on improved upper trunk, UE, and neck/head control • Improve ROM in hip extension • Improve strength of shoulder stabilizers • Lead-up for bed mobility, quadruped activities, floor-to-stand transfers • Activities in posture: holding, weight shifting, UE reaching, assumption of posture • Modified prone-on-elbows activities can be practiced in sitting (table top) and plantigrade (modified standing) positions
Quadruped	
All-fours position (hands and knees) Weightbearing at knees, through extended elbows and hands Stable posture Wide BOS Low COM	• Focus on improved trunk, LE, UE, and neck/head control • Improve strength of trunk, hip, shoulder, and elbow stabilizers • Decrease extensor tone at knees by prolonged weightbearing • Decrease flexor tone at elbows, wrists, and hands by prolonged weightbearing with elbow extended and wrist/finger extension • Promote extension ROM at elbows, wrists, and fingers • Lead-up for plantigrade activities, floor-to-standing transfers, antigravity balance control • Activities in posture: holding, weight shifting, UE reaching, LE lifts, assumption of posture, locomotion on all fours
Hooklying, Bridging	
Hooklying: supine, knees flexed with feet flat; weightbearing at feet, buttocks, and upper trunk Bridging: elevation of the pelvis with hip extension; weightbearing at feet and upper trunk Wide BOS Low COM	• Focus on improved lower trunk and LE control • Improve strength of hip extensors and abductors, ankle stabilizers • Lead-up for bed mobility, sit-to-stand transfers, standing, and stair climbing • Bridging activities: holding, weight shifting, assumption of posture, LE lifts

TABLE 2.1 Postures: Primary Focus, Potential Treatment Benefits, and Activities[a] *(continued)*	
Posture/Description	**Primary Focus/Benefits/Activities**
Sitting	
Weightbearing through trunk and buttocks, feet Can include weightbearing through extended elbows and wrist/fingers Intermediate BOS Intermediate height COM	• Focus on improved upper trunk, lower trunk, LE, and head/neck control • Important for upright balance control • Lead-up for UE ADL skills; wheelchair locomotion • Activities in posture: holding, weight shifting, UE reaching, assumption of posture
Kneeling and Half-Kneeling	
Kneeling: weightbearing through extended hips and flexed knees; trunk is upright Half-kneeling: weightbearing through one LE with hip extended and knee flexed; other limb with hip and knee flexed, foot flat on forward limb Partial upright, antigravity position Intermediate height of COM Narrow BOS, kneeling Wide BOS, half-kneeling	• Focus on improved head/neck, upper and lower trunk, and LE control • Decrease extensor tone at knees by prolonged weightbearing on flexed knees • Improve strength of hip and trunk stabilizers • Lead-up for upright balance control, standing and stepping, floor-to-standing transfers • Activities in posture: holding, weight shifting, UE reaching, assumption of posture, knee walking
Modified Plantigrade (Modified Standing)	
Standing, all-fours position: weightbearing on feet and hands (on support surface) with extended UEs and LEs Modified upright antigravity position Stable posture Wide BOS High COM	• Focus on improved head/neck, trunk, and UE/LE control in supported, modified upright posture • Decrease tone in elbow, wrist, and finger flexors by prolonged weight-bearing with extended wrists and fingers • Increase extensor ROM at elbows, wrists, and fingers • With hips slightly flexed, COM forward of weightbearing line creating an extension moment at the knee • Increased safety for early standing (four-limb posture) • Lead-up for upright balance control, standing and stepping; standing UE ADL tasks • Activities in posture: holding, weight shifting, UE reaching, LE stepping, assumption of posture
Standing	
Weightbearing through trunk and LEs Full upright, antigravity position Narrow BOS High COM	• Focus on improved head/neck, trunk, and LE control in fully upright posture • Hips and knees fully extended • Symmetrical weightbearing through both LEs • Lead-up for upright balance control, stepping, locomotion, stair climbing; standing UE ADL skills • Activities in posture: holding, weight shifting, UE reaching, LE stepping, assumption of posture

ADL, activities of daily living; BOS, base of support; COM, center of mass; I, independent; LE, lower extremity; UE, upper extremity; ROM, range of motion.

[a]Adapted from O'Sullivan.[1]

elements in improving functional performance. The therapist must accurately identify those impairments that are linked to deficits in functional performance. An inability to stand up or climb stairs may be linked to weakness of hip and knee extensors. A strengthening program that addresses these impairments can be expected to improve function. Interventions can include traditional muscle-strengthening techniques (e.g., progressive resistance training utilizing weights and open-chain exercises). Strengthening can be effectively coupled with task-specific functional activities.[20] For example, the patient who is unable to stand up independently can practice sit-to-stand first from a high seat; as the patient's control improves, the seat is gradually lowered to standard height. The patient with difficulty in stair climbing can first practice step-ups using a low, 4-inch (10.16-cm) step; as the patient's control improves, the height of the step can be increased to standard height. The activity modification reduces the overall range in which muscles must perform, making it possible for the patient to complete the activity successfully. These examples illustrate an important training principle—that is, *specificity of training*.[27] The physiological adaptations of muscles to exercise training are highly specific to the type of training utilized. Transfer effects to improved function in sit-to-stand or stair climbing can be expected to be greater when the muscle performance and neuromuscular adaptation requirements during the functional training tasks closely approximate the desired skill.

Guided Movement

During initial training, the therapist may provide manual assistance during *early* movement attempts. This can take the form of passive movements, quickly progressing to active-assistive movements. Guidance (hands-on assistance) is used to help the learner gain an initial understanding of task requirements. During early assisted practice, the therapist can substitute for the missing elements, stabilize posture or parts of a limb, constrain unwanted movements, and guide the patient toward correct movements. For example, constraining or supporting the patient to ensure an upright sitting posture and shoulder stabilization in a position of function (70 degrees of shoulder flexion) allows the patient to focus on and control early hand-to-mouth movements. This adaptation reduces the number of body segments the patient must effectively control, thereby reducing the degrees of freedom. Guided movement also allows the patient to experience the tactile and kinesthetic inputs inherent in the movements—that is, to learn the *sensation of movement*. The supportive use of hands can allay fears and instill confidence while ensuring safety. For example, the patient recovering from stroke with impaired sensation and perception can be manually guided through early weight shifts and sit-to-stand transfers. The therapist must anticipate the patient's needs and how best to provide assistance. As the need for manual guidance decreases, the

patient assumes active control of movements. The overall goal of training is active movement control and trial-and-error discovery learning. See Box 2.4 for questions to consider when using guided movements.

Verbal Instructions and Cueing

Verbal instructions prepare the patient for correct movement and assist the patient in learning what to do. The therapist needs to help the patient focus on critical task elements to maximize early movement success. Timing cues assist the patient in premovement preparatory adjustments that focus on learning when to move. For example, during sit-to-stand transfers the therapist instructs the patient: *"On three, I want you to shift your weight forward over your feet and stand up. One, two, three."* Verbal cueing during practice provides feedback and helps the patient modify and correct his or her movements. Normally, the cerebellum drives motor learning and adaptation through the use of intrinsic sensory feedback information (somatosensory, visual, and vestibular inputs). In the absence of intrinsic feedback or with an inability to correctly use intrinsic feedback, verbal cues (augmented feedback) may be necessary. The therapist needs to select critical cues and focus the patient on recognizing intrinsic error signals associated with movement or those coming from the environment. Once the movement is completed, the patient should be asked to evaluate performance ("How did you do?") and then to recommend corrections ("What do you need to do differently next time to ensure success?"). Such evaluation helps to keep the focus on active movement control and trial-and-error discovery learning. See Box 2.4

BOX 2.4 Guided Movements: Questions to Consider for Anticipating Patient Needs[1]

- What critical elements of the task are necessary for movement success?
- How can I help the patient focus on these critical elements?
- How much assistance is needed to ensure successful performance?
- When are the demands for my assistance the greatest? The least?
- How should I position my body to assist the patient effectively during the movement without interfering with the movement?
- When and how can I reduce the level of my assistance?
- What verbal cues are needed to ensure successful performance?
- When and how can I reduce the level of my verbal cues?
- At what point is the patient ready to assume active control of the movement?
- How can I foster independent practice and critical decision-making skills that allow for adaptability of skills?

for relevant questions for the therapist to consider for anticipating patient needs.

Clinical Note: The key to success in using guided movements is to promote active practice as soon as possible, providing only as much assistance as needed and removing assistance as soon as possible. As manual guidance is reduced, verbal cueing can substitute. Guidance is most effective for slow postural responses (positioning tasks) and less effective during rapid or ballistic tasks.

Red Flag: Overuse of manually guided movements or verbal cueing is likely to result in dependence on the therapist for assistance, thus becoming a "crutch." It is important not to persist in excessive levels of assistance long after the patient needs such support. Continued guidance may result in the patient becoming overly dependent on the therapist (the "my therapist syndrome"). In this situation, the patient responds to the efforts of assistance from someone new with comments such as, "You're not doing it correctly. My therapist does it this way." This is strong evidence of an overdependence on the original therapist and the assistance being given.

Motor Learning Strategies

Motor learning is defined as "a set of internal processes associated with practice or experience leading to relatively permanent changes in the capability for skilled behavior."[26(p497)] Learning a motor skill is a complex process that requires spatial, temporal, and hierarchical organization of the CNS. Changes in the CNS are not directly observable but rather are inferred from changes in motor behavior. The reader is encouraged to review the sections on Stages of Motor Learning and Measures of Motor Learning in Chapter 1: Framework for Clinical Decision-Making and Client Management.

Cognitive Stage

The overall goal during the early learning is to facilitate task understanding and organize early practice. The learner's knowledge of the skill and its critical task elements must be ascertained. The therapist should highlight the purpose of the skill in a functionally relevant context. The task should seem important, desirable, and realistic to learn. The therapist should demonstrate the task exactly as it should be done (i.e., coordinated action with smooth timing and ideal performance speed). This helps the learner develop an internal cognitive map or *reference of correctness.* Attention should be directed to the desired outcome and critical task elements. The therapist should point out similarities to other learned tasks so that subroutines that are part of other motor programs can be retrieved from memory.

Highly skilled patients who have been successfully discharged from rehabilitation can be *expert models* for demonstration. Their success in functioning in the "real world" will also have a positive effect in motivating patients new to rehabilitation. For example, it is difficult for a therapist with full use of muscles to accurately demonstrate appropriate transfer skills to a patient with C6 complete tetraplegia. A former patient with a similar level of injury can accurately demonstrate how the skill should be performed. Demonstration has also been shown to be effective in producing learning even with unskilled patient models. In this situation the learner/patient benefits from the cognitive processing and problem-solving as he or she watches the unskilled model and evaluates the performance, identifying errors and generating corrections. Demonstrations can also be filmed. Developing a visual library of demonstrations of skilled former patients is a useful strategy to ensure the availability of effective models.

During initial practice, the therapist should give clear and concise verbal instructions and not overload the learner with excessive or wordy instructions. The overall goal is to prepare the patient for movement and reduce uncertainty. It is important to reinforce correct performance with appropriate feedback and intervene when movement errors become consistent or when safety is an issue. The therapist should *not* attempt to correct all the numerous errors that characterize this stage but rather allow for *trial-and-error learning* during practice. Feedback, particularly visual feedback, is important during the early stage. Thus the learner should be directed to "look at the movement" closely. Practice should allow for adequate rest periods and focus on repeated practice of the skill in an environment conducive to learning. This is generally one that is free of distractions (closed environment) because the cognitive demands are high during this phase of learning.

Associative Stage

During the middle or *associative stage* of learning, motor strategies are refined through continued practice. Spatial and temporal aspects become organized as the movement develops into a coordinated pattern. As performance improves, there is greater consistency and fewer errors and extraneous movements. The learner is now concentrating on *how to do* the movement rather than on *what to do.*

During this middle stage of learning, the therapist continues to provide feedback, intervening as movement errors become consistent. The learner is directed toward an appreciation of proprioceptive inputs associated with the movement (e.g., "How did that feel?"). The learner is encouraged to self-assess motor performance and to recognize intrinsically (naturally) occurring feedback during the movement. Practice should be varied, encouraging practice of variations of the skill and gradually varying the environment. For example, the learner practices bed-to-wheelchair transfers, wheelchair-to-mat transfers, wheelchair-to-toilet transfers, and finally wheelchair-to-car transfers. The therapist reduces hands-on assistance, which is generally counterproductive by this stage. The focus should be on the learner's active control and active decision-making in modifying skills in this stage of learning.

Autonomous Stage

The final or *autonomous stage* of learning is characterized by motor performance that, after considerable practice, is largely automatic. There is only a minimal level of cognitive monitoring because the motor programs are so refined that they can almost "run themselves." The spatial and temporal components of movement are becoming highly organized, and the learner is capable of coordinated movement patterns. The learner is now free to concentrate on other aspects of performance, such as *how to succeed* in difficult environments or at competitive sports. Movements are largely error-free, with little interference from environmental distractions. Thus the learner can perform equally well in a stable, predictable environment and in a changing, unpredictable environment.

Training strategies begun during associative learning are continued in this final phase. The therapist continues to promote practice. By this stage, movements should be largely automatic. The therapist can introduce environmental distractions to challenge the learner. If the learner is successful at this stage, these changes will do little to deteriorate the movements. The therapist can also incorporate *dual-task training,* in which the learner is required to perform two separate tasks at one time. For example, the patient is required to walk and carry on a conversation *(Walkie-Talkie test)* or to walk while carrying a tray with a glass of water on it. The learner should be equally successful at both tasks performed simultaneously. Only occasional feedback is needed from the therapist, focusing on key errors. Massed practice (rest time is much less than practice time) can be used while promoting varying task demands in environments that promote open skills. The learner should be confident and accomplished in decision-making from repeated challenges to movement skills that the therapist has posed. The outcome of this stage of learning is successful preparation to meet the multitask challenges of home, community, and work/play environments. Table 2.2 presents a summary of the stages of motor learning and training strategies.

Feedback

Feedback is a critical factor in promoting motor learning. Feedback can be *intrinsic (inherent),* occurring as a natural result of the movement, or *extrinsic (augmented),* sensory cueing not normally received during the movement task. Proprioceptive, visual, vestibular, and cutaneous signals are types of intrinsic feedback, whereas visual, auditory, and tactile cueing are forms of extrinsic feedback (e.g., verbal cues, tactile cues, manual contacts, and biofeedback devices). During therapy, both intrinsic and extrinsic feedback are manipulated to enhance motor learning. *Concurrent feedback* is given during task performance, and *terminal feedback* is given at the end of task performance. Augmented feedback about the end result or overall outcome of the movement is termed *knowledge of results (KR).* Augmented feedback about the nature or quality of the movement pattern produced is termed *knowledge of performance (KP).* The relative importance of KP and KR varies according to the skill being learned and the availability of feedback from intrinsic sources. For example, tracking tasks (e.g., trace a star task) are highly dependent on intrinsic visual and kinesthetic feedback (KP), whereas KR has less influence on the accuracy of the movements. Knowledge of results provides key information about how to shape the overall movements for the next attempt. Performance cues (KP) that focus on task elements and error identification are not useful without KR.

Questions that guide and inform clinical decisions about feedback include:

- What type of feedback should be employed *(mode)*?
- How much feedback should be used *(intensity)*?
- When should feedback be given *(scheduling)*?

Choices about the type of feedback involve the selection of which intrinsic sensory systems to highlight, what type of augmented feedback to use, and how to pair extrinsic feedback with intrinsic feedback. The selection of sensory systems depends on specific examination findings of sensory integrity. The sensory systems selected must provide accurate and usable information. If an intrinsic sensory system is impaired and provides distorted or incomplete information (e.g., impaired proprioception with diabetic neuropathy), then the use of alternative sensory systems (e.g., vision) should be emphasized. Supplemental augmented feedback can also be used to enhance learning. Decisions are also based on the stage of learning. Early in learning, visual feedback is easily brought to conscious attention and is important. Less consciously, accessible sensory information such as proprioception becomes more useful during the middle and final stages of learning.

Decisions about frequency and scheduling of feedback (when and how much) must be reached. *Constant feedback* (e.g., given after every trial) quickly guides the learner to the correct performance but slows retention. Conversely, *variable feedback* (not given after every trial) slows the initial acquisition of performance skills but improves retention. This is most likely due to the increased depth of cognitive processing that accompanies the variable presentation of feedback. Feedback schedules are presented in Box 2.5.

It is important to provide the learner with the opportunity and time for introspection and self-assessment. If the therapist bombards the patient with augmented feedback during or immediately after task completion,

TABLE 2.2 Characteristics of Stages of Motor Learning and Training Strategies^a

Cognitive Stage Characteristics	Training Strategies
The learner develops an understanding of task, *cognitive mapping:* assesses abilities, task demands; identifies stimuli, contacts memory; selects response; performs initial approximations of task; structures motor program; modifies initial responses ***"What to do"*** decision	Highlight purpose of task in functionally relevant terms. Demonstrate ideal performance of task to establish a *reference of correctness.* Have patient verbalize task components and requirements. Point out similarities to other learned tasks. Direct attention to critical task elements. Select appropriate feedback. **Emphasize intact sensory systems, intrinsic feedback systems.** • Carefully pair extrinsic feedback with intrinsic feedback. • High dependence on vision: Have patient watch movement. • Provide KP: Focus on errors as they become consistent; do not cue on large number of random errors. • Provide KR: Focus on success of movement outcome. **Ask learner to evaluate performance, outcomes;** identify problems, solutions. Use reinforcements (praise) for correct performance and continuing motivation. **Organize feedback schedule.** • Feedback after every trial improves performance during early learning. • Variable feedback (summed, fading, bandwidth) increases depth of cognitive processing, improves retention; may decrease performance initially. **Organize practice.** • Stress controlled movement to minimize errors. • Provide adequate rest periods using distributed practice if task is complex, long, or energy costly or if learner fatigues easily, has short attention, or has poor concentration. • Use manual guidance to assist as appropriate. • Break complex tasks down into component parts; teach both parts and integrated whole. • Utilize bilateral transfer as appropriate. • Use blocked practice of same task to improve performance. • Use variable practice (serial or random practice order) of related skills to increase depth of cognitive processing and retention; may decrease performance initially. • Use mental practice to improve performance and learning; reduce anxiety. **Assess and modify arousal levels as appropriate.** • High or low arousal impairs performance and learning. • Avoid stressors, mental fatigue. **Structure environment.** • Reduce extraneous environmental stimuli and distracters to ensure attention, concentration. • Emphasize closed skills initially, gradually progressing to open skills.
Associative Stage Characteristics	**Training Strategies**
The learner practices movements, refines motor program, spatial and temporal organization; decreases errors, extraneous movements	**Select appropriate feedback.** • Continue to provide KP; intervene when errors become consistent. • Emphasize proprioceptive feedback, "feel of movement" to assist in establishing an internal reference of correctness.

(table continues on page 24)

TABLE 2.2 Characteristics of Stages of Motor Learning and Training Strategies[a] *(continued)*

Associative Stage Characteristics	Training Strategies
Dependence on visual feedback decreases, increases for use of proprioceptive feedback; cognitive monitoring decreases ***"How to do"* decision**	• Continue to provide KR; stress relevance of functional outcomes. • Assist learner to improve self-evaluation and decision-making skills. • Facilitation techniques; guided movements are counterproductive during this stage of learning. **Organize feedback schedule.** • Continue to provide feedback for continuing motivation; encourage patient to self-assess achievements. • Avoid excessive augmented feedback. • Focus on use of variable feedback (summed, fading, bandwidth) designs to improve retention. **Organize practice.** • Encourage consistency of performance. • Focus on variable practice order (serial or random) of related skills to improve retention. **Structure environment.** • Progress toward open, changing environment. • Prepare the learner for home, community, work environments.
Autonomous Stage Characteristics	**Training Strategies**
The learner practices movements and continues to refine motor responses; spatial and temporal highly organized, movements are largely error-free; minimal level of cognitive monitoring ***"How to succeed"* decision**	Assess need for conscious attention, automaticity of movements. **Select appropriate feedback.** • Learner demonstrates appropriate self-evaluation and decision-making skills. • Provide occasional feedback (KP, KR) when errors are evident. **Organize practice.** • Stress consistency of performance in variable environments, variations of tasks (open skills). • High levels of practice (massed practice) are appropriate. **Structure environment.** • Vary environments to challenge learner. • Ready the learner for home, community, and work environments. Focus on competitive aspects of skills as appropriate, e.g., wheelchair sports.

[a]From O'Sullivan SB[1] (with permission).

this will likely prove excessive and preclude active information processing by the learner. The patient's own decision-making skills are minimized, and the therapist's verbal feedback dominates. This may well explain why the patient who is undergoing rehabilitation may show minimal carryover and limited retention of newly acquired motor skills. The withdrawal of augmented feedback should be gradual and carefully paired with the patient's efforts to correctly utilize intrinsic feedback systems.

Feedback in the form of positive reinforcement and rewards is an important motivational tool to shape behavior. Helping the patient recognize and attend to successes in training goes a long way toward reducing anxiety and depression. The institutional environment and the nature of the disability contribute to feelings of *learned helplessness*. Therapists play a major role in counteracting these feelings and ensuring that the patient is motivated to succeed. This includes making sure that the patient is an active participant in all phases of the treatment planning process, including goal setting. For activity-based training to succeed, it must have meaning and relevance for the patient.

BOX 2.5 Feedback Schedules to Enhance Motor Learning[a]

- **Constant feedback:** Feedback is given after every practice trial.
- **Summed feedback:** Feedback is given after a set number of trials; for example, feedback is given after every other or every third trial.
- **Faded feedback:** Feedback is given at first after every trial and then less frequently; for example, feedback is given after every second trial, progressing to every fifth trial.
- **Bandwidth feedback:** Feedback is given only when performance is outside a given error range; for example, feedback is given if performance (gait) is too slow or too fast, but not if it falls within a predetermined range.
- **Delayed feedback:** Feedback is given after a brief time delay; for example, feedback is given after a 3-second delay.

[a]Adapted from Schmidt, R, and Lee, T.[27(pp493–501)]

Practice

A major factor that influences motor learning is *practice*. In general, the more practice that is built into the training schedule, the greater the learning. For example, the patient who practices daily in both supervised (clinic) and unsupervised settings (home or hospital unit) will demonstrate increased learning over the patient who is seen once a week in an outpatient clinic without the benefit of any additional practice incorporated into the home exercise program (HEP). The therapist's role is to ensure that the patient practices the correct movements. Practicing incorrect movement patterns can lead to *negative learning* in which faulty habits and postures must be unlearned before the correct movements can be mastered. This sometimes occurs when a patient goes home for an extended period before participating in active rehabilitation. The organization of practice depends on several factors, including the patient's motivation, attention span, concentration, endurance, and the type of task. Additional factors include the frequency of allowable therapy sessions, which often depends on hospital scheduling, and the availability of services and payment (socioeconomic factors). For outpatients, practice at home is highly dependent on motivation, family support, and suitable environment, as well as a well-constructed HEP.

Questions that guide and inform clinical decisions about practice include:

- How should practice periods and rest periods be spaced (*practice distribution*)?
- What tasks and task variations should be practiced (*practice variation*)?
- How should the tasks be sequenced (*practice order*)?
- How should the environment be structured (*closed* vs. *open*)?

Massed practice refers to a sequence of practice and rest intervals in which the rest time is *much less* than the practice time. Fatigue, decreased performance, and risk of injury must be considered when using massed practice. *Distributed practice* refers to spaced practice intervals in which the practice time is *equal to or less than* the rest time. Although learning occurs with both, distributed practice results in the most learning per training time, although the total training time is increased. Distributed practice is the preferred mode for many patients undergoing active rehabilitation who demonstrate limited performance capabilities and endurance. With adequate rest periods, performance can improve without the interfering effects of fatigue or increasing safety issues. Distributed practice is also beneficial if motivation is low or if the learner has a short attention span, poor concentration (e.g., the patient with TBI), or motor planning deficits (e.g., the patient with dyspraxia). Distributed practice should also be considered if the task itself is complex, is long, or has a high energy cost. Massed practice can be considered when motivation and skill levels are high and when the patient has adequate endurance, attention, and concentration. For example, the patient with SCI in the final stages of rehabilitation may spend long practice sessions acquiring the wheelchair skills needed for independent community mobility.

Blocked practice refers to a practice sequence organized around one task *performed repeatedly,* uninterrupted by the practice of any other task. *Random practice* refers to a practice sequence in which a variety of tasks are *ordered randomly* across trials. Although both allow for motor skill acquisition, random practice has been shown to have superior long-term retention effects. For example, a variety of different transfers (e.g., bed-to-wheelchair, wheelchair-to-toilet, wheelchair-to-tub seat) can be practiced, all within the same therapy session. Although skilled performance of individual tasks may be initially delayed, improved retention of transfer skills can be expected. The constant challenge of varying the task demands provides high *contextual interference* and increases the depth of cognitive processing through retrieval practice from memory stores. The acquired skills can then be applied more easily to other task variations or environments (promoting *adaptability*). Blocked practice will result in superior initial performance because of low contextual interference and may be required in certain situations (e.g., the patient with TBI who requires a high degree of structure and consistency for learning).

Practice order refers to the sequence in which tasks are practiced. *Blocked order* is the repeated practice of a single task or group of tasks in order with a specified number of trials (three trials of task 1, three trials of task 2, three trials of task 3: 111222333). *Serial order* is a predictable and repeating order (practicing multiple tasks in the following order: 123123123). *Random order* is a nonrepeating and unpredictable practice order (123321312). Although skill acquisition can be achieved with all three orders, differences have been found. Blocked order produces improved early acquisition and performance of skills, whereas serial and random orders produce better retention and adaptability of skills. This result is again due to contextual interference and increased depth of cognitive processing. The key element here is the degree to which the learner is actively involved in memory retrieval. For example, a treatment session can be organized to include practice of a number of different tasks (e.g., forward stepping, backward stepping, sidestepping, and stair climbing). Random ordering of the tasks may initially delay acquisition of the desired stepping movements but over the long term will result in improved retention and adaptability of skills.

Parts-to-Whole Practice

Some complex motor skills can be effectively broken down into component parts for practice. Practice of the component parts should be followed closely by practice of the integrated whole task. For example, during initial wheelchair transfer training, the transfer steps are practiced (e.g., locking the brakes, lifting the foot pedals, moving forward in the chair, standing up, pivoting, and sitting down). During the same therapy session, the transfer is also practiced as a whole. Delaying practice of the integrated whole can interfere with learning the whole task.

Clinical Note: Parts-to-whole practice is most effective with discrete or serial motor tasks that have highly independent parts (e.g., transfers). Parts-to-whole practice is less effective for continuous movement tasks (e.g., walking) and for complex tasks with highly integrated parts (e.g., fine motor hand skills). Both require

a high degree of coordination with spatial and temporal sequencing of elements. For these tasks, emphasis on the practice of the integrated whole is desirable.

Mental Practice

Mental practice is a practice strategy in which performance of the motor task is imagined or visualized without overt physical practice. Beneficial effects result from the cognitive rehearsal of task elements. It is theorized that underlying motor programs for movement are activated but with subthreshold motor activity. Mental practice has been found to promote the acquisition of motor skills. It should be considered for patients who fatigue easily and are unable to sustain physical practice. Mental practice is also effective in alleviating anxiety associated with initial practice by previewing the upcoming movement experience. Patients who combine mental practice with physical practice can increase the accuracy and efficiency of movements at significantly faster rates than subjects who used physical practice alone. Box 2.6 defines practice schedules that can be used to enhance motor learning.

Clinical Note: When using mental practice, the therapist must ensure that the patient understands the task and is actively rehearsing the correct movements. This can be assured by having the patient verbalize the steps he or she is rehearsing.

Red Flag: Mental practice is generally contraindicated in patients with cognitive, communication, and/or perceptual deficits. These patients typically have difficulty understanding the idea of the task.

Unsupervised Practice

Regularly scheduled therapy time typically does not provide the substantial amount of practice time required for

---

BOX 2.6 Practice Schedules Enhance Motor Learning[a]

- **Massed practice:** a sequence of practice and rest times in which the rest time is much less than the practice time. For example, practice is for 1 hour with a 10-minute rest.
- **Distributed practice:** a sequence of practice and rest periods in which the practice time is often equal to or less than the rest time. For example, practice is for 10 minutes with a 10-minute rest.
- **Blocked practice:** a practice sequence organized around one task performed repeatedly, uninterrupted by practice on any other task; low contextual interference. For example, three trials of task 1 are practiced (111); other tasks practiced that session are also blocked: three trials of task 2 (222), three trials of task 3 (333), and so on.
- **Serial practice:** a predictable and repeating order of practice of multiple tasks. For example, three tasks are practiced in repeating order: 123123123.

- **Random practice:** a practice sequence in which the tasks being practiced are ordered (quasi-) randomly across trials; high contextual interference. For example, three tasks are practiced in random order: 123321312.
- **Parts-to-whole practice:** a practice sequence in which the task is broken down into its component parts for separate practice; practice of the integrated whole task is then performed.
- **Mental practice:** a practice method in which performance of the motor task is imagined or visualized without overt physical practice. For example, a patient cognitively rehearses the steps of a stair-climbing sequence using an assistive device before physically practicing the skill (the sound LE leads up and the cane and affected LE follow).

---

[a]Adapted from Schmidt, R, and Lee, T.[27(pp493–501)]

skill learning. The hours the patient spends outside of therapy either on the hospital unit or at home are generally times of limited activity. The therapist needs to engage the patient and family to use this time efficiently for meaningful practice. Patient and family training in the activities to be performed on the unit or at home (HEP) is essential. Instructions should be clear, concise, and in writing. Activities should first be demonstrated and practiced in a supervised setting. The patient can be instructed to document unsupervised practice using an *activity log* in which the patient records the activity practiced, the duration (number of repetitions) of practice, and comments as needed (e.g., level of pain, dizziness, or discomfort). The therapist should evaluate activity log recordings on a regular basis. The environment should be chosen or organized to ensure success in unsupervised practice. Patient safety and adequate rest periods are critical elements. For example, standing balance exercises are often performed in the home using hand support on the kitchen counter to improve safety—hence the name "kitchen sink exercises."

Transfer of Learning

Transfer of learning refers to the gain (or loss) in the capability of task performance as a result of practice or experience with some other task.[26] Learning can be promoted through practice using contralateral extremities, termed *bilateral transfer.* For example, the patient with stroke first practices the desired movement pattern using the less-affected extremity. This initial practice enhances the formation or recall of the necessary motor program, which can then be applied to the opposite, more involved extremity. This method cannot, however, substitute for lack of movement potential of the affected extremities (e.g., a flaccid limb on the hemiplegic side). Transfer effects are optimal when the tasks (e.g., components and actions) are similar. For example, optimal transfer can be expected with practice of a UE pattern first on one side and then on the other with an identical pattern (e.g., hand-to-mouth or forward reach and grasp). Practice of dissimilar activities can lead to negative transfer or loss in the capability to perform the criterion task. Optimal transfer can also be expected with practice in similar environments. For example, practice in moving in a simulated bedroom containing a furniture arrangement similar to the patient's real-world bedroom at home.

Lead-up activities (subskills) are commonly used in physical therapy. Lead-up activities are simpler task versions or component parts of a larger, more complex task. Lead-up activities are practiced typically in easier postures with significantly reduced postural demands and degrees of freedom. Anxiety is also reduced and safety is ensured. For example, initial upright postural control of the trunk and hips can be practiced in kneeling, half-kneeling, and plantigrade before standing. The patient develops the required hip extension and abduction stabilization control required for upright stance but without the overall demands of the standing position or fear of falling. The more closely the lead-up activities resemble the requirements of the *criterion task,* the better the transfer of learning.

Structuring the Environment

Environmental context is an important consideration in structuring practice sessions. Early learning benefits from practice in a stable or predictable *closed environment.* As learning progresses, the environment should be modified to incorporate more variable features consistent with real-world *open environments.* Practicing walking only inside the physical therapy clinic might lead to successful performance in that setting *(context-specific learning)* but does little to prepare the patient for walking at home or in the community. The therapist should gradually begin to modify the environment as soon as performance becomes consistent. Some patients, however (e.g., the patient with severe TBI and limited recovery), may never be able to function in anything but a highly structured environment.

The social benefits of working in an enriched or group environment should not be underestimated. Patients admitted for rehabilitation often have difficulty working in unfamiliar and unstimulating environments. Depression and lack of motivation are the natural outcomes. Therapists should encourage patients to socially interact with others and promote participation in group classes whenever possible. An active, engaged patient is also a motivated one.

Enhancing Patient Decision-Making

As learning progresses, the patient should be actively involved in self-monitoring, analysis, and self-correction of movements. The therapist can prompt the learner in early decision-making by posing the key questions listed in Box 2.7.

The therapist should confirm the accuracy of the patient's responses. If errors are consistent, the patient's efforts

---

BOX 2.7 Guiding Questions to Promote Active Patient Decision-Making and Autonomy[1]

- What is the goal of the intended movement?
- Did you accomplish the goal? If not, does the goal need to be modified?
- Did you move as planned? If not, what problems did you encounter during the movement?
- What do you need to do to correct the problems so that you can achieve movement success?
- For complex movements, what are the component parts or steps of the task? How should the component parts be sequenced?
- What aspects of the environment led to your success (or failure) in reaching the goal of the intended movement?
- What motivates you to keep trying?
- How confident are you in your abilities to move on your own? To be safe in your home environment?

can be redirected. For example, the patient recovering from stroke with pusher syndrome (ipsilateral pushing) consistently pushes to the affected side and will likely fall if not guarded. The therapist can pose these questions: "What direction do you feel you will fall?" and "What do you need to do to correct this problem?" The therapist can also use augmented cues (e.g., tapping or light resistance) to assist the patient in correcting postural responses and in moving toward a more symmetrical posture. Developing independent decision-making skills is critical to ensuring the learning and adaptability required for community living.

Augmented Interventions and Neuromotor Approaches

During early recovery, patients with limited voluntary control may benefit from training using augmented interventions. This can consist of hands-on guided or assisted movements and facilitated movements using specific techniques (e.g., neuromuscular facilitation techniques, sensory stimulation techniques) to promote voluntary control. For example, patients with stroke or TBI who are early in recovery and have limited voluntary movement abilities are good candidates. These interventions may help the patient bridge the gap between absent or severely disordered movements and active movements. Thus they are used to "jump-start" recovery. Two popular neuromotor approaches in current use are PNF[30,31] (discussed in Chapter 3) and NDT[32,33] (discussed below). Biofeedback and neuromuscular electrical stimulation can also be used to jump-start motor recovery.

Red Flag: Patients who demonstrate sufficient recovery and consistent voluntary movement control would not benefit from augmented interventions and an intensive hands-on approach. Prolonged use of these techniques long after they are needed is counterproductive and may actually delay recovery. Rather, these patients are candidates for activity-based, task-oriented interventions that emphasize active control and effective motor learning strategies.

Neuromuscular Facilitation Techniques

A number of neuromuscular facilitation techniques can be used to facilitate, activate, or inhibit muscle contraction. These have been collectively called *facilitation techniques,* although this term is a misnomer because these techniques also include those used for inhibition. The term *facilitation* refers to the enhanced capacity to initiate a movement response through increased neuronal activity and altered synaptic potential. An applied stimulus may lower the synaptic threshold of the motor neuron but may not be sufficient to produce an observable movement response. *Activation,* on the other hand, refers to the actual production of a movement response and implies reaching a critical threshold level for neuronal firing. *Inhibition* refers to the decreased capacity to initiate a movement response through altered synaptic potential. The synaptic threshold is raised, making it more difficult for the neuron to fire and produce movement. The combination of spinal inputs and supraspinal inputs acting on the alpha motor neuron (final common pathway) will determine whether a muscle response is facilitated, activated, or inhibited. Table 2.3 presents an overview of neuromuscular facilitation techniques.

Several general guidelines are important. Facilitative techniques can be *additive.* For example, inputs applied simultaneously, such as quick stretch, resistance, and verbal cues, are commonly combined when PNF patterns are applied. These stimuli collectively can produce the desired motor response, whereas the use of a single stimulus may not. This demonstrates the property of *spatial summation* within the CNS. *Repeated stimulation* (e.g., repeated quick stretches) may also produce the desired motor response owing to *temporal summation* within the CNS, whereas a single stimulus does not. For example, stretch is used initially in the lengthened range (PNF pattern) to initiate a movement and repeatedly at midrange to ensure that a weak muscle can move into the shortened range. The response to stimulation or inhibition is unique to each patient and depends on a number of different factors, including level of intactness of the CNS, arousal, and the specific level of activity of the motor neurons in question. For example, a patient who is depressed and hypoactive or taking CNS suppressant drugs may require larger amounts of stimulation to achieve the desired response. Stimulation is generally contraindicated for the patient with hyperactivity, but inhibition/relaxation techniques are beneficial. The intensity, duration, and frequency of simulation need to be adjusted to meet individual patient needs. Unpredicted responses can result from inappropriately applying the techniques. For example, stretch applied to a spastic muscle may increase spasticity and negatively affect voluntary movement.

Neurodevelopmental Treatment

NDT is an approach developed in the late 1940s and early 1950s by Dr. Karel Bobath, an English physician, and his wife, Berta Bobath, a physiotherapist.[32] Their early work involved patients with cerebral palsy and stroke. The primary focus in treatment was on specialized handling that inhibited spastic and reflex patterns and promoted normal postural control and movements. The rationale for this approach (hierarchical theory with top-down control) has been largely refuted by more recent studies on the nervous system.

Current NDT has realigned itself with newer theories of motor control (systems theory and a distributed model of CNS control). Many different factors are recognized as

TABLE 2.3 Neuromuscular Facilitation Techniques		
Stimulus	Response	Comments
Resistance: applied manually, using body position/gravity, or mechanically	Facilitates both intrafusal and extrafusal muscle contraction; hypertrophies extrafusal muscle fibers; enhances kinesthetic awareness (muscle spindle)	With very weak muscles, use light resistance; isometric and eccentric contractions before concentric. Maximal resistance can produce overflow from strong to weak muscles within the same synergistic pattern or to contralateral extremities.
Quick stretch: to agonist	Facilitates both intrafusal and extra-fusal agonist muscle contraction *(stretch reflex)*	Optimally applied in the lengthened range. A low-threshold response, relatively short-lived; can add resistance to maintain contraction.
Tapping/repeated quick stretch: over tendon or muscle belly	Facilitates both intrafusal and extra-fusal agonist muscle contraction *(stretch reflex)*	Tapping over muscle belly produces a weaker response than over the tendon. Tapping over a muscle is used to enhance holding in a weightbearing position.
Prolonged stretch: slow, maintained stretch, applied at maximum available lengthened range	Inhibits or dampens muscle contraction and tone due to peripheral reflex effects *(stretch-protection reflex)*	Positioning; inhibitory splinting, casting; mechanical low-load weights using traction
Joint approximation: compression of joint surfaces, using manual pressure or position/gravity; weighted vest or belt	Facilitates postural extensors and stabilizing responses (co-contraction); enhances joint awareness (joint receptors)	Approximation applied to top of shoulders or pelvis in upright weightbearing positions facilitates postural extensors and stability (e.g., sitting, kneeling, or standing). Used in PNF extensor extremity patterns, pushing actions.
Joint traction: manual distraction of joints; wrist and ankle cuffs	Facilitates joint motion; enhances joint awareness (joint receptors)	Joint mobilization uses slow, sustained traction to improve mobility, relieve muscle spasm, and reduce pain. Used in PNF flexor extremity patterns, pulling actions.

contributing to loss of motor function in patients with neurological dysfunction, including the full spectrum of sensory and motor deficits (weakness, limited ROM, and impaired tone and coordination). Emphasis is on the use of both feedback and feedforward mechanisms to support and improve postural control. Postural control is viewed as the foundation for all skill learning. Normal development in children and normal functional movement patterns in all patients are stressed. The patient learns to control posture and movement through a sequence of progressively more challenging postures and activities.[33]

NDT uses *therapeutic handling techniques* to influence the quality of the motor response. Handling is carefully matched to the patient's abilities to use sensory information

and adapt movements. It includes neuromuscular facilitation, inhibition, or frequently a combination of the two. Manual contacts are used to direct, regulate, and organize movements using tactile, proprioceptive, and vestibular inputs. *Key points of control,* defined as parts of the body that are optimal for control of inhibiting or facilitating movements, are used. Focus is on directing the patient to achieve more efficient and effective postural control and movement patterns. Abnormal movements (e.g., abnormal obligatory synergies) are restricted. The therapist provides appropriate feedback for reference of correction and movement control and directs the patient's attention to meaningful aspects of the motor task. Activities are selected that are functionally relevant and varied in terms of difficulty and environmental context. Compensatory interventions (use of the less-involved segments) are avoided. The therapist also recognizes when the patient can become independent of the therapist's assistance and take over control of posture and movement. Carryover is promoted through a strong emphasis on patient, family, and caregiver education.[33] NDT is taught today in recognized training courses;[34] foundational concepts are presented in Box 2.8. Research on the effectiveness of the Bobath approach in stroke rehabilitation has not revealed any superiority of this approach over other approaches; however, methodological shortcomings of the research exist, emphasizing the need for further high-quality trials.[35,36]

Sensory Stimulation Techniques

Sensory stimulation techniques (e.g., touch, visual, auditory, olfactory inputs) can be used to improve (1) alertness, attention, and arousal; (2) sensory discrimination; and (3) initiation of movements. During task-specific practice, the therapist can cue the patient about intrinsic sensory information vital to successful completion of the task. For example, during practice of sit-to-stand, the patient can be barefoot on a sticky mat (yoga mat) to increase attention to tactile inputs from the soles of the feet. The therapist encourages the patient to pay attention to relevant sensory cues and sets up the environment so as not to distract the patient during task performance. In addition, verbal and visual feedback can be provided to reinforce sensory awareness and motor performance.

Variable sensory impairments exist among patients. For example, decreased sensory sensitivity to stimulation and to the environment may be evident in patients with TBI who are minimally conscious and exhibit low arousal. Some patients may benefit from multisensory stimulation in a highly structured and consistent manner. Only one sensory stimulus is administered at a time, and the patient is given adequate time to respond to the stimulus. During stimulation, the patient is closely monitored for changes in behavior (e.g., diaphoresis, increased or decreased muscle tone, head turning, eye movements, grimacing, or vocalizations) or changes in vital signs (e.g., changes in heart rate, blood pressure, or respiratory rate). A systematic review published by the Cochrane Library suggests that there is no reliable evidence to support or rule out the effectiveness of sensory stimulation programs for patients with brain injury.[37]

Increased sensitivity to sensory stimulation is also seen in some patients (e.g., the patient with tactile defensiveness or high arousal). Sensory stimulation techniques are contraindicated in these patients. Excess stimulation can produce undesirable responses, including generalized arousal and fight-or-flight reactions. Rather, a soothing voice; gentle, maintained contacts; slow rocking; and neutral warmth provided by wrapping (e.g., with a blanket) the patient may lower arousal levels and help to calm the patient (e.g., the patient with TBI and high levels of arousal and agitation). These are techniques every parent with a colicky child knows and utilizes to calm the crying infant.

Sensory Retraining

Select patients with sensory deficits may be candidates for sensory retraining (e.g., the patient with stroke).[37–42] Interventions include sensory reeducation, tactile kinesthetic guiding, repetitive sensory practice, and desensitization. The patient is repeatedly exposed to training tasks that require sensory identification (e.g., numbers, letters drawn on the hand or arm), discrimination (e.g., detecting size, weight, shape, temperature, and texture of objects placed in the hand), or assisted drawing using a pencil. The tasks are

---

BOX 2.8 Neurodevelopmental Treatment (NDT) Foundational Principles[a]

- NDT is based on an ongoing analysis of sensorimotor function and carefully planned interventions designed to improve function. Principles of motor control, motor learning, and motor development guide the planning process.
- Interventions focus on the patient's strengths and competencies while at the same time addressing impairments, activity limitations, and participation restrictions. Negative signs (weakness, impaired postural control, and paucity of movement) are equally important to address in treatment as positive signs (spasticity, hyperactive reflexes).
- The POC is developed in partnership with the patient, family, and interdisciplinary team.
- Treatment focuses on the relationship between sensory input and motor output.
- Therapeutic handling is the primary NDT intervention strategy. Facilitating and/or inhibitory inputs are provided to influence the quality of motor responses.

- Training is focused on specific task goals and functional skills. The task and/or environment are modified as needed to enhance function.
- Active participation by the patient is a goal and an expectation of treatment.
- A major role of the therapist is completing an accurate analysis of motor problems and development of effective solutions.
- Motor learning principles are adhered to in the therapeutic setting, including verbal reinforcement, repetition, facilitation of error awareness (trial-and-error practice), and an environment conducive to learning, engaging the patient/client/family, and ensuring motivation.
- Direct teaching of the patient/client/family/caregiver to ensure carryover of functional activities in the home and community setting is an important component of NDT.

[a]Adapted from Howle.[34]

primarily manual, using the more affected hand for intense practice. Initial presentation of stimuli may be given to the less-affected hand to provide a reference of correctness (what the stimulus should feel like). A variety of tasks can help the patient maintain attention and motivation. Tasks are modified, and progress in difficulty is based on performance. Trainers provide random verbal feedback. Outcome measures may include testing sensory modalities (e.g., light touch temperature, two-point discrimination, sustained pressure, stereognosis, kinesthesia) and upper limb functional tests (e.g., *Wolf Motor Function Test,*[43] *Motor Activity Log*[44]). In a systematic review of the literature, Doyle et al[40] found insufficient evidence to reach conclusions on the effectiveness of any intervention for sensory impairment of the UE. Borstad et al[42] found preliminary evidence suggesting neural reorganization following a sensory training program using sensory functional magnetic resonance imaging. Limited preliminary evidence was found in support of using mirror therapy for improving detection of light touch, pressure, and temperature pain; thermal stimulation for improving rate of recovery of sensation; and intermittent pneumatic compression intervention for improving tactile and kinesthetic ability.[40] Additional research is needed. Continued practice with functionally relevant tasks is necessary to maintain the positive effects of any sensory retraining program.

Biofeedback

For patients with severe motor weakness, electromyographic biofeedback (EMG-BFB) using visual or sound signals to monitor muscle activity can be used to assist the patient in regaining neuromuscular control.[45,46] Surface electromyography electrodes are commonly used for recording. Patients who exhibit weak (trace, poor, or fair) muscle grades or deficient sensory feedback systems will benefit the most. Evidence presented in a Cochrane database summary has shown EMG-BFB to have a beneficial effect when used with standard physical therapy techniques.[46] The therapist must carefully structure the use of EMG-BFB with practice of activity-based, task-oriented training. External feedback must be reduced gradually to foster use of intrinsic feedback mechanisms and promote active movement control. Postural biofeedback using platform training is discussed in Chapter 9: Interventions to Improve Standing and Standing Balance Skills.

Neuromuscular Electrical Stimulation

Neuromuscular electrical stimulation is an effective modality used to stimulate contraction in very weak muscles. Electrodes are placed directly over the muscle to be stimulated. Contraction is elicited by depolarizing motor neurons, with larger motor units and a greater number of type II fibers firing first. The motor units will continue to fire until the stimulus stops. Neuromuscular electrical stimulation has been used to reeducate muscles, improve ROM, reduce spasticity when applied to the weak antagonist,

decrease edema, and manage disuse atrophy. Electrical stimulation in patients with stroke has been shown to reduce flexor tone and posturing of the hand, improve functional grasp, and reduce shoulder subluxation.[47,48] In a Cochrane database summary, researchers concluded that electrostimulation is a potential treatment to improve recovery of movement control and functional ability after stroke. However, the findings from the review were described as inconclusive owing to methodological problems.[49]

Functional electrical stimulation uses a microprocessor to recruit muscles in a programmed synergistic sequence for the purposes of improving functional movements. Functional electrical stimulation of the peroneal nerve has been shown to be effective in assisting dorsiflexion (reducing drop foot) and in improving walking after a stroke.[50–52]

Compensatory Intervention

Compensatory intervention strategies focus on the early resumption of function by using the less-involved (sound) body segments for function. For example, a patient with left hemiplegia is taught to dress using the right UE; a patient with a complete T1-level spinal cord lesion is taught to roll using UEs, head/upper trunk, and momentum. Central to this approach is the concept of *substitution*. Changes are made in the patient's overall approach to functional tasks. A second central tenet of this approach is modification of the task and environment *(adaptation)* to facilitate relearning of skills, ease of movement, and optimal performance. For example, the patient with unilateral neglect is assisted in dressing by color coding of the shoes (red tape on the left shoe, yellow tape on the right shoe). The wheelchair brake toggle is extended and color coded to allow easy identification by the patient.

A compensatory approach may be the only realistic approach possible when recovery is limited and the patient has severe impairments and functional losses with little or no expectation for additional recovery. Examples include the patient with complete SCI and the patient recovering from stroke with severe sensorimotor deficits and extensive comorbidities (e.g., severe cardiac and respiratory compromise). The latter example suggests severe limitations in the ability to actively move and participate in rehabilitation and to relearn motor skills. Box 2.9 presents basic principles and strategies of compensatory intervention.

Red Flags: Several important precautions should be noted with use of compensatory intervention strategies. Focus on the uninvolved segments to accomplish daily tasks may suppress recovery and contribute to learned nonuse of the impaired segments. For example, the patient with stroke may fail to learn to use the involved extremities. In addition, a focus on learning component skills without practicing the integrated whole skill may result in *splinter skills* (e.g., for the patient with

---

BOX 2.9 Compensatory Intervention[a]

- The patient is made aware of movement deficiencies.
- Alternative ways to accomplish a task are considered, simplified, and adopted.
- The patient is taught to use the segments that are intact to compensate for those that have been lost.
- The patient practices and relearns the task; repeated practice results in consistency and habitual use of the new pattern.

- The patient practices the functional skill in environments in which function is expected to occur.
- Energy conservation techniques are taught to ensure that the patient can complete all daily tasks.
- The patient's environment is adapted to facilitate practice and learning of skills, ease of movement, and optimal performance.
- Assistive devices are incorporated as needed.

[a]Adapted from O'Sullivan SB.[1]

BOX 2.10 Examples of Anticipated Goals and Expected Outcomes for Patients With Disorders of Motor Function[a]

Impact of pathology/pathophysiology is reduced.
- Risk of recurrence of condition is reduced.
- Risk of secondary impairment is reduced.
- Intensity of care is decreased.

Impact of impairments is reduced.
- Alertness, attention, and memory are improved.
- Joint integrity and mobility are improved.
- Sensory awareness and discrimination are improved.
- Motor function (motor control and motor learning) is improved.
- Muscle performance (strength, power, and endurance) is improved.
- Postural control and balance are improved.
- Gait and locomotion are improved.
- Endurance is increased.

Ability to perform physical actions, tasks, or activities is improved.
- Functional independence in activities of daily living and instrumental activities of daily living is increased.
- Functional mobility skills are improved.
- Level of supervision for task performance is decreased.

- Tolerance of positions and activities is increased.
- Flexibility for varied tasks and environments is improved.
- Decision-making skills are improved.
- Safety of patient/client, family, and caregivers is improved.

Disability associated with acute or chronic illness is reduced.
- Activity participation is improved (home, community, leisure).

Ability to assume/resume self-care, home management, and work (job/school/play) is improved.

Health status is improved.
- Sense of well-being is increased.
- Insight, self-confidence, and self-image are improved.
- Health, wellness, and fitness are improved.

Satisfaction, access, availability, and services are acceptable to patient/client. Patient/client, family, and caregiver knowledge and awareness of the diagnosis, prognosis, anticipated goals/expected outcomes, and interventions are increased.

[a]Adapted from *Guide to Physical Therapist Practice*.[53]

---

stroke). Splinter skills are those that cannot easily be generalized to variations of the same task or to other environments (poor adaptability).

Anticipated Goals and Expected Outcomes

The therapist's role is to accurately determine the patient's strengths and limitations, to fully engage the patient in collaborative planning, and to develop a POC that includes goals and outcomes that match the patient's unique needs. The therapist must also determine an appropriate level of difficulty, specifying the level of intensity, frequency, and duration of treatment. Examples of anticipated goals and expected outcomes for improving motor function are presented in Box 2.10.[53]

SUMMARY

Physical rehabilitation approaches are effective in promoting recovery of motor function. In a review of studies on recovery of function after stroke, Cochrane database researchers found that no one physical rehabilitation approach was more effective than any other approach and suggested beneficial effects when the therapist selects a mixture of different treatments.[54] As patients recover, their functional abilities and needs change. Therapists must be attuned to the patient's changing status and recognize that anticipated goals and expected outcomes can be expected to change along with the interventions likely to be most effective. Interventions focused on improving functional skills and motor learning are the mainstay of rehabilitation. These interventions need to be intense enough to promote behavioral change and neural reorganization. Adaptability of skills for function in "real-world" environments must also be a focus of treatment. To that end, the functional activities practiced must be meaningful and worthwhile to the patient. Collaborating with the patient, the therapist must select those activities that have the greatest chance of success. The choice of interventions must also take into consideration a host of other factors, including the age of the patient and overall health, number of comorbidities, level of social support and availability of care, cost-effectiveness in terms of length of stay and number of allotted physical therapy visits, and potential discharge placement.

REFERENCES

1. O'Sullivan, S. Strategies to improve motor function. In O'Sullivan, S, Schmitz, T, and Fulk, G (eds): Physical Rehabilitation, ed 6. Philadelphia, FA Davis, 2014, 393–443.
2. Fraser, C, et al. Driving plasticity in human adult motor cortex is associated with improved motor function after brain injury. Neuron, 2002; 34:831.
3. Kleim, J, Jones, T, and Schallert, T. Motor enrichment and the induction of plasticity before and after brain injury. Neurochem Res, 2003; 28:1757.
4. Nudo, RJ, Plautz, E, and Frost, S. Role of adaptive plasticity in recovery of function after damage to the motor cortex. Muscle Nerve, 2001; 24:1000.
5. French, B, et al. Repetitive task training for improving functional ability after stroke. Cochrane Database of Systematic Reviews 2007, Issue 4. Art. No.: CD006073. DOI: 10.1002/14651858.CD006073.
6. Ploughman, M. A review of brain neuroplasticity and implications for the physiotherapeutic management of stroke. Physiother Can, 2002; Summer:164.
7. Liepert, J, et al. Training-induced changes of motor cortex representations in stroke patients. Acta Neurol Scand, 2000; 101:321.
8. Taub, E, et al. Technique to improve chronic motor deficit after stroke. Arch Phys Med Rehabil, 1993; 74:347.
9. Wolf, S, et al. Effect of constraint-induced movement therapy on upper extremity function 3 to 9 months after stroke: the EXCITE randomized trial. JAMA 2006; 296:2095.
10. Wolf, S, et al. The EXCITE Trial: retention of improved upper extremity function among stroke survivors receiving CI movement therapy. Lancet Neurol, 2008; 7:33.
11. Sirtori, V, et al. Constraint-induced movement therapy for upper extremities in stroke patients. Cochrane Database of Systematic Reviews 2009, Issue 4. Art. No.: CD004433. DOI: 10.1002/14651858.CD004433.pub2.
12. Hakkennes, S, and Keating, J. Constraint-induced movement therapy following stroke: a systematic review of randomized controlled trials. Aus J Physiother, 2005; 51:221.
13. Dahl, A, et al. Short-and long-term outcome of constraint-induced movement therapy after stroke: a randomized controlled feasibility trial. Clinical Rehab, 2008; 22:436.
14. Page, S, et al. Efficacy of modified constraint-induced movement therapy in chronic stroke: a single-blinded randomized controlled trial. Arch Phys Med Rehabil, 2004; 85:14.
15. Taub, E, et al. A placebo-controlled trial of constraint-induced movement therapy for upper extremity after stroke. Stroke, 2006; 37:1045.
16. Sawaki, L, et al. Constraint-induced movement therapy results in increased motor map area in subjects 3 to 9 months after stroke. Neurorehabil Neural Repair, 2008; 33:505.
17. Richards, C, et al. Task-specific physical therapy for optimization of gait recovery in acute stroke patients. Arch Phys Med Rehabil, 1993; 74:612.
18. Visitin, M, et al. A new approach to retrain gait in stroke patients through body weight support and treadmill stimulation. Stroke, 1998; 29:1122.
19. Behrman, A, et al. Locomotor training progression and outcomes after incomplete spinal cord injury. Phys Ther, 2005; 85:1356.
20. Moseley, A, et al. Treadmill training and body weight support for walking after stroke. Cochrane Database of Systematic Reviews 2005, Issue 4. Art. No.: CD002840. DOI: 10.1002/14651858.CD002840.pub2.
21. Barbeau, H, Nadeau, S, and Garneau, C. Physical determinants, emerging concepts, and training approaches in gait of individuals with spinal cord injury. J Neurotrauma, 2006; 23:571.
22. Sullivan, K, et al. Effects of task-specific locomotor and strength training in adults who were ambulatory after stroke: results of the STEPS Randomized Clinical Trial. Phys Ther, 2007; 87:1580.
23. Duncan, P, et al. Body-weight-supported treadmill rehabilitation after stroke. N Engl J Med, 2011; 364:2026.
24. Ada, L. Randomized trial of treadmill walking with body weight support to establish walking in subacute stroke—the MOBILISE Trial. Stroke, 2010; 41:1247.
25. Franceschini, M, et al. Walking after stroke: what does treadmill training with body weight support add to overground gait training in patients early after stroke?: a single-blind, randomized controlled trial. Stroke, 2009; 40:3079.
26. Kleim, JA, and Jones, TA. Principles of experience-dependent neural plasticity: implications for rehabilitation after brain damage. J Speech Lang Hear Res, 2008; 51:S225–S239.
27. Schmidt, R, and Lee, T. Motor Control and Learning, ed 5. Champaign, IL, Human Kinetics, 2011.
28. Astrand, Per-Olof, et al. Textbook of Work Physiology—Physiological Bases of Exercise, ed 4. Champaign, IL, Human Kinetics, 2003.
29. Magill, R. Motor Learning and Control, ed 9. New York, McGraw-Hill, 2010.
30. Fitts, P, and Posner, M. Human Performance. Belmont, CA, Brooks/Cole, 1967.
31. Voss, D, et al. Proprioceptive Neuromuscular Facilitation: Patterns and Techniques, ed 3. Philadelphia, Harper & Row, 1985.
32. Adler, S, Beckers, D, and Buck, M. PNF in Practice, ed 3. New York, Springer-Verlag, 2008.
33. Bobath, B. The treatment of neuromuscular disorders by improving patterns of coordination. Physiotherapy, 1969; 55:1.
34. Howle, J. Neuro-Developmental Treatment Approach. Laguna Beach, CA, Neuro-Developmental Treatment Association, 2002.
35. Pollock, A, et al. Physiotherapy treatment approaches for stroke. Cochrane Corner. Stroke, 2008; 39:519.
36. Kollen, G, et al. The effectiveness of the Bobath concept in stroke rehabilitation. What is the evidence? Stroke, 2009; 40:e89.
37. Lombardi, F, et al. Sensory stimulation for brain injured individuals in coma or vegetative state. Cochrane Database Systematic Reviews 2002, Issue 2. Art. No.: CD001427. DOI: 10.1002/14651858.CD001427.
38. Celnik, P, et al. Somatosensory stimulation enhances the effects of training functional hand tasks in patients with chronic stroke. Arch Phys Med Rehabil, 2007; 88:1369.
39. Lynch, E, et al. Sensory retraining of the lower limb after acute stroke: a randomized controlled pilot trial. Arch Phys Med Rehabil, 2007; 88:1101.
40. Doyle, S, et al. Interventions for sensory impairment in the upper limb after stroke. Cochrane Database of Systematic Reviews 2010, Issue 6. Art. No.: CD006331. DOI: 10.1002/14651858.CD006331.pub2.
41. Schabrun, SM, and Hillier, S. Evidence for the retraining of sensation after stroke: a systematic review. Clin Rehabil, 2009; 23:27–39.
42. Borstad, A, et al. Sensorimotor training and neural reorganization after stroke: a case series. JNPT 2013; 37:27.
43. Wolf, S, et al. Assessing Wolf Motor Function Test as outcome measure for research in patients after stroke. Stroke, 2001; 32:1635.
44. Uswatte, G, et al. The Motor Activity Log-28: assessing daily use of the hemiparetic arm after stroke. Neurology, 2006; 76:1189.
45. Hiraoka, K. Rehabilitation efforts to improve upper extremity function in post-stroke patients: a meta-analysis. J Phys Ther Sci, 2001; 13:5.
46. Woodford, HJ. EMG biofeedback for the recovery of motor function after stroke. Cochrane Database of Systematic Reviews 2007, Issue 2. Art. No.: CD004585. DOI: 10.1002/14651858.CD004585.pub2.
47. Kowalczewski, J, et al. Upper-extremity functional electric stimulation-assisted exercises on a workstation in the sub-acute phase of stroke recovery. Arch Phys Med Rehabil, 2007; 88:833.
48. Meilink, A, Hemmen, B, and Ham, S. Impact of EMG-triggered neuromuscular stimulation of the wrist and finger extensors of the paretic hand after stroke: a systematic review of the literature. Clin Rehabil, 2008; 22:291.
49. Pomeroy, V, et al. Electrostimulation for promoting recovery of movement or functional ability after stroke. Cochrane Database of

Systematic Reviews 2006, Issue 2. Art. No.: CD003241. DOI: 10.1002/14651858.CD003241.pub2.

50. Yan, T, Hui-Chan, C, and Li, L. Functional electrical stimulation improves motor recovery of the lower extremity and walking ability of subjects with first acute stroke: a randomized placebo-controlled trial. Stroke, 2005; 36:80.

51. Roche, A, Laighin, G, and Coote, S. Surface-applied functional electrical stimulation for orthotic and therapeutic treatment of drop-foot after stroke—a systematic review. Phys Ther Rev, 2009; 14:63.

52. Embrey, D, et al. Functional electrical stimulation to dorsiflexors and plantar flexors during gait to improve walking in adults with chronic hemiplegia. Arch Phys Med Rehabil, 2010; 91:687.

53. American Physical Therapy Association. Guide to Physical Therapist Practice, Version 3.0., Alexandria, VA, 2014. Retrieved September 9, 2014, from http://guidetoptpractice.apta.org.

54. Pollock, A, et al. Physical rehabilitation approaches for recovery of function, balance, and walking after stroke. Cochrane Database of Systematic Reviews 2014, Issue 4. Art. No.: CD001920. DOI: 10.1002/14651858.CD001920.pub3.

History and Overview

Motor function can be improved in a wide range of patients using *proprioceptive neuromuscular facilitation (PNF)*. The philosophy, principles, and techniques of this approach were initially developed by Dr. Herman Kabat, a neurophysiologist and physician, and Maggie Knott, a physical therapist, in the 1940s and early 1950s. Their early focus was on developing a hands-on treatment that could be used to facilitate effective patterns of movement in patients with neurological impairments, especially multiple sclerosis and poliomyelitis. The approach was later successfully applied to patients with musculoskeletal impairments. Dorothy Voss, also a physical therapist, joined the team in 1952. Together, they refined the practice of PNF, enhancing its functional focus. Maggie Knott and Dorothy Voss authored the first PNF book, *Proprioceptive Neuromuscular Facilitation*, in 1956 as well as two subsequent editions appearing in 1968 and 1985.[1] Adler, Beckers, and Buck are the authors of a more recent comprehensive text, *PNF in Practice*.[2]

Early on, Kabat and Knott established postgraduate training institutes, known as the Kaiser-Kabat Institutes. One of these institutes, Kaiser Permanente in Vallejo, California, still exists today. It offers 3-, 6-, and 9-month residency programs. Participants receive classroom and laboratory instruction together with individualized instruction and extensive hours of supervised patient treatment.[3] Numerous additional postgraduate courses are available and have led to worldwide adoption of PNF. In 1985 the International PNF Instructor Group was formed, leading to the formation of the International PNF Association (IPNFA) in 1990. Its members consist of instructors and persons interested in PNF and in maintaining continuity and standards in PNF instruction, practice, and research. A full range of courses and levels of instruction can be found at their website (www.ipnfa.org).[4]

Key components of PNF include:

• Emphasis on functional outcomes
• Techniques to facilitate and enhance coordinated muscle activity
• Use of developmental postures and transitions to facilitate and enhance coordinated muscle activity
• Use of synergistic patterns of movement
• Inclusion of motor learning principles to promote skilled motor behavior

Synergies represent an important organizational element of the central nervous system (CNS) that serve to stabilize performance variables.[5] With practice, synergistic performance improves. In PNF, the synergist patterns are rotational and diagonal in nature rather than straight plane movements. This is an important concept that mirrors normal movement. The overall goal is to facilitate proximal stability of the trunk for distal controlled mobility of the extremities and to improve voluntary control and coordination of muscles both within and among patterns. Extremity patterns are unilateral or bilateral placing greater emphasis on the trunk and varied in difficulty by combining them with functional activities and postures (e.g., hooklying, rolling, sitting, quadruped, kneeling, modified plantigrade, standing, and locomotion). Techniques, largely proprioceptive, are used to facilitate or enhance movement, and motor learning principles (e.g., practice, repetition, feedback) are incorporated to promote acquisition, retention, and transfer of learning of new motor skills.

Principles

Principles inherent to PNF are used to optimize the patient's ability to move (Box 3.1). Overall goals include improved function with improved motor control, strength, and endurance. The therapist engages the patient through effective use of manual contacts, verbal commands, body position and body mechanics, and visual guidance of movement. Coordinated movement and timing are enhanced through the use of resistance, stretch, irradiation and reinforcement, and traction or approximation. Each patient has unique needs that determine the appropriate use and timing of these foundational elements. The therapist must recognize how and when to apply these elements and when to withdraw them to help the patient progress to independent movements. For weak or disordered movements, the effects of applying several elements during the same exercise (e.g., resistance, stretch, dynamic verbal commands) are additive and have a cumulative effect. Contraindications to the use of PNF include many of the same impediments to exercise in general, such as significant pain, unstable joints or fractures, and unstable medical condition.

BOX 3.1 PNF Principles

Patient position: Optimal patient performance is facilitated by ensuring that the patient is in optimal alignment. This includes positioning the patient in as close to neutral alignment as possible and providing support to body segments as needed.

Muscle positioning at optimal range of function allows for maximal contractile response *(length-tension relationship)*. The greatest muscle tension is generated in midranges; weak contractile force *(active insufficiency)* occurs in the shortened ranges. The lengthened range provides optimal stretch for muscle spindle support of contraction, while the shortened range with muscle spindle unloading provides the least amount of muscle spindle support for contraction.

Note: Changing the patient's body position (e.g., supine, sitting, standing) is used to emphasize certain segments of a pattern and to alter (increase or decrease) the postural stability demands.

Indications: enhance muscle contraction and maximize postural stability

Therapist position: The therapist is positioned directly *in line* with the desired motion (with pelvis, shoulders, and lower extremities facing the direction of the movement) to optimize application of resistance. Effective positioning also reduces the work of the therapist's arms and hands by allowing the resistance to come from the therapist's own body weight during weight shifting. In extremity patterns, as the limb moves through the pattern the therapist's position and angle of pull changes to continually optimize resistance.

Indications: enhances therapist's control of patient movements, reduce therapist fatigue through effective use of body weight and position, protect the therapist

Manual contacts: Precise manual contacts (hand placements) are used to apply input over active muscles to guide movement, facilitate strength of contraction, and to provide resistance opposite the direction of movements. The sensory input allows the patient to anticipate upcoming movement demands and to provide appropriate feedforward adjustments. A *lumbrical grip* is used to provide a comfortable and secure grip and to optimize rotation resistance. This consists of the therapist's hand positioned in metacarpophalangeal flexion with fingers and thumb griping the opposite sides of the distal segment.

Indications: guide movement (during initial learning), enhance muscle contraction and synergistic patterns; enhance kinesthetic awareness of movement or position during stabilization activities

Verbal cues and commands: Verbal cues (VCs) must be clear, concise, and well timed to the patient's movements and activity demands. Excessive or wordy cues are counterproductive and can impede motor learning.

- *Preparatory VCs* ready the patient for movement (what to do). They should optimally be accompanied by demonstration and/or guided movement to ensure the patient knows the idea behind the movement (cognitive stage of motor learning).
- *Action VCs* guide the patient through the movement, helping the patient learn how and when to move (associated stage of motor learning).

Dynamic action VCs are used to enhance the strength of muscle responses and coordination of synergistic components (e.g., *"Pull up and across your face, now bend your elbow"*). *Soft action VCs* are used when relaxation is the goal (e.g., *"Move slowly back and forth"*). Timing is critical. The patient's actions must be carefully coordinated with the therapist's VCs, resistance, and manual contacts.

- *Corrective VCs* provide augmented feedback to help the patient modify movements.

Indications: guide initial movements, improve motor learning, and enhance strength of muscle contraction and synergistic actions

Patterns of movement: Normal functional movements are composed of synergistic patterns involving the muscles of the limbs and trunk. Patterns of movement are generated by the motor cortex with input from the basal ganglia and cerebellum for programming, timing, and coordination. Synergistic patterns of movement are the basis of PNF patterns.

Timing: Normal (appropriate) timing refers to the sequencing of muscle activity to ensure smooth, coordinated movement. Functional activities require proximal stability for distal mobility; thus, core stability of the trunk is a basic requirement, and sequencing of contractions occurs proximal to distal. In extremity patterns, normal timing is from distal to proximal. Distal segments (hand/wrist or foot/ankle) begin the movement, followed closely by rotation and then proximal components. Rotation continues smoothly throughout the pattern.

Appropriate resistance: Appropriate resistance (optimal resistance) facilitates muscle contraction.[6,7] Both intrafusal and extrafusal muscle fibers contract, resulting in enhanced recruitment of motor units and improved strength of contraction. Resistance is applied manually to contracting muscles and functionally through the use of gravity to all types of contractions (isotonic [concentric and eccentric] and isometric). *Light resistance* applied to weak muscles is facilitatory and is usually applied in combination with light stretch. Appropriate resistance is used to allow for a smooth and coordinated contraction. It varies according to the individual patient and is adjusted to the goals of the specific activity. Resistance is also used to promote relaxation of antagonist muscles through the effects of reciprocal inhibition. It is important to monitor the patient for breath holding (commonly seen in isometric contractions), excessive fatigue, and unwanted irradiation.

Indications: facilitates weak muscles to contract, enhance kinesthetic awareness of motion and direction, increase strength, improve motor control and motor learning

Approximation: Approximation (compression of the joints of an extremity or the spine) is used to facilitate muscle responses in extensor patterns or during stabilizing activities. It can be applied manually by compressing the joint surfaces or functionally through the use of gravity and body weight acting on the body during upright weightbearing positions (e.g., sitting, standing, bouncing on a ball). Approximation is maintained

BOX 3.1 PNF Principles (continued)

throughout the pattern or activity and is combined with appropriate resistance and stabilizing VCs (e.g., *"Hold, hold"*). When using approximation, it is important to ensure all joints, including the spine, are properly aligned.

Indications: enhance contraction of antigravity, stabilizing muscles, and enhance function in weightbearing postures for stabilization control

Traction: A traction force applied throughout the arc of motion is used to facilitate muscle responses. Traction is maintained throughout the pattern and combined with appropriate resistance and dynamic VCs (e.g., *"Pull up"*).

Indications: weakness, inability of muscles to function in mobilizing patterns (e.g., open kinetic chain movement coupled with a stabilizing core response)

Visual input: The patient uses vision as a source of feedback to guide movements and enhance responses. The patient is instructed to look at the movements as they are occurring. During extremity patterns, this includes instructing the patient to turn the head to visually follow the distal segment (e.g., hand) through to completion of the movement. A mirror can be used to provide visual input and assist with trunk alignment and movements of the head, trunk, and extremities.

Indications: enhances contraction, motor control, and motor learning

Irradiation and reinforcement: Irradiation and reinforcement is the overflow of neuronal excitation from stronger motor units to motor units that may be weaker or inhibited (Sherrington's law of irradiation).[8] The spread or expansion of muscle response from stronger muscles to weaker muscles can occur in any direction and across any segment in the body: ipsilateral, contralateral, from extremities to trunk, or from trunk to extremities. More specifically, it can occur from phasic muscles to phasic muscles, from tonic muscles to tonic muscles, and from phasic to tonic muscles. *Temporal summation* (resulting from an increase in stimuli over time) and *spatial summation* (resulting from stimuli being applied to various segments across the body) can contribute to the spread of excitation and motor unit output across muscles. Appropriate resistance is the main mechanism for securing irradiation.

Indications: enhance strength of contraction and synergistic muscle activity

Quick stretch: The elongated position (lengthened range) of muscle and the stretch reflex are used to initiate dynamic movements and facilitate existing contractions through increased motor unit recruitment. All synergistic muscles in the pattern are elongated to optimize the effects of initial stretch. Verbal cues for voluntary movement must be synchronized with the stretch to enhance volitional responses. Resistance applied to the contracting muscle maximizes the effects of stretch.

Adapted from Voss et al.,[1] Adler, Beckers, and Buck,[2] and Johnson and Johnson.[7]

Techniques

Central to PNF are a group of therapeutic *techniques,* designed to promote and enhance movement. These techniques are presented in Box 3.2.

Applying the Principles to the Movement Patterns

The principles of PNF should guide the therapist's every manual interaction with a patient. Once a movement or stabilizing posture has been identified as the goal of treatment, the therapist should select the appropriate movement pattern to execute. The patterns should always be executed in the following manner:

- Position the patient appropriately.
- Assume an appropriate therapist position with proper body mechanics.
- Passively position the body part or segment to be facilitated in proper alignment.
- Determine the proper manual contact.
- Determine whether the intervention is to be passive movement or resisted movement.
- If a resisted movement is desired, determine whether the patient's pattern is to be resisted in midrange or at lengthened range.

- If a stretch stimulus is to be used, ensure that the patient's segment is properly elongated.
- If a stretch stimulus is to be used, couple the quick elongation with the proper verbal command and appropriate resistance, being sure to emphasize the traction at the beginning of the range and throughout the movement.
- If a midrange position is selected to initiate resistance, begin with a slowly building isometric resistance and progress to either concentric or eccentric resistance.
- Always observe the whole patient to determine the effect of therapist resistance and ensure proper irradiation and reinforcement.
- Always ensure that the trunk and interconnecting joints demonstrate appropriate stability before facilitating an extremity pattern.[6,7]

Patterns of Movement

Normal motor activity occurs in synergistic and functional patterns of movement. Proprioceptive neuromuscular facilitation patterns are *spiral* and *diagonal* in character and combine motion in all three planes: flexion/extension, abduction/adduction, and transverse rotation. They closely

(text continues on page 41)

BOX 3.2 PNF Techniques

Rhythmic Initiation
General goals: promote learning of a new movement, improve intra- and intermuscular coordination, promote relaxation and independent movement
Movement training occurs in four phases.
  1. The patient is instructed to relax (*"Relax, let me move you"*). The therapist moves the patient passively through the range, establishing appropriate speed and rhythm using verbal commands.
  2. Movements are then progressed to active assisted (*"Now, help me move you"*).
  3. The patient is then asked to move independently (*"Now, move up on your own"*).
  4. Movements are resisted (*"Now, push up"*). Appropriate resistance is used during the resistive phase to enhance movement.[4] Transitions between the different phases are smooth and continuous. Rhythmic initiation typically involves unidirectional movement but can be applied in both directions to enhance reciprocal movements.
Indications: inability to relax, hypertonicity (e.g., spasticity and rigidity), difficulty initiating movement, uncoordinated movement, motor planning or motor learning deficits (e.g., apraxia or dyspraxia), communication deficits (e.g., aphasia)

Prolonged Holds
General goals: based on the clinical application of irradiation, Johnson and Saliba Johnson[7] have described and defined two neuromuscular treatment techniques based on the principle of prolonged holds and the law of irradiation: *phasic shakes* (or *phasic spread*) and *tonic spread*. Before describing these techniques of irradiation, it is important to define the terms *source* and *target segments*:

   The *source segment* is the strong or efficient segment where resistance is applied to facilitate increased neuromuscular output elsewhere.
   The *target segment* is the segment with an inefficient muscular response that will benefit from irradiation from another segment in the body.

Clinical Note: Identifying a proper source segment, patient position, and appropriate resistance will directly affect the quality and effectiveness of irradiation. It is crucial to note that if not facilitated appropriately, irradiation can lead to increased tone and an abnormal motor response.

Phasic shakes: Irradiation achieved through the application of phasic shakes involves a sustained prolonged hold of phasic muscles leading to a spread of activation to tonic (stabilizing) muscles. This utilization of a prolonged hold will often generate a tetany or isometric tremor of the phasic muscles, eliciting a "shaking" of the muscles being resisted. This is a direct result of the inability or absence of tonic or core stabilizers to produce a stabilizing contraction or dynamic stability for distal mobility. When this phenomenon is observed, the therapist continues to resist the dominant phasic muscles

until the irradiation facilitates activation of the tonic or stabilizing muscles. Once the irradiation occurs to the core stabilizers, the tetany (or observed shaking) stops and the patient is able to stabilize efficiently. For example, prolonged resistance applied to bilateral lower extremity flexion/abduction (source) will lead to the eventual fatigue of the prime movers with irradiation to the trunk stabilizers (target) and the activation of a dynamically stable core. This irradiation technique is more commonly used with orthopedic populations, given the nature and challenge of the prolonged holds.
Tonic spread: Applying a tonic spread involves using the irradiation from tonic (stabilizing) muscles of one segment to tonic (stabilizing) muscles of a different segment (e.g., irradiation from the pelvic/hip tonic stabilizers to the trunk tonic stabilizers). To facilitate an isometric (stabilizing) contraction, initial resistance to the source segment must be applied *slowly* and with a *low* load aimed at facilitating tonic fibers. As the therapist perceives a building muscular response at the *source* segment, resistance is slowly increased, allowing for further irradiation and increased motor output at the *target* segment. This technique leads to improved dynamic stability through the direct facilitation of tonic stabilizing musculature at the target segment.

Reversals of Antagonists
Description: two techniques that allow for agonist contraction followed by antagonist contraction without pause or relaxation: *dynamic reversals* and *stabilizing reversals*

Dynamic Reversals (Isotonic Reversals)
General goals: improve intra- and intermuscular coordination (smooth reversals of antagonists, rate of movement), strength, and active range of motion, endurance

   Dynamic reversals use isotonic concentric contractions of first agonists, then antagonists performed against resistance. First, the therapist resists contraction of one pattern (e.g., flexion-adduction-external rotation: *"Now, pull up and across your body"*). At the end of the desired range, a preparatory command is given to reverse direction, and the therapist switches hands to resist the opposite pattern. The patient is then instructed to move in the opposite direction (e.g., action command for extension-abduction-internal rotation: *"Now, push down and out toward me"*). The technique can be used with or without a hold at the end range of each direction. Reversals are repeated as often as necessary. If an imbalance exists, the stronger pattern is selected first, with progression to the weaker pattern. Modifications include working in a particular part of the range, progressing to full ROM (moving through increments of ROM). Initially, the patient can be asked to hold steady at the endpoint of ROM in preparation for the transition (dynamic reversals, hold): *"Now, pull up and across your body and hold."* Progression is then to no hold as the patient learns to transition smoothly between patterns. An initial stretch can be used to initiate the movement response.

BOX 3.2 PNF Techniques (continued)

Indications: impaired strength, range, and coordination; inability to easily reverse directions between agonist and antagonist; fatigue

Stabilizing Reversals (Isometric Reversals)
General goals: facilitate isometric (tonic stabilizing) contractions at the segment being resisted; improve stability, strength, intra- and intermuscular coordination, endurance, range of motion.

Stabilizing reversals use alternating isometric contractions with stabilizing holds of first agonists (*"Hold this position, and don't let me move you. Hold it."*) and then antagonists (*"Now hold this position, and don't let me move you"*) against resistance. A low load resistance is applied very slowly to a particular body part or two separate body segments. The therapist builds the resistance (combined with traction or approximation) until a strong isometric stabilizing hold is felt under both hands, indicating that the patient is able to stabilize and maintain the position.

Once a stabilizing contraction is achieved, one of the therapist's hands should begin increasing the amount of resistance with the intention to slowly take over application of resistance (control of contraction) to free the opposite hand. Throughout this transition, the verbal command continues to be *"Hold it; keep it there."* As one manual contact takes over, the opposite hand is "melting" off.

Before the therapist's hands are transitioned to placement in the opposite pattern a preparatory command is given. This sequence is repeated, with the therapist's hands moving from one body segment to the opposite body segment. If an imbalance exists, the stronger pattern is selected first, with progression to the weaker pattern.

Indications: impaired strength, stability and balance, coordination

Rhythmic Stabilization
General goals: improve stability (cocontraction of antagonists), strength, endurance, ROM, and intra- and intermuscular coordination; promote relaxation and decrease pain

Rhythmic stabilization uses isometric contractions of antagonist patterns, focusing on cocontraction of muscles. Rhythmic stabilization of the trunk utilizes resistance applied to one segment (e.g., on the anterior shoulder, the therapist's right hand pushes backward) while applying resistance to the other segment (e.g., on posterior pelvis, the therapist's left hand pulls forward). The therapist builds the resistance up slowly; no movement is allowed. Verbal commands include *"Hold, don't let me move you, hold, hold."* The therapist then shifts hands and applies resistance in the opposite direction, keeping each hand on the same section of the trunk (e.g., the therapist's right hand is placed forward on the front of the shoulder and resists the hold while the left hand is placed on the back of the pelvis and resists the hold). Verbal commands include *"Now, don't let me move you the other way, hold, hold."* An

alternative command is *"Don't let me twist you, hold, hold."* Upper trunk flexors and rotators are resisted at the same time as lower trunk extensors and rotators.

Indications: impaired strength and coordination, limitations in ROM, impaired stabilization control and balance

Repeated Stretch (Repeated Contractions)
General goals: enhance initiation of motion and motor learning, increase agonist strength and endurance, improve intra- and intermuscular coordination and ROM, reduce fatigue

Repeated isotonic contractions are performed, directed to the agonist muscles, initiated by a quick stretch and enhanced by resistance. The stretch can be performed from the beginning of the range (lengthened range) for very weak muscles or throughout the range at a point of weakness. The therapist gives a preparatory command (*"Now"*) while providing quick stretch of the muscles working in the pattern. An action command (*"Pull up and across"*) follows. The technique is repeated when the therapist notes a weakening of the contraction during a pattern (*"Again, pull up and across"*). Sufficient opportunity for a volitional effort/muscular response must be allowed before the next repeated stretch.

Indications: impaired strength, difficulty initiating movement, fatigue, and limitations in active ROM. The technique should not be applied in the presence of joint instability, pain, or injured muscle.

Combination of Isotonics
General goals: improve motor learning and improve intra- and intermuscular coordination, increase strength and ROM, promote stability, eccentric control and endurance, and improve function

Combination of isotonics utilizes concentric, isometric, and eccentric contractions of agonist muscles without loss of tension.[6,7] The limb is resisted moving through the range (concentric contraction) followed by a stabilizing contraction (holding in the position) and then an eccentric or lengthening contraction, moving slowly back to the start position; there is no relaxation between the types of contractions. Verbal commands are directed toward each phase of the movement (*"Push up." "Now, hold." "Now, slowly let me win."* or *"Slowly let it lengthen"*). The technique is typically used in antigravity activities and assumption of postures (e.g., bridging and sit-to-stand transitions).

During rolling, combination of isotonics can initially begin with an isometric hold (in sidelying), then progress to an eccentric lengthening followed by concentric shortening, with the sequence repeated through increments in ROM.

Indications: weak postural muscles, inability to eccentrically control body weight during movement transitions (e.g., sit-to-stand and stand-to-sit, poor dynamic postural control).

(box continues on page 40)

BOX 3.2 PNF Techniques (continued)

Timing for Emphasis (TE)
General goals: alter normal timing using resistance to enhance a more localized contraction and to emphasize a particular component within the pattern. For example, appropriate resistance can be used to elicit a strong contraction and allow irradiation and reinforcement to occur from strong to weak muscles within a synergistic pattern. The strong muscles can also be resisted isometrically ("locking in") while motion is allowed in the weaker muscles.

Indications: weakness, poor coordination, or both

Contract-Relax
General goals: improve ROM through facilitation, inhibition, and strengthening and relaxation of muscle groups

This facilitation stretching technique is usually performed at a point of limitation of ROM. The patient actively moves the limb in the pattern to the point of limitation using agonist contraction *("Pull your foot up, turn your leg out, and lift up and out").* The therapist then asks for a strong contraction of the range-restricting muscles (antagonists) *("Now, turn your leg in and hold").* The contraction is held for 5 to 8 seconds, enhancing relaxation through the inhibitory effects from autogenic inhibition. Voluntary relaxation and active movement then follow the hold into the new range of the agonist pattern *("Relax. Now turn and lift your leg up and out").* This action enhances relaxation through the additional inhibitory effects of reciprocal inhibition. The cycle is typically repeated several times until no additional range is obtained. The technique is best followed with active movements in the new range (e.g., repeated contractions of the agonist muscles) to maintain or enhance gains in range.

Indications: limitations in ROM. Contraindications include recent injury with inflammation and swelling, recent surgery.

Hold-Relax
General goals: improve ROM through facilitating, inhibiting, strengthening, and relaxing muscle groups.

This facilitation stretching technique is usually performed in a position of comfort and below the level that causes pain. The patient actively moves the limb in the pattern to the end of pain-free ROM (agonist contraction). A strong isometric contraction of the restricting muscles (antagonists) is resisted (providing autogenic inhibition), followed by voluntary relaxation and passive movement into the newly gained range of the agonist pattern. The therapist instructs the patient to pattern: *"Hold, don't let me move you."* This is followed by a command to *"Relax; now, let me move your leg up and out."*

Indications: limitations in passive ROM, especially with pain and contraindications including recent injury with inflammation and swelling, recent surgery

Replication (Hold-Relax-Active Motion)
General goals: improve intra- and intermuscular coordination and agonist muscle control in the shortened range and promote motor learning

The patient is positioned in the end position (shortened range) of a movement and is told *"Hold, and don't let me move you."* The isometric contraction is resisted, followed by voluntary relaxation and passive movement into the lengthened range *("Relax. Now let me move you back").* The therapist then instructs the patient to perform an isotonic contraction through the range: *"Now, push back"* into the end position again. Stretch and tracking resistance are applied to facilitate the isotonic contraction. For each repetition, increasing ROM is desired.

Indications: marked weakness and inability to sustain a contraction in the shortened range

Clinical Note: Combination of isotonics may be a more effective way to teach a new pattern. It is similar to replication, but instead of a passive movement into the range, the patient is taken there through an eccentric contraction. This allows for continued kinesthetic/proprioceptive awareness of the movement.

Resisted Gait Progression
General goals: improve coordination and timing of lower trunk/pelvis during locomotion.

Stretch, approximation, and appropriate resistance are applied manually to facilitate lower trunk/pelvic motion and progression during walking; the level of resistance is light so as to not disrupt the patient's momentum, coordination, and velocity. Resisted gait progression can also be applied using an elastic resistance band. Verbal commands include *"On three, I want you to step forward with your right foot. One, two, three, and step, step, step."*

Indications: impaired timing and control of lower trunk/pelvic segments during locomotion, impaired endurance.

Rhythmic Rotation
General goals: promote relaxation and increased range in muscles restricted by excess tone

Relaxation is achieved using slow, repeated rotations of a limb or body segment. Rotations can be passive or active. Verbal commands include: *"Relax, let me move you, back and forth, back and forth"* (passive movements) or *"Relax, roll your legs outward, now roll them inward"* (active movements). The rotations are continued until muscle tension relaxes. Movements are slow and gently progress through increased range.

Indications: relaxation of hypertonia (spasticity, rigidity) combined with passive or active ROM of the range-limiting muscles

Adapted from Voss et al,[1] Adler, Beckers, and Buck,[2] and Johnson and Saliba Johnson.[7]

resemble patterns used in normal activities and sports. Patterns are varied by changing the action of the intermediate joint (i.e., elbow or knee) or by changing the position of the patient (e.g., supine, sitting, or standing). Patterns can be unilateral or bilateral; bilateral patterns can be symmetrical, asymmetrical, or reciprocal. Motion components and primary synergistic muscle components of the PNF patterns of movement are presented in Table 3.1 for the upper extremity (UE), in Table 3.2 for the lower extremity (LE), and in Table 3.3 for the head, neck, and trunk.

Scapular Patterns

Patterns involving the scapula influence the function of the cervical and thoracic spine and the upper extremities. Both scapular motion and stability are required. Motion

TABLE 3.1 Motion Components and Primary Synergistic Muscle Components of the Four PNF UE Patterns of Movement[a]

Joint/Body Segment	Motion Components	Primary Synergistic Muscle Components
Pattern of Movement: UE Flexion, Adduction, External Rotation		
Scapula	Anterior elevation	Serratus anterior, levator scapulae, rhomboids
Shoulder	Flexion, adduction, external rotation	Pectoralis major (clavicular portion), deltoid (anterior portion), coracobrachialis, biceps brachii (long head)
Elbow	• Straight* • Flexion • Extension	• Triceps, anconeus • Biceps brachii, brachialis • Triceps, anconeus
Forearm	Supination	Supinator, brachioradialis
Wrist	Flexion toward radial side	Flexor carpi radialis
Fingers	Flexion, adduction toward radial side	Flexor digitorum superficialis and profundus, lumbricales, interossei
Thumb	Adduction, opposition	Flexor pollicis longus and brevis, adductor pollicis, opponens pollicis
Pattern of Movement: UE Extension, Abduction, Internal Rotation		
Scapula	Posterior depression, rotation and adduction (inferior angle)	Rhomboids
Shoulder	Extension, abduction, internal rotation	Teres major, latissimus dorsi, deltoid (middle, posterior), triceps (long head), teres major, subscapularis
Elbow	• Straight* • Flexion • Extension	• Triceps, anconeus • Biceps, brachialis • Triceps, anconeus
Forearm	Pronation	Pronator (teres and quadratus), brachioradialis
Wrist	Extension toward ulnar side	Extensor carpi ulnaris
Fingers	Extension, abduction toward ulnar side	Extensor digitorum longus, lumbricales, interossei
Thumb	Palmar abduction, extension	Abductor pollicis (brevis), extensor pollicis

(table continues on page 42)

TABLE 3.1 Motion Components and Primary Synergistic Muscle Components of the Four PNF UE Patterns of Movement[a] *(continued)*

Joint/Body Segment	Motion Components	Primary Synergistic Muscle Components
Pattern of Movement: UE Flexion, Abduction, External Rotation		
Scapula	Posterior elevation	Trapezius (upper, middle), levator scapulae, serratus anterior
Shoulder	Flexion, abduction, external rotation	Deltoid (anterior), biceps (long head), coracobrachialis, supraspinatus, infraspinatus, teres minor
Elbow	• Straight* • Flexion • Extension	• Triceps brachii, anconeus • Biceps brachii, brachioradialis • Triceps brachii, anconeus
Forearm	Supination	Biceps, brachioradialis, supinator
Wrist	Extension toward radial side	Extensor carpi radialis longus and brevis,
Fingers	Extension toward radial side	Extensor digitorum longus, interossei
Thumb	Extension, abduction	Extensor pollicis longus and brevis, abductor pollicis longus
Pattern of Movement: UE Extension, Adduction, Internal Rotation		
Scapula	Anterior depression, rotation, and abduction (medial angle)	Serratus anterior, pectoralis minor, rhomboids
Shoulder	Extension, adduction, internal rotation	Pectoralis major (sternal portion), teres major, subscapularis
Elbow	• Straight* • Flexion • Extension	• Triceps, anconeus • Biceps, brachialis • Triceps, anconeus
Forearm	Forearm: pronation	Pronator teres and quadratus, brachioradialis
Wrist	Flexion toward ulnar side	Flexor carpi ulnaris
Fingers	Flexion, adduction, ulnar deviation	Flexor digitorum superficialis and profundus, lumbricales, interossei
Thumb	Flexion, adduction, opposition	Flexor pollicis longus and brevis, adductor pollicis, opponens pollicis

*Straight, maintained elbow extension (i.e., straight arm pattern); LE, lower extremity; UE, upper extremity.

[a]Adapted from Voss, Ionta, and Myers,[1] and Adler, Beckers, and Buck.[2]

occurs in two diagonals: anterior elevation–posterior depression and posterior elevation–anterior depression. Patterns are typically performed in the sidelying position, although other positions (e.g., sitting, standing) may be used. Scapular patterns contribute to performance of many functional activities (e.g., rolling, reaching, and dressing).[2] (See additional discussion of scapular patterns in Chapter 4: Interventions to Improve Bed Mobility and Early Trunk Control.)

Scapular Anterior Elevation—Posterior Depression

Position: The patient is positioned in sidelying (midfrontal plane) with the head in neutral; the therapist is positioned behind the patient in line with the movement (Fig 4.16).

Anterior Elevation

Start: The scapula and glenohumeral complex is down and back in posterior depression.

TABLE 3.2 Motion Components and Primary Synergistic Muscle Components of the Four PNF LE Patterns of Movement[a]

Joint/Body Segment	Motion Components	Primary Synergistic Muscle Components
Pattern of Movement: LE Flexion, Adduction, External Rotation		
Hip	Flexion, adduction, external rotation	Psoas major, iliacus, obturator externus, pectineus, gracilis, adductor longus and brevis, sartorius, rectus femoris
Knee	With knee straight	Quadriceps
	With knee flexion	Hamstrings, gracilis, gastrocnemius
	With knee extension	Quadriceps, especially vastus medialis
Ankle/foot	Dorsiflexion and inversion	Tibialis anterior
Toes	Extension, medial deviation	Extensor digitorum, extensor hallucis
Pattern of Movement: LE Extension, Abduction, Internal Rotation		
Hip	Extension, abduction, internal rotation	Gluteus medius, minimus, maximus, biceps femoris
Knee	With knee straight	Quadriceps
	With knee flexion	Hamstrings, gracilis, gastrocnemius
	With knee extension	Quadriceps, especially vastus lateralis
Ankle/foot	Plantar flexion, eversion	Gastrocnemius, soleus, peroneus longus and brevis
Toes	Flexion, lateral deviation	Flexor digitorum, flexor hallucis
Pattern of Movement: LE Flexion, Abduction, Internal Rotation		
Hip	Flexion, abduction, internal rotation	Tensor fascia lata, rectus femoris, gluteus medius and minimus
	With knee straight	Quadriceps
	With knee flexion	Hamstrings, gracilis, gastrocnemius
	With knee extension	Quadriceps especially vastus lateralis
Ankle/foot	Dorsiflexion and eversion	Peroneus brevis and tertius
Toes	Extension, lateral deviation	Extensor digitorum, extensor hallucis
Pattern of Movement: LE Extension, Adduction, External Rotation		
Hip	Extension, adduction, external rotation	Gluteus maximus, piriformis, gemelli obturator internus, quadratus femoris, adductor magnus
Knee	With knee straight	Quadriceps
	With knee flexion	Hamstrings, gracilis
	With knee extension	Quadriceps, especially vastus medialis
Ankle/foot	Plantar flexion and inversion	Gastrocnemius, soleus, posterior tibialis
Toes	Flexion, medial deviation	Flexor digitorum, flexor hallucis

LE, lower extremity; UE, upper extremity.
[a]Adapted from Voss, Ionta, and Myers,[1] and Adler, Beckers, and Buck.[2]

TABLE 3.3 Motion Components and Primary Synergistic Muscle Components of PNF Head/Neck and Trunk Patterns of Movement[a]

Joint/Body Segment	Motion Components	Primary Synergistic Muscle Components
	Head and Neck Flexion With Rotation to Right	
Cervical	Flexion	Longus capitis, longus colli, rectus capitis anterior, platysma, sternocleidomastoid, scalenus anterior
	Rotation	*Contralateral:* scalenes; sternocleidomastoid (turns head toward opposite side), upper trapezius *Ipsilateral:* rectus capitis anterior, longus capitis, longus colli, oblique capitis inferior
	Lateral flexion	Longus colli, rectus capitis lateralis, scalenes, sternocleidomastoid (tilts head toward shoulder on the same side)
	Head and Neck Extension With Rotation to Left	
	Extension	Rectus capitis posterior, obliquus capitis superior, iliocostalis, longissimus capitis, upper trapezius
	Rotation	*Contralateral:* Multifidi and rotatores, semispinalis capitis, upper trapezius *Ipsilateral:* obliquus capitis inferior, splenius cervicis and capitis
	Lateral Flexion	Iliocostalis cervicis, longissimus capitis, obliquus capitis superior splenius cervicis and capitis, upper trapezius
	Chop to Left	
Upper extremities	Bilateral asymmetrical UE patterns	Same as for extension-abduction-internal rotation of right UE (lead arm) and extension-adduction-internal rotation of left UE
Trunk	Flexion to the left, left lateral flexion, left rotation	Left external oblique, right internal oblique, rectus abdominis
	Lift to Right	
Upper extremities	Bilateral asymmetrical UE patterns	Same as for flexion-abduction-external rotation of the left UE (lead arm) and flexion-adduction-external rotation of the right UE
Trunk	Extension to the right, right lateral flexion, right rotation	All long and short neck and upper trunk extensors, left multifidi and rotatores
	Bilateral Symmetrical Flexion-Abduction-External Rotation With Trunk Extension	
Upper extremities	Bilateral symmetrical UE patterns	Same as for flexion-abduction-external rotation of UEs, bilateral symmetrical patterns
Trunk	Extension	All long and short neck and upper trunk extensors

TABLE 3.3 Motion Components and Primary Synergistic Muscle Components of PNF Head/Neck and Trunk Patterns of Movement[a] *(continued)*

Joint/Body Segment	Motion Components	Primary Synergistic Muscle Components
	Bilateral LE Flexion With Rotation to Left	
	Bilateral asymmetrical LE patterns	Same as for flexion-abduction-external rotation with knee flexion on left and flexion-adduction-external rotation with knee flexion on right
	Trunk	Right external oblique, left internal oblique, rectus abdominis
	Bilateral LE Extension With Rotation to Right	
	Bilateral asymmetrical LE patterns	Same as for extension-adduction-internal rotation with knee extension on left and extension-abduction-internal rotation with knee extension on right
	Trunk	All long and short lower trunk extensors, right quadratus lumborum, left multifidi and rotatores

[a]Adapted from Voss, Ionta, and Myers,[1] and Adler, Beckers, and Buck.[2]

Movement: The scapula and glenohumeral complex moves up and forward toward the nose, with the inferior angle rotating away from the spine.
Verbal cues: *"Pull your shoulder up and forward. Pull."*
Manual contacts: One hand is placed on the superior/anterior aspect of the glenohumeral complex, and the other hand is placed over the first hand. Resistance is down and back.

Posterior Depression
Start: The scapula and glenohumeral complex is up and forward in anterior elevation.
Movement: The scapula and glenohumeral complex moves down and back, with the inferior angle rotating toward the spine.
Verbal cues: *"Push your shoulder down and back to me. Push."*
Manual contacts: The base (heel) of the hand is placed on the vertebral border of the scapula and lumbrical grip to control the inferior medial border of the scapula, and the other hand is placed over the first hand. Resistance is up and forward.

Scapular Posterior Elevation—Anterior Depression
Position: The patient is positioned in sidelying; the therapist is positioned above and behind the patient's head in line with the movement.

Posterior Elevation
Start: The scapula and glenohumeral complex is positioned down and forward toward the opposite hip in anterior depression.

Movement: The scapula and glenohumeral complex moves up and back.
Verbal cues: *"Push your shoulder up and back. Push."*
Manual contacts: One hand is placed on the superior/posterior aspect of the acromion and the spine of the scapula, and the other hand is placed on top. Resistance is down and forward during the last half of the arc of movement.

Anterior Depression
Start: The scapula and glenohumeral complex is positioned up and backward in posterior elevation.
Movement: The scapula and glenohumeral complex moves down and forward toward the opposite hip.
Verbal cues: *"Pull your shoulder down toward your belly button. Pull."*
Manual cues: One hand is placed posteriorly on the axillary border of the scapula, and the other hand is placed on the lateral border of the pectoralis major muscle and inferior border of the coracoid process. Resistance is up and back.

Upper Extremity Patterns

Upper extremity patterns are named for the action occurring at the proximal joint (shoulder). There are two diagonal planes of motion.

• Diagonal 1 includes the antagonist pair of patterns flexion-adduction-external rotation and extension-abduction-internal rotation.
• Diagonal 2 includes the antagonist pair of patterns flexion-abduction-external rotation and extension-adduction-internal rotation.

The intermediate joint (elbow) can be maintained in extension (straight arm pattern) or can flex or extend using intermediate pivot action. See Table 3.1 for synergistic motion components. The terms *proximal hand* and *distal hand* refer to the location of the therapist's hand placement on the patient (manual contacts). The therapist's distal hand grips the patient's hand (palmar or dorsal surface); the proximal hand grips the patient's upper arm for emphasis of the shoulder or over the forearm for emphasis of distal joints.

Clinical Note: The term *elbow straight* means that the elbow is maintained in extension throughout the pattern. The term *elbow extension* or *flexion* denotes dynamic movement from flexion into extension or extension into flexion.

UE Flexion-Adduction-External Rotation With Elbow Straight

Start position: In supine, the UE is elongated (shoulder extension, abduction, internal rotation, elbow extension, forearm pronation, wrist and finger extension).

Movement: The hand closes as the wrist and fingers flex; the forearm supinates and the shoulder moves into external rotation, flexion, and adduction; the UE moves up and across the face with the ulnar side of the hand leading; the elbow remains straight. The head turns as the eyes follow the hand, thus keeping the arm from contacting the nose (Fig. 3.1).

Verbal cues: *"Squeeze my hand, turn, and pull up and across your face, keep your elbow straight. Pull up."*

Manual contacts: The therapist's distal hand grips the palmar surface of the patient's hand with fingers on the ulnar side and the thumb on the radial side (lumbrical grip), allowing the wrist to flex toward the radial side; the proximal hand grips over the anterior-medial surface of the patient's upper arm, providing resistance opposite to the direction of movement.

UE Flexion-Adduction-External Rotation With Elbow Flexion

Start position: In supine, the UE is elongated (same as for the elbow straight pattern).

Movement: The hand closes as the wrist and fingers flex; the forearm supinates and the shoulder moves into external rotation, flexion and adduction. As the arm begins to pull up, the shoulder and elbow begin to flex together; the UE moves up and across the face with the patient's closed fist approximating the opposite ear (Fig. 3.2).

Verbal cues: *"Squeeze my hand, turn, and pull up and across your face and bend your elbow. Pull up."*

Manual contacts: Same as for the elbow straight pattern.

UE Flexion-Adduction-External Rotation With Elbow Extension

Start position: In supine, the UE is elongated (shoulder extension, abduction, internal rotation, *elbow flexion*, forearm pronation, wrist and finger extension)

Movement: The hand closes as wrist and fingers flex; the forearm supinates and the shoulder moves into external rotation, flexion, and adduction. As the shoulder flexes the elbow moves into extension (Fig. 3.3).

Verbal cues: *"Squeeze my hand, turn, and pull up and across your face and straighten your elbow. Pull up."*

Manual contacts: Same as for the elbow straight pattern.

UE Extension-Abduction-Internal Rotation With Elbow Straight

Start position: In supine, the UE is elongated (shoulder flexion, adduction, external rotation, elbow straight, forearm supination, wrist and finger flexion).

Movement: The hand opens as the wrist and fingers extend; the forearm pronates, the shoulder moves into internal rotation,

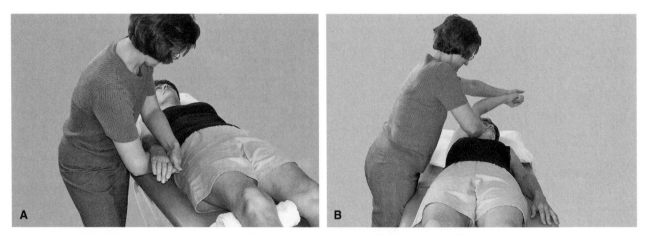

FIGURE 3.1 Supine, UE flexion-adduction-external rotation with elbow straight (A) Start position: The patient's UE is in an elongated position (shoulder extension-abduction-internal rotation, elbow extension, forearm pronation, wrist and finger extension). The therapist's distal hand is placed in the patient's palm; the proximal hand grips anterior-medial upper arm from underneath. The therapist applies initial stretch and resistance to shoulder flexors, adductors, and external rotators (proximal hand) and wrist and finger flexors (distal hand). Resistance is maintained as the UE moves through the range to the end position (B). The elbow remains extended (position unchanged) throughout the pattern.

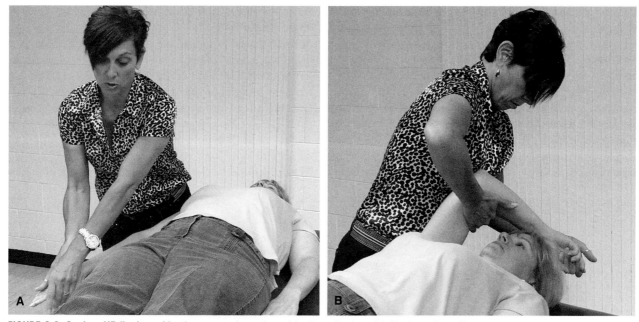

FIGURE 3.2 Supine, UE flexion-adduction-external rotation with elbow flexion (A) Start position: The UE is in the elongated position, the same as in the straight arm pattern. The therapist's manual contacts are the same as in the straight arm pattern. The therapist applies the same initial stretch and resistance as in the straight arm pattern for hand-wrist-forearm-shoulder components, with added resistance to elbow flexion after distal action (hand, wrist, forearm) and beginning rotation occurs. Resistance is maintained as the UE moves through the range to the end position (B). The elbow is fully flexed with the closed fist near the side of the head and the opposite ear.

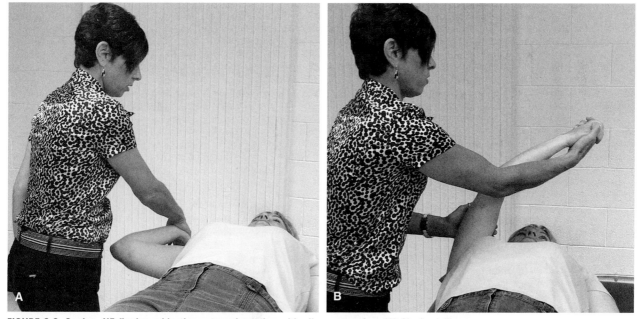

FIGURE 3.3 Supine, UE flexion-adduction-external rotation with elbow extension (A) Start position: The patient's UE is in an elongated position, and the hand-wrist-forearm-shoulder components are the same as in the straight arm pattern; the elbow is fully flexed. The therapist's manual contacts are the same as in the straight arm pattern. The therapist applies the same initial stretch and resistance for hand-wrist-forearm-shoulder components with the added resistance to elbow extensors given after distal action and beginning rotation occurs. Resistance is maintained as the UE moves through the range to the end position (B). The elbow is fully extended.

extension and abduction; the limb pushes down and out with the ulnar side of the hand leading; the elbow remains straight (Fig. 3.4).

Verbal cues: *"Open your hand, turn, and push down and out to your side. Keep your elbow straight. Push."*

Manual contacts: The therapist's distal hand grips the dorsal surface of the patient's hand with the fingers on the ulnar side and the thumb on the radial side (lumbrical grip); the proximal hand grips over the posterior-lateral surface of the patient's arm, providing resistance opposite the direction of movement.

UE Extension-Abduction-Internal Rotation With Elbow Flexion

Start position: In supine, the UE is elongated (same as for the elbow straight pattern).

Movement: The hand opens as the wrist and fingers extend; the forearm pronates and the shoulder moves into internal rotation, extension, and abduction. As the shoulder extends, the elbow moves into flexion (Fig. 3.5).

Verbal cues: *"Open your hand, turn, and push down and out to your side. Bend your elbow. Push."*

Manual contacts: Same as for the elbow straight pattern.

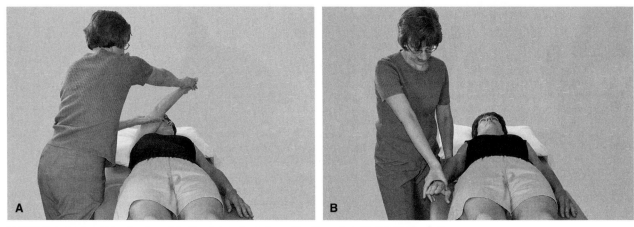

FIGURE 3.4 Supine, UE extension-abduction-internal rotation with elbow straight (A) Start position: The patient's UE is in an elongated position (shoulder flexion-adduction-external rotation, elbow extension, forearm supination, wrist and finger flexion). The therapist's distal hand grips the dorsal-ulnar surface of the patient's hand; the proximal hand applies pressure to the posterior-lateral surface of the patient's arm. The therapist applies stretch and resistance to shoulder extensors, abductors, and internal rotators (proximal hand) and wrist and finger extensors (distal hand). Resistance is maintained as the UE moves through the range to the end position (B). The elbow remains extended (position unchanged) throughout the pattern.

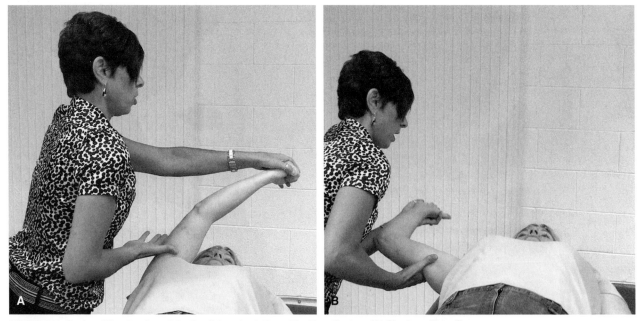

FIGURE 3.5 Supine, UE extension-abduction-internal rotation with elbow flexion (A) Start position: The patient's UE is in an elongated position, the same as in the straight arm pattern. The therapist's manual contacts are the same as for the straight arm pattern. The therapist applies the same stretch and resistance for hand-wrist-forearm-shoulder components, with added resistance to elbow flexors given after distal action and beginning rotation occurs. Resistance is maintained as the UE moves through the range to the end position (B). The elbow is fully flexed.

UE Extension-Abduction-Internal Rotation With Elbow Extension

Start position: In supine, the UE is elongated (shoulder flexion, adduction, external rotation, *elbow flexion,* forearm supination, wrist and finger flexion).

Movement: The hand opens as the wrist and fingers extend; the forearm pronates and the shoulder moves into internal rotation, extension, and abduction. As the shoulder extends, the elbow moves into extension (Fig. 3.6).

Verbal cues: *"Open your hand, turn, and push down and out to your side. Straighten your elbow. Push."*

Manual contacts: Same as for the elbow straight pattern.

> **Clinical Note:** The flexion-adduction-external rotation pattern can be remembered as the primary pattern (bringing the hand up and across the face). It can be used to promote the functional activities of feeding and grooming. The extension-abduction-internal rotation patterns (elbow straight and elbow extension) are important patterns that can be used to promote weight-bearing on an extended UE (e.g., needed for seated push-ups, transfers, or using assistive devices for gait).

UE Flexion-Abduction-External Rotation With Elbow Straight

Start position: In supine, the UE is elongated (fingers and wrist flexed with ulnar deviation, forearm pronated, elbow straight, shoulder extended, adducted, and internally rotated with the closed fist resting on the opposite hip).

Movement: The hand opens as the wrist and finger extend; the forearm supinates and the shoulder moves into external rotation, flexion, and abduction; the UE is lifted up and out with the radial side of the hand leading; the elbow remains straight (Fig. 3.7).

Verbal cues: *"Open your hand, turn, and lift your arm up and out toward me. Keep your elbow straight."*

Manual contacts: The therapist's distal hand grips the dorsal-radial surface of the patient's hand. The proximal hand grips from underneath on the anterior-lateral surface of the upper arm, providing pressure opposite to the direction of movement.

UE Flexion-Abduction-External Rotation With Elbow Flexion

Start position: In supine, the UE is elongated (same as for the elbow straight pattern).

Movement: The hand opens as the wrist and fingers extend, the forearm supinates, and the shoulder moves into external rotation, flexion, and abduction. As the shoulder flexes, the elbow moves into flexion; the open hand approximates the top of the head (Fig. 3.8).

Verbal cues: *"Open your hand, turn, lift your arm up and out toward me. Bend your elbow."*

Manual contacts: The therapist's distal hand grips the dorsal-radial surface (same as for the straight arm pattern); the proximal hand grips from underneath the upper arm on the anterior-lateral surface, providing resistance opposite the direction of movement.

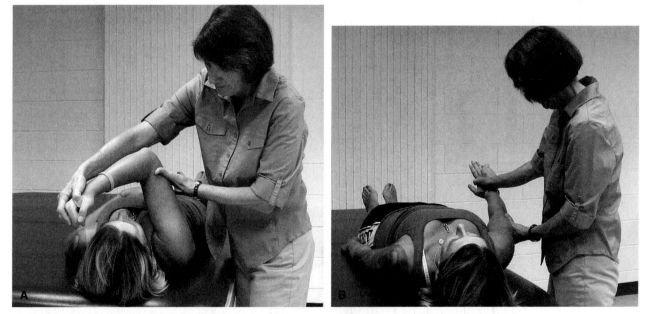

FIGURE 3.6 Supine, UE extension-abduction-internal rotation with elbow extension (A) Start position: The UE is in the elongated position with shoulder-wrist-hand components the same as for the straight arm pattern; the elbow is fully flexed. The therapist's distal grips are the same as for the straight arm pattern; the proximal hand resists using a C-grip. The therapist applies the stretch and resistance to shoulder, elbow, and hand as in the straight arm pattern, with added resistance to elbow extensors given after distal action and beginning rotation occurs. Resistance is maintained as the UE moves through the range to the end position (B). The elbow is fully extended.

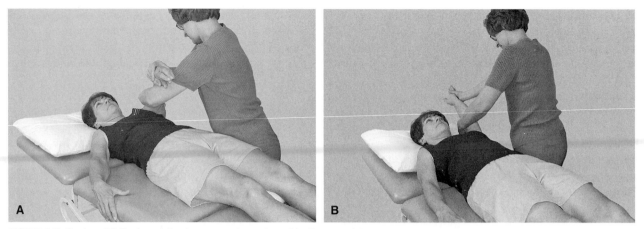

FIGURE 3.7 Supine, UE flexion-abduction-external rotation with elbow straight (A) Start position: The UE is in an elongated position (shoulder extension-adduction-internal rotation, elbow extension, forearm pronation, wrist and finger flexion). The therapist's distal hand grips the dorsal-radial surface of the patient's hand; the proximal hand applies pressure over the anterior-lateral surface of the patient's upper arm. The therapist applies initial stretch and resistance to shoulder flexors, abductors, and external rotators (proximal hand) and wrist and finger extensors (distal hand). Resistance is maintained as the UE moves through the range to the end position (B). The elbow remains extended (position unchanged) throughout the pattern.

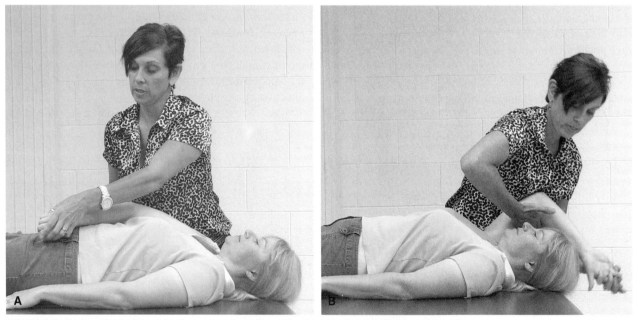

FIGURE 3.8 Supine, UE flexion-abduction-external rotation with elbow flexion (A) Start position: The UE is in the elongated position with all components the same as for the straight arm pattern. The therapist's distal grip is the same as for the straight arm pattern; the proximal hand grips the humerus from underneath. The therapist applies the same stretch and resistance as in the straight arm pattern for hand-wrist-forearm-shoulder components, with added resistance to elbow flexors given after distal action and beginning rotation occurs. Resistance is maintained as the UE moves through the range to the end position (B). The elbow is fully flexed and the forearm is touching the patient's head.

UE Flexion-Abduction-External Rotation With Elbow Extension

Start position: In supine, the UE is elongated (fingers and wrist flexed with ulnar deviation, forearm pronated, *elbow flexed on chest,* shoulder extended, adducted, and internally rotated).

Movement: The hand opens as the wrist and fingers extend, the forearm supinates, and the shoulder moves into external rotation, flexion, and abduction. As the shoulder flexes, the elbow moves into extension (Fig. 3.9).

Verbal cues: *"Open your hand and turn. Push it up and out toward me. Straighten your elbow."*

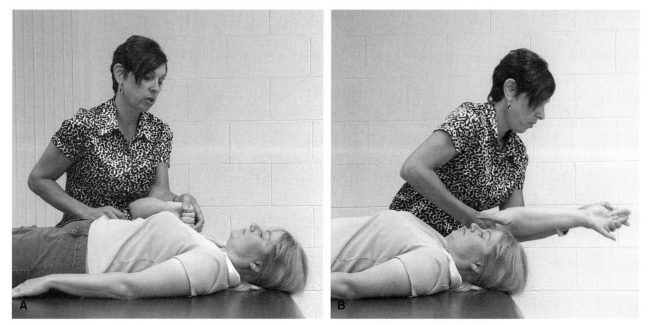

FIGURE 3.9 Supine, UE flexion-abduction-external rotation with elbow extension (A) Start position: The UE is in the elongated position with shoulder-wrist-hand components the same as for the straight arm pattern; the elbow is fully flexed. The therapist's distal grip is the same as for the straight arm pattern; the proximal hand wraps around the humerus from the medial side. The therapist applies the same stretch and resistance as in the straight arm pattern for hand-wrist-forearm-shoulder components, with added resistance to elbow extensors given after distal action and beginning rotation occurs. Resistance is maintained as the UE moves through the range to the end position (B). The elbow is fully extended.

Manual contacts: The therapist's distal hand grips the dorsal-radial surface (same as for the straight arm pattern); the proximal hand grips from underneath the upper arm on the anterior-lateral surface, providing resistance opposite the direction of movement.

UE Extension-Adduction-Internal Rotation With Elbow Straight

Start position: In supine, the UE is elongated (fingers and wrist extended, forearm supinated, elbow straight, shoulder flexed, abducted, and externally rotated).

Movement: The hand closes with wrist and finger flexion. The shoulder internally rotates, adducts, and extends, pulling the UE down and across the body toward the opposite hip, radial side of the hand leading. The elbow remains straight (Fig. 3.10).

Verbal cues: *"Squeeze my hand, turn, and pull down and across to your opposite hip. Keep your elbow straight. Pull."*

Manual contacts: The therapist's distal hand grips the palmar surface of the patient's hand. The proximal hand grips over the posterior-medial surface of the patient's upper arm, providing pressure opposite the direction of movement.

UE Extension-Adduction-Internal Rotation With Elbow Flexion

Start position: In supine, the UE is elongated (same as for the elbow straight pattern).

Movement: The hand closes with wrist and finger flexion, the shoulder internally rotates, adducts and extends, radial side of

the hand leading; as the shoulder extends, the elbow flexes, bringing the fisted hand down and across the chest (Fig. 3.11).

Verbal cues: *"Squeeze my hand, turn, and pull down and across to your chest. Bend your elbow."*

Manual contacts: The therapist's distal hand grips the palmar surface of the patient's hand; the proximal hand grips over the posterior-medial surface of the patient's arm, providing resistance opposite the direction of movement.

UE Extension-Adduction-Internal Rotation With Elbow Extension

Start position: Supine, the UE is elongated (fingers and wrist extended, forearm supinated, *elbow flexed,* shoulder flexed and abducted, and externally rotated).

Movement: The hand closes with wrist and finger flexion, and the shoulder internally rotates, then adducts and extends, with the elbow extending. The fisted hand moves down and across to the opposite hip (Fig. 3.12).

Verbal cues: *"Squeeze my hand, turn, and push down and across to your opposite hip. Straighten your elbow."*

Manual contacts: The therapist's distal hand grips the palmar surface of the patient's hand; the proximal hand grips over the posterior-medial surface of the patient's upper arm, providing resistance opposite to the direction of movement.

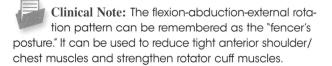 **Clinical Note:** The flexion-abduction-external rotation pattern can be remembered as the "fencer's posture." It can be used to reduce tight anterior shoulder/chest muscles and strengthen rotator cuff muscles.

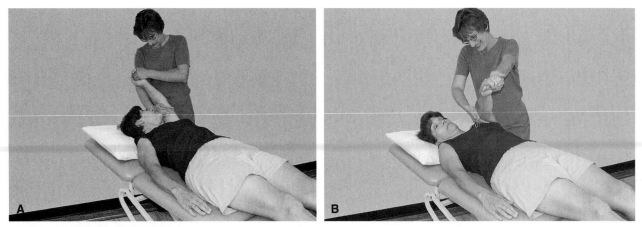

FIGURE 3.10 Supine, UE extension-adduction-internal rotation with elbow straight (A) Start position: The UE is in the elongated position (shoulder flexion-abduction-external rotation, forearm supination, wrist and finger extension). The therapist's distal hand is placed in the palm of the patient's hand; the proximal hand provides pressure to the posterior-medial surface of the patient's arm. The therapist applies initial stretch and resistance to shoulder extensors, adductors, and internal rotators (proximal hand) and wrist and finger flexors (distal hand). Resistance is maintained as the UE moves through the range to the end position (B). The elbow remains extended (position unchanged) throughout the pattern.

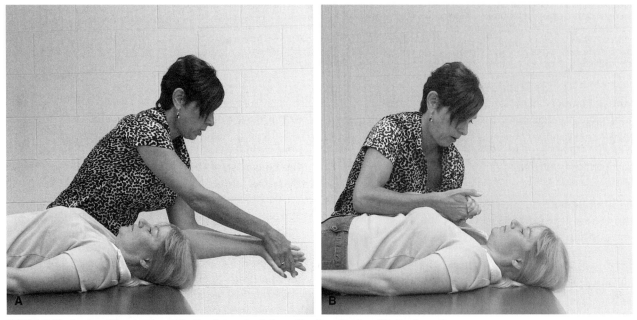

FIGURE 3.11 Supine, UE extension-adduction-internal rotation with elbow flexion (A) Start position: The UE is in the elongated position with all components the same as for the straight arm pattern; the manual contacts are the same as for the straight arm pattern. The therapist applies initial stretch and resistance to shoulder extensors-adductors-internal rotators, forearm pronators, and wrist and finger flexors, with added resistance to elbow flexors given after distal action and beginning rotation occurs. Resistance is maintained as the UE moves through the range to the end position (B). The elbow is fully flexed with the fisted hand resting on the chest.

Pelvic Patterns

Patterns involving the pelvis influence the function of the spine and the lower extremities. Both pelvic motion and pelvic stability are required. Motion occurs in two diagonals: anterior elevation–posterior depression and posterior elevation–anterior depression. Patterns are typically performed in the sidelying position, although other positions, such as standing, can be used. Pelvic patterns contribute to performance of many functional activities (e.g., rolling). Pelvic depression patterns contribute to LE weightbearing and walking. Pelvic elevation patterns contribute to walking (swing phase), stepping, stair-climbing, and leg lifting.[2] (See additional discussions of pelvic patterns in Chapter 4: Interventions to Improve Bed Mobility and Early Trunk Control and Chapter 10: Interventions to Improve Locomotor Skills.)

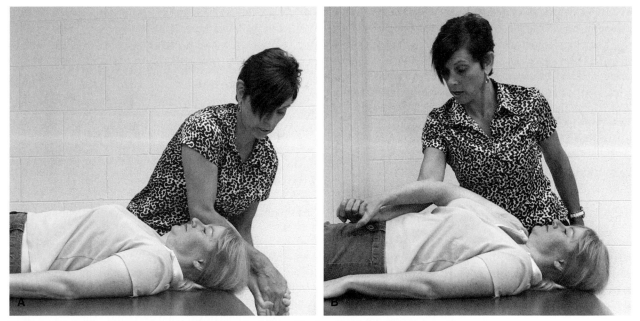

FIGURE 3.12 Supine, UE extension-adduction-internal rotation with elbow extension (A) Start position: The UE is in the elongated position with shoulder-wrist-hand components the same as for the straight arm pattern; the elbow is fully flexed. The manual contacts are the same as for the straight arm pattern. The therapist applies initial stretch and resistance to shoulder extensors-adductors-internal rotators, forearm pronators, and wrist and finger flexors, with added resistance to elbow extensors given after distal action and beginning rotation occurs. Resistance is maintained as the UE moves through the range to the end position (B). The elbow is fully extended.

Anterior Elevation—Posterior Depression

Position: The patient is positioned in sidelying with both LEs flexed to about 60 to 90 degrees if range of motion (ROM) allows; the lumbar spine is in neutral position with no lateral shear. The therapist stands (or kneels) behind the patient at the level of the thighs or knees and facing the patient's lower shoulder in line with the movement (Fig 4.16).

Anterior Elevation

Start: The pelvis positioned back and down in posterior depression.
Movement: The pelvis moves up and forward into anterior elevation; there is slight shortening (lateral flexion) of the trunk. There should be no trunk rotation.
Verbal cues: *"Pull your pelvis up and forward. Pull."*
Manual contacts: One hand is placed over the iliac crest, the other hand is placed over the first hand.

Posterior Depression

Start: The pelvis is up (elevated) and forward (anterior).
Movement: The pelvis moves down and backward into posterior depression.
Verbal cues: *"Sit into my hand. Push down and back."*
Manual contacts: The base (heel) of one hand is placed on the ischial tuberosity using a lumbrical grip; the other hand is placed over the first hand.

Anterior Depression—Posterior Elevation

Position: The patient is positioned in sidelying with the lower LE flexed to about 90 degrees if ROM allows and the upper LE in a straight knee position with the hip flexed to about 20 degrees. The therapist stands behind the patient at the level of the shoulders in the line with the movement.

Posterior Elevation

Start: The pelvis is down (depression) and forward (anterior).
Movement: The pelvis moves up and back into posterior elevation. Posterior elevation can be started as a hold in the shortened ROM with light resistance and progressed using combination of isotonics to slowly increase the range.
Verbal cues: *"Push your pelvis up and back. Push."*
Manual contacts: The base (heel) of the hand is on the iliac crest; the other hand is placed over the first hand.

Clinical Note: When performing any pelvic pattern, the therapist should ensure that the appropriate coupled motion occurs between the pelvis and the lumbar spine and that no rotation or extension of the spine is allowed.

Lower Extremity Patterns

Lower extremity patterns are named for motions occurring at the proximal joint (hip) or by one of two diagonals. Diagonal 1 includes the antagonist pair of patterns hip flexion-adduction-external rotation and extension-abduction-internal rotation. Diagonal 2 includes the antagonist pair of patterns flexion-abduction-internal rotation and extension-adduction-external rotation. The intermediate joint (knee) can be maintained in extension (straight leg pattern) or can flex or extend using intermediate pivot action. See Table 3.2 for synergistic muscular components.

The *proximal* and *distal hand* manual contacts are positioned to provide resistance over the contracting muscles and are in the direction of the movement. The therapist's distal hand grips the patient's foot (palmar or dorsal surface); the proximal hand grips the patient's thigh (anterior-medial or posterior-lateral surface) for emphasis of the hip or over the lower leg for emphasis of distal joints.

> 📋 **Clinical Notes:** The term *knee straight* means that the knee is maintained in extension throughout the pattern; the term *knee extension/flexion* denotes dynamic movement from flexion into extension or extension into flexion.

The rotations for the flexion-adduction-external rotation and extension-abduction-internal rotation LE patterns are the same as for the UE diagonal 1 patterns, whereas the rotations for the flexion-abduction-internal rotation and extension-adduction-external rotation LE patterns are opposite those for the UE diagonal 2 patterns.

LE Flexion-Adduction-External Rotation With Knee Straight

Start position: In supine, the LE is elongated (hip extension, abduction, internal rotation with knee straight and foot and ankle plantarflexion and eversion)

Movement: The toes extend, foot/ankle dorsiflexes and inverts, the knee remains straight; the hip externally rotates and pulls up and across the body, moving into hip adduction and flexion (Fig. 3.13).

Verbal cues: *"Pull your foot up, turn your heel in, keep your knee straight and pull up and across your body."*

Manual contacts: The therapist's distal hand provides resistance on the medial aspect of the dorsal foot, allowing the toes to extend; the proximal hand grips over the anterior–medial aspect of the thigh proximal to the knee.

LE Flexion-Adduction-External Rotation With Knee Flexion

Start position: In supine, the LE is elongated (same as for knee straight pattern).

Movement: The toes extend, foot/ankle dorsiflexes and inverts, and the knee flexes; the hip flexes, adducts, and externally rotates (Fig. 3.14).

Verbal cues: *"Pull your foot up and in, bend your knee, and pull up and across."*

Manual contacts: Same as for the knee straight pattern.

LE Flexion-Adduction-External Rotation With Knee Extension

Start position: In supine, the LE is elongated (hip extension, abduction, internal rotation with *knee flexion*; foot and ankle plantarflexion and eversion). The knee is flexed to 90 degrees over the side of the table.

Movement: The toes extend, foot/ankle dorsiflexes and inverts, and the *knee extends*; the hip flexes, adducts, and externally rotates (Fig. 3.15).

Verbal cues: *"Pull your foot up, now kick your foot up and across your body, and straighten your knee."*

Manual contacts: Same as for the knee straight pattern.

> 📋 **Clinical Note:** When LE flexion-adduction-external rotation is performed in sitting, the therapist is able to emphasize the knee extension portion of the pattern and the quadriceps (especially the vastus medialis) through intermediate joint action (Fig. 3.16). Verbal command: *"Pull your foot up, turn, and kick your foot up and across your other leg."*

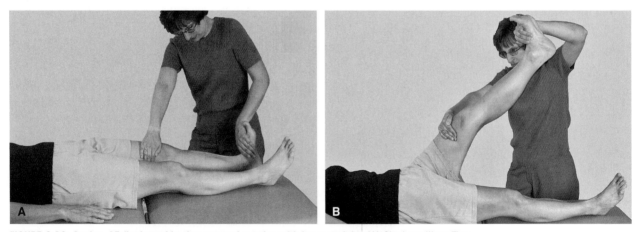

FIGURE 3.13 Supine, LE flexion-adduction-external rotation with knee straight (A) Start position: The LE is in the elongated position (hip extension, abduction, internal rotation with knee straight and foot and ankle plantarflexion and eversion). The therapist's distal hand grips the patient's dorsal-medial foot; the proximal hand applies pressure on the anterior-medial surface of the patient's thigh just proximal to the knee. The therapist applies initial stretch and resistance to hip flexors, adductors, and external rotators (proximal hand) and ankle dorsiflexors and invertors (distal hand). Resistance is maintained as the LE moves through the range to the end position (B). The knee remains extended (position unchanged) throughout the pattern.

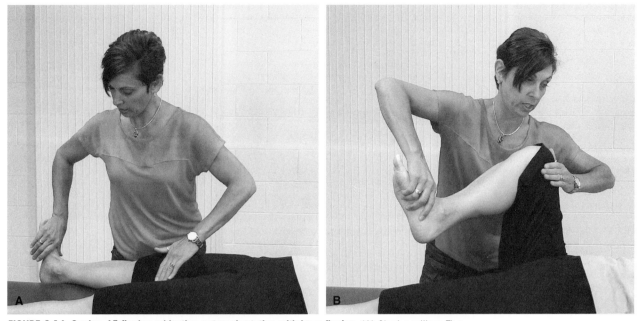

FIGURE 3.14 Supine, LE flexion-adduction-external rotation with knee flexion (A) Start position: The LE is in the same elongated position as in the straight knee pattern. The therapist's manual contacts are the same as for the knee straight pattern. The therapist applies initial stretch and resistance to hip flexors, adductors, and external rotators (proximal hand) and ankle dorsiflexors and invertors (distal hand), with added resistance to knee flexors given after distal action (foot-ankle) and beginning rotation occurs. Resistance is maintained as the LE moves through the range to the end position (B). The knee is fully flexed.

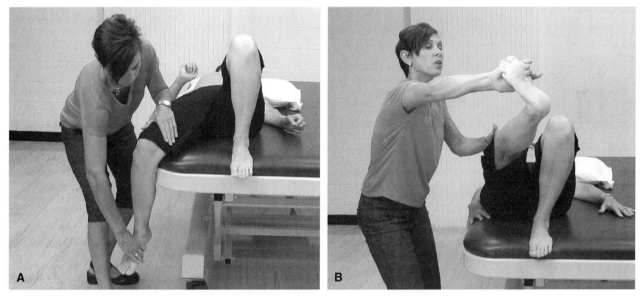

FIGURE 3.15 Supine, LE flexion-adduction-external rotation with knee extension (A) Start position: The hip-foot-ankle is in the same elongated position as in the straight knee pattern; the knee is fully flexed off the side of the table. The therapist's manual contacts are the same as for the knee straight pattern. The therapist applies initial stretch and resistance to hip flexors, adductors, and external rotators (proximal hand) and ankle dorsiflexors and invertors (distal hand), with added resistance to knee extensors given after distal action and beginning rotation occurs. Resistance is maintained as the LE moves through the range to the end position (B). The knee is fully extended. The opposite knee is flexed and foot is flat on table to stabilize the lumbar spine.

LE Extension-Abduction-Internal Rotation With Knee Straight

Start position: In supine, the LE is elongated (hip flexion, adduction, external rotation with knee straight; foot/ankle dorsiflexion and inversion).

Movement: The foot/ankle plantarflexes and everts; the hip internally rotates, extends, and abducts, pushing the foot down and out. The knee remains straight (Fig. 3.17).

Verbal cues: *"Push your foot down, turn your heel out, and push down and out toward me. Keep your knee straight."*

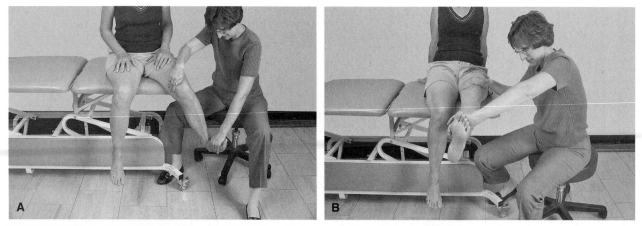

FIGURE 3.16 Sitting, LE flexion-adduction-external rotation with knee extension (A) Start position: The LE is in the same elongated position as in supine, and the knee is fully flexed. The therapist's distal hand grips the patient's dorsal-medial foot. The proximal hand applies pressure over the patient's anterior-medial thigh. The therapist applies stretch and resistance to hip flexors-adductors (proximal hand) and knee extensors and ankle dorsiflexors-invertors (distal hand). Resistance is maintained as the LE moves through the range to the end position (B). The knee is fully extended.

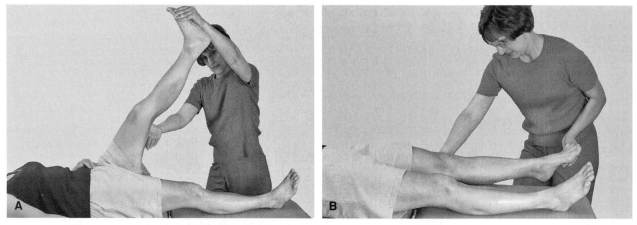

FIGURE 3.17 Supine, LE extension-abduction-internal rotation with knee straight (A) Start position: The LE is in the elongated position (hip flexion, adduction, external rotation, knee flexion, foot and ankle dorsiflexion and inversion). The therapist's distal hand grips the plantar-lateral surface of the patient's foot; the proximal hand applies pressure on the patient's posterior-lateral thigh. The therapist applies stretch and resistance to hip extensors, abductors, and internal rotators (proximal hand) and ankle plantarflexors and evertors (distal hand). Resistance is maintained as the LE moves through the range to the end position (B). The knee remains extended (position unchanged) throughout the pattern.

Manual contacts: The therapist's distal hand provides resistance on the lateral plantar surface of the foot and toes. The proximal hand provides pressure on the posterior-lateral aspect of the thigh just proximal to the popliteal space.

LE Extension-Abduction-Internal Rotation With Knee Flexion

Start position: In supine, the LE is elongated (same as for the knee straight pattern).

Movement: The foot/ankle plantarflexes and everts; the hip internally rotates, extends, and abducts, pushing the LE down and out. After the hip begins to move, the knee begins to bend, eventually flexing to 90 degrees over the side of the table (Fig. 3.18).

Verbal cues: "*Push your foot down, turn, and push your hip down and out toward me. Bend your knee.*"

Manual contacts: Same as for the knee straight pattern.

LE Extension-Abduction-Internal Rotation With Knee Extension

Start position: In supine, the LE is elongated (hip flexion, adduction, external rotation with *knee flexion;* foot and ankle dorsiflexion and inversion). The knee is flexed to 90 degrees over the other LE with the heel approximately over the other knee.

Movement: The foot/ankle plantarflexes and everts; the hip internally rotates, extends, and abducts, pushing the LE down and out. After the hip begins to move, the knee extends, with both the hip and knee extending fully at the same time (Fig. 3.19).

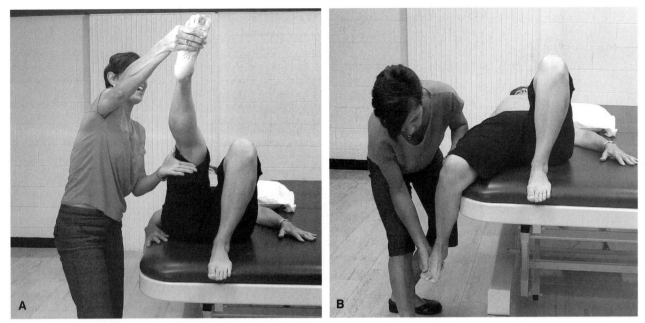

FIGURE 3.18 Supine, LE extension-abduction-internal rotation with knee flexion (A) Start position: The LE is in the same elongated position as in the straight knee pattern. The manual contacts are the same as for the straight knee pattern. The therapist applies stretch and resistance to hip extensors, abductors, and internal rotators (proximal hand) and ankle plantarflexors and evertors (distal hand), with added resistance to knee flexors given after distal action and beginning rotation occurs. Resistance is maintained as the LE moves through the range to the end position (B). The knee is fully flexed off the side of the table.

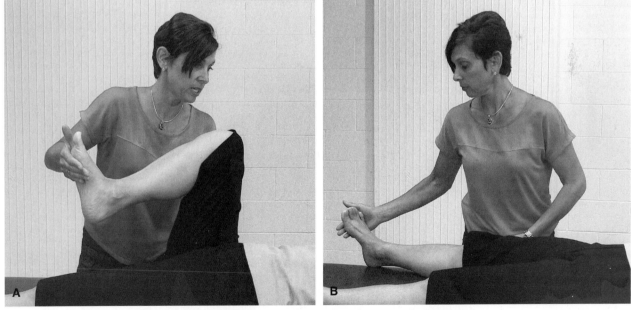

FIGURE 3.19 Supine, LE extension-abduction-internal rotation with knee extension (A) Start position: The hip-ankle-foot is in the same elongated position as in the straight knee pattern; the knee is flexed. The manual contacts are the same as for the straight knee pattern. The therapist applies stretch and resistance to hip extensors, abductors, and internal rotators (proximal hand) and ankle plantarflexors and evertors (distal hand), with added resistance to knee extensors given after distal action and beginning rotation occurs. Resistance is maintained as the LE moves through the range to the end position (B). The knee is fully extended.

Verbal Cues: *"Push your foot down. Now push your hip down and out toward me. Straighten your knee."*

Manual Contacts: Same as for the knee straight pattern.

> **Clinical Note:** When extension-abduction-internal rotation with knee flexion is performed in sitting, the therapist is able to emphasize the knee flexion portion of the pattern and the hamstrings (especially the medial hamstrings) through intermediate joint action (Fig. 3.20). Extension-abduction-internal rotation patterns (knee straight and knee extension) can be used to promote hip extension-abduction control with knee extension, which is needed for stance phase of gait and stability control.

LE Flexion-Abduction-Internal Rotation With Knee Straight

Start position: Supine, the LE is elongated (hip extension, adduction, and external rotation with knee straight and foot plantarflexed and inverted).

Movement: The foot/ankle dorsiflexes and everts; the hip internally rotates, flexes, and abducts, lifting the LE up and out. The knee remains straight (Fig. 3.21).

Verbal cues: *"Lift your foot up. Now lift your leg up and out toward me. Lift up."*

Manual contacts: The therapist's distal hand provides pressure over the dorsal-lateral surface of the foot, just proximal to the toe line to avoid restricting toe extension movement. The proximal hand provides resistance over the anterior-lateral surface of the thigh, just proximal to the knee.

LE Flexion-Abduction-Internal Rotation With Knee Flexion

Start position: In supine, the LE is elongated (same as for knee straight pattern).

Movement: The foot/ankle dorsiflexes and everts; the knee flexes as the hip internally rotates, flexes, and abducts (Fig. 3.22).

Verbal cues: *"Lift your foot up, bend your knee, and lift up and out toward me."*

Manual contacts: Same as for the knee straight pattern. Resistance to knee flexion is key to providing emphasis at the knee.

LE Flexion-Abduction-Internal Rotation With Knee Extension

Start position: In supine, the LE is elongated (hip extension, adduction, external rotation with the knee flexed over the end of the table).

Movement: The foot/ankle dorsiflexes and everts; the knee extends as the hip internally rotates, flexes, and abducts, lifting the leg up and out (Fig. 3.23).

Verbal cues: *"Lift your foot up and out, straighten your knee, and lift up and out toward me."*

Manual contacts: Same as for the knee straight pattern.

> **Clinical Note:** When LE flexion-abduction-internal rotation is performed in sitting position, emphasis can be placed on the knee extension portion of the pattern and the quadriceps (especially the lateral quads) through intermediate joint action (Fig. 3.24). The sitting position is also optimal if emphasis on the dorsiflexors

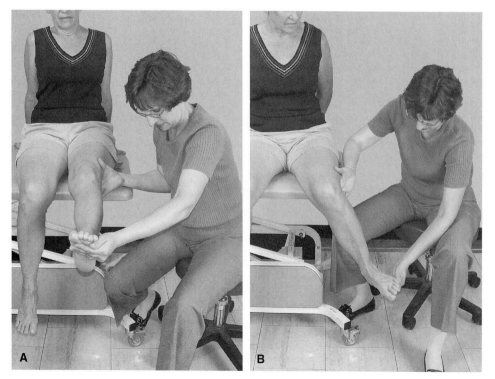

FIGURE 3.20 Sitting, LE extension-abduction-internal rotation with knee flexion (A) Start position: The LE is in the elongated position (foot-ankle-knee). The therapist's distal hand grips the plantar-lateral surface of the patient's foot. The proximal hand applies pressure on the patient's posterior-lateral thigh. The therapist applies stretch and resistance to hip abductors-internal rotators (proximal hand) and knee flexors, and ankle plantarflexors-evertors (distal hand). Resistance is maintained as the LE moves through the range to the end position (B). The knee is fully flexed.

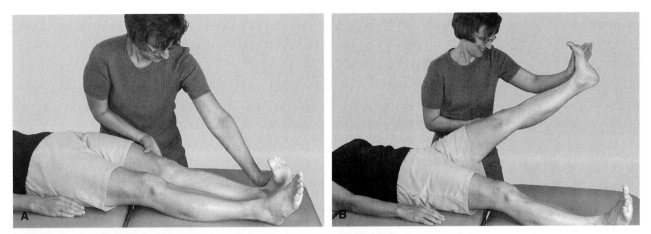

FIGURE 3.21 Supine, LE flexion-abduction-internal rotation with knee straight (A) Start position: The LE is in the elongated position (hip extension, adduction, external rotation, knee extension, foot and ankle plantarflexion and inversion). The therapist's distal hand grips the patient's dorsolateral foot; the proximal hand applies pressure on the patient's anterior-lateral thigh. The therapist applies stretch and resistance to hip flexors, abductors, and internal rotators (proximal hand) and ankle dorsiflexors and evertors (distal hand). Resistance is maintained as the LE moves through the range to the end position (B). The knee remains extended (position unchanged) throughout the pattern.

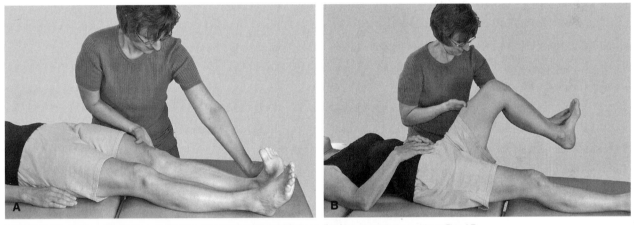

FIGURE 3.22 Supine, LE flexion-abduction-internal rotation with knee flexion (A) Start position: The LE is in the elongated position, same as for the straight knee pattern. The therapist's distal hand grips the patient's dorsal-lateral foot; the proximal hand applies pressure on the patient's anterior-lateral thigh. The therapist applies stretch and resistance to hip flexors, abductors, and internal rotators (proximal hand) and ankle dorsiflexors-evertors (distal hand), with added resistance to knee flexors given after distal action and beginning rotation occurs. Resistance is maintained as the LE moves through the range to the end position (B). The knee is fully flexed.

and evertors is needed (a common problem for many patients with ankle/foot weakness, e.g., the patient with stroke). With distal pivot action, the proximal hand can shift to the dorsal–lateral lower leg.

Verbal Cues: *"Lift your foot up and out, straighten your knee, and lift up and out."*

LE Extension-Adduction-External Rotation With Knee Straight

Start position: In supine, the LE is elongated (in hip flexion, abduction, internal rotation, knee straight, foot/ankle dorsiflexion and eversion).

Movement: The toes flex, the foot/ankle plantarflexes and inverts; the knee remains straight, and the hip extends, adducts, and externally rotates (Fig. 3.25).

Verbal Cues: *"Push your foot and toes down, turn and push your hip down and in, and keep your knee straight."*

Manual contacts: The distal hand holds the plantar surface of the foot with fingers applying resistance on the posterior-medial surface, just proximal to the toes (it is important to allow for toe flexion). The proximal hand applies pressure to the thigh on the medial-posterior side just above the popliteal space.

LE Extension-Adduction-External Rotation With Knee Flexion

Start position: In supine, the LE is elongated (same as for the straight knee pattern). The patient is positioned at the end of the table to allow full knee flexion.

Movement: The toes flex, and the foot/ankle plantarflexes and inverts. As the hip extends and pushes down into

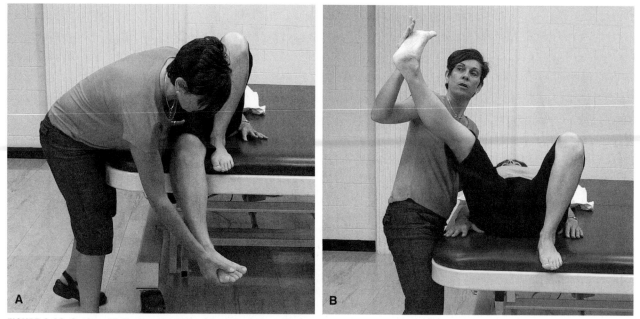

FIGURE 3.23 Supine, LE flexion-abduction-internal rotation with knee extension (A) Start position: The hip-ankle-foot is in the same elongated position as in the straight knee pattern; the knee is flexed. The therapist's distal hand grips the medial-plantar surface of the patient's foot; the proximal hand applies pressure over the posterior-medial aspect of the patient's thigh. The therapist applies stretch and resistance to hip extensors, adductors, and external rotators (proximal hand) and knee extensors, ankle plantarflexors-invertors (distal hand), with added resistance to knee extensors given after distal action and beginning rotation occurs. Resistance is maintained as the LE moves through the range to the end position (B). The knee is fully extended.

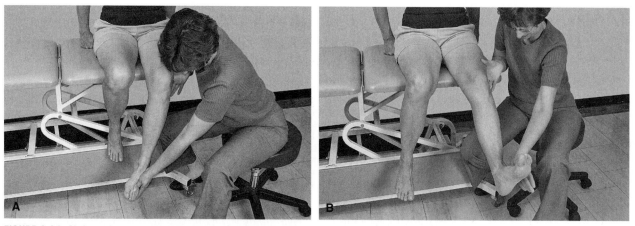

FIGURE 3.24 Sitting, LE flexion-abduction-internal rotation with knee extension (A) Start position: The hip-ankle-foot is in the same elongated position as the straight knee pattern; the knee is flexed. The therapist's distal hand grips the patient's dorsolateral foot; the proximal hand applies pressure on the patient's anterior-lateral thigh. The therapist applies stretch and resistance to hip abductors-internal rotators (proximal hand) and knee extensors, and ankle dorsiflexors-evertors (distal hand). Resistance is maintained as the LE moves through the range to the end position (B). The knee is fully extended.

adduction and external rotation, the knee flexes over the end of the table (Fig. 3.26).

Verbal cues: "*Push your foot and toes down, push your hip down and in, and bend your knee.*"

Manual contacts: Same as for the knee straight pattern.

LE Extension-Adduction-External Rotation With Knee Extension

Start position: Supine, the LE is elongated (in hip flexion, abduction, internal rotation, *knee flexion,* foot/ankle dorsiflexion and eversion).

Movement: The toes flex, the foot/ankle plantarflexes and inverts. As the hip extends and pushes down into adduction, and external rotation, the knee extends (Fig. 3.27).

Verbal cues: *"Push your foot and toes down, push down and in, and straighten your knee."*

Manual contacts: Same as for the knee straight pattern.

Head and Neck Patterns

Head/neck patterns combine flexion or extension with rotation and lateral flexion to the right or left. Synergistic muscular components are presented in Table 3.3.

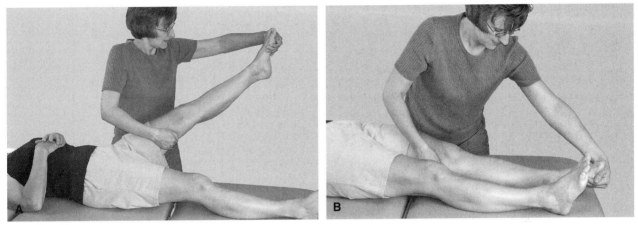

FIGURE 3.25 Supine, LE extension-adduction-external rotation with knee straight (A) Start position: The LE is in the elongated position (hip flexion, abduction, internal rotation, knee extension, foot/ankle dorsiflexion and eversion). The therapist's distal hand grips the medial-plantar surface of the patient's foot; the proximal hand applies pressure over the posterior-medial aspect of the patient's thigh. The therapist applies stretch and resistance to hip extensors, adductors, and external rotators (proximal hand) and ankle plantarflexors and invertors (distal hand). Resistance is maintained as the LE moves through the range to the end position (B). The knee remains extended (position unchanged) throughout the pattern.

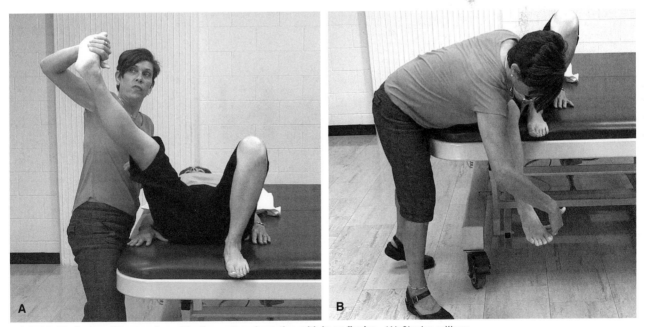

FIGURE 3.26 Supine, LE extension-adduction-external rotation with knee flexion (A) Start position: The LE is in the same elongated position as the straight leg pattern. The manual contacts are the same as for the straight leg pattern. The therapist applies stretch and resistance to hip extensors, adductors, and external rotators (proximal hand) and ankle plantarflexors and invertors (distal hand), with added resistance to knee flexors given after distal action and beginning rotation occurs. Resistance is maintained as the LE moves through the range to the end position (B). The knee is fully flexed.

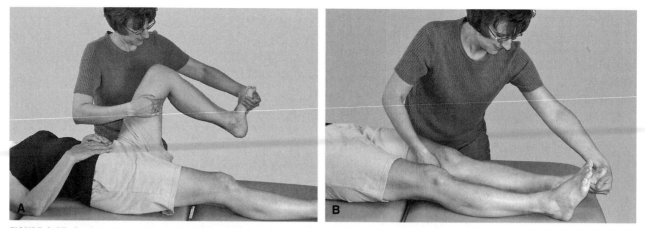

FIGURE 3.27 Supine, LE extension-adduction-external rotation with knee extension (A) Start position: The hip-ankle-foot is in the same elongated position as the straight leg pattern; the knee is flexed. Manual contacts are the same as for the straight leg pattern. The therapist applies stretch and resistance to hip extensors, adductors, and external rotators (proximal hand) and ankle plantarflexors and invertors (distal hand), with added resistance to knee extensors given after distal action and beginning rotation occurs. Resistance is maintained as the LE moves through the range to the end position (B). The knee is fully extended.

Flexion With Rotation to the Left, Extension to the Right

Start position: This pattern is typically performed sitting; it can also be performed in other positions, for example, in supine with the head resting in the therapist's hands, and the head over the edge of table. The therapist is positioned behind the patient.

Movement: The patient's head rotates to the left, and the neck flexes with rotation; the chin tucks and approximates the left clavicle (Fig. 3.28). During the extension with rotation to the right pattern (antagonistic pattern), the head rotates to the right, the neck extends with right rotation, and the chin lifts up and away (Fig. 3.29).

Verbal cues: *"Tuck your chin in, turn your head to the left, and pull it down until it touches your chest. Now turn your head to the right and lift your chin up and away from your chest."*

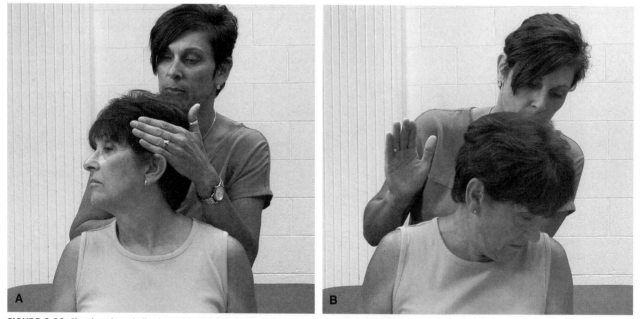

FIGURE 3.28 Head and neck flexion with rotation to the left (A) Start position: In sitting, the head is in an elongated position (rotated and extended to the right). The head rotates to the left, the neck flexes, and the chin tucks, bringing the patient's head down to the chest. Manual contacts are on the left side of the chin with the fingers pointing in the line of the diagonal and the top of the patient's head (an alternate manual contact is used with this patient with hand on left side of head due to temporomandibular joint pain). The therapist applies light stretch and resistance to head rotation and neck flexion to the left. Resistance is maintained as the head moves through the range to the end position (B).

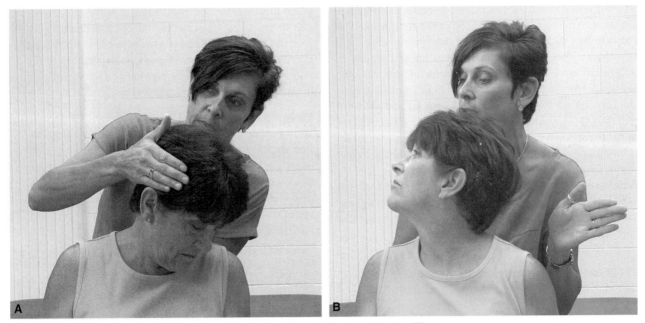

FIGURE 3.29 Head and neck extension with rotation to the right (A) Start position: In sitting position, the head is in an elongated position (rotated and flexed to the left). The head rotates to the right, the neck extends, and the chin lifts up and away. Manual contacts are on the right side of the head. The therapist applies light stretch and resistance to head rotation and neck extension to the right. Resistance is maintained as the head moves through the range to the end position (B).

Manual contacts: *Flexion:* The therapist's left hand holds along the inferior surface of the mandible and provides resistance to neck flexion, rotation, and lateral motion; the right hand rests on the posterior-lateral aspect of the skull to control rotation. *Extension:* The therapist's right hand is positioned on the right posterior-lateral surface of the occiput and provides resistance to neck extension and rotation; the left hand rests on the superior surface of the mandible. Resistance is light, and the patient is able to move the head without any strain.

Clinical Note: Flexion with rotation to the right and extension to the left patterns are performed using similar manual contacts, verbal cues (VCs), and movements to the opposite side.

Trunk Patterns

In chop/reverse chop or lift/reverse lift patterns, the UEs work together with the trunk using bilateral asymmetrical patterns. In thrust/reverse thrust patterns or bilateral symmetrical (BS) pattern, the UEs work together with the trunk using BS patterns. These patterns can be performed in supine, sitting, kneeling, or standing, depending on the patient's degree of trunk control. The more elevated the patient's center of mass and the more reduced the base of support, the greater the level of postural difficulty. Resistance is adjusted accordingly. Lower trunk bilateral asymmetrical patterns are performed in supine. Synergistic muscular components are presented in Table 3.3.

Chop (Bilateral Asymmetrical UE Extension With Neck and Trunk Flexion and Rotation to the Right (or Left) Side)

Start position: In sitting, the lead right arm is positioned in flexion-adduction-external rotation with elbow straight; the assist left arm is positioned in flexion-abduction-external rotation with the elbow flexed with the hand holding on top of the right wrist. The head is turned to the left with the eyes focused on the hands.

Movement: The head and trunk flex and rotate to the right (Fig. 3.30). The lead right arm moves down and out in extension-abduction-internal rotation with elbow straight; the assist left arm moves down and across into extension-adduction-internal rotation with elbow extension.

Verbal cues: *"Push your arms down and toward me; turn your head and look down at your hands. Reach down toward your right knee."*

Manual contacts: The therapist's manual contacts are similar to those for unilateral UE extension-abduction-external rotation pattern on the lead arm. Alternately, the distal hand can hold over the wrist assisting the hand gripping the wrist. The proximal hand can provide pressure to the patient's lateral-posterior arm or can be positioned on the patient's forehead, resisting the head and neck movement.

Reverse Chop (Bilateral Asymmetrical UE Flexion With Neck and Trunk Extension and Rotation to the Left Side)

Start position: In sitting, the lead right arm is positioned in extension-abduction-internal rotation with elbow straight; the assist left arm is positioned in extension-adduction-internal rotation with the hand holding on top of the right wrist. The head is turned with the eyes looking down at the hands.

Movement: The lead right arm moves up and across in flexion-adduction-external rotation with elbow straight; the assist left arm moves up and across in flexion-abduction-external rotation. The head and trunk extend and rotate to the left in the opposite direction of the chop (Fig. 3.31).

Verbal cues: *"Squeeze my hand, turn and pull your arms up and across your face, turn and look up at your hands. Reach up and around."*

Manual contacts: The therapist's distal hand grips the hand of the lead arm; the proximal hand is positioned on the anterior-medial surface of the lead arm (similar to placement in UE flexion-adduction-external rotation).

Lift (Bilateral Asymmetrical UE Flexion With Neck and Trunk Extension and Rotation to the Right Side)

Start position: In sitting, the lead right arm is positioned in extension-adduction-internal rotation with elbow straight; the assist left arm is positioned in extension-abduction with the hand holding underneath the right wrist. The head is turned to the left with the eyes focused on the hands.

Movement: The lead arm moves in extension-abduction-external rotation with elbow straight; the assist arm moves in flexion-adduction-external rotation. The head and trunk extend and rotate to the right (Fig. 3.32).

Verbal cues: *"Lift your arms up and out toward me, turn and look up at your hands. Reach up and around."*

Manual contacts: The distal hand grips the right hand (similar to resisting UE extension-abduction-external rotation pattern); the proximal hand provides pressure on the anterior-lateral surface of the arm (a c-grip is depicted in Fig. 3.32). Alternately, pressure can be provided on the top of the head, resisting the head and neck movement.

Reverse Lift (Bilateral Asymmetrical UE Extension With Neck and Trunk Flexion and Rotation to the Left Side)

Start position: In sitting, the lead right arm is positioned in flexion-abduction-external rotation with elbow straight; the assist left arm is positioned in flexion-adduction-external rotation with the hand holding underneath the right wrist. The head is turned to the right with the eyes focused on the hands.

Movement: The lead arm moves in extension-adduction-internal rotation with elbow straight; the assist arm moves in extension-abduction-internal rotation. The head and trunk flex and rotate to the left in the opposite direction of lift (Fig. 3.33).

Verbal cues: *"Squeeze my hand, turn, and pull your arms down and across your body. Lift and turn your head. Reach down and across."*

Manual contacts: The distal hand grips the right hand (similar to resisting UE D2E pattern); the proximal hand provides pressure on the medial-posterior surface of the arm.

📁 **Clinical Note:** The mnemonic phrases "chop on top" and "lift from underneath" are helpful when recalling how the patient's assist hand is positioned in chop and lift patterns.

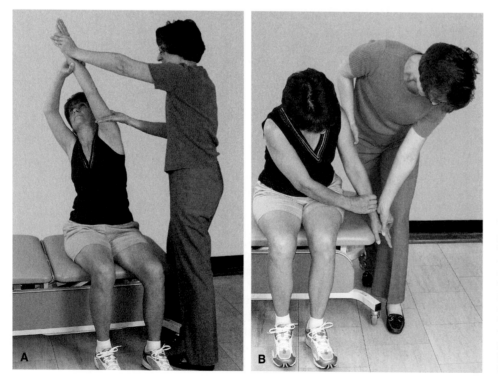

FIGURE 3.30 Sitting, chop (bilateral asymmetrical UE extension with neck and trunk flexion and rotation to the left) (A) Start position: The UEs are in an elongated position overhead (the lead left UE is positioned in flexion, adduction, external rotation; the assist right hand holds on top of the lead wrist). The therapist applies light stretch and resistance as patient's lead left UE moves down into the extension-abduction-internal rotation pattern; the assist hand maintains its hold on the wrist. The head and trunk rotate and flex to the left. Resistance is maintained through the movement, ensuring that trunk flexion with rotation and weight shift to the left side occurs (B).

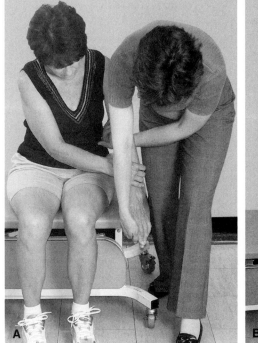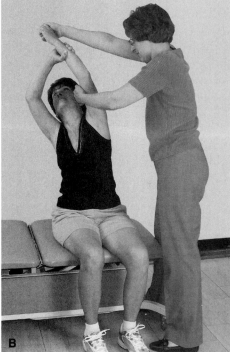

FIGURE 3.31 Sitting, reverse chop (A) Start position: The UEs are in an elongated position by the left side (the lead left UE is positioned in extension-abduction-internal rotation; the assist right hand holds on top of the wrist). The therapist applies light stretch and resistance as the patient's lead left UE moves into flexion-abduction-external rotation; the assist hand maintains its hold on the wrist. Resistance is maintained through the movement, ensuring that trunk extension and rotation with weight shift to the right side occurs (B).

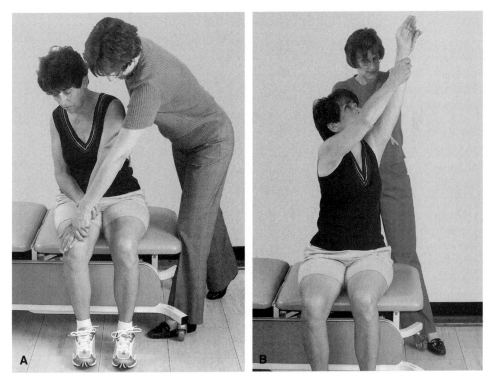

FIGURE 3.32 Sitting, lift (bilateral asymmetrical UE flexion with neck and trunk extension and rotation, to the left) (A) Start position: The UEs are in an elongated position crossing the body and positioned by the outside of the right knee (the lead left UE is in extension-abduction-internal rotation; the assist right hand holds onto the left wrist from underneath). The patient's lead left UE moves into flexion-abduction-external rotation; the assist hand maintains its hold on the wrist. The patient is instructed to open the hand, turn, and lift both UEs up and out to the side. The therapist resists the movement, ensuring that trunk extension and rotation with weight shift to the left side occurs (B).

Clinical Note: Rolling from supine to sidelying or into sidelying on elbow or moving up into sitting can best be facilitated using a chop pattern. For some patients (e.g., the patient with stroke) rolling supine to sidelying on the more affected side is best facilitated using a lift pattern that promotes the UE position flexion-abduction-external rotation with elbow extension.

Clinical Note: In sitting, the therapist selects *either* a chop or lift pattern. One is not a progression from the other, and there is no need to use both to improve dynamic stability control in sitting. Either pattern enhances upper trunk rotation with flexion/extension, weight shifting, and crossing the midline, all important activities for patients with unilateral neglect (e.g., the

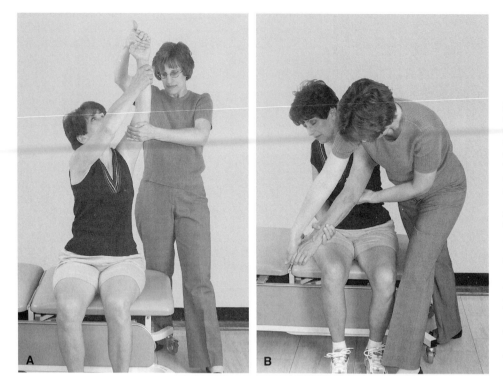

FIGURE 3.33 Sitting, reverse lift
(A) Start position: The UEs are in an elongated position (the lead left UE is in flexion-abduction-external rotation; the assist right hand holds onto the left wrist from underneath). The patient's lead left UE moves in extension-adduction-internal rotation; the assist arm maintains the hold on the wrist. The patient is instructed to close the hand, turn, and pull both UEs down and across the body. The therapist resists the movement, ensuring that trunk flexion and rotation with weight shift to the right occurs (B). Note that the therapist uses a wide BOS that allows weight shifting for continuous application of resistance throughout the pattern.

patient with stroke). These patterns can also be used to facilitate moving from heel-sitting to kneeling and reverse.

Bilateral Symmetrical UE Flexion-Abduction-External Rotation With Trunk Extension and Reversal

Start position: In sitting, both UEs are extended and adducted across the body, hands fisted (positioned in BS extension-adduction-internal rotation).

Movement: With the hands open, both UEs turn and lift up and out moving into BS flexion-abduction-external rotation. The trunk and neck extend as the patient looks up (Fig. 3.34).

Motion reversal: The UEs are appropriately resisted from underneath as they return to the start position.

Verbal cues: *"Open your hands, turn and lift up and out. Look up at your hands. Now close your hands and pull down and across your body."*

Manual contacts: The therapist resists from behind with the hands placed over the dorsal-lateral surface of the forearms or upper arms, depending on the length of the patient's arms. During the *motion reversal,* the UEs are appropriately resisted from underneath as they return to the start position.

Clinical Note: The BS flexion-abduction-external rotation patterns encourage expansion of the chest with stretching of the anterior chest muscles and strengthening of the posterior neck and trunk muscles along with rotator cuff muscles. Thus it is ideal for the patient with a functional dorsal kyphosis with forward shoulders and head (e.g., the patient with senile posture or Parkinson disease). For improved respiratory control, the patient can be instructed to slowly breathe in as the UEs elevate and slowly breathe out as they return down to the start position. For improved trunk extension control, the pattern is ideally performed in the sitting position. It can also be performed in supine or kneeling and can be used to promote transitions between heel-sitting to kneeling.

Thrust and Reverse Thrust Patterns

Start position: In sitting, both UEs are flexed and adducted to sides (shoulder adduction, elbow flexion, forearm supination, wrist and finger flexion).

Movement: *Thrust:* The hands open, the forearms pronate, and the UEs move up and across the face with the elbows extending, shoulders flexing to 90 degrees, and wrists crossing. *Reverse thrust:* The hands close, forearms supinate, elbows flex, and the UEs pull back and down to the sides (Fig. 3.35).

Verbal cues: *"Open your hands, turn, and push up and across toward me. Now close your hands, turn, pull back and down to your sides, and bend your elbows."*

Manual contacts: The therapist holds onto the lower forearm on the dorsal surface. The grips do not change with change in direction of movement.

Clinical Note: The thrust pattern is a protective pattern for the face and promotes actions of shoulder flexion and elbow extension with scapular protraction. It is useful in promoting an out-of-synergy pattern for the patient with stroke (the reverse thrust pattern should be assisted passively because it closely resembles an obligatory synergy pattern). The reverse thrust pattern is useful to promote upper trunk extension with symmetrical scapular

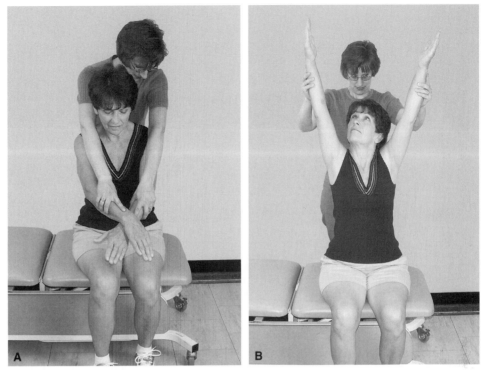

FIGURE 3.34 Sitting, UE bilateral symmetrical flexion-abduction-external rotation (A) Start position: The patient begins with both UEs extended and adducted across the body. The patient is instructed to open the hands, turn, and lift both UEs up and out, about one hand's width from the head. The therapist resists the movement, ensuring that the patient lifts both UEs up and out while extending the upper trunk (B). The therapist needs to be positioned behind the patient with both hands holding over the upper forearm or lower arm. For improved respiratory control, the patient can be instructed to breathe in deeply during flexion-abduction-external rotation, and breathe out during the reverse movement, extension-adduction-internal rotation.

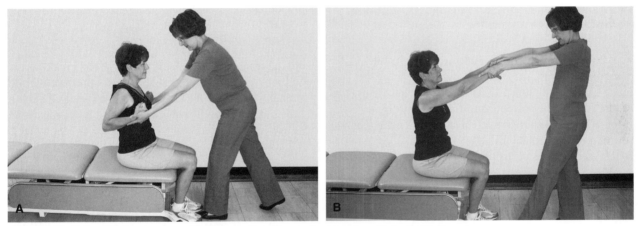

FIGURE 3.35 Sitting, UE thrust pattern (A) Start position: The patient begins with both UEs flexed and adducted, forearms supinated, hands flexed, and arms tucked close to the side. The patient is instructed to open both hands, turn, and push up and across, extending both elbows and crossing both hands in front of the face (thrust position). The therapist resists the movement and must shift weight backward to ensure that both elbows extend fully (B). During reverse thrust, the therapist resists the UEs as they flex and move back to the sides.

retraction. Functionally, it promotes a symmetrical upright sitting posture, important for the patient with slumped sitting (rounded back with forward head and shoulders).

Bilateral Asymmetrical LE Flexion With Lower Trunk Flexion and Rotation to Left (or Right)

Start position: In supine (LEs moving to the left), the LEs extended and positioned to the right with the right LE in extension-abduction-internal rotation and left LE in extension-adduction-external rotation

Movement: The LEs pull up and across the body toward the left side; the knees move into flexion with ankles dorsiflexed. In Figure 3.36, a ball is used to support the LEs in flexion to decrease the initial effort and strain on the low back.

Verbal cues: *"Feet up. Now bend both knees and swing your feet up and toward me."*

Manual contacts: The distal hand grips over the dorsal-lateral surface of both feet. The proximal hand provides pressure on the anterior-lateral surface of the nearest LE.

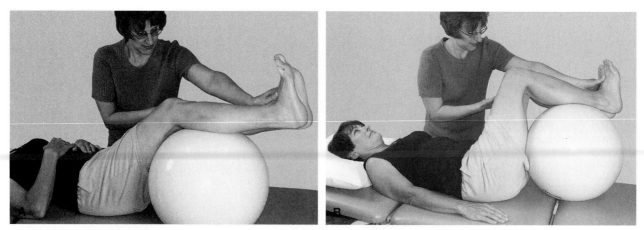

FIGURE 3.36 Supine, LE bilateral asymmetrical LE flexion, with knee flexion for lower trunk flexion (left), feet supported on ball (A) Start position: The therapist's distal hand provides pressure to both of the patient's feet on the dorsal-lateral surfaces; the proximal hand applies pressure to the patient's anterior-lateral thighs. The therapist applies stretch and resistance to both ankle dorsiflexors (distal hand) and both thighs (proximal hand) as the patient bends both hips and knees up and swings the feet up and toward the therapist (B).

Clinical Note: When the ball is not used, the proximal arm can be placed underneath the patient's thighs to provide an initial assist to lifting both legs. This activity is extremely challenging when performed from the beginning of the range, and it is important to make sure that the strain of lumbar hyperextension is avoided.

Bilateral Asymmetrical LE Extension With Lower Trunk Extension and Rotation

Start position: In supine (LEs moving to the right), the LEs are flexed and positioned to the left with right LE in flexion-adduction-external rotation and left LE is in flexion-abduction-internal rotation.

Movement: The LEs push down and across the body toward the right side; the knees move into extension with ankles plantarflexed.

Verbal cues: *"Feet down; now push down and across toward me."*

Manual contacts: The distal hand holds the plantar-lateral surface of both feet. The proximal hand provides resistance from underneath the patient's thighs.

Outcome Measures and Research Evidence

It is important to use standardized outcome measures to document the patient's improved movement abilities and outcomes of the plan of care. Measures are used to document changes in ROM, strength, and coordination (impairment level) and improved functional abilities. Instruments include the following:

Quantitative parameters:

• ROM measured by goniometry[9]
• Muscle strength measured by manual muscle test[10,11]

Qualitative parameters:

• Coordination and balance: control, speed, and steadiness[12]

Functional abilities:

• Function measured by the *Functional Independence Measure*[13,14] and other functional measures.

Research evidence on PNF is limited. As an approach to treatment that focuses on applying principles and techniques based on the individual patient's presentation, PNF does not lend itself well to the use of prescribed intervention protocols. As a result, only a small number of randomized controlled trials have studied PNF, so the overall quality of available research varies. A review of literature in 2006 by Smedes[15] revealed concentrations on specific areas, including PNF stretching techniques, stroke, gait, activities of daily living or sport performance, and vital functions. Proprioceptive neuromuscular facilitation–facilitated stretching techniques (contract-relax [CR] and hold-relax [HR]) compose by far the largest group of research studies and are reviewed here.

Some researchers have demonstrated evidence that PNF techniques are more effective than static stretching techniques in improving ROM.[16–19] Other researchers have demonstrated that PNF techniques are comparable and not more effective than static stretching.[20–23] Using a randomized control trial design, Fasen et al[24] compared four different hamstring-stretching techniques. The researchers found PNF active stretching techniques resulted in improved ROM at 4 weeks when compared with passive stretching. After 8 weeks, the passive stretch group (straight leg raise) had the greatest improvement in hamstring length. Maddigan, Peach, and Behm[25] compared three stretching techniques: PNF stretching assisted by a therapist, unassisted PNF stretching using a strap, and static stretching. All three techniques produced similar improvements in ROM along with post-stretching decrements in movement time and angular velocity. Azevedo et al[26] demonstrated similar ROM gain following a CR PNF procedure with either target stretching of the contracted muscle or stretching an uninvolved muscle distant from the target muscle. Youdas et al[27] compared two different PNF stretching techniques, HR and HR antagonist contraction (HR-AC), and found that post-stretch ROM was greater after the HR-AC procedure. Sheard and Paine[28] investigated the force of the contraction necessary to elicit positive change in ROM. They found the optimal peak force to be 64.3% of maximum voluntary isometric contraction.

Limitations in many of these studies include (1) utilization of healthy people and limited use of patient groups, (2) limited comparisons with improved functional performance, and (3) variations in methodology. What is not clear in many of the studies are the specifics of the techniques used (according to established descriptions of HR and CR techniques) and how they were applied (in diagonals or straight plane motions).

SUMMARY

This chapter has reviewed the basic concepts and components of the PNF approach, including basic principles, techniques of treatment, activities, and synergistic patterns of movement. Overall functional improvement is promoted through the use of specific principles and facilitation techniques to enhance coordinated muscle activity. Effective motor learning strategies are an important part of this approach. Extremity patterns are combined with trunk patterns to enhance postural control and improve function.

Acknowledgment: The author gratefully acknowledges the contributions of Cristiana K. Collins and Vicky Saliba Johnson in the final preparation of this chapter.

REFERENCES

1. Voss, D, Ionta, MK, and Myers, BJ. Proprioceptive Neuromuscular Facilitation: Patterns and Techniques, ed 3. Philadelphia, Harper & Row, 1985.
2. Adler, S, Beckers, D, and Buck, M. PNF in Practice, ed 3. New York, Springer-Verlag, 2008.
3. Kaiser Permanente. Post-Graduate PNF Physical Therapy Training Program. Retrieved January 2, 2014, from www.kaiserpermanente.org/facilities/Vallejo/services_overview.html.
4. International PNF Association (IPNFA). PNF from Facilitation to Participation. Retrieved January 2, 2014, from www.ipnfa.org.
5. Latash, M, and Anson, J. Synergies in health and disease: Relations to adaptive changes in motor coordination. Phys Ther, 2006; 86: 1151.
6. Saliba, VL, Johnson, GS, and Wardlaw, C. Proprioceptive neuromuscular facilitation. In Basmajian, JV, and Nyberg, R (eds): Rational Manual Therapies. Baltimore, Williams & Wilkins, 1993, 243.
7. Johnson, G, and Saliba Johnson, V. PNF 1: The Functional Application of Proprioceptive Neuromuscular Facilitation, Course Syllabus, Version 7.9, Steamboat, CO, Institute of Physical Art, 2014.
8. Sherrington, CS. The Integrative Action of the Nervous System. New Haven, Yale University Press, 1906.
9. Norkin, C, and White, J. Measurement of Joint Function, ed 4. Philadelphia, F.A. Davis, 2009.
10. Hislop, JH, and Montgomery, J. Saniels and Worthingham's Muscle Testing: Techniques of Manual Examination, ed 8. Philadelphia, Saunders (Elsevier), 2007.
11. Kendall, F, et al. Muscles: Testing and Function with Posture and Pain, ed 5. Baltimore, Lippincott Williams & Wilkins, 2005.
12. Schmitz, T, and O'Sullivan, S. Examination of coordination and balance. In O'Sullivan, S, Schmitz, T, and Fulk, G (eds): Physical Rehabilitation, ed 6. Philadelphia, F.A. Davis, 2014.
13. Guide for the Uniform Data Set for Medical Rehabilitation (Adult FIM), Version 5.0, Buffalo, NY, State University of New York, 1996.
14. Dodds, T, et al. A validation of the functional independence measurement and its performance among rehabilitation in-patients. Arch Phys Med Rehabil, 1993; 74:531.
15. Smedes, F. Is there support for the PNF-concept? A literature search on electronic databases. www.ipnfa.org/index.php/pnf-literature/open-access?download=3. Retrieved on January 6, 2014.
16. Funk, DC, et al. Impact of prior exercise on hamstring flexibility: a comparison of proprioceptive neuromuscular facilitation and static stretching. J Strength Cond Res, 2003; 3:489–492.
17. Wenos, DL, Konin, JG. Controlled warm-up intensity enhances hip range of motion. J Strength Cond Res, 2004; 3:529.
18. Weng, MC, et al. Effects of different stretching techniques on outcomes of isokinetic exercise in patients with knee osteoarthritis. Kaohsiung J Med Sci, 2009; 6:306.
19. O'Hora, J, et al. Efficacy of static stretching and proprioceptive neuromuscular facilitation stretch on hamstring length after a single session. J Strength Cond Res, 2011; 6:1586.
20. Davis, DS, et al. The effectiveness of 3 stretching techniques on hamstring flexibility using consistent stretching parameters. J Strength Cond Res, 2005; 1:27.
21. Yuktasir, B, and Kaya, F. Investigation into the long-term effects of static and PNF stretching exercise on range of motion and jump performance. J Bodyw Move Ther, 2009; 1:11.
22. Puentedura, EJ, et al. Immediate effects of quantified hamstring stretching: hold-relax proprioceptive neuromuscular facilitation. Phys Ther Sport, 2011; 12:122.
23. Chow, TP, and Ng GY. Active, passive and proprioceptive neuromuscular facilitation stretching are comparable in improving knee flexion range in people with total knee replacement: a randomized controlled trial. Clin Rehab, 2010; 24:911.
24. Fasen, JM, et al. A randomized controlled trial of hamstring stretching: comparison of four techniques. J Strength Cond Res, 2009; 23:660.
25. Maddigan, ME, Peach, AA, and Behm, DG. A comparison of assisted and unassisted proprioceptive neuromuscular facilitation techniques and static stretching. J Strength Condit Res, 2012; 5:1238.
26. Azevedo, DC, et al. Uninvolved versus target muscle contraction during contract-relax proprioceptive neuromuscular facilitation stretching. Phys Ther Sport, 2011; 3:117.
27. Youdas, JW, et al. The efficacy of two modified proprioceptive neuromuscular facilitation stretching techniques in subjects with reduced hamstring muscle length. Physiother Theory Pract, 2010; 4:240.
28. Sheard, PW, and Paine, TJ. Optimal contraction intensity during proprioceptive neuromuscular facilitation for maximal increase of range of motion. J Strength Cond Res, 2010; 24:416.

4 Interventions to Improve Bed Mobility and Early Trunk Control

CRISTIANA K. COLLINS, PT, PhD, CFMT, NCS;
VICKY SALIBA JOHNSON, PT, FAAOMPT; AND
THOMAS J. SCHMITZ, PT, PhD

Bed mobility is a basic skill that promotes independence and allows for self-care activities. Whether treating a patient with neurologic involvement, a patient who is elderly or debilitated, or a person with acute low back pain, impaired bed mobility can be a challenge for the patient, as well as family and health-care providers. Interventions focus on facilitating the most efficient and pain-free skills for moving in bed to accomplish activities such as rolling, personal hygiene, dressing, and coming to sitting in preparation for transfers or transition to standing. This chapter presents methods for examining and evaluating the key components required for bed mobility, as well as activities, techniques, and exercises that can promote improved efficiency and independence.

Interventions to Improve Control in Bed Mobility Skills

Bed mobility skills involve rolling from supine to sidelying and from sidelying to supine or prone, moving in bed (bridging and scooting), and moving from supine or sidelying to sitting. People who have efficient neurological and musculoskeletal systems utilize a variety of strategies and patterns to roll, all characterized by smooth transitions between postures. Patients with neurological involvement (e.g., stroke, spinal cord injury [SCI]), musculoskeletal impairments (e.g., severe acute disc pathology, trauma, recent surgery), or extensive weakness (e.g., chronic obstructive pulmonary disease, renal disease, chronic pain) often demonstrate difficulty with movement transitions and antigravity control.

Task Analysis

Task analysis informs development of the physical therapy plan of care (POC) and requires the therapist to address questions related to understanding three key elements: (1) the task, (2) characteristics of the individual patient, and (3) the impact of the environment on motor control strategies. Inherent to each of these components of task analysis are questions to be considered and answered by the therapist. See the discussion on task analysis in Chapter 2: Interventions to Improve Motor Function (summarized in Box 2.2).

Task analysis also allows the therapist to identify the link between the patient's inability to effectively use an appropriate movement strategy (abnormal movement) and underlying impairments. This information helps identify the need for additional examination procedures and directs and guides selection of intervention strategies. Critical to performing a task analysis is knowledge of efficient posture and movement and the ability to deconstruct a task into its component skills.

In observing human movement, it is important to note that *normal* movement such as normal gait characteristics is simply a guide to understanding what one should expect. In all functional mobility skills, one can observe great variations across the lifespan regarding what may be considered "normal" (e.g., the considerable variation in gait characteristics exhibited within a population of "normal" people). This has been referred to as the *challenge of normal* with the suggestion that, as movement specialists, physical therapists should be observing and aiming for efficiency of movement. *Efficient movement* is defined as having adequate mechanical capacity (mobility of joint, soft tissue, muscular, and neurovascular components), appropriate neuromuscular function (ability to initiate a contraction and to demonstrate adequate strength and endurance), and effective motor control (the ability to demonstrate proper movement strategies to assume and maintain a balanced posture while engaged in a functional activity with changing task demands).[1,2]

Automatic core engagement,[2] or the automatic activation of the core/stabilizing tonic muscles throughout the body, provides the dynamic stability necessary for distal mobility during the performance of a functional task. This automatic timing of the core activation, or the *anticipatory postural adjustments,* is necessary for the dynamic stability required for effective volitional movement. An insult affecting *transitional mobility, static postural control* (stability), and/or *dynamic postural control* (controlled mobility, static-dynamic control) can directly affect a patient's ability to demonstrate these strategies, leading to inefficient or dysfunctional posture and movement.

Clinical Note: Traditionally, the word *core* has been used to refer to the trunk, and the two terms are used interchangeably. However, *core* is also used more globally to include both the stabilizing muscles of the trunk and the stabilizing muscles of the interconnecting segments (pelvic and shoulder girdle). The trunk, pelvic, and shoulder girdle regions each have core stabilizers, which must work synergistically with prime movers in proper timing to provide dynamic stability for effective distal mobility.

Examination and Evaluation

The physical therapy *examination* of bed mobility skills, as for all functional tasks, includes observation and visual analysis of the task and palpation of body segments during performance in addition to data obtained from indicated tests and measures (e.g., range of motion [ROM], manual muscle test, sensory examination).

The physical therapy *evaluation,* or the interpretation of bed mobility examination data, is performed within the context of motor task requirements: mobility, stability (static postural control), controlled mobility (dynamic postural control), and skill (consistent smooth coordinated movement). This context also informs clinical decision-making to develop a POC that addresses deficits in bed mobility. Treatment interventions aimed at reestablishing these motor task requirements are based on addressing impairments in the following areas:

- Mechanical capacity (joint, soft tissue, and neural) to improve mobility
- Neuromuscular function to promote stability and controlled mobility
- Motor control to promote efficient task performance

For example, when working with a patient to improve bridging skills for the functional purpose of scooting side to side in bed, the physical therapist first assesses and treats any limitations in mechanical capacity, such as decreased hip, knee, or ankle ROM, to assure availability of the required mobility to assume the bridging position and eventually to scoot. Once in the position, neuromuscular function is addressed to assure that the patient can stabilize in the position (stability) before asking the patient to move within that position (controlled mobility). Once adequate mobility, stability, and controlled mobility are achieved, emphasis shifts to facilitating the motor control strategies necessary for efficient scooting side to side.

Interventions are selected based on identified impairments in mechanical capacity, neuromuscular function, and/or motor control. The primary goal of treatment is to restore efficient movement to optimize function. Descriptions of the proprioceptive neuromuscular facilitation (PNF) principles discussed in this chapter (patient and therapist position, manual contacts [MCs], verbal cues or commands, movement patterns, timing, appropriate resistance,[1,2] approximation, traction, visual input, irradiation and reinforcement, and quick stretch) are addressed in Chapter 3: Proprioceptive Neuromuscular Facilitation (summarized in Box 3.1). Descriptions of the specific PNF techniques (rhythmic initiation, combination of isotonics, dynamic [isotonic] reversals, stabilizing [isometric] reversals) are summarized in Box 3.2.

Postures and Techniques to Improve Bed Mobility Skills

The following sections present postures and techniques to improve early trunk control, bed mobility skills, and neuromuscular function in preparation for sitting, standing, and gait. Based on an understanding of motor task requirements and developmental progressions, general characteristics and mobility requirements of each posture or activity are described (i.e., hooklying, bridging, sidelying, and rolling). Interventions are organized by type of motor control required: *transitional mobility* (ability to move from one position to another), *static postural control* (stability), *dynamic postural control* (controlled mobility, static-dynamic control), and *skill level activities* (function). See discussion in Chapter 2: Interventions to Improve Motor Function. Patient outcomes consistent with the *Guide to Physical Therapist Practice*[3] are described as well as clinical applications and patient examples.

For all activities and application of techniques, patient position is a key element to facilitation of desired motor patterns. Initially, the patient should be positioned in as close to neutral alignment as possible, minimizing tissue tension and supporting body segments. Alignment and posture directly influence neuromuscular control. For patients who may have suffered a central nervous system insult and may be displaying the influence of primitive reflexes (Box 4.1), positioning can be used to minimize abnormal motor responses or biases.

Another important general consideration is therapist adherence to proper body mechanics to both prevent injury and to facilitate an optimal neuromuscular response in the patient. The desired patient or body segment movement is often a mirror image of the therapist's movement. As such, the therapist should be positioned directly in line with the desired movement to be facilitated (using a dynamic and wide base of support [BOS] to allow for weight shifts). With optimal positioning, the therapist's weight shifts will be proportionate to, and can facilitate, the direction and amplitude of the desired patient motion and allow for effective application of appropriate resistance.

Hooklying

General Characteristics
In hooklying, the patient is supine with both hips and knees flexed to approximately 60 degrees; feet are flat and weight bearing on the supporting surface. Movements from and within the hooklying position include bridging, scooting, and lower trunk rotation (LTR). With its large BOS and low center of mass (COM) this posture can be used to promote stability of the trunk and hips, dynamic postural control of the trunk and lower extremities ([LEs] e.g., LTR and controlled bridging), and functional skills (e.g., dressing and scooting in bed).

Active movements of the knees from side to side (LTR) involve crossing the midline and can be an important treatment activity for decreasing hypertonicity (e.g., patients

BOX 4.1 Tonic Reflexes: Impact on the Acquisition of Functional Rolling

Symmetrical tonic labyrinthine reflex (STLR): The STLR causes fluctuations in tone in infants and some patients with brain injury who are influenced by *body position* (prone versus supine). In the prone position, there is an increase in flexor tone; in supine, there is increased extensor tone. Excess extension or flexion tone impedes rolling motions. The therapist may consider initial sidelying rolling to eliminate prone or supine reflex influences.

Asymmetrical tonic neck reflex (ATNR): The ATNR causes fluctuations in tone in infants and some patients with brain injury who are influenced by *right* or *left neck rotation.* Neck rotation to one side results in extension of the UE on the side the head is rotated toward (chin side) and flexion of the opposite UE (skull side). The extended UE position that accompanies head turning to that side effectively blocks rolling. Normal head and neck (neutral) alignment should be maintained and the patient prevented from turning the head toward the side of the roll.

Symmetrical tonic neck reflex (STNR): The STNR causes fluctuations in tone in infants and some patients with brain injury that are influenced by *flexion* or *extension of the head and neck.* Head and neck flexion produces flexion of the UEs and extension of the LEs; extension of the head and neck causes extension of the UEs and flexion of the LEs. Normal head and neck (neutral) alignment should be maintained, and strategies to promote rolling that involve head and neck flexion or extension should be avoided.

with Parkinson's disease, stroke, SCI) and for patients with unilateral neglect (e.g., the patient with left hemiplegia). Lower trunk rotation should occur without accompanying upper trunk rotation or log rolling, which can be minimized by positioning the shoulders in abduction on the mat, if necessary. Patients with gluteus medius weakness (e.g., a Trendelenburg gait pattern) may benefit from hooklying and bridging activities to activate the hip abductors in this modified weightbearing position. Upper extremity (UE) positions can also be changed to alter the BOS in hooklying (e.g., difficulty is increased by folding the arms across the chest or holding the hands clasped together above the chest). For the patient recovering from stroke who demonstrates excess flexor tone in the UE, the hands-clasped position with both elbows extended and shoulders flexed to approximately 90 degrees can be used.

Clinical Note:

• Abnormal reflex activity (see Box 4.1) may interfere with assumption or maintenance of the hooklying position. In supine, the symmetrical tonic labyrinthine reflex (STLR) may cause the LEs to extend. A positive support reaction (applying pressure to the ball of the foot) may also cause the LE to extend; increased weight bearing in a heel-down position minimizing contact of the

ball of the foot may need to be adopted to decrease extensor tone.

• In hooklying, some patients may initially experience difficulty maintaining foot position (i.e., heels slide away from the buttocks). In these situations, the feet should be blocked in position (e.g., MCs from the therapist). In the presence of a positive support reaction, care should be taken not to block the feet such that pressure is applied to the ball of the foot, as this may cause the LE to extend. As mentioned, a heel-down position minimizing contact of the ball of the foot may need to be adopted to decrease abnormal tone activity.

Mobility Requirements

In hooklying, the cervical, thoracic, and lumbar spine are in neutral alignment. To effectively assume or function within the hooklying position, the patient must have appropriate hip, knee, and ankle mobility. Movement into hip and knee flexion and slight ankle plantarflexion is required. In addition, spine mobility is important for efficiently assuming the position, stabilizing, and functioning within it. Alternatively, the therapist may utilize adaptive positioning strategies to assist the patient in assuming the position.

Task Analysis

During transitions from supine into hooklying, the therapist should observe for efficient timing of movement of the trunk and LEs. Proper timing requires activating the core trunk muscles for stability together with hip flexors and hamstring activity to synergistically bring the LEs into a hooklying position.

Observing the patient assume the posture allows the therapist to assess core trunk muscle function as well as hip, knee, and ankle control. Common deficits observed during assumption of the position include:

• Arching or rotating the spine while pulling the LE into flexion (indicates lack of proximal core stability) with diminished hamstring activity and increased hip flexion activation
• Raising foot in the air with minimal knee flexion (indicates overuse of hip flexors without the synergistic support of hamstring activity)
• Extending one LE involuntarily while flexing opposite hip and knee (indicates lack of proximal core stability and an attempt to stabilize with the LE)

Interventions

ASSUMING THE HOOKLYING POSITION

To facilitate assumption of the position, the patient is instructed to initially push one heel into the supporting surface (with knee extended) while attempting to slide the opposite heel toward the buttocks. This strategy increases proximal stability to support movement of the dynamic limb. Facilitatory resistance to the hamstrings can be applied at the heel of moving limb (Fig. 4.1). In the presence of a diminished hamstring response, the patient may be instructed to dorsiflex the ankle

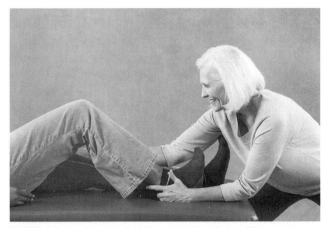

FIGURE 4.1 Facilitated (lightly resisted) unilateral hip and knee flexion in preparation for assumption of hooklying; opposite heel pushed into supporting surface to increase stability.

(or be passively positioned in dorsiflexion in the presence of weakness). Appropriate resistance may also be used to facilitate dorsiflexion. For patients with unilateral ROM limitations in hip and/or knee flexion, pillows may be used to support the extremity while the opposite LE is facilitated into position.

Stability in Hooklying

Stabilizing (holding) in the hooklying position facilitates and improves the strength of trunk muscles and hip, knee, and ankle stabilizers. For the application of holding in hooklying, the therapist guards from a half-kneeling position to one side of the patient's LEs. Manual contacts are used to assist if the patient has difficulty holding the posture initially. The patient is asked to actively hold the hooklying position. Both of the patient's knees are stable (knees are not touching), feet are in contact with the mat surface, and biomechanical alignment and symmetrical midline weight distribution are maintained. As control increases, the position of the feet can be moved more distally, decreasing the amount of hip and knee flexion. Holding is imposed at each successive repositioning of the feet as hip and knee flexion is gradually decreased. This action promotes development of selective knee control at different points in the range.

Verbal cues (VCs) for stabilization activities in hooklying include, *"Hold, keep your knees stable and feet flat, hold."*

Trunk and hip stability control (holding) are critical elements for successful functional task execution. When asking a patient to hold in hooklying, the therapist should carefully observe the activity to determine if proper alignment is being maintained with adequate stability at the trunk and LEs. Compensatory strategies (e.g., lumbar extension and pelvic rotation, LE abduction and/or external rotation [ER]) are common and should be eliminated to avoid practicing an inefficient holding pattern. Initiated in dependent postures, trunk and hip stability will eventually be progressed to upright postures and skill level activities. Trunk stability provides the foundation and support for extremity function as well as the individual's ability to interact with the environment.

Stabilizing (isometric) reversals may be used to promote stability in hooklying. The therapist is positioned diagonally in half-kneeling position to one side facing the patient. The patient is asked to hold the hooklying position while the therapist applies appropriate resistance (combined with traction or approximation, as appropriate) (Fig. 4.2). A

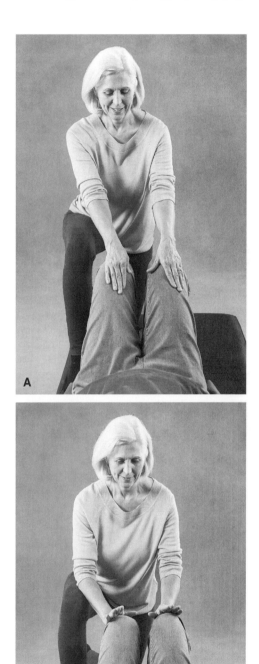

FIGURE 4.2 Stabilizing (isometric) reversals used to promote stability in hooklying can be combined with (A) traction or (B) approximation.

VC such as, *"Hold, do not let me move you,"* should be used to promote the holding response with no intent to move. The therapist's MCs can alternate between the *distal* femur on each side and the *proximal* tibia on each side (Fig. 4.3). The therapist repeats the slow, low resistance, alternating isometric contractions in various directions until the patient is able to sustain the position with adequate dynamic proximal stability. When applied across the three planes of motion, with particular emphasis on rotation, appropriate resistance will lead to a stronger response from tonic stabilizing muscles, providing improved dynamic stability control.

Comments
- Appropriate resistance is first applied in the stronger direction (to promote irradiation to weaker muscles) and then in the opposite direction.
- Initial emphasis may be placed on traction or approximation forces with progression to directional resistance.
- Once an appropriate stabilizing response is achieved, resistance is increased; approximation or traction is continued, as needed.
- Greater challenges can be imposed by gradually decreasing the amount of hip and knee flexion (e.g., from 60 to 40 to 20 degrees).
- As noted above, stabilizing (isometric) reversals may also be applied diagonally. The MCs and position of therapist vary based on the desired direction of diagonal force. For example, diagonal resistance at the knees can be applied with MCs alternating between the *distal medial* side of one knee and the *distal lateral* side of the opposite knee.

Hand placements are then reversed to resist holding in the opposite direction.
- Appropriate resistance can also be applied at the ankles/distal tibia. Distal resistance can be used to further promote stability with a focus on hamstring recruitment.
- Manual contacts should provide smooth transitions between applications of appropriate resistance in opposite directions.
- If the patient initiates a response by pushing or pulling to one side, resistance should be decreased and built slowly until the patient responds with stabilization, not pushing or pulling. This slowly developed appropriate resistance is repeated in various directions until the patient is able to sustain the position with less effort and appropriate timing.
- If weight is not evenly distributed through the feet, approximation and appropriate resistance can be used to improve weight acceptance. For example, if decreased weightbearing is demonstrated on the left, the therapist is positioned on that side. The therapist approximates through the foot and into the hip, while slowly applying appropriate resistance in a diagonal toward the upper right side of the patient's trunk.
- Unilateral holding (modified hooklying) can be practiced at various increments and decrements of hip and knee flexion ROM (Fig. 4.4).
- Appropriate resistance applied to the UEs can be used as a source of irradiation into the trunk stabilizers (Fig. 4.5).
- Elastic resistive bands can be placed around the patient's thighs to enhance proprioceptive loading and contraction of the stabilizing hip abductors.
- A small ball may be placed between the knees to promote contraction of hip adductors.

Outcomes
Motor control goal: stability (steady holding of the hooklying posture)

Functional skill achieved: improved static postural control in hooklying

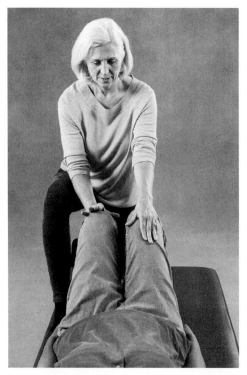

FIGURE 4.3 Applying stabilizing (isometric) reversals to promote stability in hooklying.

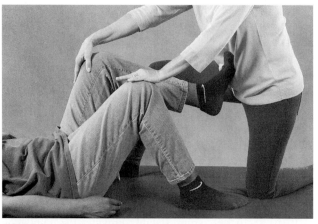

FIGURE 4.4 Holding (stability) in unilateral hooklying with alternating MCs Holding demands on the dynamic limb as the patient is asked to "*hold*" at different points in the ROM.

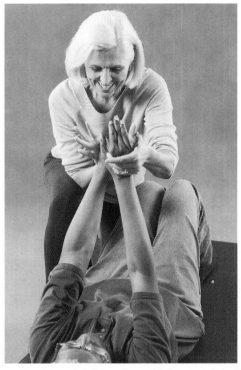

FIGURE 4.5 Applying stabilizing (isometric) reversals to UEs in hooklying to promote irradiation to trunk stabilizers.

Indications: decreased strength, diminished lower trunk stability (e.g., the patient with low back dysfunction or the patient with asymmetrical trunk control), inability to stabilize hips (e.g., the patient with abductor weakness and a Trendelenburg gait), and an inability to stabilize the knees in flexion with feet supported. Independent static postural control in hooklying is an important lead-up skill for lower trunk/pelvic stabilization during locomotion

LOWER TRUNK ROTATION IN HOOKLYING

Lower trunk rotation introduces movement to a previously static (hooklying) posture, changing the motor control demands to dynamic postural control (controlled mobility). In LTR the knees move together from side to side, a motion that elongates the trunk and allows segmental rotation, starting with the hips moving into abduction/adduction, followed by rotation of the pelvis, and finally rotation of each spinal vertebra. A reverse segmental rotation occurs with return to neutral. Rotation is then performed to the opposite side.

Rhythmic initiation can be used with LTR to teach the movement (including trunk elongation and segmental rotation) and to facilitate control for efficient movement. The patient is in hooklying with both feet flat on the mat. The therapist is half-kneeling at the base of the patient's feet. The MCs for the passive and active-assistive components are on top of the patient's knees. It is important to emphasize that prior to movement beginning at the pelvis and progressing through the spine, the hips must be released allowing the LEs to drop to the side effectively dissociating hip motion

from pelvic and spinal motion. The LTR movement then begins at the pelvis and is followed by segmental rotation of the spine. During the resistive phase of rhythmic initiation, MCs change to the medial side of one knee (closest to therapist) and the lateral side of the opposite knee (farthest from therapist) to resist both knees as they pull away. The therapist's hands must pivot to resist the complete movement of the knees down to the mat, when appropriate. This sequence is repeated with the gradual introduction of appropriate levels of resistance. The MCs then move to the opposite sides of the knees to resist movement toward the therapist.

 Clinical Notes:

- Rhythmic initiation is useful for patients with diminished control owing to weakness or increased abnormal tone. For the patient with increased tone, it may be necessary to initiate LTR with less than optimal flexion of the hips and knees. As the tone decreases, the LEs can be gradually repositioned into greater hip and knee flexion until the hooklying position is achieved.
- Patients may inappropriately perform LTR by simply allowing the knees to drop to one side allowing the pelvis to move into rotation with lumbar extension. Appropriate timing and control of the movement should be encouraged.
- An alternative application of LTR in hooklying involves positioning the patient's legs on a ball with the hips and knees flexed to approximately 70 degrees (Fig. 4.6). The therapist is half-kneeling on a diagonal to one side with MCs on the anterior aspects of the patient's legs. Using rhythmic initiation, the therapist slowly moves the ball from side to side, emphasizing a lengthening component through the trunk. This positioning eliminates tactile input to the bottom of the feet, thereby reducing the possible negative effects of a hyperactive positive support reflex. The ball also allows the patient to move from side to side easily and is an effective intervention to promote LE relaxation (e.g., for patients with multiple

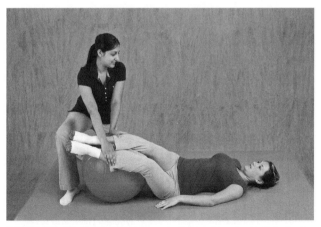

FIGURE 4.6 Hooklying, LTR using a ball (passive phase of rhythmic initiation) The patient's hips and knees are flexed and supported on the ball. Manual contacts are on the anterior aspects of the legs.

sclerosis [MS] or stroke and high levels of extensor spasticity). This positioning is also effective for decreasing strain on the lower back, if that is a concern.

Outcomes

Motor control goals: initiation of movement (mobility) and relaxation

Functional skills achieved: the movement requirements of LTR and strategies for initiating movement and relaxation

Indications: impaired function owing to hypertonia (spasticity, rigidity) and inability to initiate or control LTR

Dynamic (isotonic) reversals using isotonic contractions can be used to facilitate dynamic stability and controlled mobility during LTR. To apply dynamic reversals, the patient moves both knees together in side-to-side movements (i.e., toward the right and left, away from midline). Depending on the ROM available in the hips, pelvis, and lumbar spine, the knees may move all the way down to the mat on one side and then the other. Alternatively, movement may occur through increments of ROM. The therapist is positioned in half-kneeling slightly to one side of the patient. Appropriate resistance is applied, with the emphasis on control through repetition. The MCs alternate between the medial and lateral aspects of the distal femur (Fig. 4.7). Traction or approximation may be used to facilitate trunk muscles, ensuring that segmental spinal control is present.

The MCs are placed in the direction of movement and should allow for smooth transitions between opposing directions of movement. An isometric hold may be added at any point of weakness within the range if the need to facilitate increased motor unit output is perceived. The hold is a momentary pause (the patient is instructed to *"Hold"*); the antagonist movement pattern is then facilitated. The hold can be added in one direction only or in both directions. Verbal cues for dynamic (isotonic) reversals in hooklying

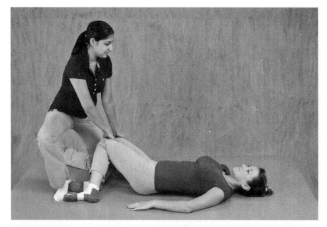

FIGURE 4.7 Lower trunk rotation, using dynamic (isotonic) reversals in hooklying Appropriate resistance is applied as the knees move in a side-to-side direction. In the example shown, manual contacts are on the *lateral* and *medial* distal femur as the knees move toward the therapist.

include, as the knees move away from the therapist, *"Pull your knees away, rolling one vertebra at a time."* The transitional cue is *"Now, reverse."* As knees move toward the therapist the cue is *"Now pull back toward me, rolling one vertebra back at a time."* If a hold (isometric contraction) is added to dynamic reversals at the end range or point of weakness, the VC is *"Hold."*

Comments

- Appropriate resistance is typically applied first in the stronger direction of movement.
- Movements begin with small-range control (e.g., one-quarter range movement in each direction) and progress through increasing ROM (increments of range) to full-range control (the knees move all the way down to the mat on each side). It is particularly important that the therapist properly facilitate (or guide) LTR to assure segmental motion while avoiding compensatory movements such as trunk extension, pelvic rotation, or non-segmental rotation.
- Initially, movements are slow and controlled, with emphasis on traction and low resistance.
- The successful application of dynamic (isotonic) reversals requires careful timing and coordination of the transitional VCs with changes in MCs between opposing directions of movement.
- Dynamic (isotonic) reversals are used to increase strength and active ROM and to promote normal transitions between opposing muscle groups.
- A smooth reversal of motion is the goal.

Outcomes

Motor control goal: controlled mobility function

Functional skills achieved: performs controlled LTR. Control of lower trunk/pelvic movements is an important prerequisite for standing and gait.

Indications: weakness and instability of the lower trunk and hip muscles, impaired coordination and timing (e.g., patients with ataxia), and limitations in ROM. Lower trunk rotation in hooklying is an important lead-up skill for upright antigravity control in standing and gait.

See Box 4.2: Student Practice Activity: Hooklying.

Bridging

General Characteristics

From the hooklying position, *bridging* involves extending the hips and elevating the pelvis from the support surface with the lumbar spine in a neutral position (initial instruction in pelvic tilting [with facilitation] may be required to identify the neutral position). Bridging is an important prerequisite requirement for moving in bed (positional changes), dressing, and for moving to the edge of the bed in preparation for sitting. It is also an important lead-up for later functional activities, such as developing sit-to-stand control, stance phase control of gait, and stair climbing.

BOX 4.2 STUDENT PRACTICE ACTIVITY: HOOKLYING

Each section of this chapter ends with a Student Practice Activity specifically designed to address the key treatment techniques and activities in that section. (Note that the section on rolling includes an additional Student Practice Activity addressing task analysis). These activities provide an opportunity to share knowledge and skills with student peers and to confirm or clarify students' understanding of the interventions. Each student in a group will contribute his or her understanding of, or questions about, the technique or treatment activity being discussed and demonstrated. Dialogue should continue until the group reaches a consensus of understanding.

Section Outline: Hooklying

ACTIVITIES AND TECHNIQUES
▲ Hooklying, stabilization (holding)
▲ Hooklying, LTR using a therapy ball
▲ Hooklying, LTR using rhythmic initiation
▲ Hooklying, LTR using dynamic (isotonic) reversals

Objective: sharing skill in the application and knowledge of treatment interventions used in hooklying
Equipment: platform mat and large therapy ball
Directions: Working in groups of four to six students, consider each entry in the section outline. Members of the group will assume different roles (described below) and will rotate roles each time the group progresses to a new item on the outline.
▲ One person assumes the role of therapist (for demonstrations) and participates in discussion.
▲ One person serves as the patient (for demonstrations) and participates in discussion.

▲ The remaining members participate in discussion and provide supportive feedback during demonstrations. One member of this group should be designated as a "fact checker" to return to the text content to confirm elements of the discussion (if needed) or if agreement cannot be reached.

Thinking aloud, brainstorming, and sharing thoughts should be continuous throughout this activity! Carry out the following activities for each item in the section outline.

1. Discuss the *activity,* including patient and therapist positioning. Consider what positional changes could enhance the activity (e.g., prepositioning a limb, hand placements to alter the BOS).
2. Discuss the *technique,* including its description, indication(s) for use, therapist hand placements (MCs), and VCs.
3. Demonstrate the activity and application of the technique by the designated therapist and patient. Discussion during the demonstration should be continuous (the demonstration should not be the sole responsibility of the designated therapist and patient). All group members should provide recommendations, suggestions, and supportive feedback throughout the demonstration. During the demonstrations, discuss strategies to make the activity either *more* or *less* challenging.

If any member of the group feels he or she requires practice with the activity and technique, the group should allocate time to accommodate the request. All group members providing input (recommendations, suggestions, and supportive feedback) should also accompany this practice.

From hooklying, bridging requires an active transition from a large to a smaller BOS with a higher COM. Greater demands are placed on the trunk, hips, and ankles for control, and on the hamstrings to maintain the knees in flexion. Bridging primarily involves the lower trunk, hip, knee, and ankle muscles. The lower trunk/hip muscles (hip abductors and adductors, and internal and external rotators) function to stabilize the hip and lower trunk while the hip extensors elevate the pelvis. The hamstrings keep the knees flexed and the feet positioned for weight bearing, and the ankle and foot muscles stabilize the feet. During bridging, the gluteus maximus is primarily responsible for hip extension because knee flexion places the hamstrings in a position of active insufficiency.

Red Flag: During elevation in bridging, the pelvis should not rotate. Patients with unilateral weakness of the gluteus maximus (e.g., the patient recovering from a hip fracture) or poor dynamic postural stability through the lower trunk (e.g., patients recovering from stroke or those with low back pain) may be unable to hold the pelvis level and the pelvis will remain lower on the weaker

side. The therapist can hold a wand or yardstick across the pelvis to demonstrate this rotation visually to the patient. Additional work on stability in hooklying and bridging such as facilitation of core trunk stabilizers, strengthening the gluteus maximus or increasing the BOS through positioning may be indicated until pelvic control improves.

The BOS in bridging may be altered to *increase* or *decrease* the challenge imposed. Initially, the activity may be made easier through positioning to increase BOS. This may be accomplished by extending the elbows, abducting the shoulders with forearms pronated and hands flat on the mat, and/or moving the feet apart. Subsequently, reducing this stabilization can increase the challenge to the patient. This is achieved by gradually adducting the shoulders (bringing the UEs closer to the trunk) with progression to the UEs folded across the chest or the hands clasped together with shoulders flexed to approximately 90 degrees and elbows extended. The therapist should note that this position may allow compensatory strategies for trunk extension as the patient may be able to utilize the latissimus muscles to lift the pelvis through closed chain shoulder extension. Inaddition, the LEs can be brought closer together, the feet may be moved farther from the buttocks (decreasing knee flexion), or static-dynamic activities maybe introduced.

Additional Considerations

- Bridging allows early weightbearing through the foot and ankle without the body weight constraints of a fully upright posture. It is an appropriate early posture for patients with motor control deficits of the trunk and LEs.
- Breath holding is common during bridging and isometric activities. This may present problems for the patient with hypertension and cardiac disability; breathing should be closely monitored. Patients should be encouraged to breathe rhythmically during all bridging activities.
- Elevating the hips higher than the head may be contraindicated for patients with uncontrolled hypertension or elevated intracranial pressures (e.g., the patient with acute traumatic brain injury).
- As with hooklying, abnormal reflex activity may interfere with assumption or maintenance of the bridging posture. Influence of the STLR may cause the LEs to extend (see Box 4.1). Pressure to the ball of the foot may elicit a positive support reaction; a heel-down weightbearing position with increased weightbearing through the heels should be adopted to inhibit this response.
- Bridging promotes selective control (out-of-synergy combination of hip extension with knee flexion) and may be indicated for patients recovering from stroke who demonstrate the influence of the mass movement synergies (when hip and knee extension may be firmly linked together with hip adduction and ankle plantarflexion).

Mobility Requirements

The bridging position requires slightly lower cervical flexion and neutral alignment of the thoracic and lumbar spine for minimal tissue tension. Mobility is required in hip extension, knee flexion, and slight ankle dorsiflexion and plantarflexion.

Task Analysis

Transition from hooklying to bridging should initiate with the pelvis in a stable neutral position with movement occurring through bilateral hip extension. The therapist may need to facilitate and ensure a neutral pelvis before initiating bridging (Fig. 4.8). When lifting the hips/pelvis into bridging, dynamic postural stability (controlled mobility) of the pelvis is required without a drop or rotation on one side. Weightbearing through the LEs should be symmetrical and comfortable. Note that while the patient moves toward hip extension from a starting position of hip flexion, bridging does not allow for hip extension past neutral without lumbar extension.

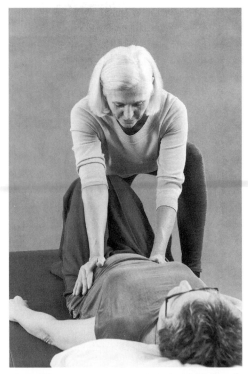

FIGURE 4.8 Facilitation of neutral pelvis before bridging For example, if a patient's resting position is a posterior or an anterior tilt, the therapist should facilitate motion into a neutral pelvis (or passively position the patient into a neutral pelvis) before working on assumption of bridging. As depicted here, MCs are slightly below bilateral anterior superior iliac spine (ASIS), facilitating/resisting movement toward a neutral pelvis (i.e., out of a posterior tilt) before transitioning from hooklying to bridging.

Interventions

TRANSITION FROM HOOKLYING TO BRIDGING

To begin bridging activities, the patient is positioned in hooklying with the hips and knees flexed to approximately 60 degrees and the feet flat on the mat. If the patient cannot achieve a foot-flat position on the mat, a folded towel can be used to provide support to promote weightbearing through the entire foot. For the patient with weakness or diminished proprioceptive awareness of the activity, the therapist can facilitate hip/pelvis elevation by placing MCs on the patient's distal thighs and pushing down (approximation) while pulling the distal thighs toward the feet (traction) (Fig. 4.9). The VC is *"Pinch your buttocks together and lift while moving your knees out over your feet."* The patient raises the hips/pelvis from the mat (concentric contraction) until the hips are extended (0 degrees or slightly less), pelvis is level, and the lumbar spine is in neutral position. For the return motion, the patient slowly controls lowering (eccentric contraction) of the hips/pelvis back down to the mat. Control of movement is the focus (collapsing back to the mat using body weight and gravity should be avoided). Tapping (quick stretch) over the gluteus maximus can be used to stimulate muscle contraction. Traction and approximation can also be performed unilaterally as needed for facilitation of the transition.

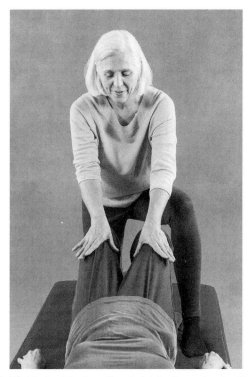

FIGURE 4.9 Hip/pelvis elevation (bridging) can be facilitated using approximation toward feet and traction through the femurs (a neurodevelopmental technique) directly away from the hips, with MCs on the distal femurs.

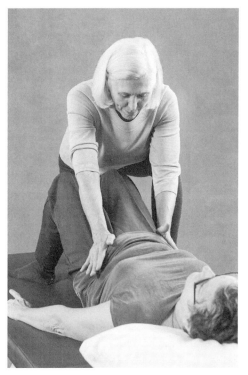

FIGURE 4.10 Applying appropriate resistance through the transition from hooklying into bridging.

Once the patient can initiate bridging without facilitation, appropriate resistance can be used to enhance the neuromuscular response and promote motor learning. Manual contacts (lumbrical grip) are on the superior (slightly medial or lateral) aspect of the pelvis, depending on the side on which the therapist is positioned. For example, if the therapist is positioned on the right side of the patient facing the patient, the right hand contact is on the medial superior aspect of the left ilium and the left hand is on the lateral superior aspect of the right ilium (Fig. 4.10). By positioning to the side of the patient, facing in a narrow diagonal in reference to the midsagittal plane, the therapist is able to effectively place greater demand on the trunk and more dynamically challenge the hips. The therapist is able to resist the hip extensors and hip adductors of one hip, and the hip extensors and abductors of the opposite hip. Applying resistance also allows the therapist to facilitate unilateral weight shifts. The VCs are *"Pinch your buttocks together and lift your pelvis,"* and progress as appropriate to, *"Lift up and over toward me."*

Combination of isotonics (COI)[1,2] utilizes appropriate resistance of concentric, isometric, and eccentric contractions without loss of tension. Against continual appropriate resistance, the patient first moves to the end range of the desired motion of lifting the pelvis up (concentric) and then holds and stabilizes (isometric) in this end position. When stability is achieved, the patient is instructed to allow the body segment to be slowly moved back to the start position

(eccentric). This is an important lead-up activity for the patient with poor eccentric control during stand-to-sit transitions. For the application of COI to bridging, the patient starts in the hooklying position. The therapist is in a half-kneeling position to one side. Bilateral MCs are on the anterior pelvis (over anterior superior iliac spines) and are applied in a diagonal direction; hand placements *do not change* during application of the technique. The hip extensors are resisted throughout. Appropriate resistance to concentric contractions is applied as the patient raises the pelvis from the mat until the hips are near extension, assuring that the lumbar spine has remained in neutral alignment (Fig. 4.11). (In attempting to overcome resistance the patient may engage lumbar extension; this is an inefficient strategy and should be avoided to prevent back injury.) When the end range is reached, appropriate resistance should continue to be applied promoting an isometric contraction as the patient holds the position. The patient then slowly lowers the pelvis back to the original start position using eccentric contractions against appropriate resistance. The VCs are *"Lift up and hold. Hold. Now slowly lower down."*

Outcomes
Motor control goal: controlled mobility
Functional skills achieved: acquires strength and control of hip extensors and abductors
Indications: weakness of hip extensors and hip abductors. Bridging is an important lead-up skill for sit-to-stand and stand-to-sit transfers and for ambulation up and down stairs.

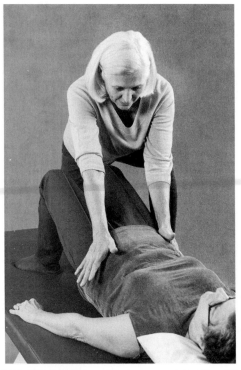

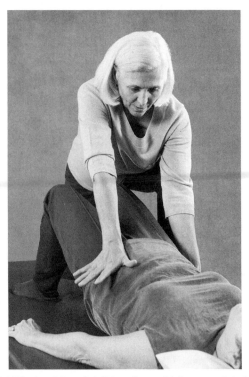

FIGURE 4.11 COI, bridging, resisted movement, holding Bilateral MCs are on the anterior pelvis and *do not change* during the application of the technique. In this illustration, appropriate resistance to concentric contractions is applied as the patient raises the pelvis (and then holds the position (isometric contraction)). *Not shown:* The patient then moves slowly back to the original start position using eccentric contractions against appropriate resistance.

FIGURE 4.12 Applying stabilizing (isometric) reversals in bridging using alternating anterior and posterior contralateral MCs at the pelvis for application of appropriate resistance to promote stability in bridging (stabilizing hold phase).

PROMOTING STABILITY (STATIC POSTURAL CONTROL) IN BRIDGING

Stabilizing (isometric) reversals can be used to facilitate stability in bridging. To apply stabilizing reversals in bridging, the therapist is positioned in half-kneeling to one side of the patient's LEs. The patient is asked to hold the bridging position while the therapist applies appropriate resistance to various points on the pelvis using the VC *"Hold, do not let me move you."* The therapist's MCs for resistance can alternate between anterior (as positioned for COI, see Fig. 4.11), posterior, medial, lateral, or contralateral anterior and posterior pelvis (Fig. 4.12). Appropriate resistance can also be applied bilaterally at distal thighs (Fig. 4.13A–C), distally at the feet, distally at the hands while held off the mat at the patient's side, or distally at clasped hands in front as if reaching for the knees. A transitional VC is provided when MCs transition to the opposing pattern of movement.

Comments

- Medial/lateral resistance applied with bilateral MCs on the lateral pelvis is effective for facilitating hip abductors and adductors.
- Therapist hand placements should provide smooth transitions between applications of appropriate resistance in opposite directions.
- The patient is not allowed to relax between contractions.

- Elastic resistive bands can be placed around the distal thighs to facilitate contraction of the lateral hip muscles (gluteus medius), further facilitating dynamic stability through irradiation.
- Appropriate resistance is built up gradually as the patient increases the force of contraction.
- If applied in a diagonal direction the resistance will facilitate an increased response of the tonic stabilizers of trunk and the pelvis and shoulder girdles.
- During any isometric contractions, the patient should be encouraged to breathe regularly.

See Box 4.3: Student Practice Activity: Bridging.

Outcomes

Motor control goal: stability of lower trunk and pelvis

Functional skills achieved: ability to stabilize the lower trunk and pelvis in all directions. These are important lead-up skills for the stabilization required during upright antigravity activities (e.g., standing and locomotion).

Indications: poor lower trunk and pelvis stability; weakness of the lower trunk, hip, and ankle muscles; impaired coordination between opposing lower trunk muscle groups

Scooting

General Characteristics

Scooting from a bridge position (also referred to as *bridge and place*) involves active lateral pelvic shifts with progression

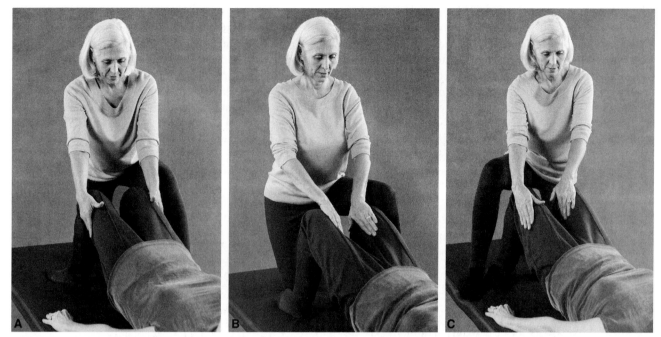

FIGURE 4.13 Applying stabilizing (isometric) reversals with alternating MCs at the distal thighs to promote stability in bridging Shown here are MCs at lateral (A), medial (B), and medial and lateral (C) aspects of the distal thighs.

BOX 4.3 STUDENT PRACTICE ACTIVITY: BRIDGING

Section Outline: Bridging
Activities and Techniques
▲ Bridging, assuming the posture using COI
▲ Bridging, stability (static postural control) using isometric reversals
▲ Scooting using rhythmic initiation
▲ Scooting using COI
▲ Scooting using dynamic (isotonic) reversals

Advanced Bridging Activities (see Appendix 4A)
▲ Bridging, single-leg lifts
▲ Bridging, alternating leg lifts, marching in place
▲ Bridging, mobile BOS using a ball, knees extended
▲ Sit to modified bridge position, movement transitions using a ball

Objective: sharing skill in the application and knowledge of treatment interventions used in bridging
Equipment Needed: platform mat and small and medium-sized balls
Directions: Working in groups of four to six students, consider each entry in the section outline. Members of the group will assume different roles (described below) and will rotate roles each time the group progresses to a new item on the outline.
▲ One person assumes the role of therapist (for demonstrations) and participates in discussion.
▲ One person serves as the patient (for demonstrations) and participates in discussion.
▲ The remaining members participate in discussion and provide supportive feedback during demonstrations. One member of this group should be designated as a

"fact checker" to return to the text content to confirm elements of the discussion (if needed) or if agreement cannot be reached.

Thinking aloud, brainstorming, and sharing thoughts should be continuous throughout this activity! Carry out the following activities for each item in the section outline.

1. Discuss the *activity,* including patient and therapist positioning. Consider what positional changes could enhance the activity (e.g., prepositioning a limb, hand placements to alter the BOS).
2. Discuss the *technique,* including its description, indication(s) for use, therapist hand placements (MCs), and VCs.
3. Demonstrate the activity and application of the technique by the designated therapist and patient. Discussion during the demonstration should be continuous (the demonstration should not be the sole responsibility of the designated therapist and patient). All group members should provide recommendations, suggestions, and supportive feedback throughout the demonstration. During the demonstrations, discuss strategies to make the activity either *more* or *less* challenging.

If any member of the group feels he or she requires practice with the activity and technique, the group should allocate time to accommodate the request. All group members providing input (recommendations, suggestions, and supportive feedback) should also accompany this practice.

to repositioning the whole body. This functional activity is important for positional changes in bed. Scooting promotes simultaneous action of synergistic muscles at more than one joint and builds on the motor control requirements of dynamic postural control (controlled mobility function) by increasing strength and control of the trunk, hip, foot and ankle, and upper body muscles.

Mobility and Stability Requirements

In addition to the mobility requirements to assume bridging, scooting requires hip abduction and adduction and internal and external rotation mobility. The ability to lengthen and shorten the lateral trunk flexors is also required for effective scooting side to side while in bridging. Reciprocal inhibition across the trunk, pelvis, and LEs is required and may need to be facilitated in a patient with increased tone and motor control deficits.

Task Analysis

To perform scooting, the patient is positioned in hooklying position. The hips are raised (bridging) and the pelvis actively shifted laterally to one side and then lowered down into the new position (Fig. 4.14). Each LE is then repositioned, followed by repositioning of the upper body in line with the new position. Scooting requires the ability to actively shift the pelvis medially and laterally from a bridged position and sufficient proximal stability and controlled

mobility function to accept weight onto one LE, then lift the opposite LE and reposition. Also required is the ability to bend the upper trunk to the side toward the new BOS and lift the thoracic cage to bring the upper body in alignment with the lower trunk and LEs. (*Note:* Weight shifting in bridging is an important lead-up activity for pelvic and LE lateral control required for gait.) Scooting allows for improved bed mobility skills and scooting to the edge of the bed in preparation for transitioning to a sitting position.

Clinical Note: Scooting is a valuable activity for the patient in the early stages of recovery from stroke. Moving the pelvis toward the more affected side stretches and elongates the trunk muscles on that side. This movement counteracts the common problem of shortening of the lateral trunk flexors on the more affected side. The patient's hands may be clasped together with the shoulders flexed and the elbows extended. This positioning effectively counteracts the common flexor and adductor posturing of the UE following stroke. Functionally, scooting in bridging will carry over to bed mobility skills such as scooting side to side and scooting to the edge of the bed before sitting up.

Interventions

Rhythmic initiation can be used to teach the patient weight shifting while maintaining the bridging position. Manual contacts are used to passively guide the pelvis into lateral weight shifts while the patient maintains active bridging. The therapist should be positioned to the side of the patient in line with the direction of movement. The weight shift is repeated. As the patient develops kinesthetic awareness and active involvement with the active-assistive motion, a progression is then made to appropriate resistance. As the technique shifts to appropriate resistance, the therapist shifts his or her body position so that the forearms are parallel to the floor and in line with the direction of the weight shift being facilitated/resisted (Fig. 4.15).

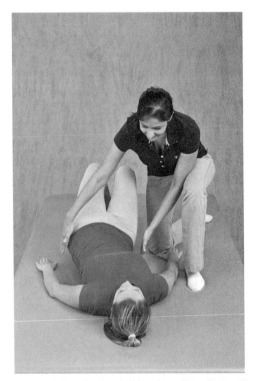

FIGURE 4.14 Scooting From a bridged position, the patient actively shifts the pelvis laterally to one side. In this example, the patient is shifting toward the left. The therapist is in guard position. *Not shown:* The patient would then lower the pelvis down to the new side position.

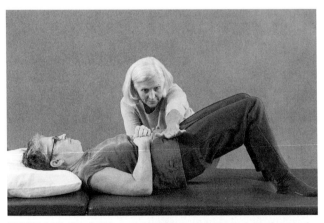

FIGURE 4.15 The lightly resisted phase of rhythmic initiation used to promote side-to-side weight shifting in bridging, in preparation for scooting Note that the therapist's forearms are parallel to the floor and in line with the direction of the weight shift being facilitated.

Combination of isotonics can also be used to promote lateral (side-to-side) weight shifts using a concentric contraction to move into a lateral weight shift, an isometric contraction at the end range, followed by an eccentric return to the beginning of the range. When using COI, remember that this is a resisted unidirectional technique and can be applied to both sides of the weight shift. As noted earlier for the technique of rhythmic initiation, therapist positioning should be in line with the direction of the lateral weight shift. The VCs are *"Lift your pelvis up, push your hips toward me. Now hold. Now slowly let your pelvis lower down."*

Dynamic (isotonic) reversals may be used to facilitate the lateral weight shift from one side to the other – a crucial component of scooting for bed mobility. The therapist's MCs and forearms are positioned in line with the resisted weight lateral shift in one direction followed by resisted movement in the opposite direction. The VCs are *"Lift your pelvis up, push your hips toward me, now push your hips away from me."*

Outcomes

Motor control goals: controlled mobility and static-dynamic control in bridging

Functional skills achieved: able to stabilize the hip/pelvis/ankle during upright antigravity activities

Indications: impaired dynamic stability (required for upright antigravity activities such as standing and locomotion)

Clinical Note: For patients undergoing active rehabilitation, advanced bridging activities may not be appropriate within the context of a progression of bed mobility activities. However, where appropriate, they have important implications as lead-up activities for upright standing, gait, and stair climbing. These advanced activities are presented in Appendix 4A on p. 94.

Sidelying

General Characteristics

The BOS in sidelying is large and the COM is low, making it a very stable posture; no upright postural control is required. Flexing either the lowermost or uppermost extremities will increase the BOS; in contrast, keeping the extremities extended reduces the BOS. Tonic reflex (STLR and asymmetrical tonic neck reflex [ATNR]) activity and related muscle tone are reduced in sidelying position (see Box 4.1). The posture may be used to increase ROM of the trunk, scapula, and pelvis, to promote the initiation of active movement, to promote trunk stability, and to encourage reciprocal trunk patterns in patients who lack upright (antigravity) control (e.g., weakness or disordered motor control).

Task Analysis

When positioning a patient in sidelying, neutral alignment should be promoted across all body segments, minimizing tissue tension and supporting body segments as needed (e.g., head and neck supported on a pillow, a pillow between the patient's legs, and a small folded towel under side of the trunk to avoid lateral flexion). To increase stability of the posture, the hips and knees may be flexed (70–90 degrees) creating an anterior BOS. Note that various levels of mobility restrictions can be accommodated to allow assumption of the sidelying position.

Interventions

PROMOTING STATIC POSTURAL CONTROL (STABILITY)

Activities are initiated in sidelying with the trunk in midrange and hips and knees positioned in 70 to 90 degrees of flexion with the UEs resting in a comfortable position at the patient's side. Stabilizing (isometric) reversals utilize stabilizing holds of antagonist patterns against appropriate resistance with emphasis on stability and not movement. Appropriate resistance is built up slowly from a low load as the patient responds to the applied force. The technique can be used to increase stability and strength. Since dynamic postural stability through the trunk is aimed at facilitation of the deeper core trunk stabilizers, the motions resisted should be those that promote reciprocal trunk activation directed at the trunk stabilizers. Resistance should be applied to opposing directions of the scapula and pelvis diagonal patterns (i.e., posterior depression of the scapula and anterior elevation of the pelvis and alternatively the reciprocal motions of these diagonals). Resistance to rotation of the upper and lower trunk in the transverse plane should be avoided because this will facilitate activation of the more superficial movers of the spine.

To apply stabilizing (isometric) reversals in the sidelying position, the therapist is positioned in line with the scapula and pelvis diagonals of anterior elevation/posterior depression (Fig. 4.16). The patient is asked to hold the position while the therapist applies appropriate resistance, beginning slowly with a low load. Resistance to isometric contractions is gradually increased until the patient's tonic stabilizers are fully

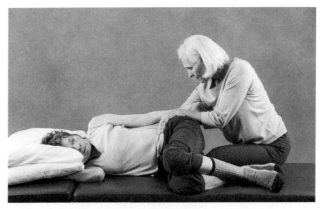

FIGURE 4.16 Applying stabilizing (isometric) reversals for stability in sidelying, beginning with appropriate resistance to left scapula posterior depression and left pelvis anterior elevation.

engaged. For example, the therapist applies appropriate resistance to end-range posterior depression of the scapula *("Hold it here")*, while appropriate resistance is simultaneously applied to anterior elevation of the pelvis *("Hold it here")*. Once the patient's maximum (appropriate) isometric response is achieved, the therapist can begin to switch input to the UE or the LE resisting the appropriate extremity diagonal patterns. The VCs for stabilizing reversals in sidelying are *"Hold, don't let me move you."* This activity should be repeated on both sides.

Comments

- Appropriate resistance should be applied first to stronger muscles to facilitate or promote irradiation to weaker muscles.
- Resistance is built up gradually as the patient increases the force of isometric hold contraction.
- During any isometric contractions, the patient should be encouraged to breathe regularly. Breath holding increases intrathoracic pressures and can produce a Valsalva effect.

Outcomes

Motor control goals: stability (static control)
Functional skill achieved: able to stabilize the trunk
Indications: weakness of the deep stabilizer muscles of the trunk; inability to stabilize the trunk

PROMOTING DYNAMIC POSTURAL CONTROL

Reciprocal trunk and extremity pattern combinations (e.g., scapula posterior depression/anterior elevation diagonal and pelvis anterior elevation/posterior depression diagonal) are deeply ingrained movement pattern combinations, developed as part of the normal developmental process and crucial to gait, the most basic and important of all functional activities. It is also often the most difficult to achieve for patients with motor control impairments involving decreased trunk control (e.g., patients with stroke, MS, Guillain Barré syndrome, SCI), increased tone or rigidity of the trunk (e.g., Parkinson's disease), or pain (e.g., low back pain). Facilitation of coordinated reciprocity (reciprocal movement) through the trunk and the extremities (i.e., dynamic postural stability for distal mobility) will result in significant improvement in bed mobility transitions (i.e., rolling) as well as achievement of sitting, scooting forward in sitting, and gait.

Rhythmic initiation can be used to teach the patient the coordinated timing and direction of reciprocal movements of the scapula and pelvis. The patient is positioned in sidelying. The therapist is behind the patient, in line with the scapula and pelvis diagonals facing the patient's head. Manual contacts are on the scapula and the pelvis. The patient is initially moved into the reciprocal combination of scapula posterior depression and pelvis anterior elevation slowly and with proper timing progressing from passive, to active assistive, to appropriately resisted and then to independent movement. This is a unidirectional technique with a passive return to the beginning of the range. The same technique can then be used for the combination of scapula anterior elevation

and pelvis posterior depression (Fig. 4.17). This is particularly useful for patients who have difficulty assuming a balanced sitting or standing position owing to shortening on one side of the trunk (e.g., the patient with stroke).

Combination of isotonics is another useful technique for promoting reciprocal combination patterns. It is effective for facilitating improved trunk control and coordination. In addition, the increased proprioceptive awareness provided by the isometric hold is useful for teaching the end range of the movement. For example, the patient moves to the end range of scapular posterior depression and pelvis anterior elevation with an isometric hold at end range, followed by an eccentric return to starting position. Appropriate resistance is applied slowly and is gradually increased. Traction should be used to facilitate the tonic stabilizers of each segment and of the trunk. The patient is instructed to move through the range against appropriate resistance and then to hold. Once an efficient isometric response is achieved, the therapist instructs the patient to *"Keep holding, but slowly let me take you back to the start position"* while eccentrically lengthening the pattern. This is also a unidirectional technique so the focus will be in one direction only. The same technique can then be used for the combination of scapula anterior elevation and pelvis posterior depression.

Clinical Note: For combination of patterns, movement may be facilitated with *timing for emphasis* by using stronger components of a pattern to facilitate weaker ones through irradiation. A maximal contraction is elicited from stronger components to allow irradiation to facilitate increased motor output in weaker components. Irradiation can be used effectively from the extremity to the trunk, from the trunk to the extremity, or from one extremity to the other. When the therapist perceives a weakness, a prolonged hold can be elicited on the stronger segment while repeated concentric contractions, facilitated by a quick stretch, can be performed and appropriately resisted on the weaker segment (techniques used for the clinical application of irradiation are described in Chapter 3: Proprioceptive Neuromuscular Facilitation, Box 3.2).

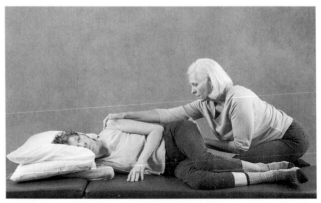

FIGURE 4.17 Rhythmic initiation to promote combination of scapula anterior elevation and pelvis posterior depression with MCs on left ischial tuberosity and superior/anterior acromion.

Dynamic (isotonic) reversals use isotonic contractions to promote active concentric movement in one direction followed by active concentric movement in the reverse direction, first with and then without relaxation. When used for reciprocal trunk patterns, this technique promotes the smooth coordinated reversal of reciprocal motions required for function (e.g., efficient gait). For example, isotonic movement is first resisted into scapula anterior elevation and pelvis posterior depression (Fig. 4.18) followed by resisted movement into scapula posterior depression and pelvis anterior elevation. Emphasis is placed on achieving the full end range of each pattern so that a concentric contraction moving in the opposite direction can be facilitated. The reversal of directions within the reciprocal pattern combination is repeated with appropriate resistance until improved control and coordination is achieved. A suggested VC for dynamic (isotonic) reversals using reciprocal patterns in sidelying position is *"Make your trunk short. Now switch and make your trunk long."*

Comments

- Reciprocal trunk patterns place great mobility demands on the spine. Graded resistance should be kept at an appropriate level for a smooth coordinated response.
- Verbal cues should be soothing, slow, rhythmic, and carefully timed with all phases of movement and facilitation (e.g., quick stretches).
- Movements may begin with small-range control and progress to larger ranges and then to full-range control.
- Initially, movements are slow and controlled using graded (appropriate) resistance; progression may include variations in speed in one or both directions.
- An isometric hold may be added in the shortened range or at any point of weakness within the range during all

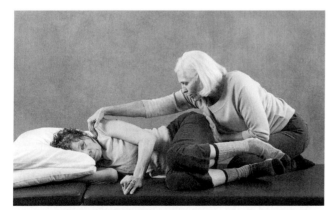

FIGURE 4.18 Applying dynamic (isotonic) reversals for reciprocal combination of pelvis and scapula Appropriate resistance is applied to left scapula anterior elevation with MC on superior/anterior acromion and to left pelvis posterior depression with MC on ischial tuberosity. *Not shown:* The motion is then reversed and appropriate resistance is applied to left scapula posterior depression with MC on inferior/medial scapula and left pelvis anterior elevation with MC on superior/anterior iliac crest.

techniques. The hold is a momentary pause (the patient is instructed to *"Hold"*) used to increase motor unit output if necessary. The hold can be added in one direction only or in both directions.

- An isometric hold may be used at the end of each reciprocal diagonal to allow the therapist time to switch MCs for reversing directions.
- Careful attention must be directed to timing the preparatory VC (such as *"and now, switch"*). This will indicate to the patient that a change in movement direction is about to take place.
- A facilitatory quick stretch can be used at the beginning of the ROM when muscles are elongated if needed to initiate the movement in the opposite direction or during a contraction at a point where weakness is perceived. Quick stretches must be timed with an immediate VC for a volitional contraction.
- In combination with rhythmic initiation for sidelying trunk reciprocation, active reciprocal extremity movements simulating arm swing and stepping movements may be performed.

Clinical Note: Reciprocal patterns of the upper and lower trunk have several important clinical implications. It is often a useful strategy for patients with stroke, who typically move the trunk as a unit without reciprocal movement of the extremities. Patients with a retracted pelvic position (commonly seen in stroke) will benefit from reciprocal trunk movement. It is also effective for patients with Parkinson's disease, who often move the trunk as a rigid unit without reciprocation of the upper and lower trunk segments, resulting in movement confined to a single plane of motion. Reciprocal trunk activity can be effective in normalizing tone, allowing more normal patterns of movement to occur.

Outcomes

Motor control goal: controlled mobility function
Functional skill achieved: ability to perform reciprocal patterns of pelvis and scapula
Indication: inability to perform smooth, coordinated reciprocal patterns of motion

See Box 4.4: Student Practice Activity: Sidelying

Rolling

General Characteristics

Rolling is an early functional activity achieved in the sequence of developmental skills. As such, it is a deeply ingrained activity that carries many of the motor control prerequisites for higher-level functional activities such as mobility of proximal and intermediate joints (e.g., scapula, shoulder, pelvis, hip, and knees); dynamic stability of the trunk; and distal controlled mobility of the extremities and head and neck. Thus, the focus of early interventions is on acquiring initial mobility and developing component skills,

---

BOX 4.4 STUDENT PRACTICE ACTIVITY: SIDELYING

Section Outline: Sidelying
Activities and Techniques
▲ Sidelying, using stabilizing (isometric) reversals
▲ Sidelying, reciprocal trunk and extremity pattern combinations (scapula posterior depression/anterior elevation diagonal and pelvis anterior elevation/posterior depression diagonal)
▲ Sidelying, rhythmic initiation
▲ Sidelying, COI
▲ Sidelying, dynamic (isotonic) reversals
Objective: sharing skill in the application and knowledge of treatment interventions used in sidelying
Equipment Needed: platform mat
Directions: Working in groups of four to six students, consider each entry in the section outline. Members of the group will assume different roles (described below) and will rotate roles each time the group progresses to a new item on the outline.
▲ One person assumes the role of therapist (for demonstrations) and participates in discussion.
▲ One person serves as the patient (for demonstrations) and participates in discussion.
▲ The remaining members participate in discussion and provide supportive feedback during demonstrations. One member of this group should be designated as a

"fact checker" to return to the text content to confirm elements of the discussion (if needed) or if agreement cannot be reached.

Thinking aloud, brainstorming, and sharing thoughts should be continuous throughout this activity! Carry out the following activities for each item in the section outline.

1. Discuss the *activity,* including patient and therapist positioning. Consider what positional changes could enhance the activity (e.g., prepositioning a limb, hand placements to alter the BOS).
2. Discuss the *technique,* including its description, indication(s) for use, therapist hand placements (MCs), and VCs.
3. Demonstrate the activity and application of the technique by the designated therapist and patient. Discussion during the demonstration should be continuous (the demonstration should not be the sole responsibility of the designated therapist and patient). All group members should provide recommendations, suggestions, and supportive feedback throughout the demonstration. During the demonstrations, discuss strategies to make the activity either *more* or *less* challenging.

---

including proximal dynamic stability and controlled mobility necessary for higher-level functional tasks. Applying extremity patterns to assist rolling carries the prerequisite requirement of sufficient ROM to position and move the extremity within the pattern. Proper positioning of the extremities is also crucial for efficient irradiation from the pattern to the trunk (or vice versa).

The supine position provides a large BOS and a low COM. Weightbearing occurs through large body segments with minimal antigravity control requirements. However, the transition from supine to sidelying, or rolling, is resisted by gravity and can be difficult for patients with increased tone or weakness in the core stabilizers. In these situations, rolling activities will begin in the sidelying position with initial focus on controlled movement toward supine or prone before moving against gravity (i.e., rolling from supine or prone into sidelying).

Task Analysis

As noted earlier, rolling is an early functional activity experienced during normal growth and development. It allows positional change and requires a synergistic movement strategy of phasic muscle activity superimposed on tonic stabilizing control (dynamic postural stability with controlled mobility). This strategy lays the foundation for upright and functional activities performed during activities of daily living. Consequently, rolling is addressed both to improve bed mobility skills and for its importance as a component skill for higher-level functional activities.

When analyzing the task of rolling, consider the following:

• Preferred strategy for rolling supine to sidelying
• Use of compensatory strategies
• How the extremities and head and neck are used to assist in rolling
• The chosen pattern for initiation of rolling
• Integration of upper and lower body segments to initiate and accomplish rolling
• Presence of pain, increased tone, or influence of tonic reflexes

See Box 4.5: Student Practice Activity: Rolling Task Analysis.

In observing and assessing the functional task of rolling, it is important to consider what constitutes an *efficient* rolling pattern. Efficient rolling is executed with associated head and neck and extremity movement, translating through pelvic and shoulder girdle control into a mass trunk flexion or elongation pattern. Patients with *less than* efficient rolling strategies utilize a segmental rolling pattern characterized by the UE/shoulder/upper trunk segment leading the activity while the LE/pelvis/lower trunk segment follows, or vice versa. In contrast, an efficient rolling pattern demonstrates integration across all body segments and is executed with the trunk rolling as a whole: both UEs/shoulders/upper trunk and LEs/pelvis/lower trunk work together with dynamic stability, proper timing, and coordination. Efficient head/neck motions are typically combined with the appropriate

Objective: to analyze rolling movements of healthy people

Procedure: Work in groups of two or three. Begin by having each person in the group roll on the mat from supine to prone and prone to supine several times in a row at normal speeds. Then have each person slow the movement down and speed the movement up, rolling in each direction.

Observe and Document: Using the following questions to guide your analysis, observe and record the variations and similarities among the different rolling patterns represented in your group.

▲ How and where is the movement initiated? Terminated?
▲ How is the movement executed?
  • Role of the trunk?
  • Use of extremity movements? Head and neck?
  • Is the pattern changed (or altered) with change of direction?
  • Is the pattern changed (or altered) with change of speed?
▲ How does rolling differ among the group members?
▲ What types of pathology or impairments might affect a patient's ability to roll?
▲ What compensatory strategies were observed?
▲ What environmental factors might constrain or impair rolling movements?

mass trunk patterns. For example, cervical flexion occurs with mass flexion for rolling toward prone, and cervical extension occurs with mass elongation for rolling back to supine. Rolling patterns may vary as a manifestation of mechanical capacity, neuromuscular function, level of motor control, general fitness level, and body weight. Patients with neurological involvement and activity limitations often demonstrate difficulty with initiating the rolling movement and moving smoothly through the full range and may demonstrate a variety of compensatory and/or less-efficient movement strategies.

Interventions

MASS TRUNK PATTERNS

Mass trunk pattern combinations (mass flexion and mass elongation) can be used to activate the tonic stabilizers of the trunk and promote control and timing of the scapula and pelvis for efficient rolling (controlled mobility on dynamic stability). Mass flexion, a combination of scapula anterior depression and pelvis anterior elevation, occurs in combination with slight trunk flexion with a shortening of the trunk (hence, the term *mass flexion*). The reverse direction, mass elongation, a combination of scapula posterior elevation with pelvis posterior depression, should occur with a return of the lumbar spine to neutral and elongation of the trunk (lumbar extension should not occur during mass elongation).

 Clinical Note: Although the mass elongation combination was originally referred to as "mass extension," the term *mass elongation*[1] was introduced to more accurately reflect the correct motion occurring through the lumbar spine.

PROMOTING MASS FLEXION AND MASS ELONGATION

Rhythmic initiation, COI, and dynamic (isotonic) reversals are effective techniques for teaching the end-range position of mass flexion or mass elongation, facilitating proper timing to promote dynamic stability for controlled mobility, improving strength and endurance of the deep tonic trunk stabilizers, and strengthening muscles of the scapula and pelvis.

ROLLING FROM SUPINE TO SIDELYING

In rolling from supine to sidelying, the effect of gravity may lead to abnormal or compensatory strategies that prevent proper timing for controlled mobility on dynamic stability. In these situations, the activity can effectively be initiated in sidelying with a progression into supine.

Clinical Note: Given the nature of opposing diagonals being combined into a mass pattern, the therapist must forego positioning in line with the diagonal and is positioned behind the patient, allowing the forearms to remain in line with each pattern being facilitated.

Combination of isotonics is an ideal technique for promoting rolling from supine to sidelying. The patient is initially positioned in sidelying at the end range of mass flexion with scapula anterior depression and pelvis anterior elevation. An isometric hold at the end range of mass flexion is facilitated with MCs on anterior coracoid for scapula anterior depression and superior/anterior ilium for pelvis anterior elevation. The MCs remain the same as the therapist progresses from an isometric hold to an eccentric contraction with lengthening away from mass flexion followed by a concentric contraction back toward mass flexion. This sequence continues building increasing ROM until the patient is able to control full eccentric lengthening and concentric shortening of mass flexion (Fig. 4.19).

The repetition through increments in ROM focuses on proper timing and coordination. The activity continues until the patient can produce an efficient mass flexion from supine transitioning smoothly into sidelying. The same activity and sequence is repeated for mass elongation moving from sidelying toward prone. As motor control, strength, and endurance improve, combined upper and LE patterns are incorporated, increasing the challenge through a longer lever arm of appropriate resistance (Fig. 4.20).

Dynamic (isotonic) reversals can be used when control in mass flexion and elongation improves. With the patient in the sidelying position (start position for mass elongation), the therapist resists (facilitates) concentric movement into mass elongation from the beginning of the range (Fig. 4.21), followed by a reversal toward concentric mass flexion, progressing toward increments in ROM until full rolling from supine to prone is achieved.

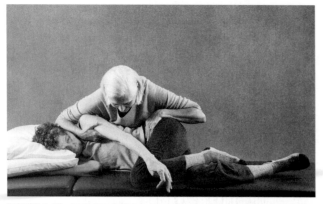

FIGURE 4.19 Applying COI for mass flexion The patient is initially positioned in sidelying position in the end range of mass flexion. The MCs are on anterior coracoid for scapula anterior depression and superior/anterior ilium for pelvis anterior elevation as the patient holds with an isometric contraction at the end range of mass flexion.

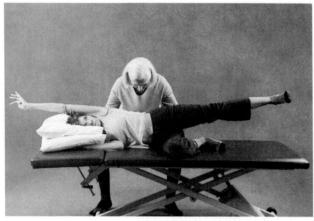

FIGURE 4.20 End range of mass elongation The left UE positioned in flexion/abduction/external rotation (FLEX/ABD/ER) with scapula posterior elevation. The MCs for application of appropriate resistance and traction are on distal/posterior/lateral humerus. The left LE is in extension/abduction/internal rotation (EXT/ABD/IR) with pelvis posterior depression. The MCs for appropriate resistance and traction are on the distal/posterior/lateral femur.

ROLLING SUPINE TO SIDELYING ON ELBOW

From supine, the patient turns and lifts the head and trunk up, moving into the sidelying-on-elbow position. The patient's lowermost UE is prepositioned with the elbow in 90 degrees of flexion in preparation for accepting weight. The therapist can promote elevation and rotation of the upper trunk by instructing the patient to reach across the body with the opposite UE (i.e., the right UE if moving toward left). To facilitate the movement, appropriate resistance can be applied to the uppermost reaching extremity using MCs distally on the UE and proximally on the anterior/superior scapula. If initial assistance is required, the therapist may place both hands on the patient's upper trunk under the axillae. The patient's uppermost UE may be prepositioned with the elbow extended and the hand placed on the therapist's shoulder

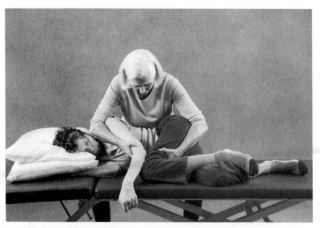

FIGURE 4.21 Mass flexion (start position for active mass elongation from the beginning of the range). Patient is in sidelying with left UE positioned in EXT/ADD/IR with scapula anterior depression and LE flexion/adduction/external rotation (FLEX/ADD/ER) with pelvis anterior elevation. For movement into mass elongation, MCs are on the distal humerus with the therapist's arm against the superior/posterior acromion for resistance to scapula posterior elevation. The opposite hand is on the distal femur with the therapist's cubital fossa cradling the ischial tuberosity to resist pelvis posterior depression. As the patient begins to move, the therapist's MCs are then positioned on the distal/posterior/lateral arm to resist and apply traction to UE FLEX/ABD/ER and on the distal/posterior/lateral thigh to resist and apply traction to LE EXT/ABD/IR. These MCs ensure that the therapist can resist the scapula posterior elevation and pelvis posterior depression through the initial part of the range, following up with appropriate resistance and traction through the extremities for the completion of mass elongation (see Fig. 4.20).

(Fig. 4.22). If needed, a small pillow or wedge may be placed under the trunk once in sidelying to minimize lateral flexion or slump. These strategies help guide movement and further promote efficient weight shift from supine to sidelying.

Rhythmic initiation may be used to promote the transition from supine to sidelying on elbow. If the goal is to instruct the patient in a coordinated and well-timed movement transition, the resisted phase of this technique is not stressed and focus is placed on the passive, active-assisted, and active phases. The MCs are placed proximally at the scapula and upper trunk or distally on the UEs. Once in the position, stabilizing (isometric) reversals can be used to promote stability within the position emphasizing the trunk and the weightbearing segment (Fig. 4.23).

Clinical Note: Patients recovering from stroke may tilt or slump laterally toward the more involved side when sitting in a chair or may demonstrate spasticity in the trunk. Such postures contribute to a loss of trunk flexibility, loss of trunk control, and poor sitting posture. Rolling into the sidelying-on-elbow position is an important activity to promote early weightbearing for dynamic stability on the more involved elbow and shoulder while promoting activation and elongation of the trunk.

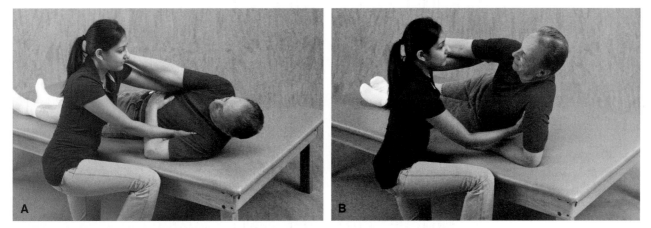

FIGURE 4.22 The therapist manually assists the patient into the sidelying-on-elbow position. (A) The patient turns and begins to lift the head and upper trunk. Note that the left UE (closest to the mat) is prepositioned in approximately 90 degrees of elbow flexion. (B) The patient then brings the elbow under the shoulder into a weightbearing position.

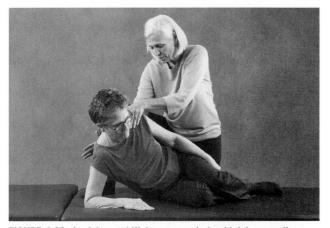

FIGURE 4.23 **Applying stabilizing reversals in sidelying-on-elbow position with MCs on right posterior inferior scapula and left anterior superior scapula** *Not shown:* Manual contacts are then moved to other body segments (pelvis, non-weightbearing UE, head, and neck) with the intention of promoting stability throughout the trunk and weight bearing segments.

From the sidelying-on-elbow position, the patient can be assisted into the prone-on-elbows posture, a very stable posture with a large BOS and low COM (Fig. 4.24). The head and upper trunk are elevated off the supporting surface, weight is distributed to the elbows and forearms, and stabilization demands are placed on the shoulder and scapulothoracic segments. The UEs are in a bilateral symmetrical position with the elbows flexed to 90 degrees and positioned directly under the shoulders; the forearms are pronated. The lower body remains in contact with the supporting surface. If lumbar extension mobility is lacking, a pillow may be placed under the lower trunk. Patients with activity limitations imposed by cardiopulmonary problems or those with high levels of abnormal UE tone may not tolerate the prone-on-elbows position well. However, some benefits of the posture can be achieved using a modification of the position (termed *modified prone on elbows*). The modification is to position the patient in sitting with the elbows bearing weight on a tabletop. An alternative

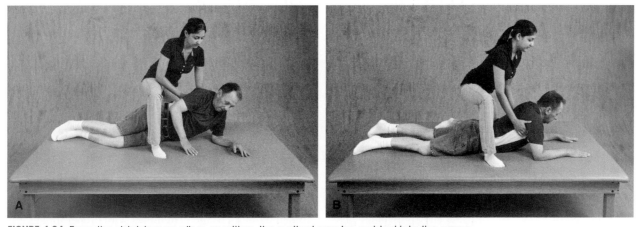

FIGURE 4.24 From the sidelying-on-elbow position, the patient can be assisted into the prone-on-elbows posture. (A) Start position: The therapist is providing support and assistance with upper trunk rotation. (B) End position: The lower trunk rotates toward prone with weight distributed to the elbows and forearms; stabilization demands are placed on the shoulder and scapulothoracic region.

while sitting on a platform mat is to position the flexed elbow on a step stool (covered with a soft towel) or other firm surface placed next to, or on both sides of, the patient for either unilateral or bilateral weightbearing at the elbow. Modified prone on elbows can also be achieved in standing, using the plantigrade position.

ROLLING: UPPER AND LOWER EXTREMITY PATTERNS

As discussed in the previous section, the scapula and pelvis play a crucial role in the ability to roll because they are direct connections between the extremities and the trunk. If dynamic stability is available through the trunk, the extremities can be engaged, creating a longer lever arm for increased ease in rolling. Thus, UE and/or LE motions occur on a dynamically stable core (a dynamic anchor for distal mobility). A variety of extremity patterns and pattern combinations can be used to facilitate rolling:

- Unilateral UE extension/adduction/internal rotation (EXT/ADD/IR) with scapula anterior depression and trunk flexion/rotation.
- Bilateral UE combination of EXT/ADD/IR with scapula anterior depression and extension/abduction/internal rotation (EXT/ABD/IR) with scapula posterior depression and trunk flexion/rotation. When a stronger (more functional) UE is used to assist the other more affected UE into the EXT/ABD/IR pattern, this combination is referred to as a *chop*.
- Unilateral LE flexion/adduction/external rotation (FLEX/ADD/ER) with pelvis anterior elevation and trunk flexion/rotation
- Bilateral LE combination of FLEX/ADD/ER with pelvis anterior elevation and flexion/abduction/internal rotation (FLEX/ABD/IR) with pelvis posterior elevation and trunk flexion/rotation
- Combination of UE EXT/ADD/IR with scapula anterior depression and ipsilateral LE FLEX/ADD/ER with pelvis anterior elevation and trunk flexion/rotation

The PNF patterns are described fully in Chapter 3: Proprioceptive Neuromuscular Facilitation.

To apply COI using an LE pattern, the patient begins in sidelying in the lengthened range of LE EXT/ABD/IR. The therapist is positioned in line with the diagonal pattern to be facilitated. The patient then moves concentrically into FLEX/ADD/ER, where an isometric hold is applied (Fig. 4.25). The patient then returns eccentrically to the starting position of EXT/ABD/IR. The ROM into LE extension and rolling back toward supine is increased slowly (increments in range) as the patient develops control. A progression is made to beginning in supine and rolling toward sidelying by moving the LE into FLEX/ADD/ER. Note that the patient's UEs may be resting in front or flexed bilaterally at the shoulder and positioned overhead. Alternatively, the upper limbs may be placed asymmetrically, with the lowermost flexed overhead and the uppermost at the side of the trunk, with the hand resting at the patient's side.

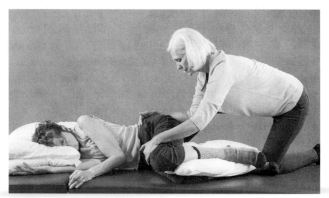

FIGURE 4.25 Applying COI to promote rolling The patient has moved concentrically into end range of LE FLEX/ADD/ER, where an isometric hold is applied. *Not shown:* Patient then eccentrically returns to start position of LE EXT/ABD/IR. The MCs are on the pelvis and distal femur.

Therapist positioning for the above activities requires that the therapist be positioned in line with the extremity diagonal being facilitated. One exception occurs when facilitating rolling through UE EXT/ADD/IR and LE FLEX/ADD/ER (mass flexion, as described in rolling supine to sidelying above). This combination of opposite diagonals does not allow the therapist to be in line with both diagonals simultaneously, so the therapist is positioned behind the patient. The therapist may also be positioned in line with one diagonal to be facilitated or resisted while the patient actively moves through the other diagonal. Given the large arcs of motion involved and the required weight shifts, these activities are best accomplished on a wide treatment table or on a floor mat.

Rhythmic initiation can be used to instruct the patient in the desired movement, to facilitate the initiation of movement, and to improve strength and coordination of the trunk and extremities.

To apply rhythmic initiation to rolling from sidelying using a single extremity pattern (either upper or LE), the therapist can use a distal (upper or LE) and a proximal (scapula or pelvis) MC for application of appropriate resistance. If using a combination of both UE and LE patterns, the MC can also be proximal or distal on each extremity.

A combination of proximal and distal MCs may also be used to facilitate missing components within a pattern. The MCs will change with application of appropriate resistance and movement through the ROM. The patient may begin in supine position moving toward sidelying and prone (higher challenge) or in sidelying moving toward prone and then progress toward starting from supine. Movement of the extremities to promote rolling is initiated passively and progressed to active assistive, then appropriately resisted. The goal is dynamic stability of the trunk followed by controlled mobility of the extremities with proper timing. This sequence is repeated with gradual increments in ROM. If necessary, a quick stretch can be used to facilitate initiation of movement in the desired direction.

Comments

- Slow sidelying passive rolling or rocking (rhythmic rotation) movements provide slow vestibular input that promotes relaxation, which is beneficial for patients with spasticity or rigidity. Rhythmic rotation is particularly effective when used with trunk counter-rotation.

- Movements begin with small-range control (e.g., one-quarter turn forward to one-quarter turn backward) and progress through increasing ROM (increments of ROM) to full-range control (from full supine to full prone position and back).

- Initially, movements are slow and controlled with emphasis on careful grading of appropriate resistance; progression is to increase speed of movement while maintaining control.

- An isometric hold may be added in the shortened range or at any point of weakness within the range to promote increased motor unit output. The hold is a momentary pause for one count when the patient is instructed to *"Hold."*

- The patient is instructed to turn the head and follow the hand with the eyes. Having the patient watch the movement promotes the use of visual sensory cues to improve movement control and promotes involvement of the head and neck, further engaging the trunk in the overall movement of rolling.

- Rhythmic initiation is ideal for initial motor learning on the use of PNF extremity patterns for rolling. As the patient achieves some control, a progression is made from active-assistive to active to resisted movement, with the end result being independent movement.

- Rhythmic initiation is also a valuable technique for the patient with stroke who is unable to initiate rolling (apraxia) and for the patient who demonstrates impaired cognition and motor learning (e.g., traumatic brain injury). The initial passive and active-assisted movements help teach the patient the desired movement. The VCs should be soothing, slow, rhythmic, and well timed with movements.

- Movement may be facilitated with *timing for emphasis* by using stronger components of a pattern to facilitate weaker ones through irradiation.

- Using PNF upper and LE patterns together with COI is effective to promote increased strength and control of the movements required for transitioning from sidelying to supine position.

Clinical Note: Neck flexion and extension patterns with rotation can also be used to promote rolling. From a sidelying (or supine) position, neck flexion and rotation is used to facilitate rolling toward prone. From a sidelying (or prone) position, neck extension and rotation is used to roll toward supine. These patterns are also described in Chapter 3: Proprioceptive Neuromuscular Facilitation.

Outcomes

Motor control goal: mobility progressing to controlled mobility

Functional skill achieved: able to roll independently from supine to prone and back

Indications: Rolling is of functional significance for improved bed mobility, preparation for independent positional changes in bed (e.g., pressure relief), and as a lead-up (component skill) for LE dressing and independent transfers from supine to sitting positions. In addition, rolling promotes trunk control and the development of functional movement patterns (e.g., coordination of extremity and trunk movement) and is a frequent starting point for mat activities for patients with significant neurological (e.g., the patient with stroke or high-level spinal cord lesion) or musculoskeletal (e.g., motor vehicle accident or trauma) involvement. Although activities are typically initiated on a platform mat, rolling must also be mastered on the surface of a bed similar to the one the patient will use at home. See Box 4.6: Student Practice Activity: Rolling.

Compensatory Movements and Strategies

The strategies outlined in the following paragraphs are used to achieve functional bed mobility when a patient does not have active movement. These are strategies often utilized by patients with complete SCIs or true weakness where a compensatory strategy is required for independent function. The therapeutic goal is function, recognizing that proper dynamic stability with controlled mobility is not available to these patients. In these situations, rolling can be assisted by prepositioning the limbs (e.g., crossing one ankle over the other) and using compensatory movements and strategies that use momentum (created by extremity movements) to facilitate movement and help propel the body through the roll. Compensatory interventions to promote rolling may begin in supine or sidelying positions and progress from small ranges to larger ranges (increments in ROM), and finally to full ROM: for example, from a sidelying position (pillows may be required initially for support), rolling first one-quarter turn forward, then backward, to one-half turns, to a full turn moving from sidelying to supine, or to prone.

- Momentum can be generated by using head and neck motions, by lifting the contralateral UE or LE (or both) up and across the body in the direction of the roll movement (e.g., for rolling to the right, the left UE and/or left LE is lifted up and across the midline of body to the right).

- Prepositioning the limbs (before movement begins) can also be used to promote rolling.
  - Upper extremities
    - From sidelying or supine, the lowermost UE (the one closest to the direction of the roll) can be flexed overhead to avoid getting it trapped under the body

BOX 4.6 STUDENT PRACTICE ACTIVITY: ROLLING

Section Outline: Rolling

Activities and Techniques

▲ Mass flexion and mass elongation patterns in sidelying position, including scapula posterior depression/anterior elevation diagonal in combination with the pelvis anterior elevation/posterior depression diagonal
- Mass flexion and mass elongation in sidelying, using rhythmic initiation
- Mass flexion and mass elongation in sidelying, using COI
- Mass flexion and mass elongation in sidelying, using dynamic (isotonic) reversals

▲ Rolling from supine to sidelying, using COI

Objective: sharing skills in application and knowledge of strategies to promote improved rolling

Equipment Needed: platform mat

Directions: Working in groups of four to six students, consider each entry in the section outline. Members of the group will assume different roles (described below) and will rotate roles each time the group progresses to a new item on the outline.

▲ One person assumes the role of therapist (for demonstrations) and participates in discussion.

▲ One person serves as the patient (for demonstrations) and participates in discussion.

▲ The remaining members participate in discussion and provide supportive feedback during demonstrations. One member of this group should be designated as a "fact checker" to return to the text content to confirm

elements of the discussion (if needed) or if agreement cannot be reached.

Thinking aloud, brainstorming, and sharing thoughts should be continuous throughout this activity! Carry out the following activities for each item in the section outline.

1. Discuss the *activity,* including patient and therapist positioning. Consider what positional changes could enhance the activity.
2. Discuss the *technique,* including its description, indication(s) for use, therapist hand placements (MCs), and VCs.
3. Demonstrate the activity and application of the technique by the designated therapist and patient. Discussion during the demonstration should be continuous (the demonstration should not be the sole responsibility of the designated therapist and patient). All group members should provide recommendations, suggestions, and supportive feedback throughout the demonstration. During the demonstrations, discuss strategies to make the activity either *more* or *less* challenging.

If any member of the group feels he or she requires practice with the activity and technique, the group should allocate time to accommodate the request. All group members providing input (recommendations, suggestions, and supportive feedback) should also accompany this practice.

- If shoulder ROM is limited, the shoulder may be adducted and the hand tucked under the hips close to the body.
- Lower extremities
  - Prepositioning the LEs with the feet/ankles crossed (described below) or positioning the hips on a pillow creating a one-quarter turn is a useful initial strategy. As the patient progresses, the pillow can be removed and the LEs uncrossed.
  - From a supine position, the LEs can be extended with the feet crossed (e.g., the patient with tetraplegia). When one foot is crossed over the other, the uppermost foot is placed in the direction of the roll. For example, in rolling toward the right, the left foot is crossed over the right (Fig. 4.26).
  - From supine position, the LE opposite the direction of the roll (e.g., the right LE if rolling toward the left) can be positioned in approximately 60 degrees of hip and knee flexion with the foot flat on supporting surface to propel the roll, pushing the body into sidelying and then further into prone (e.g., the patient with stroke). This is referred to as a *modified* hooklying position because only one LE is flexed. This LE positioning can also be used for rolling from a sidelying position (Fig. 4.27).

- From prone to supine, shoulder abduction and elbow flexion with a fisted or open hand placed on the mat can be used to help push the body into sidelying.
- The therapist's position and movements should not restrict or limit the patient's ease of movement. The therapist is positioned behind or in front of the patient to assist

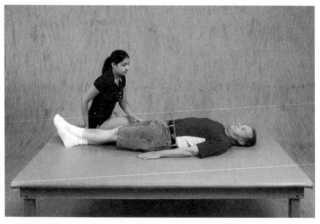

FIGURE 4.26 Patient is positioned in supine with the knees extended and the left foot crossed over the right in preparation for rolling toward the right.

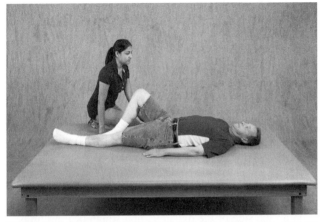

FIGURE 4.27 Patient positioned in modified hooklying The right LE is in approximately 60 degrees of hip and knee flexion in preparation for rolling to the left.

movements as needed. Patients with communication deficits (e.g., aphasia) or those who depend heavily on visual or verbal cueing benefit from being able to see the therapist positioned in front.

- Optimal use of momentum will improve function and decrease the effort required to accomplish the roll.
- The therapist should provide instructions and VCs to focus the patient's attention on key task elements and improve overall awareness of task demands.

Clinical Notes:

- In the absence of trunk or extremity strength, it is important for patients to develop compensatory strategies to achieve the functional task of rolling. However, from a therapeutic perspective it is crucial that the physical therapist focus on teaching and facilitating dynamic proximal stability for efficient distal mobility during rolling whenever possible. For example, although rolling from a position of modified hooklying (compensatory strategy) will allow the patient to complete the task, it does not promote active engagement of a stable trunk for the extremities to work from. Teaching the patient to engage the trunk as much as neurophysiologically possible by lifting the head, or bringing a UE into extension/adduction, or bringing a LE into flexion/adduction as a way to initiate the roll will promote integration of any available dynamic proximal stability with distal mobility, which is crucial for many functional activities.
- Normal postural reactions contribute to rolling. Patients who have excessive (hyperactive) symmetrical or asymmetrical tonic reflex activity (see Box 4.1) coupled

with excess tone may have difficulty rolling. Normal postural reactions that contribute to rolling in young children include body-on-body righting reactions and neck-righting reactions; these are normally integrated in the postural responses of healthy adults. In addition, supine or prone positions may be difficult or contraindicated for patients who have cardiopulmonary involvement such as chronic obstructive pulmonary disease or congestive heart failure or who have undergone recent surgical procedures involving the trunk.

- Patients recovering from stroke will require practice in rolling to both sides: over onto the *more affected side* and over onto the *less affected side* (the more difficult activity). The more involved UE can be effectively supported to keep the shoulder forward by having the patient clasp the hands together with fingers intertwined, both elbows extended, and shoulders flexed (hands-clasped position). The patient can also be taught to support the more involved shoulder in a slightly protracted position by bringing the involved hand to the opposite shoulder and placing the uninvolved hand around the posterior aspect of the involved humeral head to support the affected shoulder while rolling. This positioning allows the patient to use the uninvolved UE to initiate rolling, finishing either in sidelying or prone position with the affected shoulder in a safe and neutral position.

SUMMARY

This chapter explored interventions to improve bed mobility and early trunk control. Within the context of motor task requirements (mobility, stability, and controlled mobility), activities and techniques were presented to improve control in hooklying, bridging, sidelying, and rolling. Each of these postures or activities represents critical lead-up skills to independent bed mobility function, including positional changes, scooting, dressing, personal hygiene, and transitions from supine to sitting. The interventions presented were designed to address the overriding goal of providing patients with the most efficient, functional, and pain-free bed mobility movement strategies.

REFERENCES

1. Saliba Johnson, VL, Johnson, GS, and Wardlaw, C. Proprioceptive neuromuscular facilitation. In Basmajian, JV, and Nyberg, R (eds): Rational Manual Therapies. Baltimore, Williams & Wilkins, 1993, 243.
2. Johnson, G, and Saliba Johnson, V. PNF 1: The Functional Application of Proprioceptive Neuromuscular Facilitation, Course Syllabus, Version 7.9. Steamboat, CO, Institute of Physical Art, 2014.
3. American Physical Therapy Association. Guide to Physical Therapist Practice, Version 3.0. Alexandria, VA, American Physical Therapy Association, 2014. Retrieved March 4, 2015, from http://guidetoptpractice.apta.org.

Advanced Bridging Activities

Appendix 4A presents advanced bridging activities used to further promote dynamic postural stability required for upright antigravity activities such as standing, gait, and stair climbing.

Bridging, Single-Leg Lifts

Static-dynamic activities involve unilateral LE weightbearing in bridging. The patient raises one LE (dynamic limb) from the mat while maintaining the bridge position using the opposite LE (static limb) for support. The dynamic limb may be held steady with the hip partially flexed and the knee extended (Fig. 4A.1), or further challenges may be imposed by adding movement (e.g., alternating between partial hip flexion with knee extension to close to full hip and knee flexion). Further challenges may be imposed by removing UE support from the mat and moving the shoulders into flexion, with elbows extended and the hands clasped together.

Bridging, Alternating Leg Lifts, Marching in Place

This activity alternates static and dynamic elements between the two lower limbs. From a bridge position, marching in place (hip and knee flexion) requires lifting one LE (dynamic) off the mat using hip and knee flexion, returning it to the start position (static), and then immediately lifting the opposite LE (dynamic) in the same pattern with return to the start position (static). Patients who are unstable will demonstrate a pelvic drop on the side of the dynamic, non-weightbearing limb. A wand or yardstick can be placed across the pelvis to provide visual feedback to assist keeping the pelvis level.

Static-dynamic movements in bridging can be facilitated with tactile (e.g., tapping) or verbal cueing. Initially, increased stability of the posture may be required to free one lower limb. This may be accomplished by increasing the BOS through positioning of the UEs. As control progresses, difficulty can be increased by reducing the UE support. The speed and range of movements may be varied to increase the difficulty of the activities. Patients can work up to marching and then "running" in place or "running" from side to side. The latter activities impose considerable challenge to the bridging position and should be performed only by patients who demonstrate efficient motor control strategies with sufficient dynamic stability and controlled mobility.

Bridging, Mobile BOS Using a Ball, Knees Extended

With the patient in a hooklying position, a medium-sized ball is placed under the patient's legs. Maintaining leg position on the ball, the patient then elevates the pelvis, extending the hips and knees (Fig. 4A.2). This activity significantly increases the postural challenge of pelvic elevation because the BOS is not fixed. The patient must stabilize the legs on the ball and maintain the ball position in addition to elevating the pelvis.

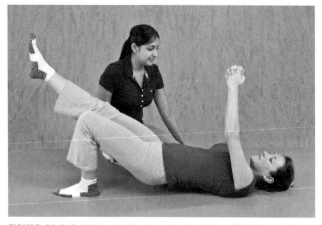

FIGURE 4A.1 Bridging, static-dynamic single-leg lifts The challenge may be increased by flexing the shoulders and extending the elbows with the hands clasped together.

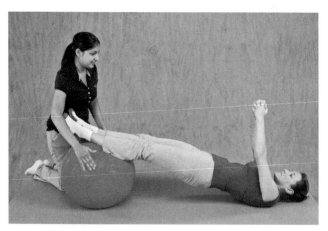

FIGURE 4A.2 Bridging using a mobile BOS to support the legs with the knees extended.

The more distally the ball is placed under the legs (toward the feet), the more difficult the activity. The hamstrings participate more fully in stabilization with the knees extended. The patient should be encouraged to use the UEs on the mat to increase the stability of the posture initially, and then reduce UE time on the mat as control increases. A progression from this activity is bridging with a mobile BOS using a small ball to support the feet with the knees flexed (Fig. 4A.3).

Sit to Modified Bridge Position, Movement Transitions Using a Ball

This advanced stabilization activity presents considerable challenge to postural control. It involves movement transition from sitting on a ball to a modified bridge position (upper trunk supported by ball). The patient begins by sitting on an appropriately sized ball. The hips and knees should be flexed to 90 degrees. The patient "walks" both feet away from the ball maintaining knee flexion while the hips move toward extension. The ball will roll upward along the center of the trunk until the head and shoulders are resting on the ball (Fig. 4A.4). The patient maintains the hips in the extended position with the pelvis level. Initially, fingertip or hand touch-down support may be necessary; as control develops, hand contact is removed. Alternatively, additional stability can be accomplished by "locking" the elbows against the ball (with elbows flexed and shoulders extended and adducted against the ball). The progression would be to the UEs folded across the chest to the more difficult position of shoulder flexion to approximately 90 degrees and elbows extended with hands clasped together.

Modified Bridge Position, Static-Dynamic Activities Using a Ball

Static-dynamic activities in a modified bridge position provide high-level challenges to postural control and should be reserved for late-stage rehabilitation (Fig. 4A.5). These challenges can include lifting one LE (the dynamic limb can move in hip flexion or knee extension) while the static limb stabilizes the body and maintains the bridge position. Alternating

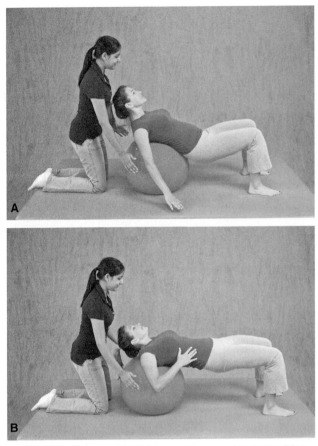

FIGURE 4A.4 Sit to modified bridge position, movement transitions using ball From a sitting position on a ball (not shown), the patient "walks" both feet away from the ball until the head and shoulders are resting on the ball. UE support may be required during early movement transitions. This may be accomplished by (A) positioning the patient's hands and fingertips for touch-down support, if needed, and (B) "locking" the elbows against the ball to increase stability.

LE lifts (marching in place) can then be performed. An additional activity while maintaining a single-limb bridge position on the ball is writing alphabet letters with the foot (or great toe) of the dynamic limb.

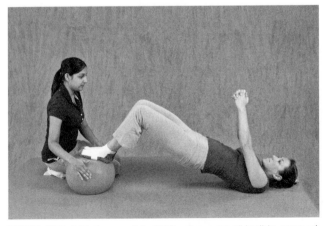

FIGURE 4A.3 Bridging, mobile BOS using a small ball to support the feet with the knees flexed.

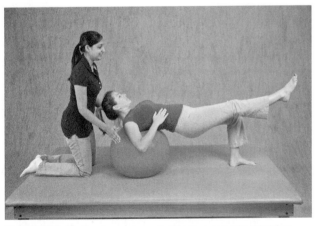

FIGURE 4A.5 Static-dynamic activities in a modified bridge position.

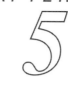

CHAPTER

5

Interventions to Improve Sitting and Sitting Balance Skills

SUSAN B. O'SULLIVAN, PT, EdD, AND
EDWARD W. BEZKOR, PT, DPT, OCS, MTC

This chapter focuses on sitting control and interventions that can be used to improve sitting and sitting balance skills. Careful examination of the patient's overall status in terms of impairments and activity limitations that limit sitting control is necessary. This includes examination of musculoskeletal alignment, range of motion (ROM), and muscle performance (strength, power, and endurance). Examination of motor function (motor control and motor learning) focuses on determining weightbearing status, postural control, and neuromuscular synergies required for static and dynamic control. It also examines use of sensory (somatosensory, visual, and vestibular) cues for sitting balance control and central nervous system (CNS) sensory integration mechanisms. Finally, the patient must be able to safely perform functional movements (activities of daily living [ADL]) in sitting and in varying environments (clinic, home, work [job/school/play], and community).

Biomechanics of Sitting

It is important to understand the foundational requirements of sitting. Sitting is a relatively stable posture with a moderately high center of mass (COM) and a moderate base of support (BOS) that includes contact of the buttocks, thighs, and feet with the support surface. The pelvis is the foundation for sitting and strongly influences postural alignment of the entire axial skeleton. A *neutral pelvic position* is optimal for sitting. This is characterized by (1) an anterior superior iliac spine (ASIS) that is level or slightly lower than the posterior superior iliac spine (PSIS) (sagittal plane) and (2) a level position of both ASISs (frontal plane). Both ischial tuberosities should be equally weightbearing. The lumbar spine has a natural lumbar lordosis accompanied by extension throughout other areas of spine. The head and trunk are vertical, maintained in midline orientation over the pelvis with a "chin-in" position of the head. During active erect sitting, the line of gravity (LoG) passes close to the axes of rotation of the head and spine. During relaxed erect sitting, the LoG is slightly anterior to these axes of rotation, whereas during slumped or slouched sitting, the LoG is well forward of these axes (Fig. 5.1).[1]

The trunk muscles actively maintain upright postural control and core stability, including co-contractions of the trunk extensors (erector spinae muscles) and flexors (abdominals). Activity of the erector spinae muscles is greatest

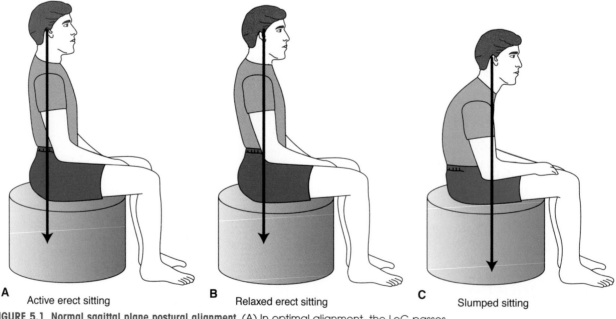

A Active erect sitting **B** Relaxed erect sitting **C** Slumped sitting

FIGURE 5.1 Normal sagittal plane postural alignment (A) In optimal alignment, the LoG passes close to the axes of rotation of the head, neck, and trunk. (B) During relaxed sitting, the LoG changes very little, remaining close to those axes. (C) During slumped sitting, the LoG is well forward of the spine and hips.

during active erect sitting as opposed to relaxed or slumped sitting.[1,2] Lower extremity (LE) muscles are important stabilizers of the trunk and pelvis. Ankle dorsiflexors (anterior tibialis) and hip flexors (iliopsoas) are activated during backward displacements of the trunk, whereas calf muscles (soleus), knee muscles (vastus lateralis, biceps femoris), and hip extensor muscles (gluteus maximus) brake forward movement of the trunk. When the feet are hanging free on a raised seat, control shifts solely to trunk and hip muscles with *limit of stability (LOS)* reached much sooner than when feet are in contact with the floor.

Common Impairments in Sitting

Although not all-inclusive, deficits in sitting can be broadly grouped into those involving pelvis and spine alignment, weightbearing, and extensor muscle weakness. Changes in normal alignment result in subsequent changes in other body segments. In a posterior pelvic tilt position, the ASIS is higher than the PSIS with flattening of the lumbar spine. If severe enough, the patient sits back, bearing weight on the sacrum (sacral sitting). This posture is associated with increased flexion of the thoracic spine (dorsal kyphosis) with a protracted (forward) head posture (Fig. 5.2). To maintain a horizontal gaze, the upper craniocervical region compensates by extending slightly. Over time, this posture results in adaptive shortening of muscles and ligaments and increased passive tension on ligaments and joints. A habitually posterior tilt posture creates a flexion torque that results in increased compression on the anterior margin of lumbar discs with overstretching of the posterior annular fibrosis and increased risk of a protruding nucleus pulposus. It also increases stress on extensor muscles in the thoracic and cervical spine, resulting in neck and back pain.[2] Posterior pelvic tilt is commonly seen in patients with weak core (trunk) muscles, limited pelvic and hip joint mobility, and limitations in ROM or hamstring muscle spasticity.

Anterior tilt of the pelvis occurs when the ASIS is lower than the PSIS, producing a pronounced lordosis in the lumbar spine. This is typically seen in patients with overall muscle weakness, especially in abdominal muscles. Anterior pelvic rotation occurs when one ASIS is farther forward than the other, causing the spine to rotate, perhaps resulting in a scoliosis curvature. Weightbearing on the ischial tuberosities is typically unequal. This posture can result from asymmetrical muscle strength and muscle tone or changes in hip joint mobility.

Lateral tilting of the pelvis occurs when one ASIS is higher on one side than the other ASIS (pelvic obliquity). This positioning creates unequal weightbearing on the ischial tuberosities and can result in a compensatory C-curve or S-curve of the spine. This curvature is seen in patients with asymmetrical muscle strength or asymmetrical muscle tone (e.g., the patient with stroke) or the patient with limited hip joint mobility. Box 5.1 summarizes common impairments in sitting.

Treatment Strategies for Improving Postural Control in Sitting

The patient begins by sitting on a firm surface with 90-degree angles at the hips and knees and LEs at normal hip-width

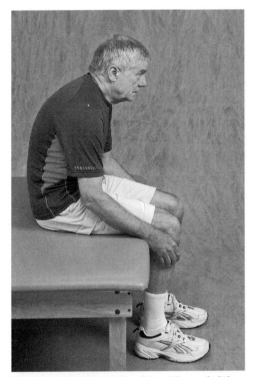

FIGURE 5.2 Abnormal alignment in sitting (slumped sitting posture) The patient exhibits a forward head position, dorsal kyphosis, flattening of the lumbar spine, and a posterior pelvic tilt.

BOX 5.1 Common Impairments in Sitting

Deficits in Pelvic Position
- *Excessive posterior tilt of the pelvis* results in flattening or reversal of the lumbar curve (slumped or *sacral sitting*) with increased flexion of the thoracic spine (dorsal kyphosis) and a protracted head position (forward head).
- *Excessive anterior tilt of the pelvis* results in increased lordosis and increased lateral rotation and abduction of the hips.

Deficits in Head/Upper Trunk Alignment
- Patients with extensor weakness typically demonstrate a *forward head position,* rounded thoracic spine *(kyphosis),* with a flattened lumbar curve.

Deficits in Seated Weightbearing
- Patients may demonstrate asymmetrical alignment with increased weightbearing on one side (e.g., the patient with stroke).

apart. Activities are selected that the patient can almost master. Progression is obtained by varying the level of difficulty. Greater challenges can be incorporated into sitting activities by:

• Modifying the BOS
• Modifying the support surface
• Varying sensory inputs
• Incorporating upper extremity (UE) or LE movements
• Challenging anticipatory and reactive balance control

See Box 5.2 for strategies to vary postural stabilization requirements and level of difficulty.

Clinical Note: A wide-based sitting posture (LEs abducted and externally rotated, UEs used for support) is a common compensatory change in patients with decreased sitting control.

Motor Learning Strategies

The therapist should instruct the patient in the correct sitting posture and demonstrate the ideal position to provide an accurate *reference of correctness.* It is important to focus the patient's attention on key task elements (e.g., neutral pelvic position, trunk extension) to improve overall sensory awareness of the correct sitting posture and position in space. Initial practice requires the patient to focus full attention on the task and its key elements. *Augmented feedback* (e.g., tapping, light resistance, and verbal cueing) can be used to focus attention on *key errors,* which are those errors that, when corrected, result in considerable improvement of performance, with other elements of the task falling into place. Tactile cues can be used to call attention to missing elements. For example, tapping on the posterior neck and/or trunk can facilitate and engage the extensor muscles. Visual cues can be utilized by having the patient sit directly in front of a mirror. A vertical line of tape applied to a plain shirt worn by the patient can help the patient recognize vertical position. Augmented feedback should also emphasize positive aspects of performance, providing reinforcement and enhancing motivation. As soon as appropriate, augmented feedback should be reduced or withdrawn.[3,4]

Attentional focus and motor learning can be improved by using appropriate verbal cues. Internal cues focus on specific body movements, such as *"Bring your head over your hips."* Research has demonstrated greater movement efficiency, automaticity, and retention when external cues are used. External cues focus on the overall goal of the movement, the outcomes. For example, *"Keep your head directly over your hips with your trunk straight and pelvis neutral."*[5,6] Suggested verbal instructions and cueing are presented in Box 5.3.

With repeated practice, the level of cognitive monitoring decreases as motor learning progresses. With an autonomous level of learning, postural responses are largely automatic, with little conscious thought for routine postural

BOX 5.2 Varying Postural Stabilization Requirements and Level of Difficulty

Base of Support
Postural control can be challenged by altering the base of support (BOS). Progression is from:

• Long-sitting to short-sitting
• Bilateral UE support to unilateral UE support to no UE support
• Hands positioned on the thighs to arms folded across the chest
• Both feet flat on the floor to no foot contact with the floor (e.g., sitting on a high seat)

Support Surface
Postural control can be challenged by altering the support surface. Progression is from:

• A firm surface (e.g., a platform mat) to a soft, compliant surface (e.g., foam or disc) or a low cushioned seat (e.g., upholstered chair).
• Sitting on a stationary, fixed support surface to sitting on a mobile surface (e.g., an inflated disc, rocker board, or therapy ball)
• Sitting with feet flat on a stationary surface to feet on a mobile surface (e.g., a small ball or roller)

Sensory Inputs
Postural control can be challenged by altering the sensory inputs. Progression is from:

• Eyes open to eyes closed
• Eyes fixed on a stationary target directly in front of the patient to head turns (e.g., up and down, side to side)
• Visual support can be increased by using a mirror to assist the patient in perceptual awareness of vertical and postural symmetry. Vertical lines improve awareness (e.g., the patient wears a vertical line drawn or taped on the front of a shirt and matches it to a vertical line taped on a mirror).
• Sitting in a chair with a back support or sitting with the back against a wall maximizes somatosensory cues and support to the trunk, while sitting on a mat or ball with no back support is more difficult.
• Sitting sideward against a wall can provide feedback about lateral alignment (e.g., the patient with stroke and pusher syndrome sits with the shoulder on the sound side against a wall). Progression is to no wall contact.
• Somatosensory inputs from the feet can be maximized by having the patient barefoot or wearing flexible-soled shoes; foot contact is maintained on the support surface; progression is to one foot contact (legs crossed) to no foot contact.

control. This level of control can be tested by using *dual-tasking,* the ability to perform a secondary task (motor or cognitive) while maintaining sitting control.[7] The patient is asked to perform a secondary motor task (e.g., pouring water from a pitcher into a glass) or a secondary cognitive task (e.g., counting backward from 100 by 7s) during sitting. Any decrement in postural control is noted.

BOX 5.3 Suggested Verbal Instructions and Cueing

Cues With an Internal Focus
- *"Sit tall. Hold your head up, chin tucked, and shoulders over your hips."*
- *"Tighten your stomach and back muscles, lift your head up, straighten your back."*
- *"Shift your weight over to your left* [or right] *hip."*

Cues With an External Focus
- *"Keep the rocker board you are sitting on steady, with your weight balanced."*
- *"Sit tall. Focus on the clock* [or other object] *directly in front of you."*
- *"Keep the inflated disk* [or ball] *you are sitting on as steady as possible."*
- *"Hold the ball straight in front of you as steady as you can."*
- *"Imagine you are a puppet with a string from the top of your head pulling you straight up."*

Red Flag: The use of mirrors to improve postural alignment is contraindicated for patients with visual-perceptual spatial deficits (e.g., vertical disorientation or position-in-space deficits seen in some patients with stroke or traumatic brain injury [TBI]).

Clinical Note: Patients who are unstable in sitting are likely to demonstrate increased anxiety and fear of falling when first positioned in sitting. It is important for the therapist to demonstrate the ability to control for instability and falls to instill patient confidence. Two therapists may be needed to assist severely involved patients (e.g., early sitting of the patient with TBI). In this situation, one therapist sits directly in front of the patient who is positioned in short-sitting on a platform mat, and one is behind the patient. A therapist positioned in front of the patient can lock his or her knees around the outside of the patient's knees and firmly stabilize them (Fig. 5.3). This action assists the patient by extending the BOS. If positioned behind the patient, the therapist can sit on a therapy ball. The ball is used to support the lumbar spine and maintain the upright posture. The patient's arms can rest on the therapist's knees for support (Fig. 5.4).

Interventions to Improve Static Control in Sitting

Static postural control (stability) is necessary to maintain upright sitting. Important factors when examining stability control include the ability to maintain correct sitting alignment and the ability to maintain the posture for prolonged times. For example, the patient who can sit for only 30 seconds

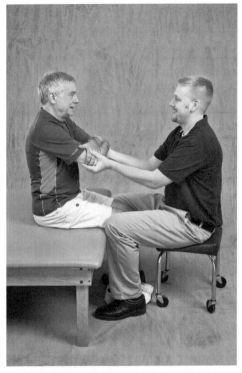

FIGURE 5.3 Early stabilization in sitting from in front The therapist stabilizes the patient from the front by locking both knees around the patient's knees. The patient's arms are cradled and held by the therapist. Note the improvement in erect posture compared with Figure 5.2.

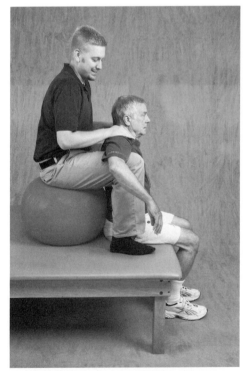

FIGURE 5.4 Early stabilization in sitting from behind The therapist stabilizes the patient from behind, sitting on a therapy ball. The ball is used to provide support to the lumbar spine. The patient's UEs are resting on the therapist's knees or can be held straight in front with hands clasped.

before losing control and falling to one side demonstrates poor sitting stability, whereas the patient who can sit for 5 minutes or longer while holding the trunk steady demonstrates good sitting stability. Other control factors frequently examined in stability control include the amount of postural sway (which should be minimal), the ability to maintain center of alignment, the ability to sit without UE support, and the ability to sit without grasping the edge of the mat or hooking the feet onto the edge of the mat by forcefully flexing the knees.

The patient is instructed to sit with the head and trunk vertical, pelvis neutral, both hips and knees flexed to 90 degrees, and feet flat on the floor. Posture is symmetrical with equal weightbearing over both buttocks and feet. Initially, one or both of the patient's UEs can be used for support as needed. The shoulder is abducted and extended, and the elbow and wrist are extended with the hand open and positioned at the side (Fig. 5.5A).

Clinical Note: The UE weightbearing position is a useful position to counteract UE flexor-adductor spasticity common in the patient recovering from stroke or TBI. Initially, the technique of slow passive movement with gentle rotations (i.e., *rhythmic rotation*) can be used to move the spastic UE into position. Additional stimulation (tapping or stroking) over the triceps can assist the patient in maintaining elbow extension. The fingers are extended with the thumb abducted (Fig. 5.5B). The dorsum of the hand can also be stroked to help keep the hand open.

Clinical Note: The patient with shoulder instability (e.g., the patient recovering from stroke who has a flaccid, subluxed shoulder) also benefits from weightbearing and compression through an extended UE. The proprioceptive loading that occurs increases the action of stabilizing muscles around the shoulder. The therapist can add additional stimulation by lightly compressing (approximating) the top of the shoulder downward while stabilizing the elbow as needed.

Clinical Note: The patient with elbow instability due to UE paralysis (e.g., the patient with a spinal cord injury (SCI) and a complete C6 tetraplegia who has no triceps function) can be assisted to maintain an extended UE position using shoulder girdle musculature. The patient first throws back the shoulder into full shoulder extension while externally rotating the shoulder and supinating the forearm. When the UE is weightbearing in this position, the patient contracts the anterior deltoids to flex the shoulder (closed chain action), which will extend the elbow. This is followed by rapid shoulder depression to maintain elbow extension. This technique will stabilize the UE in extension and external rotation. The therapist must keep in mind that this patient's fingers must remain flexed (interphalangeal flexion) during weightbearing to protect the tenodesis grasp.

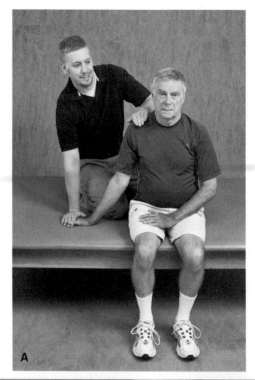

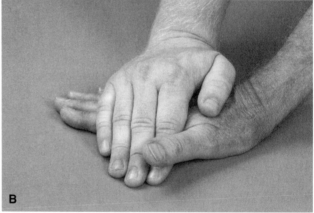

FIGURE 5.5 The patient sits with unilateral UE support (A) The patient's right shoulder is abducted and externally rotated, the elbow is extended, and the wrist and fingers are extended. The therapist assists in shoulder and hand position. This is a useful position for the patient who exhibits UE flexor-adductor spasticity. (B) Close-up of the hand position. The fingers are extended with the thumb abducted.

Varying UE and LE Support

Modifying the BOS and varying the amount of support from the UEs or LEs can be used to challenge stability control. The patient can be progressed from sitting with bilateral UE support (hand flat or fisted), to unilateral UE support, to finally no UE support. Initially both feet and thighs can be in contact with the support surface, progressing to one LE crossed over the other (only one foot in contact with the support surface) to sitting on a high table (elevated seat) with both feet off the floor and only the thighs and buttocks in contact with the support surface.

Varying the BOS: Long-sitting, Short-sitting, Side-sitting

Long-sitting is an important posture for developing initial sitting control in patients with limited sitting control, e.g., the patient with SCI and limited trunk muscles. Initially, the hands are positioned behind the patient to maximize the BOS (shoulders, elbows, and wrists are extended with base of hand bearing weight). As control develops, placing hands in front and finally at the sides of the hips varies their position and increases stability demands. Sitting then progresses to short-sitting activities, with the knees flexed over the side of a mat and feet in contact with the support surface. Adequate range of the hamstrings (90–110 degrees) is required for the patient to sit with a neutral pelvis. Decreased range in the hamstrings results in a posterior pelvic tilt with sacral sitting and overstretching of low back muscles (Fig. 5.6).

In the side-sitting position, the patient sits on one hip with the LEs flexed and tucked to the opposite side. Because this posture elongates the trunk on the weightbearing side, this is a useful activity for patients with spastic trunk muscles (e.g., the patient with stroke). When the more affected UE is weightbearing, prolonged stretch is also applied to the elbow, wrist, and finger flexors (Fig. 5.7). Alternately, both UEs can be held in front in a hands-clasped position (hands clasped together with both elbows extended and shoulders flexed).

Applying Resistance to Promote Stability

Light resistance to the head and upper trunk can be used to facilitate and engage muscles to hold. Generally, extensor muscles demonstrate greater weakness than flexor muscles. As control increases, resistance is gradually withdrawn and the patient progresses to active holding.

Clinical Note: Light approximation (joint compression) through the spine can be used to stimulate postural stabilizers; the therapist places both hands on the shoulders and gently compresses downward.

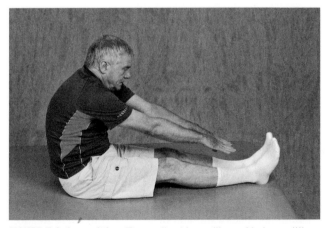

FIGURE 5.6 Long sitting The patient is positioned in long-sitting, with knees extended. This patient exhibits tight hamstrings with resultant posterior pelvic tilt, sacral sitting, dorsal kyphosis, posterior pelvic tilt, and sacral sitting.

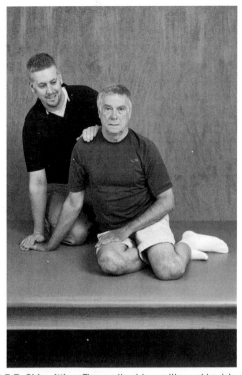

FIGURE 5.7 Side-sitting The patient is positioned in side-sitting, with knees flexed and tucked to one side. Weight is borne more on the right hip and right UE, which is extended and weightbearing. Sitting in this position places a stretch on the trunk lateral flexors, elbow, wrist, and finger flexors. This stretch can be beneficial for the patient with stroke who demonstrates spasticity and shortening in these muscles.

Approximation is contraindicated in patients with spinal deformity or an inability to assume an upright position (e.g., the patient with osteoporosis and kyphosis) and in patients with acute pain (e.g., disc pathology or arthritis). Alternatively, the therapist may have the patient sit on a ball and gently bounce up and down to activate extensor muscles and promote stability via activation of joint proprioceptors in the spine.

The proprioceptive neuromuscular facilitation (PNF) technique of *stabilizing reversals* can be used. The patient is asked to hold the sitting position while the therapist applies resistance first in one direction, then in the opposite direction. When applying medial/lateral (M/L) resistance, hand placements are on the borders of the scapula as if pushing the upper trunk sideward, away from the therapist (Fig. 5.8), then pulling the upper trunk toward the therapist. During anterior/posterior resistance, the therapist applies resistance as if pushing the upper trunk backward and then pulling the upper trunk forward toward the therapist. Manual contacts are alternated, first on one side of the upper trunk and then on the other. The resistance is built up gradually, starting from very light resistance and progressing to moderate resistance. Initially, only a small amount of motion is allowed, progressing to holding steady. Verbal cues (VCs) include *"Push against my hands and don't let me move you."* The therapist provides a transitional command (*"Now don't let me pull*

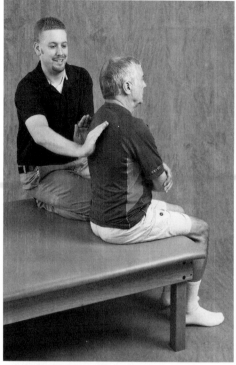

FIGURE 5.8 Sitting, holding using stabilizing reversals The patient is sitting with feet flat on the floor and the UEs folded across the chest. The therapist is applying lateral resistance while the patient allows only small-range movement and progresses to holding steady. The left hand is placed on the axillary border of scapula, while the right hand is positioned on the vertebral border of the scapula on the other side of the trunk. Hand placements are then reversed to apply resistance in the opposite direction.

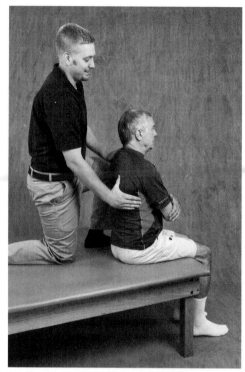

FIGURE 5.9 Sitting, holding using rhythmic stabilization The patient is sitting with feet flat on the floor and the UEs folded across the chest. The therapist is applying resistance with the left hand on the anterior upper trunk pulling backward, while the right hand is on the lower scapula pushing forward. The patient resists all attempts for movement, holding steady.

you the other way") before sliding the hands to resist the opposite muscles. This allows the patient the opportunity to make appropriate anticipatory postural adjustments. The position of the therapist will vary according to the line of force that needs to be applied.

The PNF technique of *rhythmic stabilization* can also be used. The patient is asked to hold the sitting position while the therapist applies rotational resistance to the upper trunk. One hand is placed on the posterior trunk of one side (the lower axillary border of the scapula) pushing forward, while the other hand is on the opposite side, anterior upper trunk, pulling back (Fig. 5.9). The therapist's hands then reverse for the opposite movement (each hand remains positioned on the same side of the trunk). No motion is allowed. VCs for rhythmic stabilization include *"Don't let me move you. Now don't let me move you the other way."*

Clinical Note: Interventions to promote stability are an important lead-up for many functional activities (e.g., dressing, grooming, toileting, and feeding) and for later transfer training.

Outcomes

Motor control goal: improved stability (static control) and postural alignment in sitting

Functional goal: maintain the sitting position independently with minimal sway and no loss of balance for a specific time (i.e., 3 minutes, 5 minutes)

Interventions to Improve Dynamic Control in Sitting

In sitting, dynamic postural control (controlled mobility) is necessary for moving in the posture (e.g., weight shifting, turning) or moving the limbs (e.g., reaching, lifting) while maintaining postural stability. These movements produce disturbances of the COM and require ongoing anticipatory postural adjustments in balance to maintain upright sitting. Initially, the patient's attention is directed to the key task elements required for successful postural adjustments and movement (e.g., *"Shift your weight over onto your left buttock, reach with your hand to grab the ball"*). With increased practice, the postural adjustments become more automatic.

Sitting, Active Weight Shifts

The patient is encouraged to shift weight from side to side, forward and backward, and diagonally with trunk rotation. Re-education of the LOS is one of the first goals. The patient is encouraged to shift as far as possible in any one direction without losing balance and then to return to the midline position. Initially, weight shifts are small range, but gradually the range is increased (i.e., moving through *increments of range*).

Clinical Note: Patients with ataxia (e.g., cerebellar pathology) exhibit too much movement and have difficulty holding steady (maintaining stability). Weight shifts are large to begin with and are progressed during treatment to smaller and smaller ranges (moving through *decrements of range*). Stability, or holding steady, is the final goal of this progression.

Clinical Note: Patients with excess UE flexor tone (e.g., the patient with stroke or TBI) may benefit from weight shifting forward and backward with the elbow extended and the hand open and weightbearing. The rocking promotes relaxation to the spastic muscles of the hand (wrist and finger flexors) and elbow (elbow flexors), most likely through mechanisms of prolonged stretch and relaxing effect of slow vestibular stimulation (Fig. 5.10).

A large ball can be used to facilitate weight shifting. The patient sits with shoulders flexed, elbows extended, and hands resting on a large ball placed in front. Alternately, a smaller ball can be placed on a tabletop positioned in front of the patient. The patient is instructed to move the ball slowly forward and backward and side to side. Initially, the therapist stands on the opposite side of the ball to assist in controlling the range and speed of movements. This activity has a number of benefits. The ball can provide UE support and inhibitory positioning for the patient with a spastic UE (e.g., the patient recovering from stroke). It also reduces anxiety that may occur with weight shifting forward because the patient does not feel threatened with falling forward to the floor. Movements can be easily assisted using the ball. The movements forward and backward can be used to promote increased shoulder ROM in unsuspecting patients who may be otherwise anxious about passive ROM of a tight, restricted shoulder (Fig. 5.11).

Upper trunk rotation is a difficult movement for many patients (e.g., the patient with Parkinson's disease who has difficulty with most rotation activities). With arms outstretched and hands on a large ball in front, the patient moves the ball to one side, then the other. Alternatively, the patient can be instructed to hold arms outstretched with hands clasped together and move the hands to one side, then the other. *"Turn your body and hands to one side and line them up with the clock* [or any target], *now turn to the other side."* The therapist monitors the position and directs the patient to keep the trunk erect and buttock (both ischial tuberosities) and thighs in contact with the support surface.

Clinical Note: Interventions to promote weight shifting are important lead-up activities for more advanced sitting balance activities, pressure relief, and transfers.

Active Weight Shifts Against Resistance

The PNF technique of dynamic reversals can be used. Manually graded resistance can be applied as the patient moves forward and backward (anterior-posterior shifts) or from side to side (medial-lateral shifts). The therapist alternates hand placement, first on the anterior upper trunk to resist the upper body pulling forward and then on the posterior

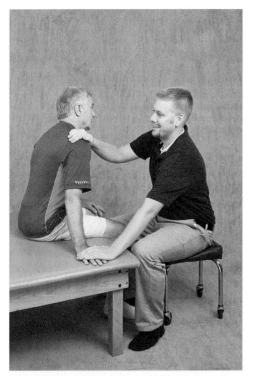

FIGURE 5.10 Sitting, weight shifting with UE support The patient is sitting with both feet flat on the floor and the right UE extended and weightbearing. The therapist is holding on top of the patient's hand to prevent finger flexion, while the right hand is on top of the shoulder applying approximation. The weight shifting enhances relaxation of the patient's right UE.

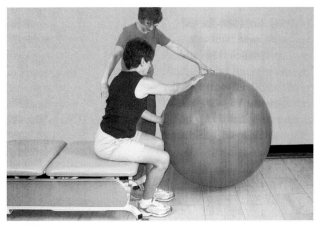

FIGURE 5.11 Sitting, weight shifting with hands on a ball The patient is sitting with both feet flat on the floor and both hands on top of a large therapy ball. The therapist instructs the patient to roll the ball over to the left. The upper trunk rotates as the patient moves the ball to that side. The activity is then repeated to the opposite side.

upper trunk to resist movement backward. To resist M/L shifts, manual contacts are on the lateral aspect of the upper trunk under the axilla and the other hand on the scapular border on the opposite side of the trunk (Fig. 5.12). It is important to avoid resisting directly on the lateral shoulders (humerus). Smooth reversals of antagonists are facilitated by well-timed VCs *("Pull away"* or *"Push back")* and a transitional cue *("Now")* to indicate the change in direction. A quick stretch is used to initiate the reverse movement. Progression is from partial-range to full-range control (moving through increments of range). Shifts may also be resisted in diagonal and in diagonal/rotational directions. A hold may be added in one or both directions if the patient demonstrates difficulty moving to one side (e.g., the patient with stroke). The hold is a momentary pause (held for one count); the antagonist contraction is then facilitated.

Voluntary Movements and Task-Oriented Practice

Active movements of the UE or LE can be used to promote dynamic postural control and anticipatory balance. Limb movements can be performed individually or in combination (e.g., bilateral symmetrical, bilateral asymmetrical, or reciprocal). The therapist can provide a target (e.g., *"Reach out and touch my hand"* or *"Throw the ball in the basket"*). Reaching movements can begin with objects placed within arm's length and progressed to beyond arm's length, requiring a weight shift. Strategies for varying practice to increase skill include increasing the distance to be reached, varying speed, reducing or altering BOS in sitting, increasing object weight and size, involving multiple extremities, and adding a time constraint. If the patient fails to demonstrate adequate postural control or begins to lose control as fatigue develops, he or she is directed to reduce the speed or range of limb movements or rest before continuing with the activities. Emphasis on task-oriented practice will enhance carryover into real-world situations and environments (e.g., pouring water from a pitcher into a glass, folding laundry). Patients should be encouraged to practice movements outside of scheduled therapy time. Using an activity diary to document outside practice is a useful tool for many patients.

Sitting with voluntary (unilateral, bilateral, or reciprocal) arm and leg movements can be used to improve trunk control, facilitate axial rotation, and improve spinal flexibility[8] and is a useful preparatory intervention for promoting functional mobility required for ambulation.[9,10] For example, the patient sits on a stationary surface (platform mat) with feet flat on the floor performing active or resisted alternate arm or leg raises. The intervention can be made more challenging by changing the speed and range of the movements, the stability of the surface, or by modifying visual inputs with eyes closed or in a busy environment. Examples of voluntary limb movements in sitting are presented in Box 5.4 and demonstrated in Figures 5.13 through 5.16.

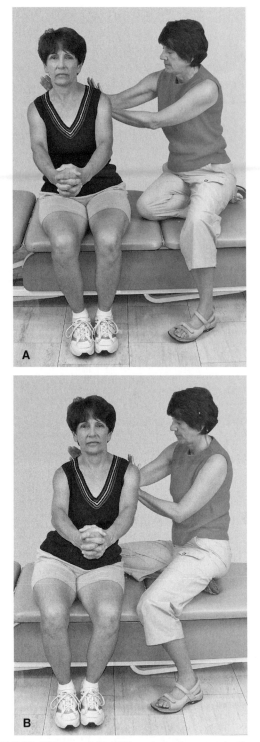

FIGURE 5.12 Sitting, weight shifting, dynamic reversals The patient practices lightly resisted weight shifting side to side. The UEs are held steady in front, shoulders flexed, elbows extended, and hands clasped together. The therapist provides light stretch and resistance to enhance movement. The patient has moved away from the therapist (not shown) and then (A) pushes back toward the therapist. The end position (B) shows the patient with weight shifted onto the left side.

BOX 5.4 Examples of Voluntary Limb Movements Performed in Sitting

Upper Extremity Activities

- Raising one or both UEs forward (shoulder flexion) or to the side (shoulder abduction); reaching for objects placed on a counter or tabletop
- Raising one or both UEs overhead; reaching for objects placed on a high shelf
- Stacking cones with the target cone moved to different locations within or slightly beyond the patient's reach (Fig. 5.13)
- Reaching down to pick up an object (e.g., cup, book) from the floor or from a small raised stool, forward or sideways (Fig 5.14)
- Using both hands to complete a task (e.g., pouring water from a pitcher into a glass; folding laundry on a tabletop; lifting a tray (Fig. 5.15)
- Ball activities: handing off the ball to the therapist and receiving return pass; throwing and catching a ball; bouncing a ball
- Tossing and catching a small ball, balloon, or small scarf
- Lifting a ball with both hands and moving it diagonally up and across the body

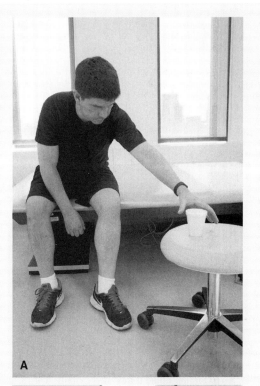

A

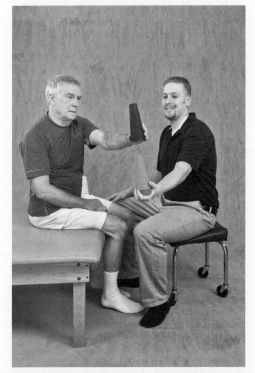

FIGURE 5.13 Sitting, reaching using cone stacking The patient practices upper trunk rotation with UE reach, grasp, and release. The therapist varies the position of the target stacking cone to vary the amount of movement and weight shifting. The patient who sits with an asymmetrical sitting position (e.g., the patient with stroke) can be encouraged to shift to the more affected side.

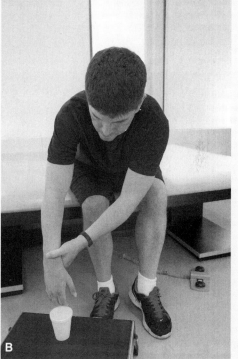

B

FIGURE 5.14 Sitting, reaching sideways in sitting The patient with stroke and right hemiparesis practices reaching down to the side to pick up a cup placed on a small stool, first with the less affected hand (A) and then with an assist to the hemiparetic hand (B).

(box continues on page 106)

BOX 5.4 Examples of Voluntary Limb Movements Performed in Sitting (continued)

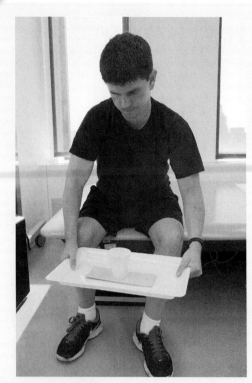

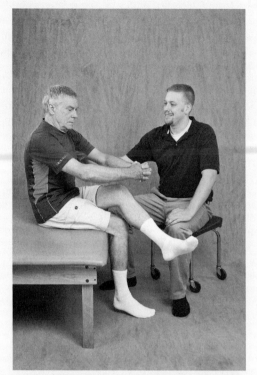

FIGURE 5.15 Sitting, lifting a tray The patient with stroke and right hemiparesis practices lifting a tray without spilling a cup of water.

Lower Extremity Activities
• Extending one knee out in front to full extension and then flexing
• Marching in place, alternating lifting one knee up, then the other
• Performing toe-offs and heel-offs, bilateral symmetrical or reciprocal
• Holding one foot off the floor and performing toe circles or "writing" the letters of the alphabet with the foot
• Alternate crossing one limb over the other, then repeating to the other side (Fig. 5.16).

FIGURE 5.16 Sitting, dynamic LE movements The patient practices crossing and uncrossing the left leg over the right. This activity requires a weight shift toward the static side and away from the side of the dynamic limb. The UEs are held steady in front, shoulders flexed, elbows extended, and hands clasped together. This forces the dynamic adjustments to occur in the lower trunk and pelvis and does not permit the patient to use an upper trunk lateral tilt.

Four-Limb Activities
• Mexican hat dance: Both UEs move reciprocally in elbow flexion and extension while both LEs move reciprocally in knee extension and flexion.

Clinical Note: The sequencing and motor control involved with reciprocal arm and leg training is beneficial for coordination difficulties seen with conditions such as cerebellar ataxia.

Resisted Limb Movements

The addition of resistance to limb movements strengthens and enhances control of the limbs (e.g., the patient with weakness following brain injury). It also serves the valuable function of directing the patient's attention to the control of limb movements and away from actions of the trunk. This helps to promote automatic control of postural mechanisms required for sitting. Resistance to the extremities can be in the form of lightweight cuffs, elastic resistive bands, pulleys, or manual resistance. The therapist typically starts with unilateral movements and progresses to combination (bilateral and reciprocal) movements. With resisted movements, the level of resistance is determined by the ability of the trunk to stabilize and maintain upright sitting, not by the strength of the UEs. If stabilization is lacking, resistance may be contraindicated and active movements should be promoted.

Unilateral PNF patterns are often used initially, when dynamic control is lacking or when one extremity is needed for weightbearing and support. As control develops, the patient progresses to more challenging bilateral patterns. Patterns that can be effectively used to challenge trunk control in sitting include chop/reverse chop (see Figs. 3.30 and 3.31) and lift/reverse lift (Figs. 3.32 and 3.33). Both involve movement of the trunk (either extension with rotation or flexion with rotation) combined with bilateral asymmetrical patterns of both UEs. In addition, there is a weight shift from one side (buttock) to the other. Emphasis is on using the combined arm movements to enhance control and range of the trunk movements. See Chapter 3: Proprioceptive Neuromuscular Facilitation for a description of patterns and techniques.

> **Clinical Note:** A chop pattern to the more involved side is useful for the patient with stroke who exhibits homonymous hemianopsia, unilateral neglect, and difficulty crossing the midline. A lift pattern toward the less affected side is useful for moving the hemiparetic UE out of a flexion synergy.

Another PNF pattern often used to develop dynamic postural control in sitting is bilateral symmetrical UE flexion/abduction/external rotation with upper trunk extension (see Fig. 3.34). This posture has the added advantage of expanding the chest and enhancing full range in trunk extension.

> **Clinical Note:** Upper extremity bilateral symmetric flexion/abduction/external rotation is a useful activity for the patient with a functional kyphosis and rounded, forward shoulders (e.g., the patient with Parkinson's disease). Respiration can be improved by telling the patient to *"Slowly breathe in"* during the flexion/abduction/external rotation and to *"Slowly breathe out"* during bilateral symmetric extension/adduction/internal rotation.

Thrust/reverse-thrust patterns can also be used to promote dynamic stability in sitting (see Fig. 3.35). The UEs move together up and across the face, with hands opening, forearms pronating, elbows extending, and shoulders flexing above 90 degrees. This is a protective pattern for the face and promotes shoulder flexion and elbow extension with scapular protraction. In withdrawal or reverse thrust, the hands close, the forearms supinate with elbow flexion, and the shoulders extend, pulling the arms back and to the sides. Holding in the reverse-thrust position (withdrawal pattern) is a useful activity to promote symmetrical scapular adduction, trunk extension, and upright trunk posture.

Outcomes

Motor control goal: improved dynamic postural control (controlled mobility)

Functional skills achieved: appropriate functional skills in sitting, allowing independence in reaching and ADL (e.g., bathing, grooming, and dressing)

Interventions to Improve Scooting

Scooting is the ability to move the body forward and backward while sitting. The key to successful scooting is the weight shift toward the stabilizing (static) side. This unweights the dynamic side before moving the pelvis forward (or backward). The UEs are held off the support surface and are not used for push-off or assisting movement. Scooting is an important lead-up activity for independent bed mobility and for independent sit-to-stand transfers (scooting forward to the edge of the seat before standing up).

Scooting in the Short-Sitting Position

The patient sits at the edge of the mat, with both feet flat on the floor. The patient practices moving forward or backward by walking on his or her buttock ("butt walking"). The therapist can initially verbally cue the movements (e.g., *"Shift your weight over to right side, now scoot forward moving your left side* [pelvis and thigh] *forward"*). The motion can be further assisted by having the therapist lift and support the thigh of the dynamic limb to reduce friction effects. Movements of the dynamic limb can also be lightly resisted at the front of the knee (manual contacts on the upper tibia, avoiding the patella) or on the posterior hip to enhance backward movement. The patient is instructed to clasp the hands together with both elbows extended and UEs held in front (Fig. 5.17), which helps to restrict side-to-side upper trunk movements and isolates the motion to the lower trunk and pelvis. The patient is instructed: *"Hold your hands together directly in front; do not let them move side to side while you are scooting."*

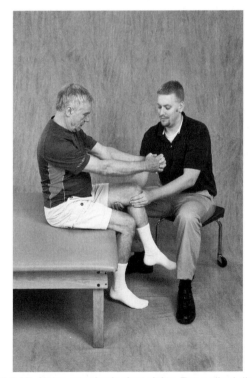

FIGURE 5.17 Sitting, scooting in short-sitting The patient sits with both hands clasped together in a forward position (elbows extended and shoulders flexed). The patient practices weight shifting to one side while moving the opposite limb forward. The therapist instructs the patient in the movements and provides some unweighting of the dynamic limb and resistance to enhance the forward movement of the limb. The patient then shifts to the other side and moves the opposite limb forward, scooting forward to the edge of the mat.

Scooting in the Long-Sitting Position

Scooting in the long-sitting position is often used for patients who initially may require the extended BOS offered by position (e.g., the patient with SCI). Adequate range of the hamstrings is necessary to prevent sacral sitting and overstretching of the low back muscles (e.g., 90- to 100-degree straight leg raising). With the patient in long-sitting position, the therapist is positioned at the patient's feet and assists the motion by holding both feet off the mat, reducing LE friction effects. The patient is instructed to shift to one side and move the opposite pelvis forward. The process is then reversed as the patient moves forward. *"I want you to shift your weight to one side and move your pelvis forward on the other side."* As in scooting in short-sitting position, the patient's hands can be held clasped in front or can be held to the sides to assist in balance while moving.

Scooting Off a High Table Into Supported Unilateral Standing

The patient sits on a high table with both feet off the floor. The patient is instructed to scoot forward to the edge of the table (Fig. 5.18A). The patient then rotates the pelvis forward on the dynamic side while extending the hip and knee on the same side. The patient places the foot on the floor, keeping the other hip resting on the table (half-sitting on the table) (Fig. 5.18 B). This activity promotes unilateral weightbearing and is a useful activity for patients who lack symmetrical weightbearing in standing (e.g., patients recovering from stroke who place most of their weight on the sound side). This activity requires the patient to stand on the more affected LE. Proper height of the treatment table is important to facilitate the correct posture, so an adjustable-height table is required for this activity.

Interventions to Improve Balance Control in Sitting

Balance is defined as the ability to maintain the COM within the BOS while controlling body alignment and orientation of the body to the environment. Balance control is achieved through the actions of a number of different body systems working together. These include the sensory systems (visual, somatosensory, and vestibular inputs as well as sensory integration actions of the CNS), musculoskeletal system (muscle synergies), neuromuscular system (postural tone; automatic postural synergies; anticipatory, reactive, and adaptive mechanisms), and cognitive/perceptual systems (internal representations, interpretation of sensory information, motor planning). *Reactive balance* control refers to the ability to maintain or recover balance when subjected to an unexpected challenge and is based on feedback-driven adjustments. These include manual perturbations (disturbances in the COM) and changes in the support surface (disturbances in the BOS), such as platform perturbations. *Postural fixation reactions* stabilize the body against an

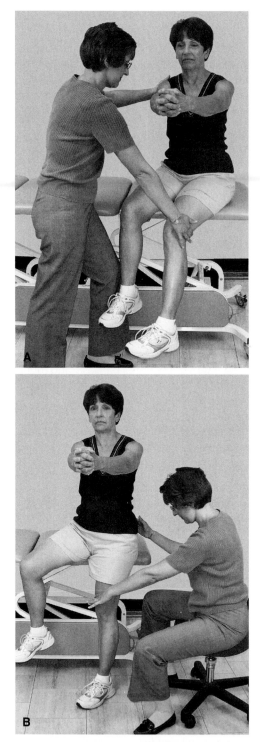

FIGURE 5.18 Sitting, scooting off a high table into unilateral standing (A) The patient sits with both hands clasped together in a forward position (elbows extended and shoulders flexed). The patient practices weight shifting to one side while moving one limb forward. The therapist instructs the patient in the movements and provides some unweighting of the dynamic limb and resistance to enhance the forward movement of the limb. The patient then shifts to the other side and moves the opposite limb forward, scooting forward to the edge of the table. (B) The patient then moves one LE into weightbearing (supported standing) while keeping the other hip on the table. The therapist provides light pressure to the quadriceps to enhance extension. An adjustable-height table is required to ensure proper standing height.

external force (e.g., a perturbation or nudge). *Tilting reactions* reposition the COM within the BOS in response to changes in the support surface (e.g., sitting on a wobble board). *Anticipatory balance* control allows the CNS to modify (preset) the nervous system in advance of voluntary movements. The central set or overall state of readiness of the CNS is influenced by feedforward adjustments based on prior instructions, prior experience, and the context of the balance experience. For example, the responses of a patient when catching a ball produces far different results if instructions included that the ball was inflated versus weighted (e.g., 3 lb [1.36 kg]). *Adaptive balance control* refers to the ability to adapt or modify postural responses relative to changing task and environmental demands. Prior experience (learning) influences a person's adaptability and shapes strategy selection.[7] Optimal function is achieved when all aspects of balance control are working during performance of self-initiated activities, during destabilization and corrective actions, and during reactive responses to prevent a fall.

Interventions selected are based on a careful examination of the systems contributing to balance control and the functional outcomes of impairments (e.g., functional performance and fall history). For most patients, balance training is a multifaceted program. It frequently begins in the sitting posture and is progressed through other upright postures that serve to increase the challenge by raising the COM and decreasing the BOS (e.g., kneeling and standing). More severely affected patients (e.g., the patient with TBI or SCI) may spend considerable time in rehabilitation working on sitting balance. For other patients who are less severely affected, sitting balance training may represent only a brief part of the balance training program, with greater emphasis placed on standing balance training. The following section offers suggested strategies and training activities in sitting.

Interventions to Promote Reactive Balance Control

The patient sits on a stationary surface (platform mat) with feet flat on the floor. The therapist provides small-range *manual perturbations* in various different directions, forward and backward, side to side, and diagonally. Manual contacts should be on the trunk, not on the shoulders or UEs. It is important to ensure appropriate postural responses. For example, with backward displacements, trunk and hip flexors are active. With forward displacements, trunk and hip extensors are active. Upper extremity protective extension reactions can be initiated if the displacements move the COM near or past the LOS and are more easily activated with sideward displacements than with anterior-posterior displacements. If patient responses are inappropriate (i.e., lack adequate countermovements or adequate timing), the therapist may need to guide the initial attempts either verbally or manually. The patient can then progress to active responses. Perturbations should be appropriate for the patient's level of control. It is important to use gentle perturbations; excessive forces are not

necessary to stimulate balance responses. The therapist can vary the BOS to increase or decrease difficulty during the perturbations. Progression is from predictable perturbations (*"Don't let me push you backward"* and *"Now don't let me pull you forward"*) to unpredictable perturbations applied with no preliminary instructions. In the former situation, both anticipatory and reactive control mechanisms are activated, whereas in the latter, primarily reactive control mechanisms are used.

Clinical Note: It is important to know the patient's capabilities and to anticipate the patient's ability to respond. Exceeding the patient's capabilities may induce anxiety and fear of falling. *Postural fixation* is the likely response to this situation and is often seen in the patient with cerebellar ataxia. It is equally important to adjust responses, increasing the level of difficulty appropriate to the patient's improving capabilities.

Promoting Balance Control Using Mobile and Compliant Surfaces

Rocker Board or Inflated Disc

Activities on a moveable surface (rocker board, inflated disc, or therapy ball) can be used to alter the patient's BOS and engage postural mechanisms. Rocker boards (equilibrium boards) are constructed to allow varying motion. The type and amount of motion are determined by the design of the board. A curved-bottom (bidirectional) board allows motion in two directions; a dome-bottom board allows motion in all directions. The degree of curve or size of the dome determines the amount of motion in any direction; motion is increased in boards with large curves or high domes. The type of board used depends on the patient's capabilities and the type and range of movements permitted.

An inflated disc is a dome-shaped cushion that is positioned under the patient while sitting. It allows limited motion in all directions (Fig. 5.19A). Challenges can be varied by changing the level of inflation (a firm disc provides a greater challenge than a soft disc) or by varying the BOS (Fig. 5.19B).

When sitting on the wobble board or disc, the patient's feet should be flat on the floor. A step or stool may be needed for patients with a shorter stature when sitting on a platform mat. Initial activities include having the patient maintain a balanced, centered, or aligned sitting position. The patient can then progress to active weight shifts, tilting the board or moving on the disc in various directions. These patient-initiated challenges explore the LOS and stimulate both anticipatory and reactive balance mechanisms.

Computerized Platform/Feedback Training

A computerized platform system can provide the patient with feedback on the center of pressure measurements. The

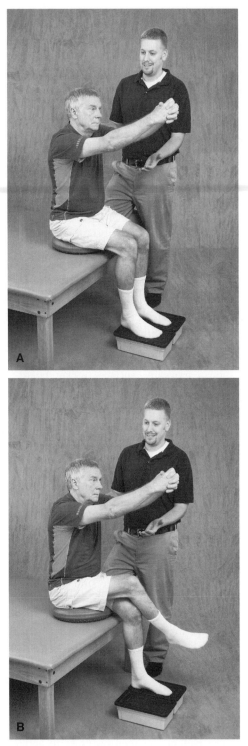

patient sits on the platform and practices holding the body steady (focus on center of alignment) and moving the body in all directions (focus on LOS). Visual feedback is provided on a monitor indicating shifts in the center of pressure. This setup is similar to computerized devices used to promote standing balance.

Ball Activities

Therapy balls can be used to promote balance responses. Sitting on the ball facilitates postural mechanisms through intrinsic feedback mechanisms (visual, proprioceptive, and vestibular inputs) and challenges reactive and adaptive postural control. The use of the ball also adds novelty to rehabilitation programs and can be easily adapted to group classes. Patients may feel initially insecure and should be carefully guarded. The therapist may sit directly behind the patient, shadowing the patient's body with his or her own (Fig. 5.20), or the therapist can stabilize from the front. If the patient is very insecure, the ball can initially be positioned on a floor ring that prevents the ball from moving in any direction. A ball that is slightly underinflated and positioned on a soft floor mat will roll less easily than a fully inflated ball positioned on a tile floor. Initially the therapist can provide manual cues, manual assistance, or

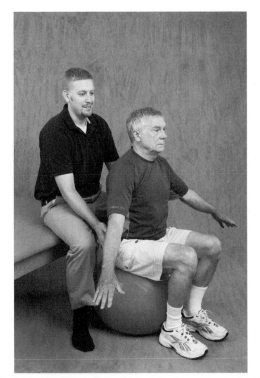

FIGURE 5.20 Sitting on ball, holding Initially, as the patient sits on a therapy ball, the therapist can shadow and support the patient from behind by sitting on a mat (for maximum security) or on another ball. The therapist maintains both hands near the patient's hips but does not hold onto the patient or the ball. The patient is instructed to maintain a steady position on the ball. Both UEs are held out to the sides in a low guard position, with hips and knees flexed to 90 degrees and feet apart.

FIGURE 5.19 Sitting on an inflated disc, holding The patient sits on an inflated disc with both feet flat on a small step. (A) The hands are clasped together in a forward position (elbows extended, shoulders flexed). The therapist instructs the patient to maintain a steady posture (centered alignment). (B) The patient then is instructed to maintain balance while crossing the right leg over the left, a movement that reduces the patient's BOS and increases the challenge to balance.

VCs to guide the patient in the correct movements or to stabilize the patient. As control develops, active control is expected, and the therapist assumes a hands-off approach.

Choosing the right size ball is important to ensure proper sitting posture. When the patient sits on the ball, the hips and knees should be flexed to 90 degrees *(the 90-90 rule)* with knees aligned over the feet. Feet should be flat on the floor and positioned hip-width apart. Guidelines for choosing the correct ball size based on patient height are presented in Box 5.5.

Clinical Note: Patients with restricted hip flexion during sitting (e.g., the patient with a new total hip replacement) will benefit from using an oversized ball to decrease the angle of the hip. Patients who are overweight or obese may require a larger ball that has a greater surface area.

Static Ball Activities

Initially, the patient is instructed to maintain a neutral position in sitting (toes and knees pointing forward, feet hip-width apart, knees aligned over the feet, pelvic neutral position). The patient is instructed, *"Sit tall and hold steady; don't let the ball roll in any direction."* Sitting off to one side will result in instability and movement off the ball. Approximation in the form of gentle bouncing can be used to assist upright posture. Initially, the hands can rest on the knees (a position of maximum stability). As control develops, the patient is instructed to hold the UEs up (e.g., in a forward position with the shoulders flexed, elbows extended, and the hands clasped together) (Fig. 5.21A). Alternatively, the patient can hold the arms out to the sides with shoulder abduction and elbow extension (Fig. 5.21B). This allows the UEs to assist in balancing while on the ball. The patient can also be instructed to focus on a visual target, which can enhance stabilizing responses.

Dynamic Ball Activities

Dynamic ball activities should be attempted only after the patient achieves static control. As previously discussed, the addition of trunk and limb movements requires anticipatory balance control as well as reactive control. Examples are provided in Box 5.6 and depicted in Figures 5.22 through 5.32.

Clinical Note: It is important for the patient to actively stabilize the upper body during pelvic motion training, preventing any attempts to move by

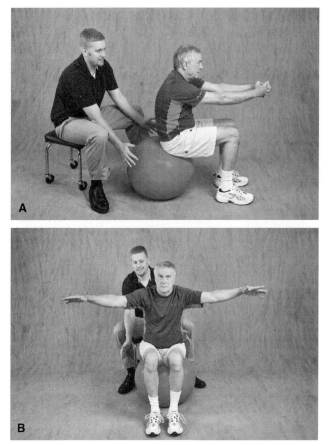

FIGURE 5.21 Sitting on ball, holding (A) The patient maintains steady sitting on the ball while holding both hands clasped together in a forward position (elbows extended and shoulders flexed). (B) For added balance control, the UEs can be held with shoulders abducted out to the sides and elbows extended.

tilting the upper trunk. This can be achieved by having the patient maintain both UEs steady (e.g., holding both hands clasped together or holding a second ball). The patient is instructed, *"Hold your upper body steady. Keep your hands straight ahead on the target in front of you."*

Clinical Note: Ball activities should be monitored closely and modified to ensure patient safety. The therapist should be attentive and utilize appropriate guarding techniques. For some patients (e.g., the patient with TBI and cerebellar ataxia), this may require utilizing a safety belt or an overhead safety harness. Such precautions allow the patient with significant balance challenges to practice without manual assistance.

Red Flag: Patients with vestibular insufficiency may experience increased dizziness, nausea, or anxiety during activities on the therapy ball. Such patients should be monitored carefully for such changes during the activity and the level of challenge decreased to tolerable levels. For some severely involved patients, ball activities may be contraindicated.

BOX 5.5 Guidelines for Ball Size

Patient Height	Recommended Ball Size
Less than 5 ft, 0 in	45 cm
5 ft, 0 in.–5 ft, 7 in.	55 cm
5 ft, 8 in.– 6 ft, 3 in.	65 cm
More than 6 ft, 3 in	75 cm

(text continues on page 115)

BOX 5.6 Dynamic Ball Activities

Pelvis and Trunk Activities
- *Anterior/posterior pelvic shifts.* The patient rolls the ball forward and backward using anterior and posterior pelvic tilts, holds briefly, and then returns to neutral pelvic position (Fig. 5.22).
- *Lateral weight shifts.* The patient rolls the ball from side to side (Fig. 5.23) with M/L pelvic shifts, holds briefly, and then returns to neutral pelvic position.
- *Pelvic clock.* The patient rotates the ball in a full circle by using pelvic actions, first clockwise and then counterclockwise.
- *Lateral trunk rotation.* The patient extends both UEs out to the sides, rotates (twists) as far as possible to the left, returns to midline, and then twists to the right; these rotations can be combined with head/neck rotations ("look arounds"). Trunk rotations can also be performed holding a small ball (Fig. 5.24); rotations can also be performed diagonally.
- *Diagonal trunk rotation.* The patient lifts a small ball positioned on the floor or on a small stool to the side up and across the body to the other side.

Upper Extremity Movements
- *UE lifts.* The patient raises one UE to the forward horizontal position or overhead, and then returns; this can be repeated with the opposite UE
- *UE bilateral symmetrical lifts.* The patient performs an overhead reach with extended elbows (Fig. 5.25A) or with elbows flexed (Fig. 5.25B). Both patterns provide a pectoral stretch, expanding the chest and promoting upper trunk extension.

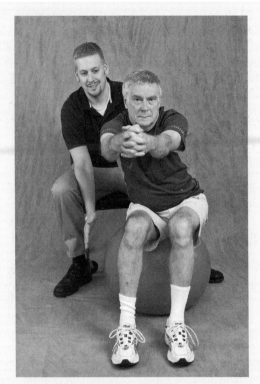

FIGURE 5.23 Sitting on ball, lateral pelvic shifts The patient sits on a ball, holding both hands clasped together in a forward position (elbows extended and shoulders flexed). The head, upper trunk, and UEs are held steady. The therapist instructs the patient to roll the ball from side to side, moving the ball to the side using pelvis movements (lateral tilts).

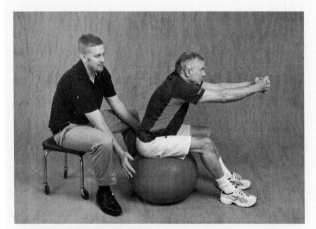

FIGURE 5.22 Sitting on ball, anterior-posterior pelvic shifts The patient sits on a ball, holding both hands clasped together in a forward position (elbows extended and shoulders flexed). The head, upper trunk, and UEs are held steady. The therapist instructs the patient to roll the ball forward and backward, moving the ball by using pelvic movements (backward or posterior pelvic tilts and forward or anterior pelvic tilts).

- *UE circles.* The patient holds both UEs out to the sides and rotates first forward (clockwise) and then backward (counterclockwise).
- *Catching and throwing a ball.* The patient practices passing and catching or throwing a ball against a target and catching (Fig. 5.26A and B). Feet can be positioned flat on floor or on an inflated disc to increase the challenge to balance (Fig. 5.27).

Lower Extremity Movements
- *Knee lifts.* The patient lifts one LE up into hip flexion, holds briefly, and then returns to neutral position; can be repeated with the other limb.
- *Marching in place (alternate knee lifts).* The patient marches rhythmically in place, first slowly and then with increasing speed.
- *Marching in place with contralateral UE/LE lifts.* The patient raises the right UE and the left knee, lowers them, and then repeats with the left UE and right knee (Fig. 5.28).
- *Knee extension.* The patient straightens the knee and holds the foot out in front for three counts and

BOX 5.6 Dynamic Ball Activities (continued)

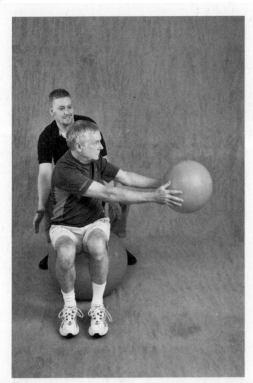

FIGURE 5.24 Sitting on ball, head and trunk rotation The patient practices head and trunk rotation to the left while holding a small ball and maintaining sitting stability. The patient then twists to the other side, moving the ball as far as possible in the new direction.

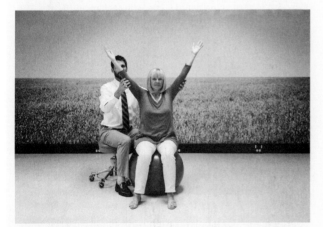

FIGURE 5.25 Sitting on ball, bilateral symmetrical overhead reach with extended elbows This pattern provides a pectoral stretch, expands the chest, and promotes symmetrical upper trunk extension.

then returns (Fig. 5.29). This activity can progress to reciprocal opposite knee and elbow extension (Fig. 5.30).

- *Knee extension with ankle movements* (circles, or writing letters of the alphabet in space with the dynamic foot).

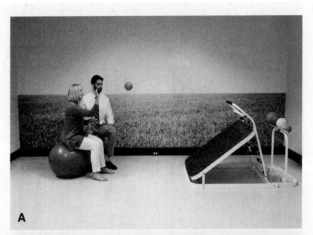

A

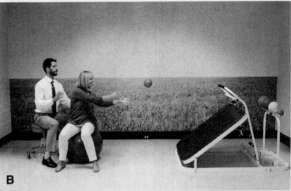

B

FIGURE 5.26 Sitting on ball, throwing and catching a small ball The patient practices throwing and catching a small ball bounced off a target while maintaining sitting stability (A). The therapist varies the direction of the throw by having the patient turn to one side and throw and catch the ball (B).

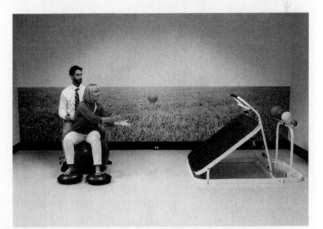

FIGURE 5.27 Sitting on ball, throwing and catching a ball bounced off a target while maintaining sitting stability Challenge to dynamic balance is increased by having both feet positioned on inflated discs.

(box continues on page 114)

BOX 5.6 Dynamic Ball Activities (continued)

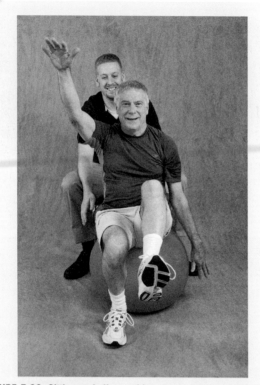

FIGURE 5.28 Sitting on ball, marching The patient practices marching (alternate hip and knee flexion movements) while maintaining stable sitting on the ball. These movements are combined with reciprocal UE movements (shoulder flexion and extension). This is a four-limb movement pattern that requires considerable dynamic stability while sitting on the ball.

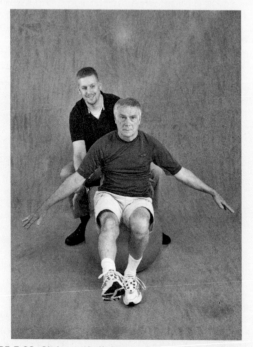

FIGURE 5.29 Sitting on ball, knee extension The patient practices lifting one foot up and extending the knee while maintaining stable sitting on the ball. The UEs are held out to the sides in a guard position. The activity can be progressed by having the patient trace letters or numbers with the dynamic foot.

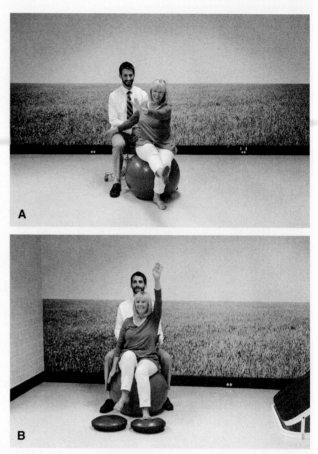

Figure 5.30 Sitting on ball, LE lifts with reciprocal UE lifts The patient practices extending one knee with opposite UE lift, foot in contact with floor **(A)** or flexing the hip with opposite UE lift, foot positioned on mobile disc **(B)**.

- *Side steps.* The patient moves the LE out to the side into hip abduction and knee extension (Fig. 5.31), holds briefly, and then returns. This activity can progress to hip abduction with the knee flexed, moving down into unilateral kneeling while half-sitting on the ball (a modified half-kneeling position).
- *Heel lifts and toe-offs.* The patient lifts both heels off the floor while keeping the toes in contact, and then reverses and lifts both toes off the floor while keeping the heels in contact with the floor. Activity can be progressed to reciprocal lifts.
- *Kicking a ball.* A small ball is rolled toward the patient, who then kicks it back to the therapist.

Four-Limb Activities
- *Jumping jacks.* The patient raises both UEs overhead, claps the hands, and returns hands to the start position (along sides of ball). This activity is combined with bouncing on the ball and alternating reciprocal knee extension and flexion (Fig. 5.32).

BOX 5.6 Dynamic Ball Activities (continued)

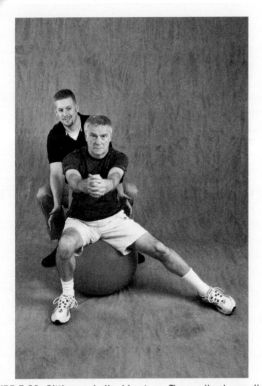

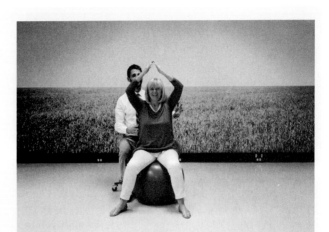

FIGURE 5.32 Sitting on ball, jumping jacks The patient practices jumping jacks, raising both UEs overhead and clapping hands while performing alternate reciprocal hip abduction/adduction of both LEs.

FIGURE 5.31 Sitting on ball, side steps The patient practices stepping out to the side, moving one LE into hip abduction with knee extension while maintaining stable sitting on the ball. The UEs are held with both hands clasped together in a forward position (elbows extended and shoulders flexed).

Promoting Adaptive Balance Control

Adaptive balance control can be enhanced by modifying or changing task or environmental demands. Examples are presented in Box 5.7.

Outcomes
Motor control goal: improved sitting balance control
Functional skills achieved: demonstrates appropriate functional balance skills in sitting, allowing for independence in ADLs

Seated Integrative Medicine Exercises

Integrative medicine combines ancient wisdom and current best practice to provide patient-centered care that considers the health of the entire person, including spirit, mind, and body, and emphasizes wellness and preventive medicine. Integrative medicine is defined by The Consortium of Academic Health Centers for Integrative Medicine as "the practice of medicine that reaffirms the importance of the relationship between practitioner and patient, focuses on the whole person, is informed by evidence, and makes use of all

appropriate therapeutic approaches, health-care professionals, and disciplines to achieve optimal health and healing."[11]

The clinical benefits of mind/body exercise are well documented.[12–14] Tai chi and yoga are examples of engaging and fun integrative exercises that can be utilized in the rehabilitation setting. These exercises may be performed in a 1:1 clinician-to-patient ratio or in group classes. Individualized treatments allow manual cues and VCs to be tailored to the specific needs of the patient and permit close guarding for patients at risk for falls. Group classes provide an environment rich with opportunities for socialization and support.

Seated Tai Chi

Tai chi is an ancient Chinese martial art form of slow, mindful movements and postures that emphasize body awareness, flexibility, strength, and balance. Current and emerging research demonstrates the profound functional and psychosocial impact this exercise style can have on patients with movement disorders. The functional benefits of tai chi include improved balance, improved functional mobility, and increased walking endurance.[15–17]

There are many psychosocial benefits of tai chi, including pain and stress reduction.[18,19] Chronic debilitating

BOX 5.7 Strategies to Promote Adaptive Balance Control

- **Modify the support surface and somatosensory inputs:** Change from sitting on a platform mat to sitting on a dense foam pad to an inflatable disc to a ball; change surface under feet from a sticky mat (yoga mat) to a tile floor to an inflatable disc to both feet on a small ball.
- **Modify visual input:** Change from eyes open to eyes closed.
- **Modify the BOS:** Change from feet wide apart to feet together to one leg crossed to feet on a mobile surface (inflated disc or ball); change from UEs supporting to no support (e.g., UEs held in front, out to the sides, or folded across the chest).
- **Modify limb movements:** Progress from unilateral to bilateral limb movements to combinations of limb movements (e.g., four-limb activities); modify the direction and range of movements); add/vary the amount of resistance.
- **Modify the activity:** Increase the speed, range, number of repetitions.
- **Pace the activity:** Use an external rhythmic timing device (e.g., a metronome or personal listening device with a specific music beat).
- **Use dual-tasking:** Add a secondary motor or cognitive task (e.g., sitting while holding a tray with a glass of water on it or counting backward by 3s from 100).
- **Modify the environment:** Progress from a closed environment (e.g., quiet room with no distractions needed for some patients with TBI) to an open environment (busy treatment area or gym) to simulated home environment.

---

diseases are known to create a burden of illness on patients as well as family members and caregivers.[20] Programs that encourage social participation and involvement of family members, friends, and caregivers are associated with improved health and well-being for both the patient and support partner in addition to improved patient compliance and continued exercise adherence after structured exercise programs are completed. A tai chi "buddies" program with combined classes for patients with Parkinson's disease and their support partner, usually a family member or friend, resulted in both the patient and support partner reporting improved physical, psychological, and social benefits.[12] Appendix 5A: Seated Tai Chi Sequence provides a sample tai chi exercise routine appropriate for patients unable to perform standing exercises because of joint pain, weakness, or balance issues. The routine emphasizes seated weight shifts, balance, flexibility, and strength training. The routine can be performed as part of an individual treatment session or a home exercise plan (HEP), or in a group setting to facilitate socialization.

Seated Yoga

The practice of yoga was developed in India as a means of connecting the physical, mental, and spiritual body. There are many different styles of yoga. Most combine a sequence of physical postures (called asanas) and controlled respirations (the practice called pranayama) that emphasize alignment, flexibility, strength, balance, and breath awareness. The benefits of yoga exercise have been shown in a variety of patient conditions.[21–26] Appendix 5B: Seated Yoga Sequence for Late Parkinson's Disease, provides a sample seated yoga exercise routine designed to improve a patient's posture, flexibility, and core stability. The routine can be performed as part of an individual treatment session or HEP, or in a group setting to facilitate socialization.

Outcome Measures of Sitting Ability

It is important to use standardized outcome measures to document the patient's sitting ability and outcomes of the plan of care. Some measures are disability specific, for example, the *Mobility Scale for Acute Stroke Patients,*[27] and the *Postural Assessment for Stroke Patients.*[28,29] Others are generic and in general use; one of the most commonly used measures in rehabilitation is the *Functional Independence Measure.*[30,31] In evaluating which instruments to use, it is important to understand the parameters being measured, which can include:

- *Descriptive parameters:* the patient's level of dependence or independence (the amount of assistance the patient requires); difficulty, fatigue, or pain; fluctuations by time of day; level of medication; environmental influences
- *Quantitative parameters:* the amount of time the patient is able to maintain the sitting posture and the time required to complete an activity in sitting (e.g., trunk or extremity movements)
- *Qualitative parameters:* steadiness in maintaining posture; steadiness in response to altering the BOS; use of handhold support to maintain posture; ease in weight shifting and extremity movements; overall coordination of movements; ability to accept challenges and maintain posture

Table 5.1 presents standardized outcome measures of sitting ability.

Student Practice Activities

The Student Practice Activities in Box 5.8 focus on task analysis of sitting. Student Practice Activities in Box 5.9 focus on techniques and strategies to improve sitting and sitting balance control. Student Practice Activities in Box 5.10 present selected clinical problems and patient data and require students to practice clinical decision-making regarding the interventions.

(text continues on page 120)

TABLE 5.1 Outcome Measures of Sitting Ability

Measure	Specific Items
Berg Balance Test (BBT)[32–35]	Sit-to-stand Sitting unsupported
Trunk Control Test[36]	Sitting edge of bed Feet off floor Supine-to-sit
Duke Mobility Skills Profile[37]	Sitting unsupported Sitting reach to take object Rising from chair Bed-to-chair
Trunk Impairment Scale[38]	Static sitting Lateral lean Lateral pelvic tilt Trunk rotation
Postural Assessment for Stroke Patients (PASS)[28,29]	Sitting without support, feet on floor Supine-to-sit Sit-to-supine Sit-to-stand Stand-to-sit
Mobility Scale for Acute Stroke Patients[27]	Supine-to-sit Sitting unsupported Sit-to-stand
Fugl-Meyer Assessment-Balance Subscale[39–41]	Sitting unsupported
Rivermead Mobility Index[42,43]	Supine-to-sit Sitting unsupported Sit-to-stand
Motor Assessment Scale[44]	UE activities in supported sitting
Modified Functional Reach[45]	Distance of forward reach in sitting
Performance Oriented Mobility Assessment-Balance Subscale (POMA)[46]	UE activities in supported sitting Distance of forward reach in sitting
Function in Sitting Test (FIST)[47]	Static sit Reach forward Pick item up off floor Lateral reach with uninvolved UE Lateral reach with involved UE Pick up item from behind with uninvolved UE Sit with eyes closed Anterior nudge Posterior nudge Anterior scooting Lateral nudge Pick up item from behind with involved UE Lift involved foot off floor Posterior scooting (2 in.) Lateral scooting (2 in.) Shake head "no"

(table continues on page 118)

TABLE 5.1 Outcome Measures of Sitting Ability *(continued)*

Measure	Specific Items
Functional Independence Measure (FIM)[30,31]	Bathing Dressing Toileting Transfers: bed chair, wheelchair, toilet, tub, shower
Barthel Index[48,49]	Bathing Dressing Toilet transfers Bed-to-chair transfers

---

BOX 5.8 STUDENT PRACTICE ACTIVITY

Task Analysis of Sitting

OBJECTIVE: To provide practice opportunities for developing skill in task analysis of sitting

EQUIPMENT NEEDS: Adjustable-height platform mat or treatment table and a dome-shaped wobble board

DIRECTIONS: Work in groups of two or three. Begin by having each person in the group sit on the mat, first in short-sitting (knees flexed, feet flat on the floor) and then in long-sitting (knees extended). Then have each person practice weight shifts to the LOS in both postures. Finally, have each person sit on a dome-shaped wobble board placed on a hard sitting surface. Have each person practice sitting centered on the board (no tilts); then have each person sit on the wobble board with reduced BOS (one leg crossed over the other; sitting on a high seat without contact of the feet on the floor).

OBSERVE AND DOCUMENT: Using the following questions as a guide, observe and record the variations and similarities observed among the different sitting patterns represented in the group.

▲ What is the person's normal sitting alignment?
▲ What changes are noted between short- and long-sitting postures?
▲ During weight shifts exploring LOS, are the shifts symmetrical in each direction?
▲ When sitting on a wobble board, how successful is the person at maintaining centered alignment on the board (without touch-down support)? What is the position of the UEs? What changes are noted when one leg is crossed over the other? When both feet are off the ground using a high seat?
▲ What types of pathology/impairments might affect a patient's ability to sit?
▲ What compensatory strategies might be necessary?
▲ What environmental factors might constrain or impair sitting? What modifications are needed?

BOX 5.9 STUDENT PRACTICE ACTIVITY

Techniques and Strategies to Improve Sitting and Sitting Balance Control

▲ Sitting, holding
  • Stabilizing reversals
  • Rhythmic stabilization
▲ Sitting, weight shifts, cone stacking
▲ Sitting, weight shifts, dynamic reversals
▲ Sitting, application of PNF UE patterns, using dynamic reversals
  • Chop and reverse chop
  • Lift and reverse lift
  • Bilateral symmetrical thrust and withdrawal
  • Bilateral symmetrical flex/abdomen (abd)/external rotation (ER), rhythmic initiation
▲ Sitting, manual perturbations

▲ Sitting, ball activities
  • Pelvic shifts (anterior-posterior, side to side, pelvic clock)
  • UE lifts (unilateral, bilateral symmetrical, bilateral asymmetrical, reciprocal with marching)
  • LE lifts (hip flexion, knee extension, with ankle circles or writing letters, side steps, heel lifts, toe-offs)
  • Head and trunk rotation (lateral rotations, diagonal rotations)
  • Marching in place (contralateral UE and LE lifts)
  • Jumping jacks (bouncing with UE lifts overhead)
  • Catching and throwing a ball (inflated ball, weighted ball); batting a balloon
  • Kicking a rolling ball

BOX 5.9 STUDENT PRACTICE ACTIVITY (continued)

▲ Dual-task activities: simultaneously sitting on the ball and pouring a glass of water; counting backward from 100 by 7s
▲ Scooting in short-sitting or in long-sitting, assisted
▲ Scooting off a high table into modified standing

OBJECTIVE: To provide practice opportunities for developing skill in interventions designed to improve sitting and sitting balance control.

EQUIPMENT NEEDS: Platform mat, treatment table, therapy balls, cones, balloons, water pitcher, and glass

DIRECTIONS: Working in groups of four to six students, consider each entry in the section outline. Members of the group will assume different roles (described below) and will rotate roles each time the group progresses to a new item on the outline.

▲ One person assumes the role of therapist (for demonstrations) and participates in discussion.
▲ One person serves as the patient (for demonstrations) and participates in discussion.
▲ The remaining members participate in discussion and provide supportive feedback during demonstrations. One member of this group should be designated as a fact-checker to return to the text content to confirm elements of the discussion (if needed) or if agreement cannot be reached.

Thinking aloud, brainstorming, and sharing thoughts should be continuous throughout this activity! Carry out the following activities for each item in the section outline

1. Discuss the *activity,* including patient and therapist positioning. Consider what positional changes could enhance the activity (e.g., prepositioning a limb, hand placements to alter the BOS).
2. Discuss the *technique,* including its description, indication(s) for use, therapist hand placements (manual contacts), and VCs.
3. Demonstrate the activity and application of the technique by the designated therapist and patient. Discussion during the demonstration should be continuous (the demonstration should not be the sole responsibility of the designated therapist and patient). All group members should provide recommendations, suggestions, and supportive feedback throughout the demonstration. During the demonstrations, discuss strategies to make the activity either *more* or *less* challenging.

If any member of the group feels he or she requires practice with the activity and technique, the group should allocate time to accommodate the request. All group members providing input (recommendations, suggestions, and supportive feedback) should also accompany this practice.

BOX 5.10 STUDENT PRACTICE ACTIVITY

Selecting Appropriate Interventions to Improve Sitting Control

OBJECTIVE: Based on selected clinical problems and patient data, practice clinical decision making skills by selecting appropriate therapeutic interventions for improving sitting control.

The significant findings from a physical therapy examination are presented for each case.

Case 1: Patient With Traumatic Bilateral Transfemoral Amputations Secondary to a Motor Vehicle Accident

ROM: BLE hip ext -0-5
Manual Muscle Test: BLE gluteus maximus 3+/5, gluteus medius 3+/5, I abdominals 3/5
Posture: Anterior pelvic tilt with excessive lumbar lordosis
Balance: Modified Functional Reach Test = 7 inches
Function: Patient demonstrates multiplanar instability in sitting. Progress with prosthetic gait training is impeded by strength, ROM, postural, and balance deficits.

INTERVENTIONS:
1.
2.
3.

DIRECTIONS: Based on the clinical information provided, select and list three appropriate therapeutic interventions for that patient. Interventions chosen should be those that would be employed during the first three therapy sessions.

Case 2: Patient With Stroke (Right Cerebrovascular Accident)
ROM: Left (L) shoulder ER 0°–5°, abd 0°–50°; L hip ER 0°–5°, abd 0°–15°
Manual Muscle Test: L shoulder ER 3/5, abd 3/5; L gluteus maximus 3/5
Posture: L shoulder subluxation with flexor add spasticity; L hip internal rotation (IR) and add spasticity
Balance: Function in Sitting Test = 2/4 reach forward, 0/4 pick item up off the floor, 1/4 lateral reach with involved UE
Function: Lateral instability and slumped to L side with eating

INTERVENTIONS:
1.
2.
3.

(box continues on page 120)

BOX 5.10 STUDENT PRACTICE ACTIVITY (continued)

Case 3: Patient Is an Active Duty Army Soldier Who Suffered Second- and Third-Degree Burns Over 70% of His Body From an Improvised Explosive Device. Currently Intubated With Supplemental Oxygen

ROM: BUE, BLE, and trunk present with significant ROM limitations throughout.
Manual Muscle Test: Soleus 3+/5, biceps femoris 3+/5, gluteus maximus 3+/5
Posture: Forward flexed spine
Balance: Berg Balance Test = 0/4 transfer sitting to standing and 0/4 sitting unsupported, feet on floor
Function: Decreased intercostal chest expansion, decreased tidal volume, and poor secretion clearance

INTERVENTIONS:
1.
2.
3.

Case 4. Patient With Parkinson's Disease

ROM: BUE shoulder flex 0°–110°, ER 0°–20°, BLE straight leg raise 0°–70°, hip IR 0°–10°, ER 0°–20°
Manual Muscle Test: Erector spinae strength 2/5
Posture: Functional kyphosis, sacral sitting
Balance: Barthel Index = feeding 5/10, grooming 0/5, dressing 5/10
Function: Decreased trunk rotation, lack of head trunk dissociation; moderate assist sitting at edge of bed to put on socks and shoes; unable to put on seatbelt independently

INTERVENTIONS:
1.
2.
3.

Key: abd, abduction; add, adduction; BLEs, both lower extremities; BUEs, both upper extremities; ext, extension; ER, external rotation; flex, flexion; IR, internal rotation; L, left; R, right.

SUMMARY

This chapter has presented the requirements for sitting and sitting balance control. Interventions that promote static and dynamic control as well as reactive, anticipatory, and adaptive balance skills have been addressed. Ensuring patient safety while progressively challenging control using a variety of exercises and activities is key to improving functional performance.

Sound clinical decision-making will help identify the most appropriate activities and techniques to improve sitting and sitting balance skills for an individual patient. Many of the interventions presented in this chapter will provide the foundation for developing a home exercise plan (HEP) to improve function. Although some of the interventions described clearly require the skilled intervention of a physical therapist, many can be modified or adapted for inclusion in a HEP for use by the patient (self-management strategies), family members, or others who are participating in the patient's care.

REFERENCES

1. Levangie, P, and Norkin, C. Joint Structure & Function, ed 5. Philadelphia, F.A. Davis, 2011.
2. Neumann, D. Kinesiology of the Musculoskeletal System, ed 2. St. Louis, Mosby Elsevier Science, 2009.
3. Schmidt, R, and Lee, T. Motor Control and Learning: A Behavioral Emphasis, ed 5. Champaign, IL, Human Kinetics, 2011.
4. Magill, R. Motor Learning and Control: Concepts and Applications, ed 9. New York, McGraw-Hill, 2011.
5. Wulf, G. Attentional focus and motor learning: a review of 15 years. Int Rev Sport Exer Psychol, 2013; 6:77.
6. Sturmberg, C, et al. Attentional focus of feedback and instructions in treatment of musculoskeletal dysfunction: a systematic review. Manual Ther, 2013; 18:458.
7. Shumway-Cook, A, and Woollacott, M. Motor Control—Translating Research Into Clinical Practice, ed 4. Baltimore, Lippincott Williams & Wilkins, 2012.
8. Schenkman, M, et al. Exercise to improve spinal flexibility and function for people with Parkinson's disease: a randomized, controlled trial. J Am Geriatr Soc, 1998; 46:1207–1216.
9. Hass, C, et al. Concurrent improvements in cardiorespiratory and muscle fitness in response to total body recumbent stepping in humans. Eur J Appl Physiol, 2001; 85:157–163.
10. Page, S, et al. Resistance-based, reciprocal upper and lower limb locomotor training in chronic stroke: a randomized, controlled crossover study. Clin Rehabil, 2008; 22:610–617.
11. The Consortium of Academic Health Centers for Integrative Medicine. About us. Retrieved on July 6, 2014, www.imconsortium.org/about/home.html.
12. Klein, P, and Rivers, L. Tai chi for individuals with Parkinson's disease and their support partners: program evaluation. J Neurol Phys Ther, 2006; 30:22–27.
13. Raub, J. Psychophysiologic effects of hatha yoga on musculoskeletal and cardiopulmonary function: a literature review. J Altern Complement Med, 2002; 8:797–812.
14. Wang, C, Collet, J, and Lau, J. The effect of tai chi on health outcomes in patients with chronic conditions: a systematic review. Arch Internal Med, 2004; 164:493–501.
15. Hackney, M, and Earhart, G. Tai chi improves balance and mobility in people with Parkinson's disease. Gait Posture, 2008; 28:456–460.
16. Hackney, M, et al. Effects of tango on functional mobility in Parkinson's disease: a preliminary study. J Neurol Phys Ther, 2007; 31:173–179.
17. Li, F, et al. Tai chi-based exercise for older adults with Parkinson's disease: a pilot-program evaluation. J Aging Phys Act, 2007; 15:139–151.
18. Esch, T, et al. Mind/body techniques for physiological and psychological stress reduction: stress management via tai chi training—a pilot study. Med Sci Monit, 2007; 13:CR488–CR497.
19. Ghaffari, B, and Kluger, B. Mechanisms for alternative treatments in Parkinson's disease: acupuncture, tai chi, and other treatments. Curr Neurol Neurosci Rep, 2014; 14:451.
20. Hodgson, J, Garcia, K, and Tyndall, L. Parkinson's disease and the couple relationship: a qualitative analysis. Fam Syst Health, 2004; 22:101.
21. Ebnezar, J, et al. Effect of an integrated approach of yoga therapy on quality of life in osteoarthritis of the knee joint: a randomized control study. Int J Yoga, 2011; 4:55–63.
22. Ebnezar, J, et al. Effect of integrated yoga therapy on pain, morning stiffness and anxiety in osteoarthritis of the knee joint: a randomized control study. Int J Yoga, 2012; 5:28–36.

23. Ebnezar, J, et al. Effects of an integrated approach of hatha yoga therapy on functional disability, pain, and flexibility in osteoarthritis of the knee joint: a randomized controlled study. J Altern Complement Med, 2012; 18:463–472.

24. Garfinkel, M, et al. Yoga-based intervention for carpal tunnel syndrome: a randomized trial. JAMA, 1998; 280:1601–1603.

25. Evans, S, et al. Impact of iyengar yoga on quality of life in young women with rheumatoid arthritis. Clin J Pain, 2013; 29:988–997.

26. Tekur, P, et al. Effect of short-term intensive yoga program on pain, functional disability and spinal flexibility in chronic low back pain: a randomized control study. J Altern Complement Med, 2008; 14:637–644.

27. Simondson, J, Goldie, P, and Greenwood, K. The mobility scale for acute stroke patients: concurrent validity. Clin Rehabil, 2003; 17:558–564.

28. Benaim, C, et al. Validation of a standardized assessment of postural control in stroke patients: the Postural Assessment Scale for Stroke Patients (PASS). Stroke, 1999; 30:1862.

29. Pyoria, O, et al. Validity of the postural control and balance for stroke test. Physiother Res Int, 2007; 12:162.

30. Guide for the Uniform Data Set for Medical Rehabilitation (Adult FIM), Version 4.0, Buffalo, NY, State University of New York, 1993.

31. Dodds, T, et al. A validation of the Functional Independence Measurement and its performance among rehabilitation in-patients. Arch Phys Med Rehabil, 1993; 74:531.

32. Berg, K, et al. Measuring balance in the elderly: preliminary development of an instrument. Physiother Can, 1989; 41:304.

33. Berg, K, et al. Measuring balance in the elderly: validation of an instrument. Can J Public Health, 1992; 83:S7.

34. Berg, K, Wood-Dauphinee, S, and Williams, J. The balance scale: reliability assessment with elderly residents and patients with an acute stroke. Scand J Rehabil Med, 1999; 27:27.

35. Blum, L, and Korner-Bitensky, N. Usefulness of the Berg Balance Scale in stroke rehabilitation: a systematic review. Phys Ther, 2008; 88:559–566.

36. Hsieh, C, et al. Trunk control as an early predictor of comprehensive activities of daily living function in stroke patients. Stroke, 2002; 33:2626–2630.

37. Duncan, P. Duke Mobility Skills profile. Durham, NC, Center for Human Aging, Duke University; 1989.

38. Verheyden, G, Nieuwboer, A, Mertin, J. The Trunk Impairment Scale: a new tool to measure motor impairment of the trunk after stroke. Clin Rehabil, 2004; 18:326–334.

39. Fugl-Meyer, A, et al. The post-stroke hemiplegic patient: a method for evaluation and performance. Scand J Rehabil Med, 1975; 7:13.

40. Fugl-Meyer, A. Post-stroke hemiplegia assessment of physical properties. Scand J Rehabil Med, 1980; 63:85.

41. Gladstone, D, Danells, C, and Black, S. The Fugl-Myer assessment of motor recovery after stroke: a critical review of its measurement properties. Neurorehabil Neural Repair, 2002; 16:232.

42. Collen, F, et al. The Rivermead Mobility Index: a further development of the Rivermead Motor Assessment. Int Disabil Stud, 1991; 13:50–54.

43. Duncan, P, Jorgensen, H, and Wade, D. Outcome measures in acute stroke trials: a systematic review and some recommendations to improve practice. Stroke, 2000; 31:1429–1438.

44. Carr, J, et al. Investigation of a new motor assessment scale for stroke patients. Phys Ther, 1985; 65:175–180.

45. Tsang, Y, and Mak, M. Sit-and-reach test can predict mobility of patients recovering from acute stroke. Arch Phy Med Rehabil, 2004; 85:94–98.

46. Tinetti, M. Performance-oriented assessment of mobility problems in elderly patients. J Am Geriatr Soc, 1986; 34:119.

47. Gorman, S, et al. Development and validation of the Function in Sitting Test in adults with acute stroke. J Neurol Phys Ther, 2010; 34:150–160.

48. Granger, C, et al. Stroke rehabilitation analysis of repeated Barthel Index measures. Arch Phys Med Rehabil, 1979; 60:14.

49. Mahoney, F, and Barthel, D. Functional evaluation: The Barthel Index. Maryland State Med J, 1965; 14:61.

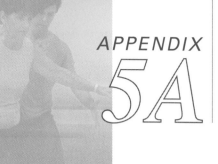
Seated Tai Chi Sequence

Preparation

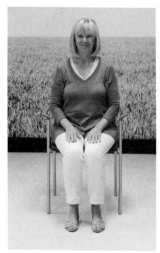

Start perch sitting (body at front of chair), sitting tall and relaxed with feet together.

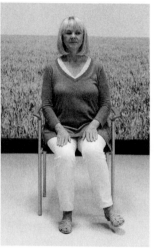

Shift weight right and step left leg out to side.

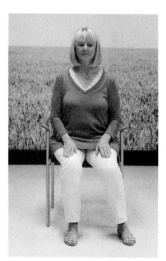

Sit with feet shoulder width apart.

Raise Hands

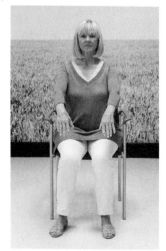

With soft arms leading with wrists, arms float up.

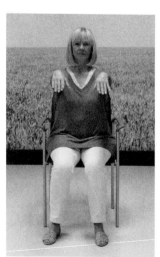

Hands rise to shoulder height.

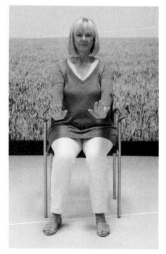

Hands float down to rest on thighs.

Hold Ball

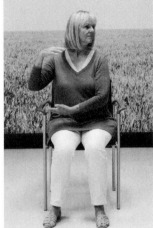 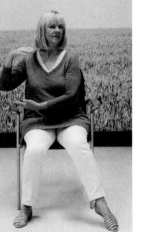 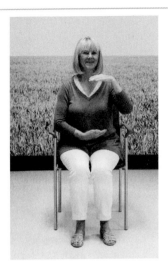

Hold ball on right with slight trunk rotation to right. Look left.

Step left leading with toe.

Step right foot in. Hold ball on left.

Repeat Hold Ball Sequence to Opposite Side

Part the Wild Horse's Mane

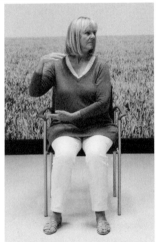 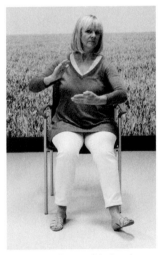 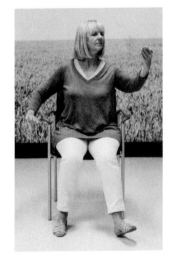

Hold ball on right with slight trunk rotation to right. Look left.

Step left leading with heel. Hands pass over one another as if parting a horse's mane.

Continue to flow arms apart and shift left.

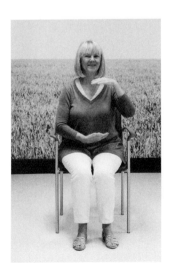

Step right foot in. Hold ball on left.

Repeat Part the Wild Horse's Mane Sequence to Opposite Side

(continues on page 124)

Single Whip

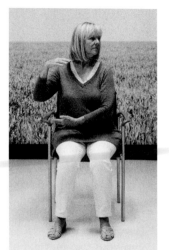

Hold ball on right with slight trunk rotation to right. Look left.

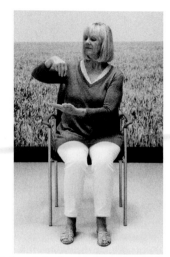

Relax right hand downward, fingertips touching thumb.

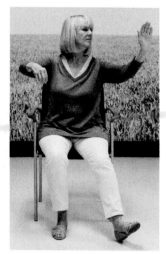

Lift weight from left heel and pivot on ball of foot while extending right arm out to side. Step to left and sweep left hand (palm in) across face, rotate palm away from face and extend left arm.

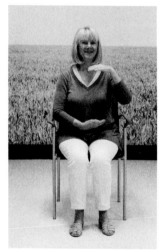

Step right foot in. Hold ball on left.

Repeat Single Whip Sequence to Opposite Side

Closing Position

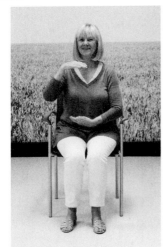

Hold ball on right. Feet shoulder width apart.

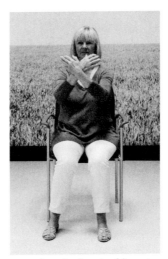

Cross wrists in front of heart, palms facing in.

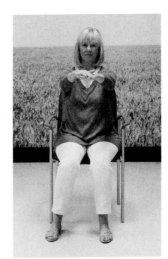

Uncross wrists extending elbows.

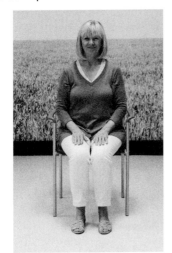

Arms float down with palms resting on thighs. Step in and sit tall and relaxed.

Developed by Edward W Bezkor, DPT, OCS, MTC. Adapted from Li, F. Transforming traditional Tai Ji Quan techniques into integrative movement therapy—tai ji quan: moving for better balance. J Sport Health Sci, 2014;3(1): 9–15.

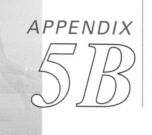

APPENDIX

5B

Seated Yoga Sequence for Late Parkinson's Disease

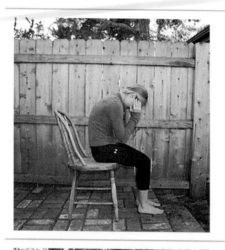

Chair Cat Pose (Marjaryasana)

1. Start perch sitting (body at front of chair), sitting tall and hands on the side of your head.
2. As you exhale, round your spine toward the back of the chair, bring your shoulders and head forward while bringing your elbows together. Hold for 5 seconds.

Chair Cow Pose (Bitilasana)

As you inhale, arch your back and look up to the sky. Open your chest and spread your elbows wide. Hold for 5 seconds.

Chair Gate Pose (Parighasana)

1. Start sitting tall with your right hand on the chair and left arm raised to the sky, palm facing in.
2. Inhale deeply.
3. As you exhale, side-bend your torso to the right and look up to your left hand. Hold for 5 seconds.
4. Repeat on the opposite side.

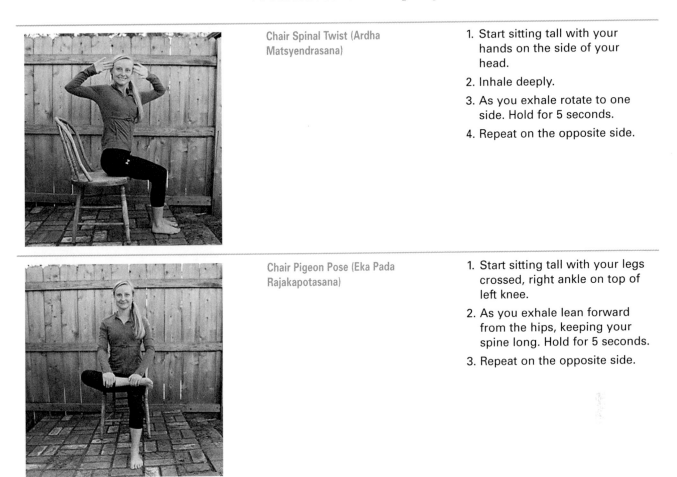

Chair Spinal Twist (Ardha Matsyendrasana)

1. Start sitting tall with your hands on the side of your head.
2. Inhale deeply.
3. As you exhale rotate to one side. Hold for 5 seconds.
4. Repeat on the opposite side.

Chair Pigeon Pose (Eka Pada Rajakapotasana)

1. Start sitting tall with your legs crossed, right ankle on top of left knee.
2. As you exhale lean forward from the hips, keeping your spine long. Hold for 5 seconds.
3. Repeat on the opposite side.

Developed by Edward W Bezkor, DPT, OCS, MTC. Adapted from yoga asanas by Yogi Swatmarama, compiler of the Hatha Yoga Pradipika in 15th century CE." Reference: *Hatha Yoga Pradipika*. Yoga Publications Trust, 2000, ISBN 978-81-85787-38-1

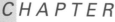

6

Interventions to Improve Intermediate Trunk and Hip Control: Kneeling and Half-Kneeling Skills

THOMAS J. SCHMITZ, PT, PhD

This chapter focuses on interventions to improve intermediate trunk and hip control using kneeling postures. Kneeling offers the benefit of achieving improved trunk and hip control without the demands required to control the knee and ankle. Inherent to these upright, antigravity postures are important prerequisite requirements for standing. For example, kneeling postures are particularly useful for developing initial upright postural control and for promoting hip extension and abduction stabilization control required for standing. By eliminating the demands of upright standing, patient anxiety and fear of falling are typically diminished. Kneeling activities also provide important lead-up skills for independent floor-to-standing transfers.

The postures addressed in this chapter are *kneeling* (Fig. 6.1A) and *half-kneeling* (Fig. 6.1B). In kneeling, both hips are extended, with bilateral weightbearing occurring primarily at the knees and upper tibia, with the legs and feet resting on the support surface. This creates a wider base of support (BOS) than that seen in standing but not as wide as

seen in half-kneeling. In half-kneeling, one hip remains extended, with weightbearing at the knee and upper leg; the opposite hip and knee are flexed to approximately 90 degrees, with weightbearing occurring at the foot placed forward on the supporting surface. In kneeling postures, height of the center of mass (COM) is intermediate.

Clinical Note: Patients with significant cerebellar dysfunction and ataxia (e.g., the patient with traumatic brain injury [TBI] or cerebellar degeneration) benefit from practice in these more stable postures. For these patients, kneeling and half-kneeling are functionally important as transitional activities in preparation for upright standing.

Kneeling

In kneeling, the COM is intermediate; it is higher than in supine or prone positions and lower than in standing. The BOS is influenced by the relative length of the leg and foot and is positioned largely posterior to the COM. Thus, this

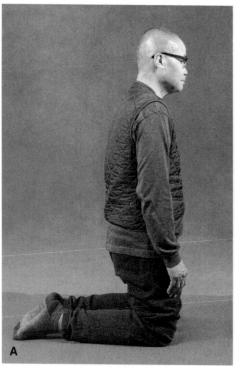
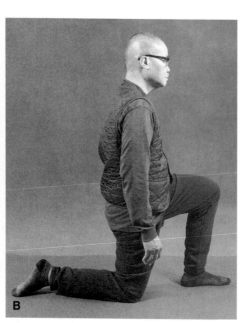

FIGURE 6.1 (A) Kneeling posture. Both hips are extended, with bilateral weightbearing on the knees and legs; the BOS is narrow. (B) Half-kneeling posture. One hip is extended, with weightbearing on the knee and leg. The opposite hip and knee are flexed to approximately 90 degrees with slight abduction; the foot is forward and placed flat on the support surface. The BOS is wide and angled on a diagonal between the posterior and anterior limbs.

posture is more stable posteriorly than anteriorly. Owing to this relative anterior instability, trunk and hip extensors must compensate for any forward shift in the COM. This is an important safety issue: If the patient does not have the ability to compensate (e.g., has trunk and hip extensor weakness), anterior displacement may cause the patient to fall forward.

Kneeling involves head, trunk, and hip muscles for upright postural control. The head and trunk are maintained vertically in midline orientation with normal spinal lumbar and thoracic curves. The pelvis is level in horizontal orientation. Weightbearing in kneeling is through the hips and on the knees and legs. Both hips are extended with the knees flexed to approximately 90 degrees. This position represents an advanced lower extremity (LE) pattern (initiated during bridging) of hip extension with knee flexion required for gait (i.e., terminal phase of stance).

General Characteristics

- The relatively low COM (compared with standing) makes kneeling a safe posture for initially promoting upright trunk and hip control. If the patient inadvertently loses control, the distance to the mat is small; with contact guarding from the therapist, a fall would be unlikely to result in injury.
- Compared with standing, the degrees of freedom are reduced. In kneeling, control of the knee or foot and ankle is not required to maintain upright trunk and hip control.
- Prolonged positioning in kneeling provides strong inhibitory influences (inhibitory pressure on patellar tendon) acting bilaterally on the quadriceps. It is therefore a useful intervention to dampen hypertonicity for patients with LE extensor spasticity.
- Owing to the inherent inhibitory influences of the posture, kneeling may be an important intervention to immediately precede standing and gait activities for the patient with LE extensor spasticity and a scissoring gait pattern.

📁 **Clinical Notes:**

- Patients with strong abnormal flexor synergy influence (e.g., the patient with stroke) will have difficulty maintaining the hip in extension; the tendency will be to recruit hip flexors with knee flexors. In this situation, the therapist may use manually guided (active assistive) movement to assist with hip extension.
- For the patient whose foot pulls strongly into dorsiflexion when positioned in kneeling, a small pillow or towel roll may be placed under the dorsum of the foot to relieve pressure on the toes.
- For the patient with limitations in plantarflexion range of motion (ROM), the ankle/foot may be positioned over the edge of a platform mat.
- Patients who experience knee discomfort and knee pain from prolonged positioning may benefit from kneeling on a more resilient surface such as folded towels or a high-density foam cushion placed under both

knees. An alternative is to incorporate several shorter time intervals in kneeling over the course of a treatment session to avoid or reduce the discomfort.

⊘ **Red Flag:** Kneeling may be contraindicated in some patients, such as those who have rheumatoid arthritis or osteoarthritis affecting the knee, patients with knee joint instability, or patients recovering from recent knee surgery.

Prerequisite Requirements

Before using kneeling exercises, the therapist must consider several important requirements for assuming the posture. Hip extension ROM is necessary; if limitations exist (e.g., hip flexion contractures), the patient's ability to achieve the needed hip extension will be compromised. Sufficient strength of the trunk and hip extensor muscles is necessary to keep the head and trunk upright and the hips extended. This is particularly important given the relative anterior instability inherent in the posture. Although kneeling provides an important opportunity for improving posture and balance control, adequate stability (static postural control) is needed for initial maintenance of the upright posture.

Interventions to Improve Intermediate Trunk and Hip Control in Kneeling

Kneeling: Assist-to-Position

Assist-to-position movement transitions (physical assistance provided by therapist) into kneeling can be effectively accomplished from a heel-sitting position with the patient's hands resting on a ball in front (Fig. 6.2A). The therapist is positioned behind the patient to assist with movement into hip extension with application of approximation force once in upright kneeling (Fig. 6.2B). Alternatively, the patient and therapist may both be positioned heel-sitting facing each other. Therapist hand placements are on the posterior upper trunk passing under the axilla and on the contralateral posterior hip/pelvis, allowing the therapist to assist with lifting the trunk into the upright position as well as with moving the patient's hips toward extension. The patient's hands may be supported on the therapist's shoulders, which assist in guiding the upper trunk in the desired direction of movement. The verbal cue (VC) is *"Lift up, bring your hips forward and move up into kneeling."*

Kneeling: Holding

Early interventions typically focus on stability (static postural control). Recall that static postural control is the ability to maintain (hold) a posture with the COM over the BOS with the body at rest (no motion). The patient is kneeling, actively holding the posture. Initially, attention is directed toward postural alignment. The head and trunk are upright (vertical) and symmetrical (midline orientation) with normal spinal lumbar and thoracic curves; the pelvis is level. Both hips are extended with the knees flexed to approximately 90 degrees. Symmetrical weightbearing occurs at the knees

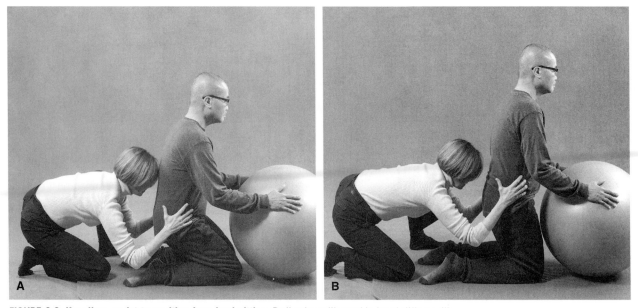

FIGURE 6.2 Kneeling, assist-to-position from heel-sitting Patient positioned in heel-sitting with hands supported on a ball in front. (A) Therapist assists movement transition from behind with (B) application of approximation force (stability) once posture is assumed.

positioned in a comfortable kneeling base width (i.e., distance between knees). The legs and feet are supported posteriorly on the mat surface; the ankles are plantarflexed.

To promote stability in kneeling, the therapist may guard from a half-kneeling position facing the patient. Manual contacts (MCs) are used as required to guard or to assist if initial holding of the posture is difficult. Effective hand placements include the posterior upper trunk passing under the axilla and on the contralateral posterior hip/pelvis. Alternatively, each of the therapist's hands may be cupped around the lateral aspect of the pelvis on both sides. The patient's hands may be supported on the therapist's shoulders. If the therapist is guarding from behind with MCs on the pelvis, the patient's hands may be resting on a ball in front (see Fig. 6.2B). As control increases, MCs are removed. The patient's bilateral hand placement on the therapist's shoulders (or ball) is reduced from bilateral to unilateral and then to touch-down support as needed. For touch-down support, the therapist continues half-kneeling in front of the patient with elbows flexed, forearms supinated, and hands open to provide support as needed while postural stability is established (a ball in front can also be used for touch-down support). VCs are used to encourage holding the position and promote upright postural alignment and even weight distribution (*"Hold; keep your head and trunk upright and weight evenly distributed on knees"*).

Clinical Note: During initial holding in kneeling, the patient with weakness and instability may benefit from using upper extremity (UE) support. As mentioned, this can be accomplished using a ball or by vertically positioning a small bolster (or stool) in front

of the patient for weightbearing support on the forearms or hands (shoulders flexed and elbows extended). Alternatively, the patient's hands can be placed on a large ball positioned in front for support (Table 6.1, Fig. 1) or on bolsters (or stools) placed on each side of the patient. A wall or wall ladder next to a mat can also be used effectively for this purpose.

Applying Resistance to Promote Stability

The proprioceptive neuromuscular facilitation (PNF) technique of stabilizing (isometric) reversals can be used to promote stability. Resistance is applied to opposing muscle groups within a relatively static kneeling posture.

The patient is asked to maintain the kneeling position as resistance is applied to small-range isotonic contractions alternating between agonist and antagonist muscle groups (Fig. 6.3). Only very limited movement is allowed, progressing to stabilizing (holding) in the posture. The MCs shift throughout the application of this technique. The manual input should always be a combination of resistance with approximation or resistance with traction. To promote stability, the linear resistance is less with the approximation or traction being the primary input. Resistance is typically applied first in the stronger direction of movement (agonists) until the patient's maximum is reached. Once the patient is fully resisting with agonists, one hand continues to resist while the opposite hand is positioned to resist the antagonists. When the antagonists begin to engage, the other hand is also moved to resist antagonists. The goal is sustained holding.[1] The VCs are used to indicate the direction of resistance (*"Hold, don't let me push you backward, hold"*) and a change in direction with a transitional cue (*"Now don't let me pull you forward"*).

TABLE 6.1 Ball Activities to Enhance Posture and Balance Control in Kneeling

A. Static Postural Holding
Focus is on postural alignment and even weight distribution during active holding while maintaining the COM over BOS). Hands are resting on ball in front (start position) and knees are in symmetrical stance position (Fig. 1).

B. Weight Shifting
For medial/lateral weight shifting in kneeling, the patient actively shifts the pelvis from side-to-side. Anterior/posterior shifts are accomplished by rolling the ball forward (Fig. 2) and backward. For diagonal shifts, the knees are in a step position. Progression is from small to larger ranges (increments in ROM), and finally to full ROM.

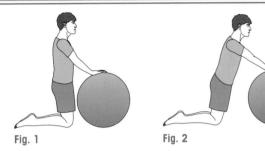

Fig. 1   Fig. 2

C. Static Dynamic Control
This activity requires maintaining the kneeling posture with reduced extremity support. It begins with freeing a single UE (Fig. 3) or LE with progression to simultaneously freeing one UE and one LE (Fig. 4).

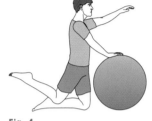

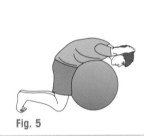

Fig. 3   Fig. 4

D. Trunk Extension
From kneeling, the trunk is flexed forward to rest on the ball with hands placed behind the head (Fig. 5). The trunk is then extended (Fig. 6). If this activity initially proves too challenging, it can begin with hands placed on the ball, progressed to arms folded across chest, and finally to hands behind the head.

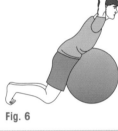

Fig. 5   Fig. 6

E. Hip and Knee Extension
From a kneeling position, the trunk is flexed forward with forearms resting on a ball (Fig. 7). The ball rolls forward slightly as the hips and knees are extended (Fig. 8). Initially feet and elbows are wide apart (large BOS) and progressively brought closer together (smaller BOS).

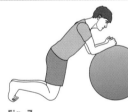
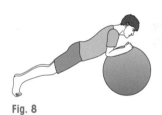

Fig. 7   Fig. 8

F. Trunk, Hip, Knee Extension (hands on ball)
From kneeling, the trunk is flexed forward on a ball with hands positioned to each side (Fig. 9). The elbows extend as the trunk, hips, and knees are extended (Fig. 10). Progression is from feet and hands apart (large BOS) to feet and hands closer together (smaller BOS) to elimination of UE support (see below).

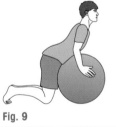
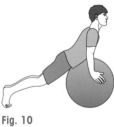

Fig. 9   Fig. 10

G. Trunk, Hip, Knee Extension (hands free)
From kneeling, the trunk is flexed forward on a ball with shoulders flexed and elbows extended (Fig. 11). The trunk, hips, and knees are then extended (Fig. 12). Alternatively, the arms may be held across chest, hands placed behind head, or holding a weighted wand grasped with both hands. The feet are initially apart and gradually brought closer together.

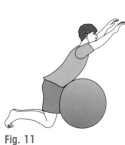
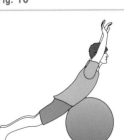

Fig. 11   Fig. 12

(table continues on page 132)

TABLE 6.1 Ball Activities to Enhance Posture and Balance Control in Kneeling *(continued)*

H. Forward Roll

This activity begins in kneeling with shoulders flexed, elbows extended, and fisted or clasped hands resting on ball in front (Fig. 13). As the ball is moved forward, the shoulders are further flexed and hips move toward extension (Fig. 14). Focus is on alignment and control of the trunk and pelvis. Progression utilizes increments in ROM advancing to full ROM as ball is moved farther away from body.

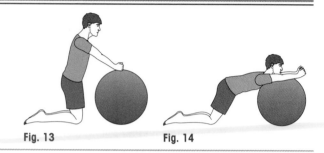

Fig. 13   **Fig. 14**

I. Kneeling on Ball

Beginning next to a wall or in the corner of a room, this activity first uses bilateral support with progression to unilateral UE support (Fig.15). Further progression is to using no UE support (Fig. 16), to active UE movements (unilateral to bilateral in multiple directions, e.g., balloon tapping), and then to resisted UE movements (e.g., holding a weight; unilateral [Fig. 17] to bilateral [Fig. 18]). Trunk rotation can be accomplished using a wand held across the shoulders (Fig. 19).

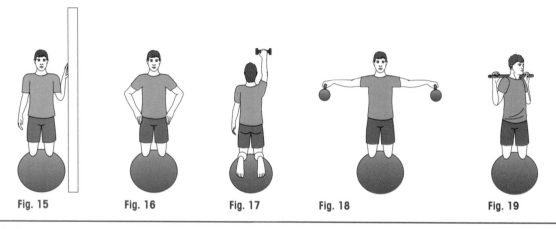

Fig. 15   **Fig. 16**   **Fig. 17**   **Fig. 18**   **Fig. 19**

Note: During activities in kneeling, elastic resistive bands placed around distal thighs will increase proprioceptive feedback and facilitate contraction of the lateral hip muscles (gluteus medius).

The PNF technique of rhythmic stabilization can also be used. The patient is asked to hold the kneeling position without moving (isometric contractions) as resistance is applied simultaneously to opposing muscle groups (e.g., upper trunk flexors and lower trunk extensors [Fig. 6.4] *or* upper trunk extensors and lower trunk flexors; trunk rotators are also activated). With bilateral MCs, resistance is built up gradually as the patient responds to the applied force. Although no movement occurs, resistance is applied as if twisting or rotating the upper and lower trunk in opposite directions. No relaxation occurs as the direction of resistance is changed. The goal is cocontraction of antagonists. The verbal cue is *"Don't let me move you, hold, hold; now don't let me move you the other way."*

Outcomes

Motor control goals: stability (static postural control)
Functional skill achieved: Patient is able to stabilize during upright kneeling

Comments

• During initial activities in kneeling, the patient with instability will benefit from additional support provided by placing hands on the therapist's shoulders or other supportive surface (e.g., therapy ball [see Fig. 1 in Table 6.1], small bolsters, or high stools).

• Elastic resistive bands can be placed around the distal thighs to increase proprioceptive input and facilitate contraction of the lateral hip muscles (gluteus medius).

• Light approximation can be given to the top of the shoulders or the pelvis to increase stabilizing response.

• The patient may be positioned with the knees in the step position (with one knee slightly in front of the other) and resistance applied on a diagonal.

• Kneeling is an important lead-up activity to upright stance in modified standing and standing.

Kneeling: Weight Shifting

Dynamic postural control (controlled mobility) allows for movement within a posture. Weight shifting in kneeling involves ongoing postural adjustments owing to displacement of the COM over the BOS. The knees (distal segment) are fixed while the pelvis (proximal segment) is moving. Joint approximation and stimulation of proprioceptors further enhance joint stabilization (cocontraction). Because the kneeling posture must be stabilized while moving, weight shifting improves dynamic balance. Ongoing postural adjustments become more automatic with practice.

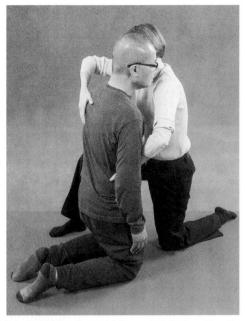

FIGURE 6.3 Stabilizing (isometric) reversals in kneeling The therapist's hands are positioned to apply approximation to the pelvis in a posterior/inferior direction while resisting and applying traction to scapula posterior depression with manual contact on the posterior/inferior/medial border of the scapula. Note that the posterior BOS is comparatively large. *Not shown:* The MCs can then be repositioned (1) to apply traction and resistance to anterior scapular depression; (2) to the UEs for resistance using any of the diagonal patterns; or (3) to the head/neck to promote stability throughout the trunk and the weightbearing extremities. Note that traction and approximation are the primary vectors of input through the MCs, and resistance is relatively light given the minimal anterior BOS.

Active reaching activities can be used to promote weight shifting in all directions or in the direction of instability (e.g., the patient with hemiplegia). The therapist provides a target (*"Reach out and touch my hand"*) or uses a functional task such as stacking cups or folding towels to promote reaching. With the hands on a large ball placed in front, the patient can also practice moving the ball forward and backward or diagonally (Table 6.1, Fig. 2), which is useful for patients requiring improved shoulder flexion ROM.

Applying Resistance to Promote Weight Shifting

The PNF technique of dynamic (isotonic) reversals can be used to provide resistance during weight shifting. The therapist is positioned in kneeling or half-kneeling directly or diagonally in front of patient. The MCs are on the pelvis. Movement may be assisted (guided) for several repetitions to ensure that the patient knows the desired movements. Relatively light resistance is used during weight shifting. Alternatively, MCs are on the pelvis/contralateral upper trunk or bilaterally on the upper trunk.

For medial/lateral weight shifts, as the patient shifts *away* from the therapist (positioned diagonally in front), resistance is applied to the side of the pelvis furthest from therapist. Without relaxation, movement is then reversed and resistance is applied to the side of the contralateral pelvis as the patient shifts *toward* the therapist. Verbal cues identify the direction of movement and alert the patient to an approaching change in direction. (*"Pull away from me; now, push back toward me."*) Dynamic (isotonic) reversals are used to increase strength and active ROM and to promote normal transitions between opposing muscle groups. A smooth reversal of motion is the goal.

For diagonal weight shifts, the patient is kneeling with the knees in step position (one knee is advanced in front of the other, simulating a step length). Resistance is applied to the pelvis as the patient shifts diagonally forward over the

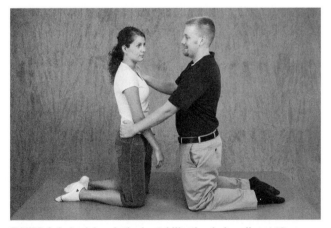

FIGURE 6.4 Applying rhythmic stabilization in kneeling MCs are on the anterior upper trunk/shoulder to resist the upper trunk flexors and rotators; the other hand is positioned on the posterior pelvis to resist the lower trunk extensors and rotators. *Not shown:* MCs are then reversed so that one hand is on the posterior upper trunk/shoulder to resist upper trunk extensors, and the other hand is on the contralateral anterior pelvis to resist lower trunk flexors.

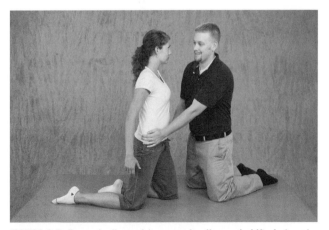

FIGURE 6.5 Dynamic (isotonic) reversals, diagonal shifts in kneeling In step position, the patient alternates between shifting weight diagonally over the forward knee (shown here) and backward over the posterior knee. Resistance is applied to active concentric movement in each direction without relaxation.

knee in front and then diagonally backward over the opposite knee (Fig. 6.5). The VC is *"Shift backward and away from me; now shift forward and toward me."*

For patients lacking control in pelvic rotation, the diagonal shifts are combined with rotation. The patient is kneeling with the knees in step position. Resistance is applied at the pelvis as the patient shifts weight diagonally forward onto the knee in front while rotating the pelvis forward on the opposite side. This is followed by a diagonal weight shift backward onto the posterior knee while rotating the pelvis backward. The VC is *"Shift forward and twist; now shift backward and twist."*

With some patients, the upper trunk may move forward (or backward) as the pelvis rotates forward (or backward), producing an ipsilateral trunk pattern. Having the patient cross the arms and support them on the therapist's shoulders will promote isolation of pelvic motion (Fig. 6.6). The patient is instructed to keep both elbows straight and move only the pelvis forward and backward during the weight shifts. The therapist's shoulder support for the crossed arms "locks" the upper trunk in place and promotes isolated pelvic motion. Alternatively, a wall adjacent to a platform mat may provide UE support.

Comments
- Weight shifting and pelvic rotation in kneeling are important lead-up skills for the weight transfers and pelvic motion needed for normal gait.
- Movements begin with small-range control and progress through increasing ROM (increments of ROM) to full-range control.
- If an imbalance of strength exists, resistance is applied first in the stronger direction of movement.
- Initially, movements are slow and controlled, with emphasis on careful grading of resistance.

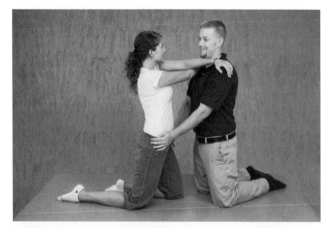

FIGURE 6.6 Dynamic (isotonic) reversals, diagonal shifts with pelvic rotation The patient shifts weight diagonally forward onto the knee in front while rotating the pelvis forward on the opposite side and then diagonally backward onto the posterior knee while rotating the pelvis backward. In this example, the patient's upper limbs are crossed, with hands supported on the therapist's shoulders and elbows extended to prevent movement of the upper trunk (dissociated from pelvic movement).

Outcomes
Motor control goal: dynamic postural control
Functional skill achieved: patient is able to weight shift independently in kneeling position

Movement Transitions: Heel-Sitting or Side-Sitting and Kneeling

Movement between heel-sitting or side-sitting and kneeling is an important lead-up activity for the patient with poor eccentric control who has difficulty sitting down slowly or going down stairs slowly. As with transitions between sitting and standing, forward trunk flexion (i.e., instructing the patient to lean forward) is important to ensure success in assuming the upright kneeling position. The therapist should encourage the patient to control lowering of the body slowly rather than "plopping" or collapsing down.

Applying Resistance to Promote Movement Transitions
Movement transitions are made from bilateral heel-sitting (buttocks make contact with the heels), up into the kneeling position, and reverse. The PNF technique of combination of isotonics (COI)[2,3] can be used to provide resistance during the movement transitions. The patient is heel-sitting with hands resting on a ball in front. The therapist is diagonally behind the patient, with MCs at the pelvis (Fig. 6.7A). Alternatively, the therapist may be heel-sitting diagonally in front with the patient's arms held forward with hands clasped. The MCs *do not change* during application of the technique.

The patient initially flexes the trunk forward and moves up into kneeling (concentric phase) by extending both hips to achieve full upright extension (Fig. 6.7B). The patient then holds the kneeling position against resistance (isometric phase). When stability is achieved, the movement transition is reversed. The patient then flexes the trunk forward (shifting the COM anteriorly) and controls lowering (eccentric phase) as the hips and knees flex until the buttocks make contact with the heels. VCs are directed toward each phase of the movement (*"Push up." "Now, hold." "Now, go down slowly."*).

Clinical Note: For patients who require a more gradual assumption of the heel-sitting position or those who find it difficult to get up from the full heel-sitting position, a small ball may be placed between the feet for the patient to sit on (Fig. 6.8). This will decrease the range of movement required (compared with full range heel-sitting).

The PNF technique of COI[2,3] can also be used to provide resistance during movement transitions from side-sitting up into kneeling and reverse. The patient is side-sitting with the UEs positioned in shoulder flexion, both elbows extended, and hands clasped together and supported on one of the therapist's shoulders (Fig. 6.9). The therapist is in front of the patient with MCs on the anterior pelvis (hand placements *do not change*). The patient first moves from side-sitting up

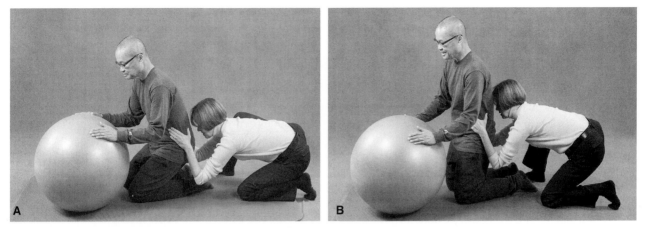

FIGURE 6.7 Applying combination of isotonics for movement transitions between bilateral heel-sitting and kneeling position. (A) From heel-sitting, concentric movement is resisted as the patient moves up toward kneeling. (B) Once in the kneeling position, the patient holds against continued resistance. *Not shown:* From kneeling, eccentric movement is resisted as the patient returns to heel-sitting.

into kneeling (concentric phase) and then stabilizes (holding phase) in the kneeling position. When stability is achieved, the patient then flexes and rotates the lower trunk toward one side and controls lowering of both hips down into a side-sitting position (eccentric phase). The trunk elongates on one side; the patient must rotate the head and upper trunk slightly to keep the UEs in position on the therapist's shoulder. Verbal cues are directed toward each phase of the movement: *"Push up." "Now, hold." "Now, go down slowly."*

Red Flag: Patients with weak hip extensors or decreased lower trunk/hip flexibility may not be able to move down into, or up from, the full side-sitting position. In these situations, the patient can be

instructed to move through the available ranges only or to sit on a cushion or firm bolster placed to the side to decrease the range of excursion and provide a platform for sitting.

Clinical Note: Moving from kneeling to side-sitting is a useful treatment activity for the patient with decreased lower trunk/pelvic mobility (e.g., the postacute patient with low back dysfunction or the patient recovering from stroke with spasticity or shortening of lateral trunk flexors). For patients with stroke, side-sitting on the more affected side lengthens the trunk side flexors and may lessen spasticity in the trunk. Hands are clasped together in front.

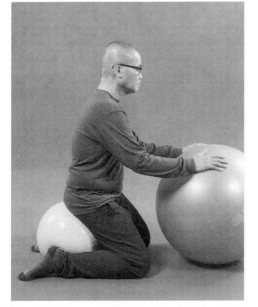

FIGURE 6.8 Heel-sitting on ball A small ball placed between the patient's feet may be used to provide a more gradual assumption of the heel-sitting position.

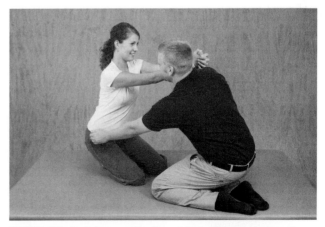

FIGURE 6.9 Applying combination of isotonics for movement transitions between side-sitting and kneeling position The patient is in the starting side-sitting position. *Not shown:* Continual resistance is applied as the patient first moves up into kneeling (concentric phase) and then stabilizes (holding phase) in the kneeling position. When stability is gained, against uninterrupted resistance, the patient slowly controls movement back to the side-sitting position (eccentric phase).

Comments

- Several repetitions of assisted or guided movement may be indicated to ensure the patient knows the desired movement transition.
- Resistance is variable in different parts of the range. As the patient moves from heel-sitting or side-sitting toward kneeling, resistance is minimal through the early and middle range where the effects of gravity are maximal. Resistance then builds up by the end of the transition to kneeling, as the patient moves into the shortened range to emphasize hip extensors. In the reverse movement, resistance is greatest initially, as the patient starts to move down into heel-sitting or side-sitting, and minimal during middle and end ranges, where the maximum effects of gravity take hold.
- If difficulty is experienced in achieving full hip extension in kneeling, the therapist may verbally cue the patient or provide resistance to the front of the hips.

Movement transitions between heel-sitting and kneeling can be performed with bilateral symmetrical UE PNF patterns using the technique of dynamic (isotonic) reversals. The patient is heel-sitting, with the head in midposition and the trunk in neutral alignment. The therapist is standing directly behind with the LEs positioned to provide a dynamic BOS (Fig. 6.10A); MCs are on the distal arms. To begin, the patient's UEs are positioned in the extension-adduction-internal rotation (EXT/ADD/IR) pattern with the shoulders adducted and internally rotated, the elbows extended with forearms pronated, and the hands closed and crossed (see Fig. 6.10A). Using dynamic reversals and the UE flexion-abduction-external rotation (FLEX/ABD/ER) pattern, continuous resistance is applied during transition into kneeling as the patient's hands open and the shoulders move toward FLEX/ABD/ER with forearm supination and wrist and finger extension (Fig. 6.10B). The VC is *"Open your hands, turn, and lift arms up and out toward me and lift up into kneeling."* The patient then returns to heel-sitting with the arms moving back down into EXT/ADD/IR. The VC is

"Make a fist, turn, and pull down and across your body, moving down into sitting on heels." Upper trunk extensors are recruited as the patient moves up into kneeling and upper trunk flexors as the patient moves down into heel-sitting.

The PNF lift (FLEX/ABD/ER) and reverse lift (EXT/ADD/IR) patterns and the PNF technique of dynamic (isotonic) reversals can also be used to promote movement transitions between heel-sitting and kneeling. The patient is heel-sitting; the therapist is standing behind and to the side with the LEs positioned to provide a dynamic BOS. To begin, the patient's *lead* limb is positioned in the reverse lift (EXT/ADD/IR) pattern across the body (shoulder adduction and internal rotation with forearm pronation and hand closed). The hand of the *assist* limb grasps underneath the wrist of the lead limb (Fig. 6.11A). The therapist's MC is on the lead UE using a loose hand (not tight) grasp to allow rotation through the movement. Using the lift pattern, the head and trunk extend and rotate as the patient moves from heel-sitting up into kneeling, bringing the *lead* limb into FLEX/ABD/ER with forearm supination and hand open (Fig. 6.11B). The VC is *"Lift your arms up and out toward me; turn and look up at your hands as you move into kneeling."* Resistance to the concentric movement in opposing patterns is continuous, with a VC (*"Reverse"*) used to mark transitions between the lift and reverse-lift.

Together with neck flexion and trunk rotation (opposite direction of lift), the lead limb then moves back down into EXT/ADD/IR as the patient assumes heel-sitting. The VC is *"Close your hand, turn, and pull your arms down and across your body and move into heel-sitting."*

The emphasis of this movement transition is recruitment of the upper trunk rotators, extensors (toward kneeling), and flexors (toward heel-sitting). It also involves crossing the midline, making it a useful activity for patients with unilateral neglect (e.g., the patient with stroke). These activities are also important lead-up skills for the assumption of an upright stance position (floor-to-standing transfers). The chop and reverse chop patterns may also be used.

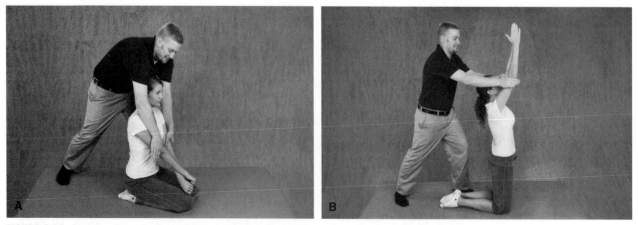

FIGURE 6.10 Applying dynamic (isotonic) reversals for movement transitions between bilateral heel-sitting and kneeling position (A) Start position: heel-sitting with UEs in the EXT/ADD/IR pattern; (B) end position: kneeling with UEs in the FLEX/ABD/ER pattern.

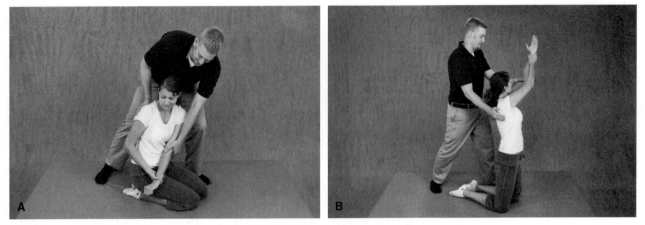

FIGURE 6.11 **Applying dynamic (isotonic) reversals for movement transitions between bilateral heel-sitting and kneeling position using PNF reverse lift and lift patterns** (A) **Reverse lift pattern:** the lead limb is positioned in EXT/ADD/IR with the patient in heel-sitting position in preparation for transition into kneeling. (B) **Lift pattern:** the lead limb moves toward (FLEX/ABD/ER) as the patient moves up into kneeling.

Clinical Note: When movement transitions are combined with UE PNF bilateral symmetrical FLEX/ABD/ER or lift patterns, careful grading of resistance is required because muscle strength is not constant throughout the ROM. Resistance should not limit the patient's ability to accomplish the movement transition into kneeling. Initially, to instruct the patient in the desired movement, the UEs may be passively moved or guided (active-assistive) through the patterns before resistance is applied. At first, movements are slow and controlled, with emphasis on the grading of resistance. For patients who demonstrate weakness, active movements against gravity (no manual resistance) may be the appropriate starting point. The therapist can subsequently initiate application of light resistance, with increased resistance as the patient approaches full kneeling.

Outcomes

Motor control goals: dynamic postural control
Functional skill achieved: patient is able to assume the kneeling position independently

Kneel-Stepping and Kneel-Walking

Kneel-stepping requires weight shifting onto one knee (stance) with contralateral hip hiking and forward pelvic rotation to advance the dynamic (swing) knee forward. The movement is then reversed as the patient practices a step backward using the same dynamic limb. Verbal cues include *"Shift your weight over onto your right knee. Now step forward with your left knee,"* and *"Now shift back over your right knee and step back."* To enhance pelvic rotation, light stretch and resistance can be applied as the dynamic knee steps forward and backward. Lateral sidestepping can also be practiced.

In kneeling-walking, the patient moves forward or backward using small steps with weightbearing on the knees. The therapist is kneeling directly in front and moves with the patient. If the patient is initially unstable, the hands may be placed on the therapist's shoulders (for light support) with a progression to no UE support. The MCs are on the pelvis to provide tactile cues while the patient practices combining weight shifting and pelvic rotation with forward and backward kneel-walking. Light stretch and resistance can be applied to promote pelvic rotation as well as approximation to promote stabilizing responses.

A progression is made to resisted kneel-walking (resisted progression). The MCs are on the pelvis to apply appropriate resistance [2,3] and facilitate movement. Resistance, stretch, and approximation are used to promote weight acceptance, pelvic rotation, lower trunk motion, stability (stance knee), and forward (or backward) progression. As the patient kneel walks forward, the therapist kneel walks backward in time with the patient's movements (Fig. 6.12). Alternatively, resisted progressions can be accomplished with the patient's hands on a ball in front with the therapist behind. Resistance is applied at the pelvis (Fig. 6.13A) with a progression to the ankles (Fig. 6.13B). A backward kneel-walking progression is also practiced. A key element of application is careful grading of resistance. In general, resistance to kneel-walking is relatively light (facilitatory) to encourage proper timing of the pelvic movements but also not to disturb the momentum, coordination, and velocity of movement. Movement against resistance and overall timing of kneel-walking can be facilitated with appropriate VCs: *"Step forward* [or backward] *against my resistance starting with your right* [or left] *knee and step, step, step...."*

Comments
- Providing verbal or tactile cues can enhance the timing and sequence of motion.
- Weight shifting with pelvic rotation is stressed.
- Kneel-walking is a lead-up activity for bipedal (upright) walking.

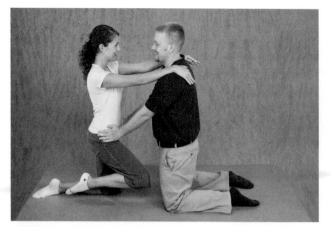

FIGURE 6.12 Resisted forward progression in kneeling (kneel-walking) with patient and therapist facing each other Appropriate resistance is applied to forward progression by placing both hands on the pelvis. MCs are on the anterior (forward) or posterior (backward) pelvis. Resistance is light so as not to disturb the patient's timing, momentum, and coordination. Approximation can be applied down through the top of the pelvis to assist in stabilizing responses as weight is taken on the stance limb.

Red Flag: Safety is always a high priority when interacting with a patient or client. Although interventions confined to a padded mat surface with the therapist in a protective guard position provide considerable inherent safety, some situations require additional precautions. Use of a guarding (transfer) belt may be warranted during early movement transitions (e.g., heel-sitting to kneeling) and during forward or backward progressions such as kneel-walking. Reinforced-fabric guarding belts with hook-and-loop fasteners are relatively inexpensive and easy to don. They not only provide improved overall safety but also enhance patient confidence when first progressing to activities that involve a higher COM and decreased BOS.

Clinical Note: Kneel-walking is an activity that is generally limited to a small number of patients. Patients with bilateral LE extensor spasticity may benefit from practice in kneel-walking (e.g., the patient with TBI or cerebral palsy). Inhibition is provided to the knee extensors while the patient is free to practice the elements needed for trunk and hip control. Patients with incomplete paraplegia and intact hip control (e.g., cauda equina injury) may also benefit from kneel-walking as a lead-up activity to gait. Assistive devices (e.g., bilateral mat crutches) can be appropriately sized for this activity. Kneel-walking is generally not used with many older patients and is contraindicated for patients with significant arthritic changes of the knee or other knee pathologies.

Outcomes

Motor control goal: skill

Functional skill achieved: patient is able to move independently in kneeling by using a reciprocal trunk and limb pattern

Strategies to Improve Balance Control in Kneeling

Some of the activities already presented provide initial interventions for improving balance control in kneeling. However, patients who demonstrate significant impairments in dynamic postural responses may be unable to control kneeling posture stability and orientation when movement of body segments is superimposed. Selection of interventions is based on evaluation of data obtained from tests and measures and identification of impairments contributing to the imbalance.

Strategies to improve balance in kneeling begin with several activities already presented: static holding (Fig. 6.14A) with progression to weight shifting (Fig. 6.14B) and functional reaching activities in all directions (dynamic postural control). *Static postural control* (stability) is necessary for maintaining the upright kneeling posture. *Dynamic postural*

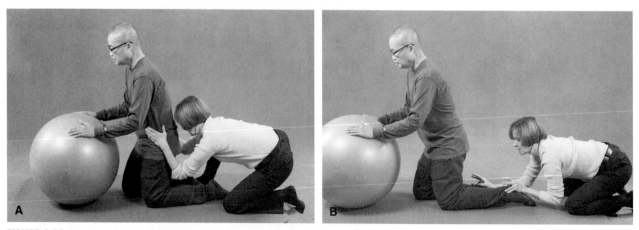

FIGURE 6.13 Resisted forward progression can be accomplished with the patient's hands supported on a ball in front with appropriate resistance applied at the (A) pelvis and (B) heels. While advancing, the patient moves the ball forward.

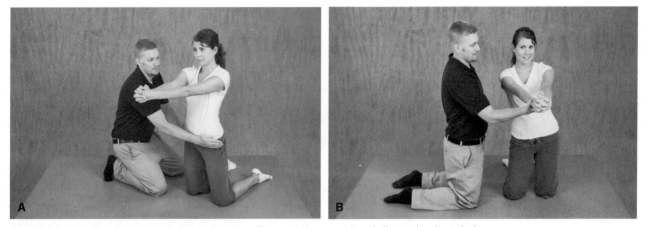

FIGURE 6.14 (A) **Kneeling, active holding of posture** This activity promotes static postural control (stability). If required, MCs may be placed at the pelvis to assist holding the position. Alternatively, MCs may be used to apply approximation through top of pelvis to promote stability.
(B) **Kneeling, medial/lateral weight shifts** This activity promotes dynamic postural control, as the kneeling posture must be stabilized during weight shifting. If required, MCs may be used initially to promote relative midline positioning of UEs during weight shifting.

control is required to control movements performed in the kneeling posture (weight shifting and reaching). Stability (Table 6.1, Fig. 1), weight shifting (Table 6.1, Fig. 2), and weight shifting combined with reaching (Table 6.1, Figs. 3 and 4) can also be promoted using a therapy ball.

Anticipatory balance control is needed for preparatory postural adjustments that accompany voluntary movements. Examples of activities that challenge anticipatory balance include practicing postural sway in all directions with gradual trajectory increments, "look-arounds" (turning the head with trunk rotation), and UE reaching ("reach-arounds"). Practicing balance in the posture can also be progressed from eyes open to eyes closed.

Reactive balance control is needed to make adjustments in response to changes in the COM or changes in the support surface. Reactive balance in kneeling can be challenged using manual perturbations that disturb the patient's COM or activities that disturb the patient's BOS such as kneeling on a compliant surface (BOSU dome, inflated disc, dense foam cushion), a tilting surface (e.g., tipper [rocker] board), or on a therapy ball (Table 6.1, Figs. 15–19). Reactive balance control allows for rapid and efficient responses to environmental perturbations required during transitions from kneeling to standing, while maintaining standing posture, and while walking.

Manual perturbations initiated by the therapist involve gentle displacement of the COM from over the BOS. Perturbations require that the patient provide a direction-specific movement response to return the COM over the BOS (state of equilibrium). To begin, the patient is kneeling on a stationary mat surface. The therapist is kneeling next to the patient (therapist positioning relative to patient will change based on the direction of perturbations). The MCs alternate between a guard position and application of displacing forces (MC perturbations) to the trunk. During initial use of perturbations or devices that challenge reactive control, a guarding belt may be warranted.

An important consideration is to ensure that the patient develops an understanding of the limits of stability (LOS) and is using appropriate responses relative to the direction of displacement. With posterior displacements in kneeling, hip and trunk flexor activity is required. With forward displacements, hip and trunk extensor activity is required. Lateral displacements require head and trunk inclination to the opposite side. Rotational displacements (twisting and displacing the trunk) require combinations of trunk movements. Protective extension of the UEs will be initiated if the displacements move the COM beyond the LOS. If patient responses are inadequate or lacking, the therapist may intervene with verbally and/or manually guided practice of initial attempts at direction-specific movement responses. Intervention is also necessary if movements are abnormal or excessive (e.g., excessive use of UEs to manage displacement instead of using core trunk muscles). The patient is then progressed to practice of active movements.

Clinical Note: Perturbations should be appropriate for the patient's available ROM and speed of control. It is important to use gentle disturbances with varied, asymmetrical MCs (tapping or nudging the patient out of position). Violent perturbations (pushes or shoves) are never appropriate. They place the patient "rigidly on-guard," defeating the purpose of the activity, and they are not necessary to stimulate balance responses. The therapist can vary the patient's BOS to increase or decrease the relative challenge of the activity (e.g., moving the knees further apart or closer together).

An inflated disc can be used to change the BOS. The patient is kneeling on an inflated disc with knees comfortably apart and ankles plantarflexed and feet supported on the mat or floor. The UEs may be positioned with shoulders flexed to approximately 90 degrees, elbows extended, and hands clasped together (Fig. 6.15). The therapist is kneeling

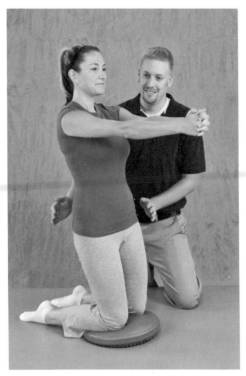

FIGURE 6.15 Kneeling on an inflated disc Initially, the patient holds the position (holding the disc steady). *Not shown:* A progression is then made to patient-initiated active weight shifts in different directions (e.g., anterior/posterior and medial/lateral).

or half-kneeling to the side of the patient in a guard position. Initially, the patient holds the position by maintaining a balanced or centered kneeling position (holding the disc steady). A progression is then made to patient-initiated active weight shifts, shifting in different directions to stimulate balance responses (e.g., medial/lateral, anterior/posterior). These patient-initiated challenges to balance stimulate both *feedforward* (anticipatory adjustments in postural activity) and *feedback-driven* (response-produced information)

adjustments to balance. A progression can be made to a higher inflated dome (e.g., a BOSU dome) to increase the challenge. With a higher dome, the knees are the primary support; the feet are not in contact with the support surface (reducing the BOS).

The BOS can also be changed using a therapy ball. A therapy ball can be used in kneeling to improve trunk, hip, knee, and UE strength and control (Table 6.1, Figs. 5 to 14) and to improve balance and stabilizing responses of the hip and trunk muscles (Table 6.1, Figs. 15 to 19). Another useful ball activity to improve strength and trunk muscle response is movement transitions from prone to heel-sitting. For this transition, the therapist is standing next to the patient in a guard position; if contact guard is required, MCs are on the pelvis. The patient begins in quadruped position over a ball that is large enough to support the patient's upper trunk. The patient then "walks" forward on the hands until the ball is positioned under the thighs (Fig. 6.16A). The patient then fully flexes both hips and knees, bringing the knees up toward the chest and the ball underneath the legs. The patient is now heel-sitting on the ball in a tucked position with the UEs extended and weightbearing on the mat or floor (Fig. 6.16B). The movements are reversed to return to the start position. The therapist can initially assist the patient into the tucked position by manually stabilizing and/or lifting the pelvis. Progression is to active movement control. A progression of this activity is to have the patient bring both knees up into a tucked position to one side (knees moving on a diagonal toward one shoulder as if moving toward a side-sitting position on the ball). The progression of interventions to improve intermediate trunk and hip control using the kneeling posture is summarized in Table 6.2.

Outcomes
Motor control goals: dynamic postural control
Functional skill achieved: patient demonstrates functional balance in the kneeling position
Indication: impaired dynamic postural responses

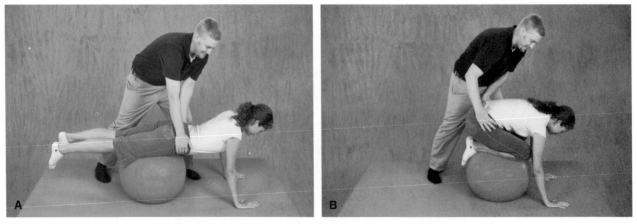

FIGURE 6.16 Prone to kneeling from a quadruped position over a ball (not shown) (A) The patient then moves forward on the hands causing the ball to move toward the thighs and the hips and knees to extend. (B) Once the ball is under the thighs, the patient flexes both hips and knees to bring the ball under the legs.

TABLE 6.2 Progression of Interventions to Improve Intermediate Trunk and Hip Control and Patient Indications	
Progression of Interventions Using Kneeling Posture	**Patient Indications**
• Assist-to-position (physical assistance) • Upper extremities used initially for support • Gradual reduction of assistance, UE support, and VCs	Inability to assume kneeling posture
• Holding: assisted to active • Resisted holding: stabilizing (isometric) reversals, rhythmic stabilization	Diminished static postural control (stability)

• Weight shifting
  • Medial/lateral
  • Diagonally
  • Diagonally with pelvic rotation
• Resisted: dynamic (isotonic) reversals
• Active reaching
	Postural muscle weakness and incoordination; inability to transition between opposing postural muscle groups

• Movement transitions between heel-sitting or side-sitting and kneeling
  • Resisted: combination of isotonics[2,3]
• Movement transitions between heel-sitting and kneeling using bilateral symmetrical UE PNF patterns (EXT/ADD/IR and FLEX/ABD/ER)
  • Resisted: dynamic reversals
• Movement transitions between heel-sitting and kneeling using UE PNF lift (FLEX/ABD/ER) and reverse lift (EXT/ADD/IR) patterns
  • Resisted: dynamic (isotonic) reversals
	Postural muscle weakness, inability to eccentrically control body weight during movement transitions, poor dynamic postural control

• Kneel-stepping and kneel-walking (forward and backward)
  • Light stretch and manual resistance: promote pelvic rotation on swing knee
  • Approximation: promote stabilizing responses on stance knee
• Resisted: kneel-walking (forward and backward)
  • Resisted: light (facilitatory)
  • Stretch (pelvic rotation)
  • Approximation (stability)
	Impaired timing, coordination, or control of pelvis and lower trunk segments

Note: Kneel-walking is a lead-up activity for bipedal (upright) walking.	
• Active holding and weight shifting • Postural sway in all directions with gradual trajectory increments to limits of stability • Upper extremity reaching in all directions • Manual perturbations • Kneeling on compliant surface (e.g., inflated disc, foam) • Kneeling on tilting surface (e.g., tipper [rocker] board) • Kneeling on therapy ball (see Table 6.1, Figs. 15–19)	Impaired balance control

Note: Interventions to improve balance can be progressed from eyes open to eyes closed.

Red Flag: Some kneeling activities using a ball are very challenging and require a great deal of lower trunk flexibility and postural control. It is important to observe the patient's responses carefully and use appropriate safety precautions and guarding strategies.

Practice and Feedback

Practice and feedback are critical to motor learning.[4,5] The therapist's selection of practice strategies and feedback mechanisms will directly affect the outcomes of interventions designed to improve intermediate trunk and hip control using kneeling postures. Initially, a verbal or visual *reference of correctness* should be provided to the patient. This will focus attention on the key elements of the posture and enhance sensory feedback about the correctness of the posture and movements performed within it.

An important consideration is that integrating practice and feedback is highly *patient-specific*. For example, a patient with significant multisystem involvement, such as a TBI, will require very different approaches to practice and feedback than will a patient who sustained a trimalleolar ankle fracture. Multiple factors must be considered when developing a feedback plan, such as the *mode* (type of feedback), *intensity* (how much should be used), and *scheduling* (when it will be given). Other important feedback elements include the patient's stage of motor learning (cognitive, associated, or autonomous), motivation, and attention span, and whether feedback will be *intrinsic* (provided by the actual movement) or *extrinsic,* also called *augmented* (provided by external sources such as VCs or MCs).

An essential element of practice is to ensure that the patient is correctly practicing the desired kneeling posture and/or movement within the posture. Faulty practice results in faulty outcomes that may need to be unlearned before the desired posture or movement can be learned. Other critical elements of practice include *distribution* (intervals of practice and rest), *variability* (what tasks are practiced), *order* (sequencing of tasks), and *structuring of the environment* (closed versus open). See Chapter 2: Interventions to Improve Motor Function, for a discussion of strategies to enhance motor learning.

Half-Kneeling

In half-kneeling, the COM is the same as in kneeling (intermediate); however, the BOS is wider and on a diagonal between the posterior and anterior limbs. One hip remains extended, with weightbearing on the stance limb; the opposite hip and knee are flexed to approximately 90 degrees with slight abduction, and the foot is placed flat on the support surface (see Fig. 6.1B). Compared with kneeling, the position imposes greater weightbearing and stability demands on the hip of the stance limb. The posture can also be used to promote ankle-stabilizing responses and movements of the forward limb as well as increase proprioceptive input through the foot.

General Characteristics

The half-kneeling posture is more stable than kneeling. Half-kneeling involves head, trunk, and hip muscles for upright postural control. The head and trunk are maintained on the vertical in midline orientation, with normal spinal lumbar and thoracic curves. The pelvis is maintained in midline orientation with the hip fully extended on the posterior stance limb. As with kneeling, *static postural control* (stability) is necessary to maintain upright posture. *Dynamic postural control* is necessary to control movements performed in the posture (e.g., weight shifting or reaching). *Reactive balance control* is needed to make adjustments in response to changes in the COM (perturbation) or changes in the support surface (tilting). *Anticipatory balance control* is needed for preparatory postural adjustments that accompany voluntary movements.

Clinical Notes:

- Holding the posture and weight-shifting activities in half-kneeling provide an early opportunity for partial weightbearing on the forward foot; the position can also be used to effectively mobilize the foot and ankle muscles (e.g., for the patient with ankle injury).
- As in kneeling, prolonged compression provides inhibitory influences on the stance-side quadriceps; there is no inhibitory pressure on the quadriceps of the forward limb.
- The asymmetrical limb positioning (one stance limb and one forward limb with foot flat) can be used to disassociate (break up) symmetrical limb patterns. Half-kneeling is a useful activity for the patient with cerebral palsy.
- As with kneeling, half-kneeling may be contraindicated in some patients, such as those who have rheumatoid arthritis or osteoarthritis affecting the knee, patients with knee joint instability, or patients recovering from recent knee surgery.

Interventions to Improve Intermediate Trunk and Hip Control in Half-Kneeling

HALF-KNEELING: ASSIST-TO-POSITION

Assist-to-position movement transitions into half-kneeling can be effectively accomplished from a kneeling position. This movement transition is an important lead-up skill to independent floor-to-standing transfers. From a kneeling position, the patient brings one limb up into the forward position with the hip and knee flexed and the foot placed flat on the mat. The opposite stance knee remains in a weightbearing position. The therapist is half-kneeling in front with the patient's hands resting on the therapist's shoulders (Fig. 6.17). MCs are on the pelvis on the stance limb and posterior thigh of the dynamic limb. The therapist may assist weight shifting toward the stance limb by gently rotating the pelvis backward on that side. This partially unloads and facilitates movement of the forward limb into position. Placing the patient's hands on the therapist's shoulders (for light support) reduces the postural stability demands during initial

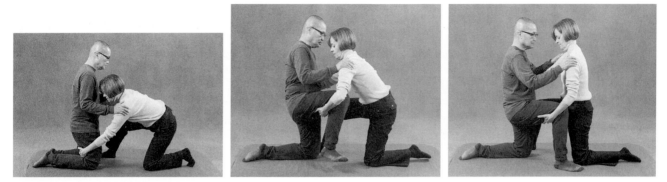

FIGURE 6.17 Half-kneeling, assist-to-position from kneeling On stance side, manual contact is on the pelvis to assist weight shifting toward that side with application of approximation force. The opposite hand assists from under the thigh of the dynamic limb.

practice. A progression is made to no UE support. Practice in assuming half-kneeling should include alternating the LEs between the stance and forward position. Verbal cues are used to guide weight shift onto the stance knee and forward movement of the opposite knee with foot placement on supporting surface (*"Shift your weight onto the left* [or right] *knee and bring the right* [or left] *knee up and place your foot flat on the mat"*).

Half-Kneeling: Holding

This activity focuses on static postural control (stability) in half-kneeling. The patient is in half-kneeling, actively holding the posture with weight equally distributed between the posterior stance knee and the foot of the forward limb. Postural alignment is maintained with the head and trunk upright and the COM kept over the BOS with the body at rest (no motion).

When the patient is practicing holding in half-kneeling, the therapist is in half-kneeling in front of the patient in a *reverse mirror-image* position (patient and therapist use opposite limbs for the stance and forward positions). Manual contact on the stance side is on the posterior upper trunk passing under the axilla and on the lateral hip/pelvis on the forward limb side. Alternatively, each of the therapist's hands may be cupped around the lateral aspect of the hip/pelvis on both sides. To reduce the postural stability demands during initial practice, the patient's hands may be positioned on the elevated forward knee for support. Alternatively, both hands may be placed on the therapist's shoulders for light support. A progression is made to using only one hand, then to touch-down support as needed, and finally to no UE support. As with kneeling, to provide touch-down support, the therapist remains in front of the patient with elbows flexed, forearms supinated, and hands open to provide support as needed while static postural control is established. Verbal cues are used to encourage holding the position with upright head and trunk posture and even weight distributed between the stance knee behind and the foot in front: *"Hold, keep your head and trunk upright and weight evenly distributed between your knee behind and your foot in front."*

Applying Resistance to Promote Stability

The PNF technique of stabilizing (isometric) reversals can be used to promote stability. Since the BOS in half-kneeling is on a diagonal, resistance is used only in the direction of the BOS. Resistance is applied on a diagonal to opposing muscle groups within a relatively static half-kneeling posture. For application of stabilizing (isometric) reversals with anterior/posterior resistance, the patient is asked to hold the half-kneeling position. The therapist is also half-kneeling, facing the patient. Manual contacts reverse between the *anterior* and *posterior* aspects of the pelvis. A transitional VC is used to indicate a change in direction. Resistance is applied to the pelvis, first as if pushing the pelvis diagonally backward toward the posterior stance knee (Fig. 6.18A), then reversed, as if pulling the pelvis frontward toward the forwardly placed limb. The goal is sustained holding. Verbal cues are used to encourage holding, indicate the direction of resistance (*"Hold, don't let me push you backward and over your knee, hold"*) and a change in direction with a transitional cue (*"Now, don't let me pull you forward and over your foot"*). The challenge of this activity may be progressed by placing the foot of the forward limb on an inflated disc (Fig. 6.18B). This increases the control demands imposed on the forward knee and ankle. The PNF technique of rhythmic stabilization can also be used to promote stability in half-kneeling. MCs are on the posterior pelvis on one side pulling forward, the other hand is on the anterior contralateral upper trunk, pushing backward. The VC is *"Don't let me move you* [twist you]—*hold, hold; now don't let me move you* [twist you] *the other way, hold."*

Outcomes

Motor control goals: stability (static postural control)
Functional skill achieved: patient is able to stabilize independently in the half-kneeling position

Half-Kneeling: Diagonal Weight Shifting

The patient performs active weight shifts diagonally over the forward limb and then diagonally backward over the stance limb.

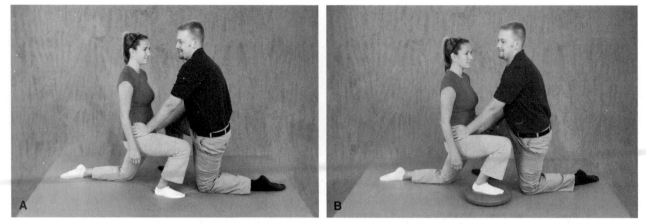

FIGURE 6.18 Applying stabilizing (isometric) reversals in half-kneeling (A) The patient is asked to maintain the position. The therapist's MCs are positioned to apply posteriorly directed resistance as if pushing the pelvis diagonally back toward the posterior stance knee (appropriate resistance is used sufficient to prevent movement). *Not shown:* Hand placements are then reversed to the posterior aspects of the pelvis to apply anteriorly directed resistance as if pulling the pelvis frontward toward the forwardly placed limb. (B) A progression is made to placing the forward foot on an inflated disc.

Applying Resistance to Promote Diagonal Weight Shifting

The PNF technique of dynamic (isotonic) reversals can be used to promote diagonal weight shifting. The patient and therapist are half-kneeling. The therapist is diagonally in front of the patient (reverse mirror image position). Continuous resistance is applied to concentric movement as the patient's weight shifts diagonally frontward over the forward limb and foot and then diagonally backward over the stance limb without relaxation. The MCs change position between the anterior and posterior pelvis to apply resistance to both forward and backward diagonal movement. The goal is to achieve a smooth transition between opposing muscle groups. Verbal cues are used to identify direction of weight shifts and to alert the patient to an approaching change in direction (*"Pull away from me; now, push back toward me"*).

Half-Sitting/Half-Kneeling

Half-sitting/half-kneeling on a ball can be used to promote static-dynamic control. The patient sits on a medium-sized ball with the hips and knees flexed to 90 degrees and the feet flat on the floor. The therapist is kneeling or half-kneeling to the side and slightly behind the patient. The patient shifts weight over toward one side, partially unweighting one limb for dynamic movement. The patient moves the partially unweighted limb down into the half-kneeling position and shifts weight onto this knee. The ball is still underneath (partially supporting) the patient as the patient assumes the half-sitting/half-kneeling position (Fig. 6.19). The movements can then be reversed to return to a centered sitting position on the ball. The challenge to static-dynamic control may be increased by having the patient practice alternate movements, moving down into half-kneeling on one side, then to sitting, and then to half-kneeling on the other side. The positioning of the patient's UEs can also be used to alter the challenge imposed, beginning with hands placed on the elevated forward knee for support, then to arms folded across the chest, and finally positioned with both elbows extended, shoulders flexed to 90 degrees, and hands clasped together (see Fig. 6.19).

Outcomes

Motor control goals: dynamic postural control
Functional skill achieved: improved static-dynamic control during weight shifting in half-kneeling position

Movement Transitions: Half-Kneeling to Standing

For assisted movement transitions from half-kneeling to standing, the patient and therapist are facing in half-kneeling.

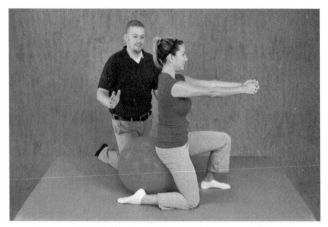

FIGURE 6.19 Half-sitting/half-kneeling position on a ball Start position: sitting on ball (not shown). The patient shifts weight to one side on the ball, unweighting the opposite dynamic limb for movement into kneeling. Shoulders are flexed with elbows extended and hands clasped together. Progression is made to alternating movements into half-kneeling on one side, then to sitting on the ball, and then to half-kneeling on the opposite side.

The patient's hands are resting on the therapist's shoulders with MCs initially at the pelvis of the stance limb and distal thigh of dynamic limb. The patient begins to shift weight forward onto the stance limb (Fig. 6.20A), then flexes and rotates the trunk, transferring weight diagonally forward over the foot of the forward limb (Fig. 6.20B). The patient then moves toward the standing position by extending the hip and knee (Fig. 6.20C). During final phase of movement, both MCs are at the pelvis.

A progression can be made to the therapist positioned behind the patient in guard position. The patient is half-kneeling with the hands supported on the elevated forward knee to assist with the rise to standing by pushing off (Fig. 6.21). The UEs can also be held with elbows extended, shoulders flexed to 90 degrees, and hands clasped together. This positioning assists with the forward transition of weight over the anterior

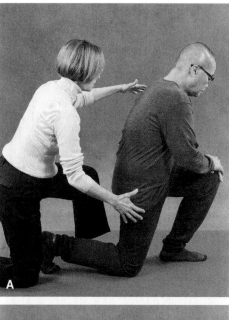

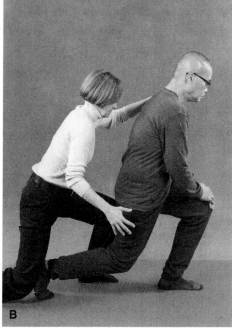

FIGURE 6.21 Movement transition, half-kneeling to standing The therapist is in a guard position behind the patient. (A) The patient shifts weight diagonally forward over the foot of the forward limb. (B) The patient then pushes off with the hands supported on the forward knee and moves up toward standing by extending the hip and knee. *Not shown:* The patient then places the feet together in upright standing.

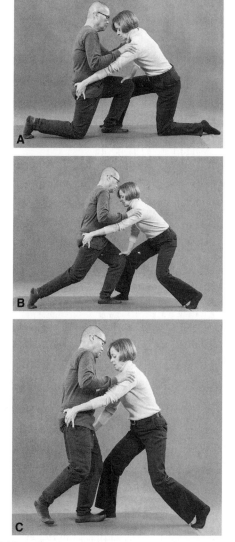

FIGURE 6.20 Assisted movement transition, half-kneeling to standing Note that MCs during early phases of movement are at the pelvis (stance limb) and distal thigh (dynamic limb) and transition to bilateral pelvis as patient approaches upright standing.

limb. This transition can also be practiced with a chair or low table in front of the patient. With the hands supported on the chair or table in front, the patient then comes up into standing using both UEs for weightbearing and push-off. A progression is made to unassisted movement transitions from half-kneeling to standing with no UE support.

Note: Practicing movement transition from half-kneeling to standing is generally a late-stage activity undertaken after the patient achieves control in standing and walking. Functionally, this activity is important to ensure that the patient who falls will be able to return to standing independently.

Outcomes

Motor control goal: dynamic postural control
Functional skill achieved: patient is able to independently accomplish movement transitions from floor to standing

Student Practice Activities

Box 6.1 is a student practice activity that focuses on analysis of treatment interventions in kneeling postures. Box 6.2 presents a student practice activity addressing selection and application of treatment interventions in kneeling postures.

BOX 6.1 STUDENT PRACTICE ACTIVITY: ANALYSIS OF TREATMENT INTERVENTIONS IN KNEELING POSTURES

OBJECTIVE: Analysis of treatment interventions to improve postural stability and reactive balance control in kneeling and half-kneeling

EQUIPMENT NEEDS: Platform mat, large ball, and inflatable disc (e.g., BOSU)

STUDENT GROUP SIZE: Four to six students

1. Using a platform or floor mat, each member of the group should alternate between the kneeling and half-kneeling postures; while in each position, practice holding for at least 45 seconds. Next, repeat the same activity, but now superimpose a gentle postural sway in all directions (medial/lateral, anterior/posterior, and diagonally). During the postural sway, start with small-range movements and work toward increments of range. Be careful to maintain the trajectory of postural sway within your LOS. While transitioning between postures, focus your attention on the postural stability demands required of each position. When the activity is complete, convene the whole group to compare and contrast your individual perceptions of the relative stability of each posture.

Guiding Questions
▲ Which posture was most stable?
▲ Within each posture, which directions of postural sway did you feel were *most* and *least* stable?

2. Again alternate between the kneeling and half-kneeling postures and focus your attention on postural stability demands. Within each posture, alter the UE positions as follows (hold each UE position for a minimum of 20 seconds): (1) resting at sides, (2) folded across chest, (3) shoulders abducted to 90 degrees with elbows extended, and (4) shoulders flexed to 90 degrees with elbows extended and hands clasped together. Alter the visual input from eyes open to eyes closed. When the activity is complete, convene the whole group to compare and contrast your individual experiences with altering the UE position and the visual input.

Guiding Questions
▲ What did you learn about changes in postural stability demands when altering the UE position?

▲ Within a given posture, which UE positions provided the *greatest* and *least* challenge to stability?
▲ What did you learn about changes in postural stability demands when altering the visual input from eyes open to eyes closed?
▲ What insights did this activity provide that can be applied clinically?

3. This activity involves applying manual perturbations (gentle nudges) and observing reactive balance control. Recall that manual perturbations initiated by the therapist involve gentle displacement of the COM from over the BOS. Reactive balance control allows for rapid and efficient responses to environmental perturbations required during standing and walking. One or more group members will assume the role of subject. One member will serve as the therapist for the application of perturbations. The subject will begin in kneeling position with an inflated disc (or BOSU dome) under the knees. The therapist will also assume a kneeling position. The therapist's MCs alternate between a guard position and application of displacing forces (manual contact perturbations) to the trunk. If more than one person is serving as a subject, the therapist should provide gentle anterior, posterior, and lateral perturbations to the trunk of each subject *individually* (*not* simultaneously) to allow careful observation of movement responses.

Guiding Questions
▲ What movement responses were used to return the COM over the BOS? Were the movements direction-specific?
▲ Were any UE protective extension responses noted? If they were, what does this indicate about the position of the COM with respect to the BOS?
▲ With posterior displacements, what muscle groups were activated (this question requires input from subjects)?
▲ With forward displacements, what muscle groups were activated?
▲ What compensatory responses were observed during lateral displacements?

BOX 6.2 STUDENT PRACTICE ACTIVITY: SELECTION AND APPLICATION OF TREATMENT INTERVENTIONS IN KNEELING POSTURES

OBJECTIVE: To share knowledge and skills in the selection and application of treatment interventions in kneeling postures based on patient indications

EQUIPMENT NEEDS: Platform or floor mat, large ball, inflatable disc, and tilting surface (e.g., tipper [rocker] board)

STUDENT GROUP SIZE: Four to six students

Directions: Below are four patient indications that may be addressed using kneeling postures.

Patient Indications:

a. Inability to assume kneeling posture
b. Postural muscle weakness, inability to eccentrically control body weight during movement transitions, poor dynamic postural control
c. Impaired balance control
d. Trunk and hip extensor weakness

For each patient indication:

1. Without discussion, each group member will *individually* select and document his or her intervention(s) choices to address the patient indication under consideration. This will include:
   • The posture or activity selected, including patient and therapist positioning.
   • If appropriate, the technique selected for application of resistance, including its description, rationale for use, therapist hand placements (MCs), and instructions and/or VCs provided to patient.
   • How the selected intervention may be progressed.

2. All group members convene to share, compare, and contrast the interventions selected. Thinking aloud, brainstorming, and sharing thoughts should be continuous until a consensus is reached. More than one intervention may be appropriate to address a single patient indication. To confirm elements of the discussion (if needed) or if agreement cannot be reached, a return to chapter content is warranted to support or refute ideas generated.

3. The selected intervention(s) will then be demonstrated. Each student in a group will contribute his or her understanding of, or questions about, the intervention being demonstrated. Again, dialogue should continue until a consensus of understanding is reached. Members of the group will assume different roles (described below) and will rotate roles each time the group progresses to a new patient indication.
   • One person assumes the role of therapist and participates in discussion.
   • One person serves as the subject/patient and participates in discussion.
   • All remaining group members participate in discussion and provide feedback after the demonstration.

4. A discussion follows the demonstration. All group members should provide recommendations, suggestions, and supportive feedback about the demonstration. Particularly important is discussion of how the intervention(s) demonstrated will then be progressed.

SUMMARY

This chapter explores interventions to improve intermediate trunk and hip control using kneeling and half-kneeling postures. These postures provide a unique opportunity to enhance intermediate *static postural control* (stability) and *dynamic postural control* (static-dynamic control) without superimposing the control requirements of upright standing. Kneeling and half-kneeling are important postures for developing critical lead-up skills required for standing and locomotion, including pelvic rotation, static and dynamic upright postural control, reactive and anticipatory balance control, and reciprocal trunk and limb patterns. The inherent patient safety provided by the relatively low COM and reduced degrees of freedom of these postures (compared with standing) enhances their importance as effective transitional postures between prone progressions and upright standing.

REFERENCES

1. Adler, S, Beckers, D, and Buck, M. PNF in Practice: An Illustrated Guide, ed 3. New York, Springer, 2008.
2. Saliba, VL, Johnson, GS, and Wardlaw, C. Proprioceptive neuromuscular facilitation. In Basmajian, JV, and Nyberg, R (eds): Rational Manual Therapies. Baltimore, Williams & Wilkins, 1993, 243.
3. Johnson, G, and Saliba Johnson, V. PNF 1: The Functional Application of Proprioceptive Neuromuscular Facilitation, Course Syllabus, Version 7.9, Steamboat, CO, Institute of Physical Art, 2014.
4. Shumway-Cook, A, and Woollacott, M. Motor Control–Translating Research Into Clinical Practice, ed 4. Baltimore, Lippincott Williams & Wilkins, 2012.
5. Schmidt, RA, and Lee, TD. Motor Control and Learning: A Behavioral Emphasis, ed 5. Champaign, IL, Human Kinetics, 2011.

CHAPTER 7

Interventions to Improve Transfer Skills

GEORGE D. FULK, PT, PhD, AND COBY NIRIDER, PT, DPT

The ability to transfer from a seated position to standing *(sit-to-stand [STS] transfer)* or to another surface is an essential skill that many people who receive rehabilitation services need to reacquire after an injury or illness. Being able to transition from bed to wheelchair and from sitting to standing places the person in a position to begin locomotion and improves interaction with the environment. Although there are various types of transfers, the ability to transfer from a seated surface to standing (and back again) (Fig. 7.1) is the most basic and provides the foundation for other types of transfers. A person who cannot bear weight through his or her lower extremities (LEs) and stand (e.g., a person with a complete spinal cord injury [SCI]) may transfer from one surface to another (e.g., wheelchair) using a sit-pivot technique (Fig. 7.2). This chapter examines various training strategies that can be used to enhance a person's ability to perform these vital transfer skills.

Task Analysis

Task analysis using critical observation skills serves as the foundation for examining how the patient performs the task[1] and for developing task-oriented interventions to improve the patient's ability to transfer. Analyzing how the patient performs the movement in combination with an examination of underlying body structure and function impairments allows the therapist to determine what factors may be causing the difficulties in performance. With this information, the therapist can then develop a plan of care (POC) designed to enhance motor learning and improve the patient's performance.

Overview of Biomechanics

It is important to have a good understanding of the normal biomechanics of the STS and sit-from-stand motion. The therapist uses this information as part of the task analysis to compare how the patient is performing the task and to identify possible impairments that may be causing the functional limitations observed. Sit-to-stand is commonly broken down into two phases: *pre-extension* and *extension*.[2] The pre-extension phase involves a forward or horizontal translation of body mass, and the extension phase involves a vertical translation of body mass. The point

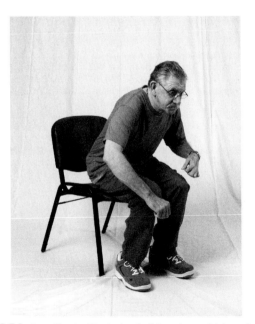

FIGURE 7.1 A patient with stroke (left hemiparesis) transfers from sitting to standing.

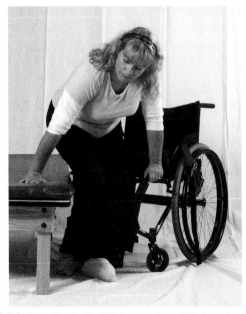

FIGURE 7.2 A patient with T12 incomplete SCI transfers from a wheelchair to a mat.

when the thighs come off the sitting surface (thigh off) is the transition between the two phases. This breakdown into two distinct phases is done to organize the clinical analysis of the movement. Normally, the movement occurs in one smooth motion.

Initially, most of the body mass is resting on the thighs and buttocks in a stable sitting posture (Fig. 7.3A). During the pre-extension phase, the upper body (head and trunk) rotates forward at the hip joints and the lower legs rotate forward over the ankle joints (dorsiflexion) (Fig. 7.3B). Once the trunk and head rotate forward, causing the body mass to translate horizontally, the extension phase begins with extension at the knees closely followed by extension at the hips and ankles.[2] The thighs then raise

off the seat (Fig. 7.3C). During the extension phase, the greatest muscle force occurs to lift the body mass up off the sitting surface. During the rest of the extension phase (Fig. 7.3D), the hips, knees, and ankles continue to extend to bring the body to an upright posture.

During the pre-extension phase (see Fig. 7.3B), the iliopsoas and tibialis anterior are the primary muscles activated to propel the body mass forward. The trunk extensors and abdominal muscles contract isometrically to stabilize the trunk while it rotates forward at the hips. During the extension phase (see Fig. 7.3D), the hip (gluteus maximus), knee (rectus femoris, vastus lateralis, and vastus medialis), and ankle extensors (gastrocnemius and soleus) are activated to lift the body up to standing.

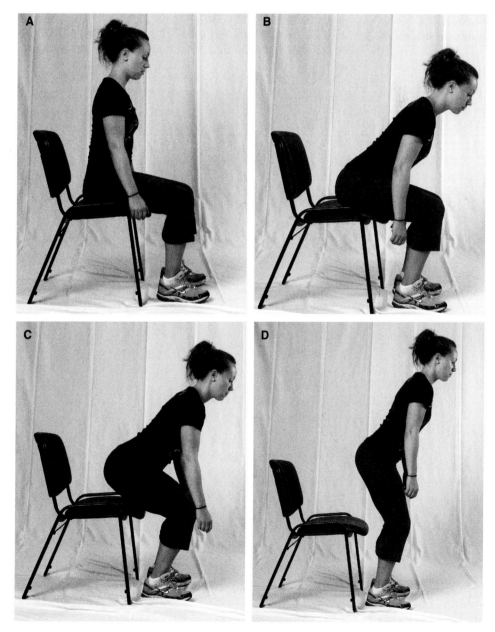

FIGURE 7.3 (A) Initial sitting posture before transferring to standing. Note that the upper trunk is erect and the pelvis is in a neutral position. (B) During the pre-extension phase, the body mass is shifted horizontally as the trunk rotates forward at the hips and the lower legs rotate forward at the ankles. Keeping the upper trunk extended and the pelvis in neutral is important for translating the body mass horizontally over the feet. (C) The extension phase begins as the thighs come off the seating surface. (D) During the extension phase, the hips and knees extend to bring the body to a standing position.

People generally utilize two basic strategies to transfer from sitting to standing: *momentum-transfer strategy* and *zero-momentum strategy*.[3] The momentum-transfer strategy involves initially generating forward momentum by flexing forward at the hips quickly as the trunk and head translate in a horizontal direction (flexion at the hips) causing the center of mass (COM) to shift toward and over the feet. The trunk extensor muscles then contract eccentrically to brake the horizontal motion. This is followed by a strong concentric contraction of the extensor muscles of the LEs to lift the body vertically.

The zero-momentum strategy entails forward flexion of the trunk until the COM is within the base of support (BOS) of the feet. Then there is a vertical lift of the body mass into a standing position. The zero-momentum strategy is more stable than the momentum-transfer strategy but requires greater muscle force to perform. People with LE weakness who utilize this strategy may also require armrests to push off of with their upper extremities (UEs). The momentum-transfer strategy requires less force because the

body is in motion as the legs begin the lift. However, there is a trade-off with stability because the person is less stable during the transition period.

The motion (angular displacement) of transitioning from standing to sitting is similar to the motions that occur during STS, only in reverse.[4] However, the timing and type of muscle contraction are different. While transitioning from standing to sitting, the body mass is moving backward and downward. Flexion of the hips, knees, and ankles is controlled by eccentric contraction of the LE extensor muscles. Additionally, the patient cannot directly see the surface upon which he or she is about to sit.

Task Analysis of Sit-to-Stand and Sit-From-Stand Transfers

Movement tasks can generally be broken down into four stages: *initial conditions, initiation, execution,* and *termination* (Table 7.1).[1] Critically examining the initial conditions includes the patient's posture and the environment in which the

TABLE 7.1 Task Analysis for Sit-to-Stand and Sit-From-Stand Transfers and Common Difficulties Exhibited/Encountered

Four Stages of Transfer Task	Elements of Task Analysis	Common Difficulties Exhibited by Patients with Neurological Disorders
Initial Conditions	• Starting posture • Environment conditions	• Initial foot placement too far forward (e.g., decreased ankle ROM) • Sitting in posterior pelvic tilt position • Increased thoracic kyphosis • Sitting too far back on the seating surface • Seat surface too low or too soft
Movement Initiation	• Timing • Direction	• Delay in initiation • Multiple attempts to initiate movement • Movement initiated too quickly • Direction of movement not efficient
Movement Execution	• Direction • Speed • Smoothness • Weight shift • Vertical lift • Balance	• Lack of strength/power • Muscle activation not in optimal sequence (e.g., begin extending too early) • Forward weight-shift not complete • Anterior weight-shift by thoracic flexion instead of hip flexion • Too much weight-shift onto less affected side • Speed too slow, does not build sufficient momentum to assist with extension phase • Fear of falling
Movement Termination	• Timing • Stability • Accuracy	• Over- or undershoot movement termination • Unsteady on completion of movement transition

motor task is being performed. Common abnormalities in posture that may impact the ability to transfer from STS include:

- Asymmetrical weightbearing (Fig. 7.4)
- Sitting with a posterior pelvic tilt causing an increased thoracic kyphosis (Fig. 7.5)
- Incorrect placement of the feet (Fig. 7.6)

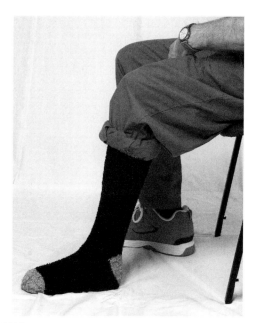

FIGURE 7.6 The patient does not place the left foot back far enough. This will make it difficult to translate the body mass horizontally during the pre-extension phase and to effectively utilize the left LE to push up during the extension phase. The inability to position the foot farther posterior could be caused by a contracture of the gastrocnemius-soleus complex or hamstring weakness.

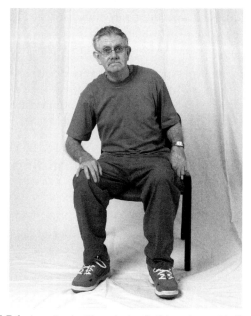

FIGURE 7.4 A patient with a stroke (left hemiparesis) sits with weightbearing primarily on the less affected (right) side.

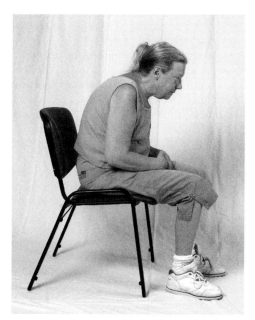

FIGURE 7.5 A patient with stroke (right hemiparesis) sits with an increased thoracic kyphosis and posterior pelvic tilt. This makes it difficult to translate the body mass horizontally during the pre-extension phase. When the patient extends to attempt to stand up, most of the body mass will be too far posterior. This will either cause the patient to lose balance posteriorly and fall back as she attempts to stand or require increased effort and strength to come to standing.

The environmental context of the transfer should also be examined. This includes the seating surface (firm or cushioned), height of the seating surface, the floor surface (tiled or carpeted), lighting conditions, presence or absence of seat armrests and backrest, and other environmental distracters such as noise. Also consider the goal of the movement or the context in which the movement is performed. Performance may vary depending on the patient's overall goal. For example, a patient may perform STS differently when asked to do so in a therapy setting as opposed to at home in the kitchen in preparation for cooking.

After examining the *initial conditions,* the therapist should observe how the patient performs the movement task. This includes the *initiation, execution,* and *termination* of the transfer.

- **Initiation.** During the initiation phase, the timing (e.g., whether the patient requires multiple attempts to begin the movement) and direction of the initial movement should be noted. Common issues during initiation of the STS transfer include delayed initiation and initiation of the movement in the wrong direction.
- **Execution.** The speed and direction of movement, the coordination of movement between different body segments, as well as balance and weight-shifting ability are all elements that impact performance and should be critically analyzed during the execution phase. Common issues that occur during the execution of the movement, which may cause difficulties or the inability to successfully transfer, include weakness, inability to fully shift weight forward (Fig. 7.7), sequencing errors in the movement pattern

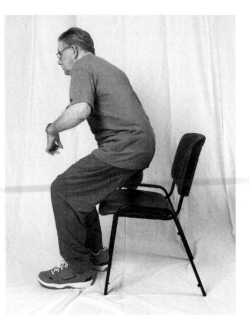

FIGURE 7.7 The patient with stroke (left hemiparesis) has not shifted his weight forward enough during the pre-extension phase. He compensates for this by using his right UE to push up from the chair.

(e.g., inability to halt forward momentum and convert to vertical movement), slowed pace, uneven weight distribution, and inability to maintain balance while moving.

- **Termination.** Common issues that occur during the termination phase of the transfer include inability to stop the transfer at the appropriate place and time (overshooting or undershooting) and inability to maintain balance upon completion. In these cases, the patient may need to take a step (i.e., use a stepping strategy) upon reaching standing to establish the COM within the BOS.

Although it is not possible to exactly replicate the effects of different types of patient impairments on the STS and sit-from-stand transition in healthy people, the student practice activity in Box 7.1 may provide further insight into some of the difficulties that patients may encounter.

Sit-to-Stand and Sit-From-Standing: Intervention Strategies

Information gained from the task analysis and examination of body structure and function and knowledge of the patient's

---

BOX 7.1 STUDENT PRACTICE ACTIVITY: TASK ANALYSIS OF SIT-TO-STAND AND SIT-FROM-STAND

OBJECTIVE: Analyze STS transfers of healthy people.

EQUIPMENT NEEDS: Use normal-height chair without armrests, chair with a low seat surface without armrests, off-the-shelf (prefabricated) ankle-foot orthotic, and a small ball.

DIRECTIONS: Work in groups of two to three students. Members of the group will perform different practice items (described below) and will rotate roles each time the group progresses to a new practice item.

▲ One person assumes the role of subject and participates in discussion.
▲ The remaining members participate in task analysis of the activity and discussion and provide supportive feedback during demonstrations. One member of this group should be designated as a "fact checker" to return to the text content to confirm elements of the discussion (if needed) or if agreement cannot be reached.

Procedure/Guiding Questions
1. Sit-to-stand/sit-from-stand transfers from a normal-height chair (seat surface approximately 17.5 in. [44.45 cm] from the floor) without armrests three to five times
   a. What is the subject's initial sitting alignment?
   b. Which strategy was used?
   c. What is the correct timing, direction, smoothness?
   d. Is appropriate postural stability and balance present during and at end of movement?
2. Sit-to-stand/sit-from-stand transfers from a low seat surface (less than 16 in. [40.64 cm] from the floor) three to five times
   a. Did the strategy change compared to a normal-height chair?
   b. What was different about the movement pattern used?
   c. Did it require more or less effort?

3. Sit-to-stand transfers from a normal-height chair without armrests under three different starting conditions: 90-degree angle between thighs and trunk (sitting erect), trunk flexed forward 30 degrees, and trunk flexed forward 60 degrees
   a. What differences were observed in the movement patterns used to transfer to standing between the three different starting positions?
   b. Which starting position required the least effort to transfer to standing?
   c. Which starting position was the most steady at termination of the transfer?
4. Sit-to-stand/sit-from-stand transfers from a normal-height chair without armrests with a small ball (6 to 8 in. [15.25 to 20.32 cm] diameter) that is partially inflated under one foot
   a. How was the movement pattern used in this transfer different from one used without a ball under one foot?
   b. Was postural stability altered during or at the end of the transfer?
   c. Which LE provided more force during the transfer?
5. Sit-to-stand/sit-from-stand transfers from a normal-height chair without armrests with one foot behind the knee (in approximately 15 degrees of dorsiflexion) and the other foot in four different positions: 15 degrees of dorsiflexion (same as the other foot; Fig. 7.8A), neutral ankle position (ankle directly under the knee), 15 degrees of plantarflexion (foot out in front of the knee; Fig. 7.8B), and with a prefabricated ankle-foot orthosis (Fig. 7.8C)
   a. How was the movement pattern different among the four conditions?
   b. Which condition required the most effort?
   c. Which LE provided the most force in each of the conditions?

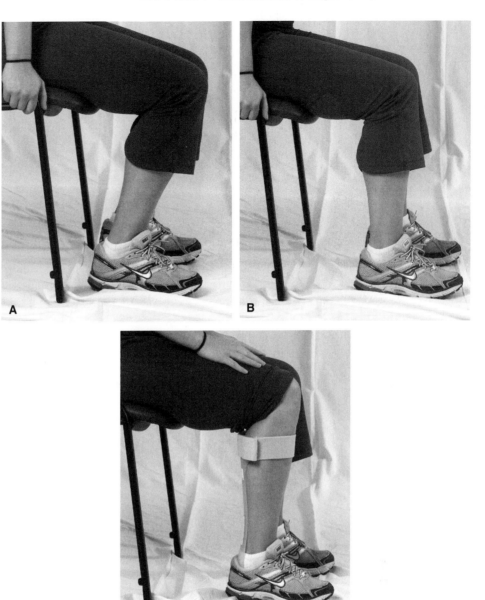

FIGURE 7.8 Sit-to-stand/sit-from-stand transfers with varying ankle positions: (A) 15-degree ankle dorsiflexion, (B) 15-degree ankle plantarflexion, and (C) with an off-the-shelf ankle-foot orthosis.

goals will allow the therapist to design a comprehensive and effective intervention program. Intensive and task-oriented rehabilitation strategies are necessary to induce use-dependent neurological reorganization to enhance motor and functional recovery.[5,6] Incorporating strategies to enhance motor learning (see Chapter 2: Interventions to Improve Motor Function) combined with intensive, task-oriented interventions provide the foundation for the POC.

Sit-to-Stand Transfers

Environment

During the initial stage of motor learning (cognitive stage), the therapist should set up the transfer practice environment to allow the patient to succeed while minimizing compensatory movement strategies. This usually entails the use of a firm, raised surface. A high-low mat (Fig. 7.9) is ideal for initial practice sessions. It allows the therapist to set the height at a point that is challenging for the patient, but not so challenging that the patient cannot successfully complete the transfer without excessive compensatory movements. Additionally, the intervention sessions should be carried out in a quiet, closed environment that is fully lighted. Verbal cues can be used to provide *knowledge of results* and *knowledge of performance,* but these should be faded over time or summarized after a certain number of trials. Verbal cues can also be used to direct the patient's attention to the task or overall movement goal. It may be more beneficial for patients with certain neurological diagnoses (e.g., patients with sensory motor cortex stroke) if verbal cues are used sparingly. Another method employed for these populations is to practice activities that disguise the target movement within a secondary "movement goal." An example of this might be encouraging a client to reach and

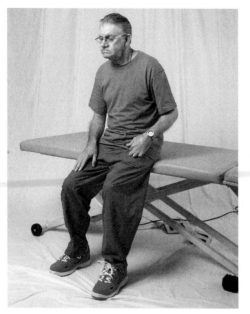

FIGURE 7.9 A high-low treatment table (or mat) may be used to vary the height of the seating surface. As the patient improves, the table can be lowered to make it more challenging.

retrieve objects placed ahead far enough that an STS movement is required to retrieve them (e.g., reaching to retrieve a cup on a countertop).

During the later stages of motor learning (associative and autonomous), as the patient's ability to perform the movement improves, the environment should be set up to more realistically reflect conditions that are likely to be encountered in the home and community. Although the environment should be made more realistic, it should still be shaped to allow the patient to succeed and then gradually be made more challenging. Specific intervention strategies can include using various seating surfaces (Fig. 7.10A–C) and an open environment where there are more external distracters. Verbal cues should be minimized at these later stages of learning. If difficulties are encountered, the patient should be encouraged to problem-solve to identify where or what the problem is.

Clinical Note: Initially, a firm sitting surface at appropriate height (usually higher than normal) should be used. Progression is to a standard seat height and then to various types of sitting surfaces (e.g., sofa, bed, toilet, stool). The environment should be progressed from a closed to an open environment.

Posture

An erect sitting posture on the edge of the seating surface, with weight evenly distributed, pelvis in a neutral position and feet behind the knees (ankle in approximately 15 degrees of dorsiflexion) (Fig. 7.11) is the ideal starting posture. Limitations in ankle range of motion (ROM) may reduce the ability to position the feet. In such situations, stretching the

gastrocnemius-soleus complex and/or performing joint mobilization to stretch the joint capsule may be indicated. Stretching can be done in both sitting and standing (Fig. 7.12A–C). The stretch should be held for at least 30 seconds and repeated 5 to 10 times. Patients should be educated to perform these stretches independently so they can be practiced multiple times a day. If the patient does not have sufficient hamstring strength to position the feet, a task-oriented strengthening program can be implemented. A towel under the foot can be used to reduce friction, or a small skateboard can be used (Fig. 7.13) as part of a task-specific strengthening program. Tape on the floor can be used to provide a target for the patient to position the foot.

Chapter 5: Interventions to Improve Sitting and Sitting Balance Skills provides a variety of interventions designed to enhance sitting posture and balance that can be used to improve initial sitting posture for transfers. As mentioned, the ideal sitting posture includes an erect, extended upper trunk, pelvis in neutral alignment, and the feet placed behind the knee (ankle in approximately 15 degrees of dorsiflexion).

Executing the Movement

The initial motion in transferring from sitting to standing is the forward translation of the upper body by flexing at the hips. Patients who sit with a posterior pelvic tilt (sacral sitting) and increased thoracic kyphosis and who have a fear of falling when leaning forward, may try to bring their body weight forward by increasing thoracic kyphosis as they flex the hips. This brings the head forward, but does not effectively translate the body mass horizontally (Fig. 7.14). From this position, it is difficult to transfer to standing because much of the body weight is too far posterior and the person can only see the floor.

An important element of practice is moving the upper body forward over the feet (i.e., hip flexion with upper trunk extended). Having the patient cross the arms in front while guided to flex forward at the hips assists in keeping the upper trunk extended and minimizes upper trunk flexion (Fig. 7.15). Alternatively, the patient's arms can be supported on a rolling tray table that can be guided forward and backward (Fig. 7.16) or on a large exercise ball (Fig. 7.17). Care should be taken to protect the integrity of the shoulder joint when performing these interventions, particularly with patients who have experienced stroke and have a subluxed shoulder. This can be done by manually supporting the joint from underneath if necessary (Fig. 7.18).

The therapist should never assist by pulling on the upper arm. The patient's feet may also need to be stabilized initially so that the lower leg rotates forward over the foot. As the patient progresses, assistance from the therapist is lessened and eventually removed.

Red Flag: The therapist should use caution when handling the shoulder to prevent joint trauma.

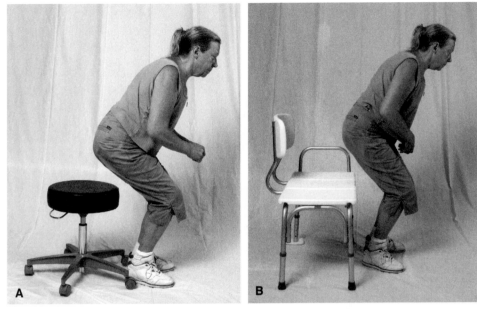

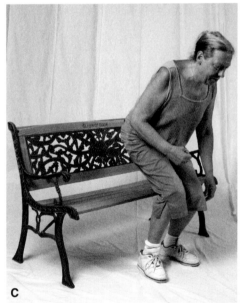

FIGURE 7.10 Practicing sit-to-stand/sit-from-stand transfers using a variety of seating surfaces will better simulate a patient's home and community environment.

As described above, during the initial stages of learning a higher seating surface (e.g., high-low mat) can be used; this is particularly useful with weak patients. A higher surface encourages weightbearing on the weaker limb and minimizes compensatory overloading of the stronger limb. For patients who require physical assistance due to weakness, the therapist can push downward and slightly posterior through the knee (Fig. 7.19). This action will also help stabilize the foot. Forward translation of the trunk can be guided with the other hand placed at the pelvis or upper trunk. Therapist positioning should not block anterior rotation of the lower leg (Fig. 7.20).

A visual target should be provided for the patient to focus on while pushing to stand up. The target should be in front and at eye level (when standing). Using a target helps the patient keep the upper trunk extended when the weight is shifted forward, provides a sense of postural alignment and vertical orientation, and discourages looking down at the feet.

Other strategies to increase loading on the more affected LE include:

- Placing the less affected LE slightly ahead of the more affected LE
- Placing the less affected LE on a small block (Fig. 7.21)
- Using a force platform to provide visual feedback about the amount of weightbearing on both LEs
- Performing simple reaching tasks to the more affected side during STS transitions ("reach and stand")

Comments

- A higher surface may be used initially for patients with weakness to promote symmetrical weightbearing.

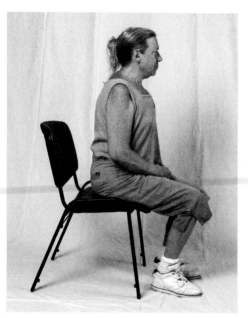

FIGURE 7.11 Positioning the ankles slightly posterior to the knee will allow the patient's weight to be translated horizontally during pre-extension.

- Manual assistance provided to the more affected knee will assist with extension.
- Therapist positioning should not block forward weight translation when assisting/guarding.
- A visual target can be used to promote upper trunk extension.

Repetitive Practice and Strengthening

Ample opportunity to practice a functional task is extremely important to enhancing motor learning and retention of the skill within the patient's environment. This is also true for transfers. Repetitive practice (11 to 14 times a day) of STS transfers has been shown to improve the ability to transfer independently without UE assistance and to increase both quality of life and physical mobility in people with stroke who are undergoing inpatient rehabilitation.[7] A key component of any intervention strategy designed to improve the ability to transition between sitting and standing should include multiple practice repetitions.

Strength training in people with stroke increases strength of the more involved LE and improves self-reported function and level of disability.[8] Lower extremity strength training can be achieved through task-oriented movements and progressive resistance using weights. In general, strengthening exercises should be done two to three times per week. Patients should perform two to three sets of 8 to 12 repetitions at their 10-repetition maximum.

Red Flag: During any standing exercises, patients at a risk of falling should be closely supervised and may need to stand next to a wall or a rail or other object to assist with balance. Light-touch down support (fingertip support) is preferred.

Task-oriented strengthening interventions in standing can include partial wall squats, step-ups and step-downs (Fig. 7.22), and mini-lunges (Fig. 7.23) (see also Chapter 9: Interventions to Improve Standing and Standing Balance Skills). Progressive resistance training can be done with ankle weights, weights with pulleys, or isokinetic machines and can include leg presses (unilateral or bilateral), squats on a Total Gym, knee flexion and extension, and standing hip extension and abduction with ankle weights.

Comments
- Repetitive practice is essential to motor learning.
- Strength training can be done through task-oriented movements or progressive resistance training with weights.

Stand-to-Sit Transfers

During practice sessions, the stand-to-sit component of the transfer should also be emphasized. One way to do this effectively is to have the patient control the descent from standing. The patient practices stopping in mid-descent on cue and either holding the position for a short time (1 to 3 seconds) or pushing back up to standing. The range and speed of descent can be varied according to the patient's ability. The patient can also be asked to sit slowly and come right back up to standing as soon as the sitting surface is felt. These intervention strategies will improve eccentric control while transitioning from standing to sitting.

Skill Practice

Once patients have mastered the basic skill of transferring and are in the associative and autonomous stages of motor learning, interventions should be designed to promote skill acquisition. A "transfer course" can be set up that requires the patient to transfer to and from many types of seating surfaces in a random order. The course can be set up such that the patient must walk a short distance to the different seating surfaces (Fig. 7.24 and see Video 7.1). Video 7.1 (available online at Davis*Plus*) depicts a patient with traumatic brain injury performing a variety of task-specific transfer interventions in a transfer circuit.

To progress the complexity of the task to better reflect the patient's real-world environment, a dual- or multitask paradigm can also be introduced. In this scenario, the patient is required to hold an object while practicing transfers. Either unilateral or bilateral use of the UE can be incorporated. For example, the patient may be asked to hold a cup (Fig. 7.25A) or hold a tray filled with one or more objects (Fig. 7.25B) while transferring. The patient can also be asked to perform a cognitive task such as subtracting serial 7s from 100 or provide the names of animals that start with a given letter. To make it more challenging, the patient can be asked to perform both the UE task and cognitive task at the same time while practicing the movement pattern.

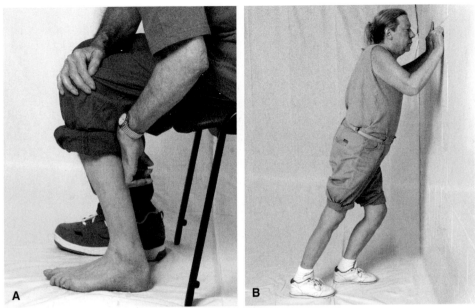

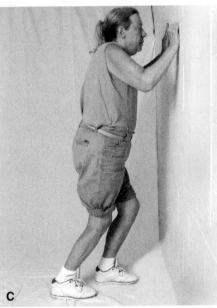

FIGURE 7.12 Both the soleus and gastrocnemius muscles should be stretched: (A) sitting soleus stretch, (B) standing gastrocnemius stretch with knee extended, (C) standing soleus stretch with knee flexed.

Speed of movement can also be an important task variable to modify during training. For example, the *sit-to-stand test* (described below in Outcome Measures of Transfer Ability) can be used during practice sessions to promote not only greater speed of movement but also greater attention to the task given the competitive nature of the test. Done across sessions, this may not only inform clinical decisions but also serve as behavioral reinforcement for the client.

Other environmental conditions can be modified as well. The floor surface can be changed to a thick carpet or dense foam. The lighting can be changed so the patient is practicing transfers in a low-light or no-light environment, similar to what would occur when a person gets up in the middle of the night to use the bathroom. Different noises can be introduced as a distracter. As with intervention strategies utilized early on, repetitive practice is key to enhancing motor learning.

Comments
• Practice should include random transferring to and from a variety of seating surfaces.
• Other motor and cognitive tasks may be incorporated when practicing.
• Practice strategies should include modifications to the environment, including lighting and floor surface.

Transfers To and From a Wheelchair

During the initial stages of rehabilitation, particularly while in the acute care or rehabilitation hospital settings, patients often use a wheelchair for mobility purposes when they are not in therapy. Some patients, especially those with cognitive impairments or those who have never used a wheelchair,

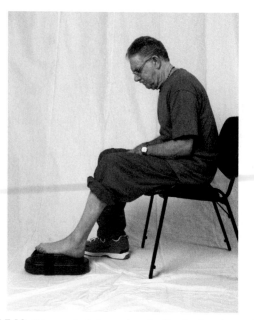

FIGURE 7.13 Using a skateboard under the foot reduces friction between the foot and the floor, making it easier for the patient to initially practice placing the foot in the correct position. The patient could also practice this activity independently as a component of a home exercise program.

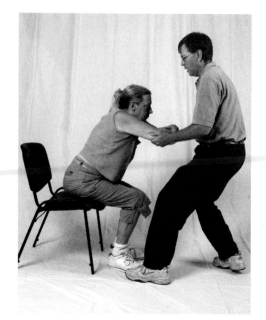

FIGURE 7.15 With the patient's UE crossed in front, the therapist guides forward translation during pre-extension while the patient maintains upper trunk extension as the lower trunk rotates forward at the hips.

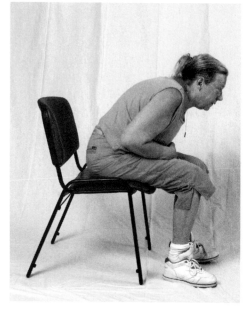

FIGURE 7.14 The patient has brought her head forward by increasing thoracic kyphosis and posterior pelvic tilt. The patient would likely lose her balance posteriorly and fall backward into the seat if she attempted to stand up from this position.

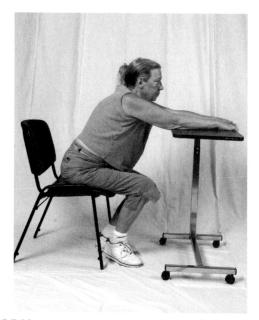

FIGURE 7.16 A tray table can assist with practicing maintaining upper trunk extension while the lower trunk rotates forward at the hips in preparation for effectively translating body mass horizontally during the pre-extension phase.

may be unable to correctly sequence the steps needed to safely position the wheelchair for transfers. In these cases, it may be appropriate to write down the sequence of steps necessary to transfer safely and tape it to the armrest of the patient's wheelchair. Although it may need to be adapted to the cognitive abilities and circumstances of the individual patient, a sample list might look like this:

1. Position wheelchair
2. Manage wheel locks
3. Manage footrests
4. Scoot to edge of wheelchair
5. Feet apart and behind knees

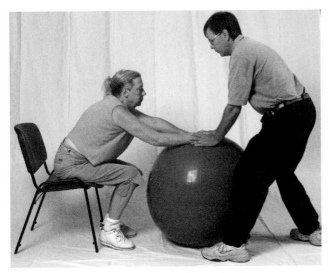

FIGURE 7.17 A therapy ball can assist the patient in learning how to effectively translate the body mass horizontally during the pre-extension phase by keeping the upper trunk extended while the trunk rotates forward at the hips.

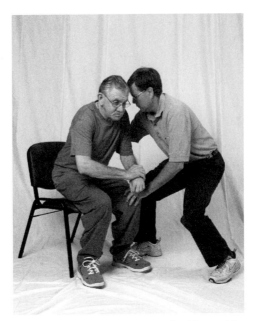

FIGURE 7.19 The therapist assists the patient by pushing down and slightly posteriorly through the knee. This will help stabilize the foot and provide assistance to extend the knee. The opposite hand is used to guide the trunk forward.

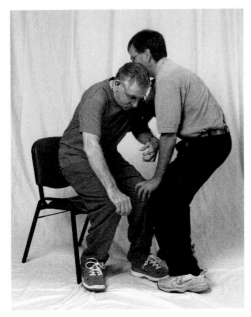

FIGURE 7.18 This patient with stroke (left hemiparesis) has a subluxed shoulder, which is manually supported by the therapist. The patient should never be assisted to standing by pulling on the shoulder joint.

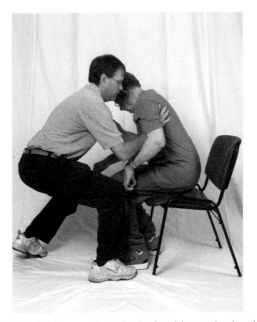

FIGURE 7.20 While providing physical assistance to stand up, the therapist should not stand so close to the patient as to block forward rotation of the trunk and lower leg. Shown here is appropriate positioning for assisting STS translation.

6. Sit tall with back straight
7. Lean forward with nose over toes
8. Push to stand up using armrests
9. Turn 90 degrees toward other surface and feel surface on the back of legs
10. Sit down slowly and safely

A similar generic list can be developed for use with all STS transfers, without the information about managing the wheelchair, as a way to remind the patient of the necessary steps.

Sit-Pivot Transfers

People who use a wheelchair as their primary method of mobility in their home and community, such as those with SCI, multiple sclerosis, or spina bifida, often must transfer in and out of the wheelchair using only the UEs (*sit-pivot transfer*). For a person with a complete SCI, the level of

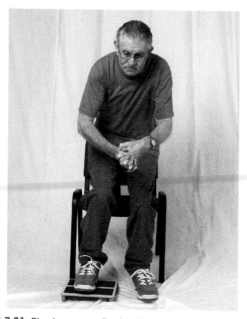

FIGURE 7.21 Placing a small raised surface (e.g., a block or step) under the less involved LE forces the patient to place additional weight on the more involved LE. This helps strengthen the more involved LE and reduces reliance on the less involved LE to provide the necessary force to stand.

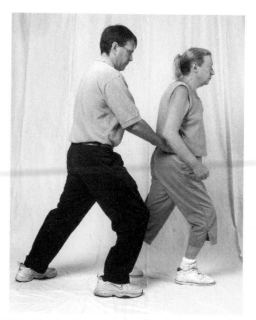

FIGURE 7.23 **The patient practices partial lunges** The length of the forward step and the amount of knee and hip flexion during the lunge can be increased as the patient's strength increases. Practice has direct functional carryover to improved stair and curb climbing.

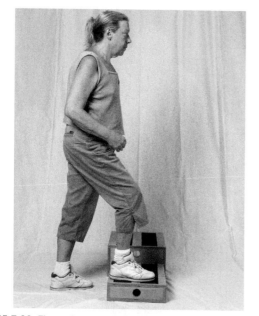

FIGURE 7.22 **The patient practices step-ups** The height of the step can be increased as the patient's LE strength increases. Practice has direct functional carryover to improved stair and curb climbing.

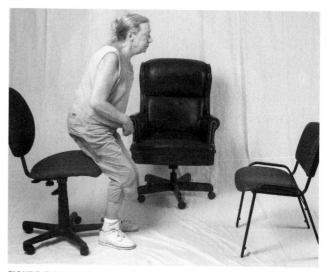

FIGURE 7.24 A "transfer course" can be set up in a circular, semicircular (shown here), or linear arrangement using a variety of seating surfaces. The transfer course should be arranged such that the patient must walk a short distance between the different seating surfaces. This activity will promote development of transfer skills required in the patient's home and community and enhance motor learning.

injury generally dictates the functional capacity for transfers. The lower the level of injury, the easier and more diverse the transfers will be. Factors other than level of preserved motor function will also impact the ability to independently perform sit-pivot transfers. These include body weight, spasticity, pain, ROM, and anthropometric characteristics.

A person with a complete C6 level SCI (American Spinal Injury Association [ASIA] A) has preserved rotator cuff muscles, deltoids, and biceps, as well as partial innervation of teres major, pectoralis major, and latissimus dorsi, which provides the strength to perform most sit-pivot transfers between even surfaces independently. Without triceps function, the elbow joint can be stabilized in extension by

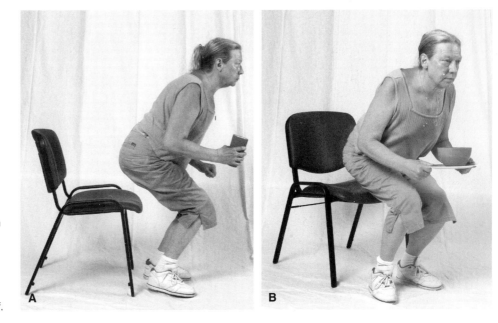

FIGURE 7.25 Transferring to standing while holding (A) a glass of water or (B) a plate with objects on it. Dual-task performance challenges the patient's control to prevent the contents from spilling from the glass or plate. This also serves to make the transfer more automatic as the patient's attention is on holding the glass or plate and not on the act of the transfer itself.

positioning the shoulder in external rotation, the elbow and wrist in extension, and the forearm in supination. To accomplish this, the patient first tosses the shoulder into extension with the forearm supinated. Once the base of the hand is in contact with the mat, the humerus is flexed to cause the elbow to extend because the arm is in a closed kinetic chain. The patient learns to control the elbow in extension in the closed chain by contracting the anterior deltoid, shoulder external rotators, and pectoralis major. The patient should avoid locking the elbow if possible because doing so may cause joint damage with multiple repetitions. To lift the trunk and hips from this position to transfer, the patient protracts and depresses the scapulae. The fingers should be flexed to preserve the tenodesis grip whenever weightbearing, and the wrist should be in neutral or close to neutral whenever possible.

Overview of Biomechanics

Unlike STS transfers, there is very little research regarding how people with SCI (or other similar disorders) perform sit-pivot transfers to and from their wheelchairs. Perry and colleagues[9] identified three components to the sit-pivot transfer: preparatory phase, lift phase, and descent phase. During the *preparatory phase,* the trunk flexes forward, leans laterally, and rotates toward the trailing arm (Fig. 7.26A). The *lift phase* starts when the buttocks lift off the sitting surface and continues while the trunk is lifted halfway between the two surfaces (Fig. 7.26B). The *descent phase* denotes the period when the trunk is lowered to the other seated surface from the halfway point until the buttocks are on the other surface (Fig. 7.26C).

The preparatory phase includes shifting the body weight from the buttocks onto the hands by flexing the trunk forward so that the shoulders are in front of the hands.[10] The ability to flex the trunk forward so that the shoulders are in front of the hands is a key component of the movement. The trailing hand is placed close to the upper thigh, anterior to the hip joint. The leading hand is placed farther away from the upper thigh to provide a space into which the buttocks and thighs can transfer. The upper trunk rotates toward the trailing hand, away from the target transfer surface. Initially this may be difficult because patients often want to see the surface they are transferring toward.

In the lift phase, the trunk and hips are lifted off the seating surface. The lower trunk is shifted in a medial lateral direction toward the leading hand. The upper trunk rotates toward the trailing hand. During the descent phase, the trunk and hips continue to be lifted off the seating surface and the trunk continues to rotate toward the trailing hand while the body is lowered onto the seating surface. Peak force generated at the trailing hand generally occurs right before the buttocks are lifted off the seating surface and while the buttocks are in the air for the lead hand.[10] Greater force is generated by the trailing than the lead UE, suggesting that the weaker UE or one that has a painful shoulder should be the lead.[9,10]

Precautions and Lead-Up Skills

Many people who use a sit-pivot transfer to and from their wheelchair are at risk of developing skin breakdown. During transfers, shearing forces on the skin should be avoided. Patients should be instructed to lift up their body instead of sliding along the surface. Multiple small lifts and pivots are better than sliding along the surface. Early in a rehabilitation program, individuals with traumatic SCI may have orthopedic precautions that include avoiding excessive stress on healing, unstable fracture sites in the spine. These precautions need to be strictly adhered to. As mentioned earlier, people with a C7 level SCI injury and above should keep their fingers flexed when weightbearing on their hands, using an extended wrist and elbow to preserve tightness in the longer finger flexors to maintain the ability to use a tenodesis grasp.

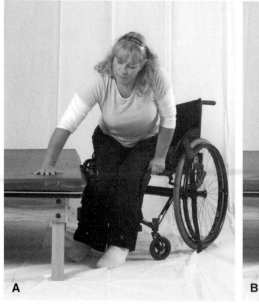

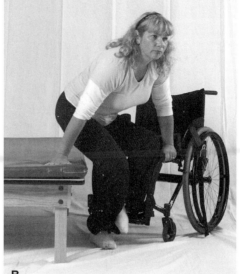

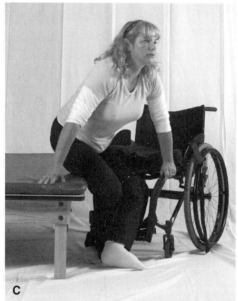

FIGURE 7.26 Sit-pivot transfer from wheelchair to mat (A) During the preparatory phase, the individual with incomplete SCI (T6) has the trailing hand on the wheelchair and the lead hand on the surface to which she is going to transfer. She flexes trunk and begins to rotate the upper trunk toward the trailing hand. (B) During the lift phase, momentum from the forward trunk flexion and rotation with triceps extension and scapular depression serve to lift the trunk and pelvis off the wheelchair. (C) During the descent phase, eccentric muscle contraction serves to lower the body to the mat.

Many lead-up skills are required in preparation for transferring in or out of a wheelchair, and they are presented in Table 7.2.

Red Flag: Shearing forces should be avoided during transfers to prevent skin breakdown. Orthopedic precautions should be carefully followed to avoid excessive force at healing, unstable spinal fracture sites.

Strategies and Activities

Very little, if any, research has been conducted that examines effective intervention strategies for developing skill in performing sit-pivot transfers. The interventions presented here are based on task-oriented balance and strengthening strategies. Multiple movement strategies should be practiced; no one technique will work for every patient. Slight variations in hand placement, foot placement, or direction of trunk flexion/rotation may allow an individual patient to become independent or perform the transfer more efficiently. Patients should be encouraged to problem-solve and experiment to find a technique that is efficient and safe.

Independence and self-confidence with short-sitting balance is the most critical prerequisite skill necessary for independent sit-pivot transfers. Patients who are not confident in their ability to maintain a safe sitting posture are not likely to be able to develop the proper technique and skills necessary to transfer independently and safely. If patients do not feel safe and confident in short-sitting, then they are not going to be confident in their ability to move from one surface to another in a sitting position.

Sitting balance training for patients with SCI and adequate range of the hamstrings should initially begin in

TABLE 7.2 Lead-Up Skills for Transferring to and from Wheelchair	
Lead up Skill	**Comments**
Position wheelchair	Wheelchair should be positioned at a 20 to 30 degree angle from the target transfer surface. Casters positioned backward will provide more stability to the wheelchair.
Set wheel locks	Different wheel locks are available (push to lock, pull to lock, or scissor locks).
Remove and replace arm rests	Armrest styles vary; some may swing-away, others may need to be removed completely.
Remove and replace leg rests	Some patients transfer by keeping their feet on the footplate; others remove the leg rests and place their feet on the ground. To provide stability, the thighs should be parallel or angled slightly higher in relation to the surface the patient is transferring to.
Manage transfer board	Patients with higher level SCI may require a transfer board to transfer in and out of the wheelchair safely and independently.
Manage lower extremities	This includes moving LEs on and off footplates and positioning appropriately.
Manage body position in wheelchair	Scooting to the edge of the seating surface and ability to position the buttocks in front of the wheel are important lead-up skills.

long-sitting (this is a more stable posture) but quickly progress to short-sitting. However, an important precaution when in the long-sitting position is to avoid overstretching low back muscles and hamstrings. For patients with midthoracic level and higher SCI, tightness in the low back muscles can provide lower trunk and pelvic stability in sitting. Patients should maintain approximately 90 degrees (but not more) of passive straight-leg-raise ROM.

Initially, static short-sitting balance activities should be practiced, then progressed to dynamic short-sitting activities; finally, patients should identify, test, and feel comfortable with their limits of stability (LOS) in short-sitting. When performing short-sitting balance interventions, the therapist should closely supervise and assist when necessary so the patient can begin to gain confidence with his or her balance ability. As the patient improves, the therapist should provide less assistance and progress the intervention so that it is more challenging. Intervention activities to promote short-sitting balance (i.e., to improve static and dynamic sitting control) are discussed in Chapter 5: Interventions to Improve Sitting and Sitting Balance Skills. Intervention activities specific to improving stand-pivot transfers include:

- Actively leaning backward, forward, and to left and right to the patient's LOS. The patient must be closely supervised and assisted when necessary during this activity for safety and to prevent a fall.
- Sitting push-ups (with or without push-up bars). As described above, a key component of the movement is flexion at the hips with an erect spine (Fig. 7.27).
- Sitting push-up with scoot to left and right. The head and trunk should lean forward and rotate away from the direction of the scoot.

Activities in prone and quadruped are beneficial to strengthen key muscles necessary for sit-pivot transfers. Prone-on-elbows activities may be beneficial, especially for patients without active triceps to strengthen scapular depressors required to lift the body during a transfer. Suggested activities in prone-on-elbows and quadruped include:

- Prone-on-elbows push-ups (Fig. 7.28)
- Prone-on-elbows scapular retraction (Fig. 7.29)

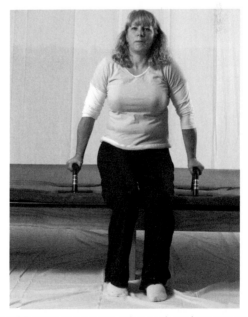

FIGURE 7.27 Seated push-ups using push-up bars are more challenging in short-sitting compared with long-sitting due to the smaller anterior BOS and lack of lengthened hamstrings providing pelvic stability.

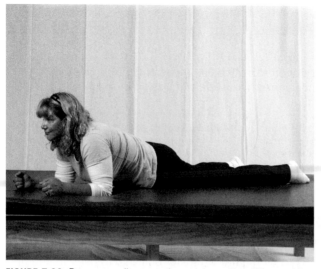

FIGURE 7.28 Prone-on-elbow push-ups strengthen the serratus anterior. As a progression, push-up height may be increased by instructing the patient to tuck the chin while lifting and rounding out the shoulders and upper thorax.

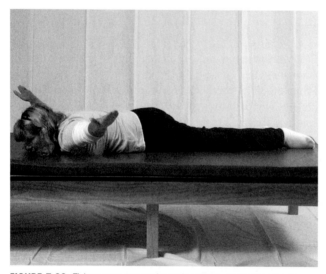

FIGURE 7.29 This prone scapular retraction exercise can be used to strengthen the middle and lower trapezius and rhomboid muscles.

- Prone-on-elbows scapular retraction with downward rotation
- Push-ups in quadruped, although the therapist may need to support the lower trunk (either manually or with a ball) to avoid excessive lumbar lordosis in patients with midthoracic level and higher SCI

Transfer Skill

Once the patient has confidence in short-sitting balance, transfer training should focus on learning the transfer skill. Developing skill with the transfer technique is more important than strength. Proper technique requires less strength and will lessen repetitive forces on the UE joints in the long-term, reducing the risk of developing overuse injuries.

To begin practicing the transfer the therapist should initially set up the environment in an optimal manner so the patient can focus on learning the transfer skill. This entails positioning the wheelchair at a slight angle to the transfer surface, using a firm surface that is the same height as the wheelchair, removing footrests, engaging the wheel locks, and assisting the patient with scooting to the edge of the wheelchair. Preliminary set up of the environment during early training will encourage success by conserving patient energy and allowing all attention to be focused on learning the actual transfer. An important goal of training is to set up the environment and intervention so that it is challenging for the patient but also so the patient can be successful and gain confidence with the transfer skill.

The initial position of the patient should be similar to a tripod. The lead hand is farther away from the body and positioned on the edge of the mat, with the shoulder in slight internal rotation. The trail hand is close to the patient's body. The patient's buttock is the middle of the tripod. The patient leans the trunk and head down and forward to weight the UEs while rotating away from the end surface being transferred to (rotate toward the trail hand). The combination of the forward/downward lean to weight the UEs and protraction of the scapulae cause the lower body to lift up. The rotation of the upper trunk and head toward the trail hand causes the lower body to rotate toward the lead hand (the surface the patient is transferring to). The patient ends the transfer with the body near and slightly behind the lead hand and the head rotated toward the trail hand (Fig. 7.30).

The therapist should be seated in front of the patient on a stool that rotates or slides to optimally facilitate the transfer. One of the therapist's hands (the one closest to the surface the patient is transferring to) should be on the posterior aspect of the patient's shoulder and slightly along the lateral aspect of the scapula. This hand facilitates the patient's diagonal trunk motion (forward/downward and rotation away from the surface the patient is transferring to). The therapist's other hand is slightly under the patient's buttocks with the forearm/wrist along the outer aspect of the patient's hip on the patient's trail hand side. This hand assists with the lifting and provides balance support (Fig. 7.31).

Comments

- Confidence and independence in short-sitting are critical.
- Skill is more important than strength.
- Instruct in head-hips relationship: The head and upper trunk move in the opposite direction of the pelvis and legs. For example, when the patient is transferring to the left, the head should move forward, downward, and to the right to facilitate the lower body lift and movement toward the left.
- Ensure flexion at the hips with trunk maintained as erect as possible.
- Set up the environment for success.

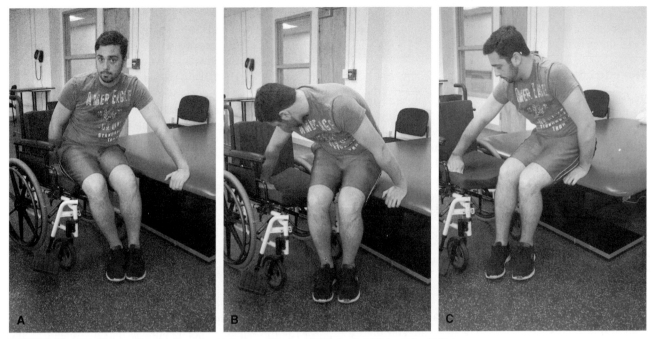

FIGURE 7.30 (A) Initial position for transfer. Note how the lead UE is in slight internal rotation and the patient's LEs are positioned such that the trunk is slightly rotated. (B) The patient flexes forward at the hips rotating the trunk toward the trail UE, which assists with the lift. (C) The patient completes the transfer with his body near the lead UE and head rotated toward the trail UE.

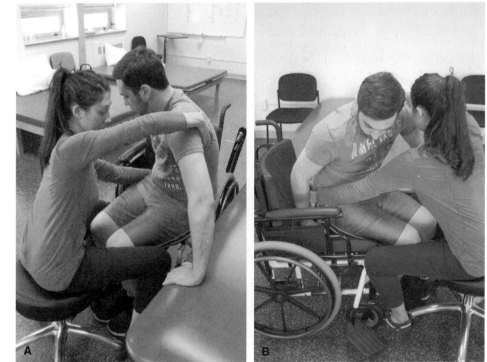

FIGURE 7.31 (A) One of the therapist's hands is positioned on the patient's posterior shoulder along the lateral aspect of the scapulae. This hand guides the patient's trunk and head flexion and rotation. Note how the therapist's LEs are positioned such that she can guide the direction of the transfer with her knees. (B) The therapist's opposite hand is on the hip/buttocks near the patient's trail hand. This hand placement provides trunk/balance support and assists lift if necessary.

- Preposition the body in an optimal manner: lead hand further from the body on the surface transferring to with the shoulder in slight internal rotation and forearm in pronation, trail hand close to the hip, feet on the floor, and trunk slightly rotated away from the surface transferring to.

- The trail UE does the most work, so if one UE is weaker or painful, set up the transfer so that the weaker or painful UE is the lead limb.
- This is a new motor task for patients so practice should be intense and multiple transfers should be performed in

one session to promote motor learning. The learning environment should be set up to be challenging but such that the patient can experience success.

Transfer Surfaces

Patients should also practice transferring to a variety of surfaces at varying heights compared with their wheelchair. These include a sofa, toilet, bathtub, shower chair, and car. The technique used to transfer to these surfaces is the same as that described above. When there is a large difference between the heights of the wheelchair and the target transfer surface, the patient must generate more momentum and force with even greater forward flexion and rotation of the trunk and head to achieve enough lift to raise the buttocks up onto the higher surface (Fig. 7.32). When transferring to a lower surface, the patient must learn to control the descent.

Floor-to-Wheelchair Transfers: Intervention Strategies

The ability to transfer out of a wheelchair and onto the floor and back is an important skill. It allows the patient to perform many important activities such as getting into a pool and playing with children on the floor. Although the patient may not plan on it, it is likely that he or she will fall out of the wheelchair at some point. The ability to transfer back into the wheelchair is essential when this happens. There are two basic floor-to-wheelchair techniques: *forward approach* and *sideward approach*. If possible, the casters of the wheelchair should be positioned backward to provide a longer wheelbase to the wheelchair, making it more stable.

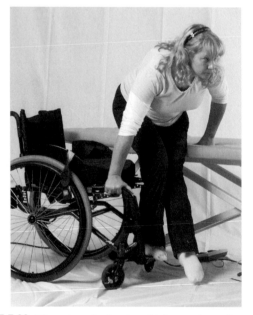

FIGURE 7.32 When transferring to a higher surface, the patient must flex forward and rotate even more than usual to generate sufficient momentum to lift the body up onto the higher surface.

Forward Approach

Initially, the person is side-sitting on one hip in front of the wheelchair. The knees are between and slightly in front of the casters; one hand is on the floor and one on the edge of the wheelchair (Fig. 7.33A). The person lifts the buttocks off the floor by pushing down with both hands, rotates the head down toward the hand by the hip, and comes up into a kneeling position facing the wheelchair (Fig. 7.33B). From the kneeling position, the person pushes down on the seat, wheels, or armrests of the wheelchair with both hands to lift the body up as high as possible to raise the buttocks higher than the seat (Fig. 7.33C). If armrests are available, pushing down on them will provide greater leverage and lift the body up higher. Once the buttocks are as high as possible, the person initiates trunk rotation while letting go with one hand, then continues to rotate the trunk and turns to land sitting in the wheelchair (Fig. 7.33D).

Sideward Approach

This technique requires a great deal of skill and hamstring flexibility, but does not require as much strength as the other two techniques. To start, the person sits diagonally in front of the wheelchair at a slight angle with one hand on the seat of the wheelchair and one on the floor (Fig. 7.34A). The person next lifts the buttocks up onto the edge of the seat by rotating the head and upper trunk down and away from the wheelchair (toward the hand on the floor) (Fig. 7.34B). This motion must be done quickly and forcefully to lift the buttocks up onto the front edge of the wheelchair. Then the person moves the buttocks back into the wheelchair onto the seat before lifting the head up. Next, the person places the hand that is on the floor onto the leg and "walks" it up the limb until he or she is sitting upright in the wheelchair (Fig. 7.34C).

Strengthening to Improve Transfer Skills

Strengthening key muscle groups using cuff weights, elastic resistive bands, free weights, pulleys, or other exercise equipment is also an important component of a comprehensive intervention program. Patients should perform two to three sets of 8 to 12 repetitions at their 10-repetition maximum. Key muscle groups to target are the elbow extensors, pectoralis major, deltoids, shoulder external rotators, scapular depressors, and serratus anterior.

Outcome Measures of Transfer Ability

It is important to use standardized outcome measures to document the patient's transfer ability. One of the most commonly used methods of measuring transfer ability is the transfer section of the *Functional Independence Measure (FIM)*.[11,12] The FIM measures the amount of

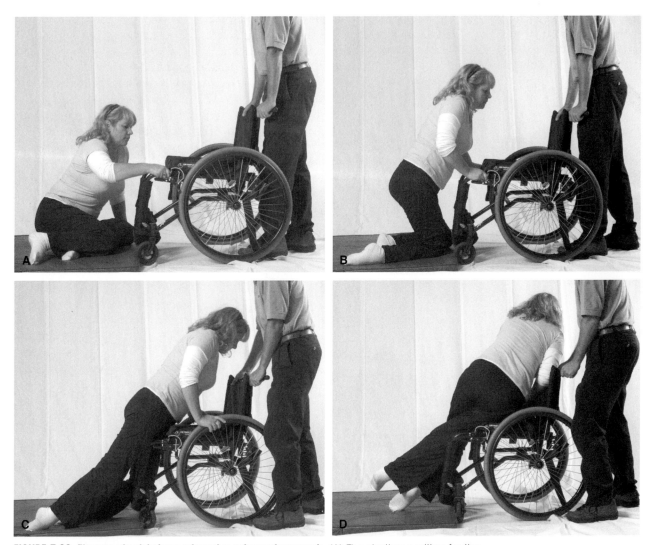

FIGURE 7.33 Floor-to-wheelchair transfer using a forward approach (A) The starting position for the forward approach is side-sitting in front of the wheelchair, with one hand on the floor and one on the wheelchair. (B) Next, the patient lifts herself into a kneeling position facing the wheelchair. (C) The patient lifts herself as high as possible, using the wheels or armrests on the wheelchair and then (D) rotates her body to turn into a sitting position in the wheelchair.

physical assistance a person requires to transfer on a 7-point ordinal scale. Scores range from a 1 (total assistance) to 7 (independent). Other standardized outcome measures that contain a component that examines a patient's ability to transfer include the *Motor Assessment Scale*,[13] the *Berg Balance Scale*,[14,15] *Wheelchair Skills Test*,[16,17] and the *Rivermead Motor Assessment*.[18] All of these tests are to some degree based on the amount of assistance the person requires and the quality of the movement. Another method

of measuring transfer ability is the *sit-to-stand test*.[19–22] There are two basic variations of this test: One measures the amount of time it takes the patient to transfer five times in succession from sitting to standing, and the other measures how many times the patient can transfer from sitting to standing in 30 seconds. The *Spinal Cord Independence Measure (SCIM)*[23,24] was designed specifically for people with SCI and assesses transfer ability as well as other aspects of function.

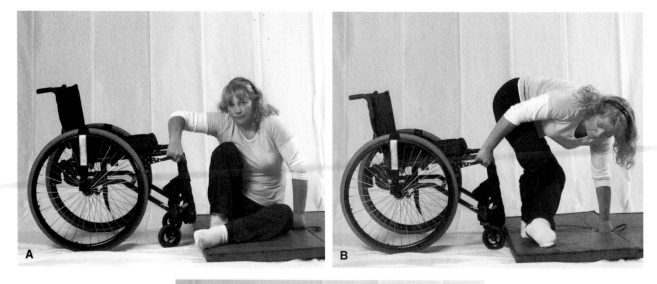

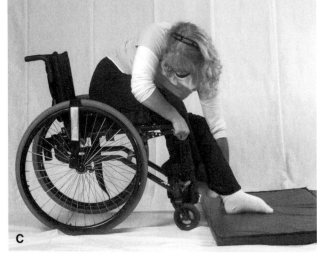

FIGURE 7.34 Floor-to-wheelchair transfer using a sideward approach (A) The starting position for the sideward approach is sitting diagonally in front of the wheelchair with one hand on the floor and one on the wheelchair. (B) The patient lifts the buttocks up off the floor by flexing the head and trunk down toward the hand on the floor while pushing down with that hand. This motion assists in lifting the buttocks off the floor and into the wheelchair. (C) The hand that is on the floor is moved onto one leg (partially obscured) and the patient "walks" the hand up the limb to bring the trunk up to a sitting position. Alternatively, the patient can use the hand on the floor together with the one on the wheelchair to quickly push up to bring the trunk to a sitting position.

SUMMARY

This chapter has presented strategies for developing and implementing a POC designed to improve transfer ability. Task analysis serves as the foundation for analyzing functional movement patterns. The results of the task analysis are used to develop task-oriented interventions. The environment and task should be shaped to challenge the patient, enhance motor learning, and promote neuroplastic changes. Repetition is also an important component of the POC.

REFERENCES

1. Hedman, LD, Rogers, MW, and Hanke, TA. Neurologic professional education: linking the foundation science of motor control with physical therapy interventions for movement dysfunction. Neurol Rep, 1991; 20:9–13.
2. Shepherd RB, and Gentile, AM. Sit-to-stand: functional relationship between upper body and lower limb segments. Hum Move Sci, 1994; 13:817–840.
3. Schenkman, M, et al. Whole-body movements during rising to standing from sitting. Phys Ther, 1990; 70:638–648.
4. Kralj, A, Jaeger, RJ, and Munih, M. Analysis of standing up and sitting down in humans: definitions and normative data presentation. J Biomech, 1990; 23:1123–1138.
5. Harvey, RL. Motor recovery after stroke: new directions in scientific inquiry. Phys Med Rehabil Clin N Am, 2003; 14(suppl. 1):S1–5.
6. Nudo, RJ. Functional and structural plasticity in motor cortex: implications for stroke recovery. Phys Med Rehabil Clin N Am, 2003; 14(suppl. 1):S57–S76.
7. Barreca, S, et al. Effects of extra training on the ability of stroke survivors to perform an independent sit-to-stand: a randomized controlled trial. J Geriatr Phys Ther, 2004; 27:59–64.

8. Ouellette, MM, et al. High-intensity resistance training improves muscle strength, self-reported function, and disability in long-term stroke survivors. Stroke, 2004; 35:1404–1409.

9. Perry, J, et al. Electromyographic analysis of the shoulder muscles during depression transfers in subjects with low-level paraplegia. Arch Phys Med Rehabil, 1996; 77:350–355.

10. Forslund, EB, et al. Transfer from table to wheelchair in men and women with spinal cord injury: coordination of body movement and arm forces. Spinal Cord, 2007; 45:41–48.

11. Stineman, MG, et al. The Functional Independence Measure: tests of scaling assumptions, structure, and reliability across 20 diverse impairment categories. Arch Phys Med Rehabil, 1996; 77:1101–1108.

12. Ottenbacher KJ, et al. The reliability of the functional independence measure: a quantitative review. Arch Phys Med Rehabil, 1996; 77:1226–1232.

13. Carr, JH, et al. Investigation of a new motor assessment scale for stroke patients. Phys Ther, 1985; 65:175–180.

14. Berg, KO, et al. Measuring balance in the elderly: validation of an instrument. Can J Pub Health, 1992; 83(suppl. 2):S7–S11.

15. Berg, K, Wood-Dauphinee, S, and Williams, J. The Balance Scale: reliability assessment with elderly residents and patients with an acute stroke. Scand J Rehabil Med, 1995; 27:27–36.

16. Kirby, RL, et al. The wheelchair skills test: a pilot study of a new outcome measure. Arch Phys Med Rehabil, 2002; 83:10–18.

17. Kirby, RL, et al. The wheelchair skills test (version 2.4): measurement properties. Arch Phys Med Rehabil, 2004; 85:794–804.

18. Lincoln, N, and Leadbitter, D. Assessment of motor function in stroke patients. Physiotherapy, 1979; 65:48–51.

19. Bohannon, RW, et al. Five-repetition sit-to-stand test performance by community-dwelling adults: a preliminary investigation of times, determinants, and relationship with self-reported physical performance. Isokinetics Exer Sci, 2007; 15:77–81.

20. Bohannon, RW. Reference values for the five-repetition sit-to-stand test: a descriptive meta-analysis of data from elders. Percept Motor Skills, 2006; 103:215–222.

21. Eriksrud, O, and Bohannon, R. Relationship of knee extension force to independence in sit-to-stand performance in patients receiving acute rehabilitation. Phys Ther, 2003; 83:544–551.

22. Bohannon, RW. Sit-to-stand test for measuring performance of lower extremity muscles. Percept Mot Skills, 1995; 80:163–166.

23. Catz, A, et al. SCIM—spinal cord independence measure: a new disability scale for patients with spinal cord lesions. Spinal Cord, 1997; 35:850–856.

24. Dawson, J, Shamley, D, and Jamous, M. A structured review of outcome measures used for the assessment of rehabilitation interventions for spinal cord injury. Spinal Cord, 2008; 46:768–780.

Interventions to Improve Wheelchair Skills

GEORGE D. FULK, PT, PhD, AND
JENNIFER HASTINGS, PT, PhD, NCS

For people who have spinal cord injury (SCI) and others who use a manual wheelchair as their primary means of locomotion, the ability to propel and maneuver over and around various obstacles and terrains in their home and community is essential for functional independence, community participation, and quality of life.[1,2] To propel a manual wheelchair independently in the home and community environments, riders need to be able to perform basic wheelchair mobility skills such as propulsion, door management, emergency egress, wheelies and be able to ascend and descend steep hills, ramps, and curbs. Optimal wheelchair configuration, which allows for the ideal rider positioning, and appropriate technique while performing these skills is important for energy efficiency, injury prevention, and safety. Physical therapists should also employ appropriate teaching strategies to promote motor learning.

Wheelchair Configuration

A wheelchair for a person who will use it for full-time mobility should be custom specified.[3] For those who will use it for more than short-duration intermittent transport, the wheelchair should be correctly measured for seat width, seat depth, backrest height, and footrest length. After sizing, configuration should be determined. Configuration establishes the dynamic stability of the wheelchair and the rider. The configuration required depends upon the disability and ability of the rider.

If the user is a part-time walker, the wheelchair should be configured to make sit-to-stand transfers easiest to accomplish. In this case, the wheelchair is best configured with swing-away or flip-up footrests to allow the feet to be positioned with knee flexion and an anterior tibial inclination. Often, a slightly higher seat height is also advantageous.

If the user will be propelling the wheelchair with his or her feet, the wheelchair seat needs to be lower to the ground and the seat depth slightly shorter. The footrest should be removable and will need to be set slightly shorter than the user's legs to allow ground clearance when in use. A chair that will be frequently pushed by a caregiver should include push handles and be set up with a slightly longer wheelbase and larger casters. This wheelchair may also have a higher backrest with a posterior bend

in the canes (vertical tubular bars supporting the backrest) to create a slight recline at the top to allow better posture and comfort for the rider.

The wheelchair that will be propelled by the rider independently for community mobility should be set up for optimal push mechanics and dynamic stability. There is a fundamental difference in the configuration needs of a person without innervated trunk muscles compared with someone who has innervated trunk muscles. People who have lower extremity (LE) amputation or lumbar paralysis will be best seated in a wheelchair with a minimal seat angulation (angle above horizontal): generally, approximately 5 degrees or 0.08 slope (Fig. 8.1A). The backrest should support the low back, providing lumbar support but not interfering with upper extremity (UE) motions or trunk rotation.

For the person with trunk paresis or paralysis, the inclination of the seat should be greater, approximately 14 degrees above horizontal (0.25 slope) with an acute seat-to-backrest inside angle (i.e., less than 90 degrees).[4] The backrest will be low, supporting the lumbar spine, and will not interfere with UE function. Optimal backrest height is adjusted to the level of T10 and should be vertical or no more than 5 degrees behind vertical (Fig. 8.1B). It should be noted that when the backrest is reclined too far posterior to upright vertical (beyond 5 degrees), the chair becomes unstable to the rear and the rider is more likely to sit with a posterior pelvic tilt, which further compromises push mechanics.

To optimize push mechanics, the seat height (including cushion height) should be such that the rider can easily reach the rear wheels with sufficient arc for a long propulsive stroke without excessive shoulder extension or elevation. The arc of push is also affected by the position of the rear axle in the horizontal plane. A more forward axle placement improves hand access to the rear half of the wheel, making it easier for the rider to perform wheelies. Changing the rear axle placement (or the caster placement) will affect the wheelbase. A longer wheelbase is more stable and tracks better, keeping the wheelchair on a straighter course when propelling forward, but is harder to turn and harder to lift the front end (e.g., performing a wheelie). Conversely, the stability of a longer wheelbase makes traversing up steep inclines easier. For curb ascent the shorter wheelbase makes lifting into a wheelie easier. Literature regarding UE protection[3,5] suggests that the

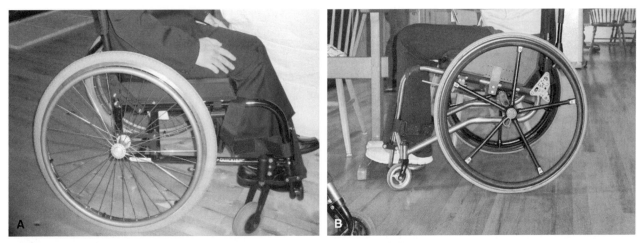

FIGURE 8.1 Wheelchair configuration (A) Wheelchair with 5-degree seat angulation; (B) wheelchair with 14-degree seat angulation with vertical backrest.

most axle-forward position that the rider can handle (and maintain good balance) is generally the best. Positioning the axle so that it aligns or is slightly forward of the shoulder when the rider is sitting fully upright is a good starting position. This is balanced with the amount of rearward tilt (inclination above horizontal) of the seat provided by the difference between the front and rear seat to floor heights. A rule of thumb is that when the rider is sitting fully upright, the axle should align between the tip of the fingers and the palm of the hand with the arm hanging relaxed.

The important point with alignment and wheelchair configuration is that the arc of push can be accomplished without shoulder hyperextension or elevation and excessive wrist motion. A rear seat to floor height that is too low will require extreme range of motion (ROM) during propulsion creating the potential for musculoskeletal injury. A rear seat to floor height that is too high also increases risk of injury because it imposes a short pushing arc requiring increased frequency of push stroke.

Caster size also affects wheelchair mobility. In general, the smaller the caster, the less roll resistance, but the more difficulty maneuvering terrain obstacles. The larger casters (6 to 8 in. [15.24 to 20.32 cm]) interfere with good foot positioning and are generally not recommended for independent propulsion with arms or feet.

Propulsion

The stroke required to propel a wheelchair can be divided into two phases: push and recovery. The push phase occurs when the user's hands apply force through the handrims to propel the wheelchair. The recovery phase occurs when the user's hands are off the handrim and are being repositioned for the next push phase. The motion pattern for the push phase is constrained by movement of the wheelchair handrim. For the recovery phase, four common movement patterns have been

identified: *arcing, semicircular, single looping,* and *double looping.*[6]

- Arcing pattern: The hand closely follows the wheelchair handrim in the reverse direction from the push (i.e., shoulder extending) to bring the hand back for the next push.
- Semicircular pattern: The hand drops under the wheelchair handrim as the shoulder extends to bring the hand back to prepare for another push.
- Single-looping pattern: The hand loops above the wheelchair handrim as the shoulder extends to bring the hand back for the next push.
- Double-looping pattern: The hand initially comes above the handrim after the push and loops back down under the handrim as the shoulder continues to extend to bring the hand back for the next push (Fig. 8.2).

The semicircular and the double-looping patterns provide the best shoulder mechanics and the longer push arcs. However, evidence has not shown clearly if one type of stroke pattern is more efficient or more likely to reduce the risk of UE injury than another.[7] A primary goal when teaching wheelchair propulsion skills is to use a pattern that minimizes the risk of UE injury. To do this the wheelchair should be optimally configured (see above), and the rider should avoid having the joints of the UE at the extreme ranges of motion throughout the push and recovery phases (i.e., extreme shoulder extension and internal rotation at the start of the propulsion cycle).[8]

The therapist should demonstrate the proper propulsion technique, emphasizing joint positioning to minimize UE injury. Riders with impaired UE sensation and strength may initially require manual cues and guidance with placing their hands in the correct position on the handrims and initiating a push. The casters of the wheelchair should be positioned in the trailing position (i.e., so that the wheelchair is ready to propel forward), and the therapist may need to provide a slight push forward to the wheelchair to

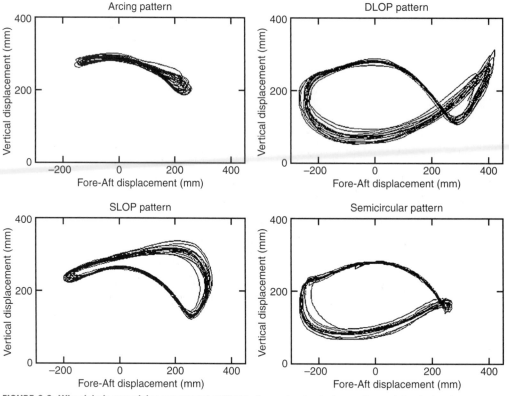

FIGURE 8.2 Wheelchair propulsion movement patterns Four classic stroke patterns (clockwise from upper left): arcing, DLOP, semi-circular, and SLOP. The arcing and SLOP patterns were classified as over-rim propulsive strokes while the semi-circular and DLOP patterns were classified as under-rim propulsive strokes.
Abbreviations: DLOP, double-looping over propulsion; SLOP, single-looping over propulsion. Reprinted with permission from Kwarciak et al. Redefining the manual wheelchair stroke cycle: identification and impact of nonpropulsive pushrim contact. Arch Phys Med Rehabil, 2009; 90:20–26.

create the initial forward momentum. Riders with limited UE function may benefit from plastic-coated handrims, foam-coated handrims (Fig. 8.3A), rubber tubing wrapped around the handrims, or projections on the handrims (Fig. 8.3B). These will provide an improved grip on the handrims and increased leverage for propulsion. Handrim projections are not recommended for community mobility. (See Box 8.1: Special Considerations for Patients with Limited Hand Function.)

Another useful teaching tool is to have a peer mentor wheelchair user be a part of the intervention session. Having a person with a similar injury demonstrate the different techniques in a skillful manner is extremely valuable. This is true when teaching all of the wheelchair skills described in this chapter.

To propel the wheelchair forward, the rider reaches back and loosely grasps the wheelchair handrims (Fig. 8.4), then pushes forward, releasing the handrim after the hands have passed in front of the hips. A more open grip that covers the tire and handrim provides better control but may lead to skin irritation on the hand. Too strong a grip and release on the handrims may slow down the wheelchair and lead to epicondylitis. Riders should practice reaching back on the handrims to initiate the stroke and pushing far forward on the handrims. The pushing stroke should be in a forward

direction and long. A well-configured wheelchair will allow the rider to reach back on the handrims to initiate the push, avoiding shoulder hyperextension and elevation of the scapula. Riders should be taught to maintain the shoulder in midrange in relation to internal and external rotation and the wrist and forearm in midrange throughout the stroke cycle. Patients with limited or no hand function can propel the wheelchair by pushing with their palms inward against the lateral aspect of the handrims (i.e., squeezing the handrims) and then pushing forward. For such patients, a handrim with high-friction coating is recommended. An appropriately configured wheelchair will also provide a measure of trunk and pelvic stability, allowing riders who have trunk paresis or paralysis to be relatively stable as they propel the wheelchair.

Propelling the wheelchair backward is done in a similar manner. Instead of reaching back on the handrims to start, the rider reaches forward on the handrims and pulls back. Riders without the ability to grasp the handrim will place their palms on the wheels behind their hips and push backward by extending their elbows and depressing their scapulae. Alternatively, this rider can hook the inside of the handrim with wrist extension and pull upward and back with a biceps action. Turning a wheelchair in a tight

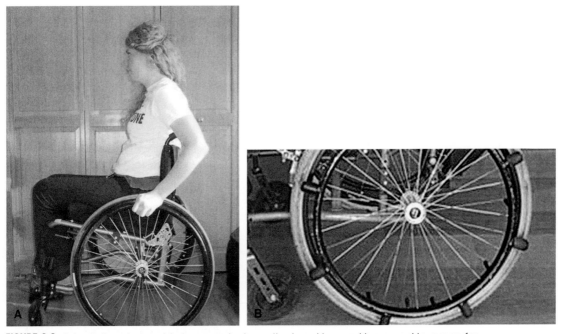

FIGURE 8.3 Adaptations to provide improved grip on the handrims and increased leverage for propulsion. (A) Rider with impaired hand function using foam-coated handrims; (B) projections on handrims.

BOX 8.1 Special Considerations for Patients With Limited Hand Function

The most important consideration when developing a plan of care for a person with limited hand function (e.g., a person with a C-6 SCI) is that people with this impaired function can effectively develop functional wheelchair skills. People with cervical SCI who use a manual wheelchair report a higher quality of life than those who rely on powered mobility.[2]

• Do not assume someone cannot do these skills because of limited hand function.
• Skills that require power moves such as ascending a 4-inch curb or higher from a stopped position, or propelling up very steep hills, or moving in a wheelie over rugged terrain will typically take full grip strength, but otherwise the wheelchair skills in this chapter are accessible to riders with impaired hand function.
• Impaired sensation needs to be considered and protection is essential.
• Gloves are a key piece of equipment. Most people with tetraplegia will be able to independently don and doff a fingerless mitt-type glove with hook and pile closure. A high-friction and protective surface that covers the palm and distal portion of the wrist is ideal.
• Do not configure the wheelchair in a manner that creates spaces between the wheels and the frame in which hands can become stuck.
• Handrims should be high friction and mounted close to the wheel or with the space between the handrim and the wheel filled.

• "Quad knobs" or "handrim projections" should be avoided when prescribing an ultralight wheelchair and for use in community mobility. Although these devices do allow a rider with impaired hand function better ability to initiate movement of a stopped wheelchair, they are very unsafe in community mobility. With impaired hand sensation, they make controlling speed or slowing a wheelchair difficult and potentially dangerous.
• Wheel locks should be clear of the propulsion arc when unlocked.
• When the rider does not have triceps function he or she will benefit from rear wheels that are more forward and a wheelchair configuration that places the seat deeper in the wheels. This configuration allows the primary movers of propulsion to be the biceps and anterior deltoid. Careful balance of the wheelchair configuration between providing dynamic balance for the rider and optimal positioning for propulsion is required.
• Anti-tip devices can provide stability while allowing optimal wheel position.
• If a custom wheelchair frame can be acquired, then a *longer* frame with a steep footrest angle will place the casters more forward and weight the front end of the wheelchair to allow improved propulsion mechanics without instability.

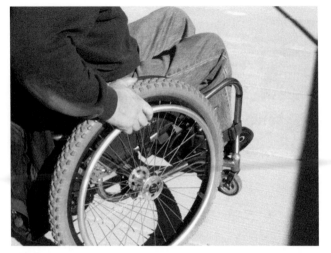

FIGURE 8.4 Grasping wheelchair handrim in preparation for propelling forward with a loose, open grip.

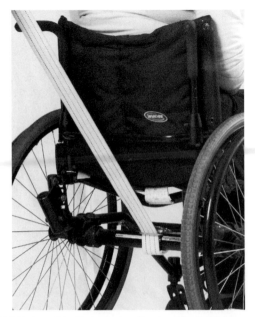

FIGURE 8.5 A gait belt securely attached to the frame of the wheelchair can be used to spot (guard) riders as they practice wheelies and other wheelchair skills.

radius or a quick turn is a combination of a forward push with one hand and a backward push with the other. With a larger radius or slower turn, the rider can apply greater or lesser force to the handrim that is on the outside of the turn (greater) or the inside of the turn (less). To turn a wheelchair that is moving, the rider applies a braking action to the handrim on the inside of the turn. This slows down the inside wheel in relation to the outside wheel, causing the wheelchair to turn. A moving turn indoors can also be done by reaching out with the hand on the inside of the turn and lightly touching or sliding the hand along the wall or doorway surface with the hand behind the rear axle. Practice is necessary to learn when to apply pressure on the wall/doorway and how much pressure to apply and to estimate the speed at which the wheelchair is travelling. If the turn is taken too soon (or too late) or too much (or too little) pressure is applied or the timing is not correct, the wheelchair will turn too quickly (or not quickly enough).

For successful motor learning to occur when teaching any wheelchair skill, the therapist should initially make sure the rider feels safe sitting in the wheelchair by closely supervising and guarding the rider. If the rider fears becoming unstable, it will be difficult for him or her to reach for the handrims and push the wheelchair, roll down a ramp, or "pop" a wheelie. To ensure the safety of the rider while practicing wheelchair skills the therapist is positioned behind the wheelchair. With a gait belt looped through the frame of the wheelchair, the therapist (Fig. 8.5) holds the gait belt in one hand and positions the other hand anterior to the patient's shoulder. Positioning the hands in this manner allows the therapist to prevent the rider from falling out of the wheelchair in the anterior direction and prevents the wheelchair from tipping over backward. Alternately, the posterior hand can be placed on the wheelchair push handle (if one is available) instead of using a gait belt (Fig. 8.6).

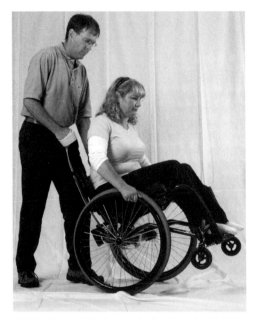

FIGURE 8.6 The therapist demonstrates how to safely spot a rider performing wheelies. Using a gait belt securely attached to the frame of the wheelchair, the therapist can pull up on the gait belt to prevent the rider from tipping over backward. The hand on the push handle of the wheelchair can help the rider maintain the wheelie.

Door Management

Basic forward, backward, and turning skills are prerequisite for opening a door, propelling through a doorway, and closing a door. There are a variety of doorway configurations and door handles. Doors can open toward or away from the rider. Doors can be free swinging or with resistance due to a self-closing mechanism. The difficulty of releasing the latch depends on the type of latch mechanism, which can be a bar, a handle with or without a thumb latch, a knob, or a lever. The basic techniques described below will need to be adapted depending on the specific environment. The easiest door to maneuver is a free-swinging door, and this should be the first task for training.

Propelling Through a Doorway With a Door That Opens Away From the Rider

The rider approaches the door at a slight angle with the rear wheels closer to the door hinges and reaches out to open the door latch with the hand that is closest to the door, keeping the opposite hand on the wheel. Maintaining the hold on the doorknob, the rider propels the outside wheel to turn the wheelchair into the doorway. The rider can then push the door open and use both hands to propel through the doorway. For a heavy self-closing door with a bar latch, the rider reaches across his or her body, as far as possible away from the hinges, to push the bar. This push position has the greatest leverage and offers the least resistance for pushing open the door. If the door is heavy or resists opening, the rider grasps the doorframe with the opposite hand and pulls the wheelchair through the doorway while the other hand pushes the door further open. The rider can also use the front end (i.e., footrest) of the wheelchair to assist with pushing open the door as he or she propels through the doorway. However, extreme caution should be used with this technique to prevent skin breakdown and injury to the toes and feet. Video 8.1 (available on Davis*Plus* at www.fadavis.com) depicts a rider propelling through a doorway that opens away from the rider.

For doors that do not close automatically, the rider can turn the wheelchair slightly toward the door after entry and push the door closed. Alternately, once the rider is through the doorway he or she can turn around to face the door and push it closed, with the wheelchair at a slight angle to the doorway (angling the wheelchair will prevent it from rolling backward as the door is pushed closed).

Propelling Through a Doorway With a Door That Opens Toward the Rider

When the door opens toward the rider, the key is to have the door swing past the rider to allow entry. If the door is in a wide hallway, this is more easily done by approaching at an angle to the doorway on the side of the door opening (side of lever, doorknob, or other opening mechanism). The rider grasps the lever and pulls open the door far enough so the front end of the wheelchair fits through the opening, optimally to the point just past the rear axle of the wheelchair, then propels with the latch-side hand to move the front of the wheelchair inside the doorway. The hand that opened the door returns to the wheelchair handrim and propels the wheelchair the rest of the way through the doorway.

When the door is heavy or has a self-closing mechanism, the technique is altered slightly by using the doorframe to assist. The initial approach is the same: release the latch with the hinge-side hand, then the other hand (latch side) reaches out for the doorframe. Placing the hand here can help stabilize the rider's trunk and provide leverage if necessary while opening the door (pushing against the doorframe with that UE, while the other pulls the door open). As the rider pulls the door open far enough so the front end of the wheelchair fits through the opening, the hand on the doorframe assists by pulling the wheelchair through the doorway. When necessary, the rider removes the hand closest to the door hinges from the handrim to push the door open as he or she propels through the doorway. Although it is not ideal, if it is a self-shutting door the rider can use the front end of the wheelchair (i.e., footrests) to assist with maintaining the door open as he or she propels through the doorway. This technique should again be done with caution to prevent injury to the toes and foot that may strike the door. Video 8.2 (available on Davis*Plus* at www.fadavis.com) depicts a rider propelling through a doorway with a door that opens toward the rider.

A free-swinging door will have to be closed by reaching back with the hand that is closest to the door hinges and pulling the door closed while rolling through the doorway. Alternately, once through the doorway, the rider can turn to face the door and pull it closed while propelling the chair backward. In this case the rider reaches for the door lever with the hand that is closest to the door hinges. The other hand can reach for the doorframe closest to the lever. This hand can assist in stabilizing the trunk and push to assist in backward propulsion of the wheelchair as the rider closes the door with the other hand. Video 8.3 (available on Davis*Plus* at www.fadavis.com) depicts a rider closing a door that closes toward the rider.

When teaching these skills, the therapist should review safety issues such as not grasping the door edge to prevent finger injury when the door closes and using caution when using the front end of the wheelchair to assist with opening the door. The tasks should be sequenced for difficulty to build upon success. In general, away-opening doors are easiest and free-swinging doors are easier than those with auto-closure. The therapist should set up the practice environment so that the rider is challenged when practicing the skill but not make it so difficult that the rider cannot complete the task. For example, if the rider cannot reach all the way to the lever to open the door initially, the physical therapist can start with the door partially open or place tape over the latch mechanism. Parts of the entire skill can also be practiced. For example, the rider can start with the door partway open and have one hand on the handrim and the other on the doorframe and practice pulling or propelling the wheelchair through the doorway. As the rider becomes more proficient in these skills, the therapist can set up the practice environment so the rider practices going through a variety of door types in terms of weight, width, entry and exit space in regard to the door, handles, small thresholds, and other such characteristics.

Emergency Egress

Everyone who uses a manual wheelchair should be able to instruct others to assist him or her down a flight of stairs. Ideally, wheelchair riders can take themselves down a flight of stairs independently when there is at least one railing available. As most fire escape stairwells are required to have a railing, it is a good place to master this skill.

As a starting point for emergency egress, it is important to learn how to do a single curb with assist up and down. The single curb down is similar to stairs with assistance and no railing. To go down, the rider approaches the curb backward and aligns the rear wheels evenly along the edge of curb. The therapist stands off the curb facing the back of the wheelchair. The rider then leans forward and grabs the forward aspect of the rear wheels. The therapist should stand in stride position and lean forward to brace the top of the backrest (for lower backrests the assistant should be farther away, making it easier to lean into the lower backrest). With coordinated effort, the rider rolls the rear wheels off the curb while the therapist stabilizes. Once the rear wheels are on the street surface the rider can continue to back off to drop casters or do a slight wheelie and turn 90 degrees to clear the curb.

The single curb assist up in the forward position is the reverse of this maneuver. The curb is approached forward and then the casters are lifted up onto the curb with assist if needed. The rider then grips the top of the wheels and leans forward to propel rear wheels up over the curb while the physical therapist provides assistance from behind with a forward (and slightly upward) push on the backrest. This is not a "lift"! The assisting force is diagonal to aid the wheels in rolling up over the curb. Video 8.4 (available on Davis*Plus* at www.fadavis.com) depicts a rider ascending a curb with assistance.

Stairs

The basic maneuver for emergency egress is as follows: descent is with the rear wheels first with the rider leaning forward toward casters; the chair is rolled down the stairs one step at a time with hands sliding down the railing(s). When masterfully done, the casters will only lightly contact each step as the wheelchair is rolling down the edge of the stairs in a balanced position. More commonly, the casters will come down somewhat forcefully on each step, and if the footrest is forward of the casters, the footrest may hit or scrape as well. It is important to maintain control of the wheelchair and not allow it to move too fast. This will keep the rider in the seat. Furthermore, the rider should maintain the wheelchair in a position with both rear wheels even, so that the descent is straight down the steps with no rotation of the chair.

The easiest technique is when there are two railings available and the stairwell is narrow enough so that the rider can hold both rails at once. The rider approaches the stairs, turns around so that the chair is centered in the stairway with

rear wheels 3 to 4 in. (7.62 to 10.16 cm) forward of the edge of the first step. The rider then places hands on both railings in a pronated grip with hands approximately level to shoulders; while leaning forward slightly, the rider pushes the wheelchair rearward so that the wheels roll off the step. Sliding the hands slightly down the railing, the process is repeated. Once mastered, the movement down the stairs can be a continuous roll after pushing off from the second step with the hands sliding down the railing. At the bottom the options are for the rider to push back off the last step and let the casters fall to ground (rider leans forward) or lift into a wheelie and either back off the final step or turn 90 degrees to clear the step, then set casters to floor.

With a single railing the technique is the same with the following modification. The rider positions the wheelchair near the railing side of the stairway approximately 4 to 6 in. (10.16 to 15.24 cm) away from the side. He or she grabs the railing with the rail-side hand in a pronated grip, reaches across body with the far-side hand, and grips the railing with a supinated grip. The rider should resist the temptation to hug into the railing because this will make the wheelchair uneven and cause rotation of the wheels or even lifting of the outside wheel. The rider uses the two arms as a counterpoint to control the wheelchair position during descent. Most riders will find it easier to make the first step while holding the railing only with the rail-side hand and having the outside hand on the wheelchair rear wheel to help wheel off the first step, then while balancing in this position, the rider's outside hand should be moved over to the railing.

Either of these techniques can be assisted by an able-bodied person who is downstairs from the wheelchair. The assistant should be in stride with feet covering at least two steps and not on the same step the wheelchair is moving to. The assistant braces the chair by leaning into backrest to slow the rolled descent and ensure speed control and that there is no possibility of rearward flipping. Assistants can further stabilize themselves by having one hand on the railing. Video 8.5 (available on Davis*Plus* at www.fadavis.com) depicts a rider descending stairs with one railing with a therapist assisting.

To teach these techniques, the therapist plays the role of the assistant as described above. Ideally, the therapist can demonstrate the skills or provide a peer video demonstration.

In the event that there is no railing on either side, stairs can be descended with an able-bodied assistant who is positioned downstairs from the rider. The technique is the same, but in this case the rider leans forward and keeps the hands on the rear wheels to provide braking. After positioning the rear wheels close to the top of the steps and leaning forward as far as possible onto the thighs, the rider pulls the wheels back to roll off the stair edge, then controls speed with a braking grip. The assistant is in contact during this initial maneuver and ensures the chair is moving with wheels in symmetry. The assistant moves, then the wheelchair moves, then the assistant, and so forth. If possible the assistant can brace against the wall for extra stability.

Wheelies

Although wheelchair accessibility has improved over recent years with the availability of curb cutouts and ramps, there are still many areas of the community that are not easily accessible with a wheelchair. The ability to perform a wheelie (Fig. 8.7) is an essential skill for negotiating curbs, descending steep ramps or hills, and traversing uneven terrain. The type of wheelchair and its configuration have an impact on how easy or difficult it is to attain a wheelie. Achieving a wheelie in a heavier wheelchair is more difficult. The position of the axle also impacts the ease of attaining a wheelie. An axle that is more forward, so that the rider's center of mass (COM) is behind the axle, makes the wheelchair less stable and more likely to tip, thus making it easier to assume a wheelie. A wheelchair is more stable with the axle plate positioned farther back, but this configuration makes it more difficult to attain a wheelie.

To accomplish a wheelie, the rider reaches back on the handrim, with hands behind the backrest, and quickly pushes forward to lift the front casters off the ground, rotating the chair approximately 45 degrees in space. The ability to maintain a wheelie should be learned in conjunction with attaining a wheelie. Both of these skills are important precursors to more advanced wheelie skills such as ascending and descending curbs and propulsion on uneven terrain. The therapist should assist the patient into the *balance point,* in which the front casters are off the ground with the wheelchair in equilibrium (i.e., the wheelchair is not going to tip over backward or forward [onto the casters]). The initial

balance point should be that which corresponds to the rider sitting fully against the backrest; if the rider leans forward off the backrest, a higher wheelie position is required, which requires greater skill. Once in the wheelie, the rider should be able to bend or straighten the arms while lightly gripping the handrim for balance correction.

For the rider to learn balance in a wheelie, he or she must experience balance control and the sway of the wheelchair that limits stability in a wheelie. An important first step in this process is for the rider to actively push and pull on the handrim while in a wheelie to feel the balance point and experience how to correct tipping too far backward or forward. A push forward will cause the casters to lift up, while a pull backward will drop the casters toward the ground. This latter maneuver is an important safety technique, and the rider should learn it early to understand how to control the wheelchair. The rider should also actively move the head and upper trunk forward and backward to learn the effect on wheelchair equilibrium. Leaning forward causes the casters to drop, whereas leaning backward raises the casters off the ground. The rider then requires practice maintaining the balance point by slightly pushing or pulling on the handrims and leaning forward and backward.

Dynamic, or moving, wheelies require that the rider allow the handrims to slide backward or forward within his or her grasp. The rider should understand that his or her hands on the handrims are what provides control and should be instructed to never completely let go of them.

When teaching wheelies, it is essential to ensure safety by appropriately guarding and supervising the rider as described earlier. Riders may be fearful of falling and reluctant to practice wheelies. The therapist must reassure the patient that he or she will not allow the rider to fall. Initially, when the rider is learning how to pop the wheelie, the therapist may need to manually assist the rider into the balanced wheelie position by pulling back on the push handles of the wheelchair.

There are two approaches to facilitate learning how to maintain a balanced wheelie position while practicing. In one approach the physical therapist taps the rider on the anterior or posterior trunk/shoulder area. This provides a tactile cue as to which direction the rider should shift the trunk to rebalance the wheelie. For example, if the rider begins to lose balance in a posterior direction (the casters are lifting further off the ground), the therapist taps the anterior trunk/shoulder to provide a tactile cue for the rider to lean forward and pull back on the handrims. If the rider is losing balance in the anterior direction (the casters are dropping toward the floor), the therapist taps the posterior trunk/shoulder to cue the rider to lean back and push forward on the handrims.

In another approach to facilitate learning, the therapist nudges the rider on the anterior or posterior trunk/shoulder area to move the rider back into the balance zone of the wheelie. For example, if the rider begins to lose balance in a

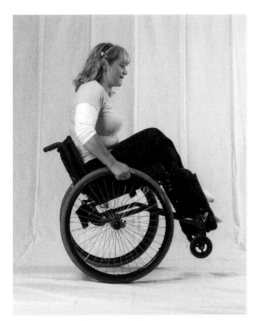

FIGURE 8.7 Maintaining a wheelie involves balancing with the front casters off the ground. Note the position of the rider's hands on the handrims near her hips. This position allows for greater control of the wheelie than with the hands either far forward or backward on the handrims.

posterior direction (the casters are lifting further off the ground) the therapist nudges the posterior trunk/shoulder in an anterior direction, which moves the rider back into the balance zone of the wheelie and prevents the rider from tipping over backward. If the rider is losing balance in the anterior direction (the casters are dropping toward the floor), the therapist nudges the anterior posterior trunk/shoulder in a posterior direction, which moves the rider into the balance zone of the wheelie and prevents the rider from tipping over forward. In both approaches, the therapist can also provide verbal cues as to which direction to pull or push the handrims.

Wheelies While Traversing Uneven Surfaces

When propelling a wheelchair on uneven surfaces (e.g., gravel, grass) there is a possibility of tipping the wheelchair over in a forward direction. On these types of surfaces, the casters can get stuck in a divot or stopped by a small object (e.g., a rock), causing the wheelchair to tip forward. Being able to propel the wheelchair forward while maintaining a wheelie can minimize this risk and allow the rider to propel the wheelchair independently over a variety of terrains. Video 8.6 (available on Davis*Plus* at www.fadavis.com) depicts a rider propelling a wheelchair on uneven terrain in a wheelie.

To propel the wheelchair forward while maintaining the wheelchair in its balance point, the rider practices leaning forward while in a wheelie (causing the wheelchair to tip forward), then pushes the handrims forward to bring the wheelchair back to the balance point. When learning this maneuver, the patient should be instructed to use a firm grip on the propulsion aspect but to allow the handrims to slide within his or her grip ("sliding grip") during the recovery aspect of the stroke. As the patient becomes more skilled, he or she can glide farther forward with each push of the handrims. Using similar techniques, the patient can learn to propel the wheelchair backward (same technique only in reverse) and turn while maintaining a wheelie (similar to making a tight turn on all four wheels—pulling backward on one handrim and pushing forward on the other).

On some uneven surfaces it may be easier to pop up into a wheelie for only a brief time (not maintain the wheelie) and push forward. The patient then crosses the surface in a series of short wheelies while pushing forward (Fig. 8.8).

Box 8.2 Student Practice Activity: Wheelie Training Progression presents activities to promote learning of both static and dynamic wheelie skills and how to teach these skills to riders.

Steep Hills and Ramps

Descent

The best way to maneuver steep descents is in a wheelie. The wheelie actually stabilizes the rider's position in the

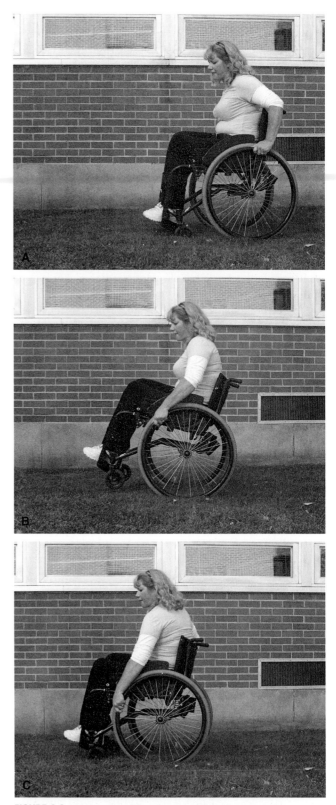

FIGURE 8.8 While propelling the wheelchair over uneven ground (A), the rider performs a continuous series of wheelies (B, C) to prevent the front casters from catching and causing the wheelchair to tip over forward.

BOX 8.2 STUDENT PRACTICE ACTIVITY: WHEELIE TRAINING PROGRESSION

OBJECTIVE: Safely and successfully teach basic wheelchair skills to a novice rider

EQUIPMENT: Any manual wheelchair but ideally an ultralight manual wheelchair with wheel locks that do not interfere with propulsion arc and a rear axle aligned with or forward of the shoulder of the rider

DIRECTIONS: Work in pairs, or optimally with a third observer who is critiquing the student therapist. Remember, you are working on mastery of *teaching* wheelchair skills; your ability to teach someone else is more important than your own ability to perform the skills.

▲ One person assumes the role of the wheelchair user (the rider).
▲ One person assumes the role of the therapist.

Key Points

▲ To safely guard, the therapist stands behind the wheelchair, with one foot forward of the other, allowing the forward leg to catch any backward tip. One hand grasps the push handle, and one hand is positioned over the shoulder of the rider in the wheelchair (contact is made only if necessary). For a rigid frame wheelchair without push handles, a strap on the rigidizer bar underneath the seat can be used; the strap should be loose so it does not affect balance.
▲ Wheelie practice should only be done with close guarding. Don't allow practice to proceed with an anti-tip device in place; it should be rotated upward or removed. The rider should not be allowed to rest on the anti-tip device.

Static and Dynamic Wheelie Skills

1. **Static balance in wheelie**
   • The therapist guards from behind and places the rider into the wheelie position.
   • The rider is instructed that proper hand placement is on top of the wheel with shoulders and elbows in slight flexion to allow pushing or pulling of the wheel to correct for balance.
   • The rider works on maintaining balance in the wheelie position.
2. **Hand control**
   • The rider is placed in the wheelie position and directed to pull the wheels back sharply (casters will fall to ground).

• The rider is placed in the wheelie position and directed to push the wheels forward sharply (the wheelchair will tip backward).
• The rider's hands should remain on the wheels and should not move on or off the wheel to "chase" the balance point.

3. **Pop into wheelie balance**
   • The rider grips the wheel posterior to the axle and pushes forward sharply.
   • The rider pops up the front casters to achieve a balanced wheelie position.
   • The therapist encourages the rider to experiment with the wheelie height. For example, when resting against the backrest, the balance point is achieved with the casters closer to the ground; when leaning forward off the backrest, the balance point is achieved with the casters farther from the ground.
   • Once the rider is able to pop up to balance position, emphasis is on maintaining this position.

GOAL: Maintain static balance in a wheelie for 5 minutes in a 2 ft² space.

Note: The rider is encouraged to work on dynamic wheelie skills (below) before mastering the 5-minute static wheelie.

4. **Dynamic balance within wheelie**
   • Wheeling forward
   • Wheeling backward
   • Balancing in a wheelie position using one hand only
   • Turning 360 degrees
   • Wheeling around corners
   • Wheeling down inclines (the rims are allowed to slide through hands for control of speed)

GOAL: Maintain dynamic balance for 10 minutes without losing the wheelie

5. **Rolling wheelie**
   • With the wheelchair gliding freely (i.e., no hand contact after push), the rider pops up into a low wheelie on the therapist's verbal cue. There is no attempt to balance in the wheelie, just a low caster lift and an immediate push onto the front half of the rear wheel for follow-through.
   • Once the glide to wheelie to follow-through has been mastered, the rider practices the same approach over a 2 in. curb, striving for glide to wheelie to follow-through over the curb.

wheelchair, allowing gravity to hold the rider into the seat rather than creating a forward falling force. The height of the wheelie is influenced by the slope of the hill: the steeper the hill, the higher the wheelie. The rider approaches the hill and lifts into a wheelie and then allows the handrims to slide through the grip to control the speed and height of the wheelie. The most difficult aspect of descending steep inclines is the transition at the bottom. When the hill ends,

rearward momentum can cause a backward tip just at the base of the hill. To avoid this, the rider should slow down and gently come out of the wheelie at the base of the hill.

Speed control is important. If the rider is moving too fast or feels like he or she is losing grip, the rider should stop and rest. To do this, the rider brakes hard on one side, allowing the other wheel to slide so that the wheelchair turns 90 degrees to the hill. This position can be maintained with little effort, but if the hill is very steep, the rider must lean the shoulders up the hill to keep from flipping over sideways down the hill. To resume movement, casters are turned back down the hill. Continuing in a slalom type pattern is usually the best way to descend safely.

If the rider has not mastered the wheelie, the challenge of descending a steep incline is keeping the trunk from falling forward while maintaining a reasonably slow speed. Gripping or braking on the wheels will tend to add to the forward gravity force and loss of trunk balance. This issue is particularly vexing for those with greater trunk paresis or paralysis. The key to stabilizing the trunk is to use the adduction strength of the UEs. Before the descent the rider should sit up tall in the wheelchair and squeeze the backrest uprights with the inside of the upper arms, hugging the elbows inward. The hands are free to control the handrims. Those with impaired hand function are advised to hook the inside of the handrim and pull upward (biceps power) for the speed control.

When the rider is not in a wheelie, the transition at the bottom of the slope is dangerous and can cause forward falls. It is imperative to approach the transition slowly and, if possible, lean back or do a small caster lift at the transition to avoid catching the footrest or casters. For an abrupt transition it is good to stop perpendicular to the hill right at the transition, allow one caster and rear wheel to make the transition, then turn off the hill with the other wheels.

Clinical Note: The maneuver just described above, whether in a wheelie or not, requires good wheel control, and therefore slick handrims can be dangerous. Hot weather can also cause handrims to become excessively hot and frequent rest breaks or gloves are required.

The guarding for traversing hills is similar to that for learning wheelies: The therapist is positioned behind the wheelchair with a front and rear guarding hand position. Skill acquisition should start on a small incline of short distance. It is imperative that the therapist keep pace with the wheelchair, so teamwork is key. The steepness of the incline should be increased rather than the length. Once the rider has learned the general technique and the rest position, he or she can generalize the technique for longer descents.

Ascent

The issue with going up inclines is keeping the casters down and not flipping over backward. If the hill is long, the rider needs to take rests. The same turn (90 degrees) should be used for a rest position as with descent, but the rider's stronger side, if the rider has one, should be on the downhill side during the rest.

The most important preparation for propelling up long or steep inclines is for the rider to reposition the buttocks to the rear of the chair. With mastery, this can be done when approaching the hill using a small lift and forward head lean. For patients just learning the skill or who have less wheelchair confidence, it is necessary to stop just before the incline and purposefully lift and move the buttocks rearward. This position shift causes forward trunk instability on level surfaces but is what provides added wheelchair stability when going up the incline. The rider needs to be able to lean more forward from the hips. The rider should feel like he or she will lose balance and fall forward onto the thighs. The rider will not fall, because he or she will "catch" trunk stability with the short, frequent push on the handrims as the wheelchair is propelled up the incline. The arc of push should be on the front top half of the wheel. Once the top is attained, it is imperative to reposition pelvis in proper position so that the rider is seated with good stability and optimal push mechanics. Video 8.7 (available at http://davisplus.fadavis.com) depicts riders with limited UE function ascending a ramp.

Note: All video segments cited in this chapter are listed in Box 8.3.

To assist learning how to propel up an incline, the therapist is positioned downhill from the rider. In addition to providing verbal cues, the therapist can assist by preventing the wheelchair from rolling backward during the recovery phase of the push.

Curbs

Performing wheelies is the easiest and most efficient method of ascending and descending a curb.

Ascent

There are two basic methods of ascending a curb: (1) powering up the curb from a stop and (2) popping up the curb on the go while moving. The first method does not require as much skill with wheelies, but it requires much more strength. Some riders do not have the strength to perform this technique. To start this skill, the rider propels the wheelchair up to the front edge of the curb, pops a wheelie, and pushes slightly forward while in the wheelie so that the front casters rest on the top of the curb with the rear wheels on the

---

BOX 8.3 Videos Available on Davis*Plus* (www.fadavis.com)

Video 8.1: Rider propelling through a doorway with a door that opens away from the rider
Video 8.2: Rider propelling through a doorway with a door that opens toward the rider
Video 8.3: Rider closing door that closes toward him
Video 8.4: Ascending single curb with assistance
Video 8.5: Rider descending stairs with one rail with therapist spotting/assisting
Video 8.6: Rider propelling wheelchair on uneven terrain in a wheelie
Video 8.7: Riders with limited upper extremity function ascending a ramp

surface below but not touching the curb (Fig. 8.9). In this position the rider reaches back and places his or her hands at the 12 o'clock position on the handrims and then drives the hands forcefully forward toward the ground while simultaneously throwing the head and trunk forward. The momentum from the push rolls the back wheels up onto the curb.

To ascend a curb on the go, the patient pops a wheelie while moving forward just before reaching the curb. This lifts the front casters so they are up on top of the curb. As the rear wheels make contact with the curb, the patient pushes forward on the handrims and leans the head and trunk forward. The forward momentum of the wheelchair (it is moving forward throughout this task) rolls the back wheels up onto the curb (Fig. 8.10). The key aspect of this task is the skill and timing required to perform the wheelie. The rider must be able to pop a wheelie while moving forward and must accurately time the wheelie. If the wheelie is popped too soon, the casters will fall back down and won't clear the curb, and the front end of the wheelchair will hit the curb. If the wheelie is too late, the rear wheels will hit the curb while in a high wheelie, and this causes a tendency to flip the chair over backward. In both of these instances, the rider is in danger of falling from the chair. Because the wheelchair is moving forward continuously, the on-the-go technique does not require as much strength as does the other method. However, more skill with popping a wheelie is required. This skill should be practiced initially without a curb so that a wheelie can be obtained on command while moving in a steady glide down a hallway.

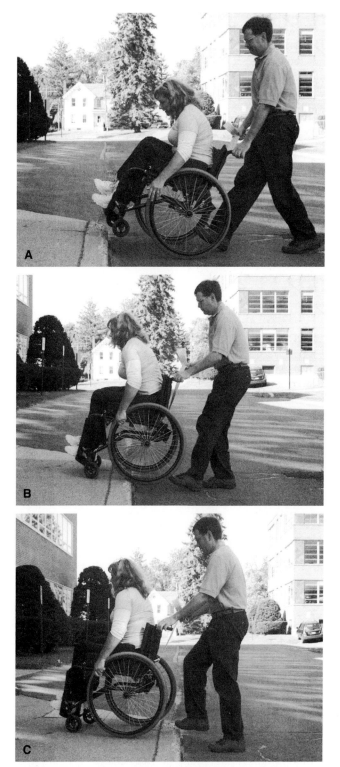

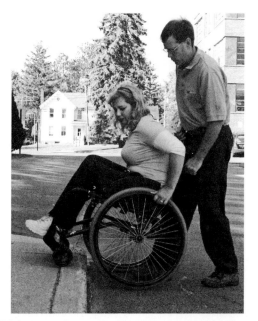

FIGURE 8.9 Ascending curbs: The rider pops a wheelie up the curb from a stopped position. Being able to ascend a curb from a stopped position without forward momentum requires a great deal of skill and upper body strength. The rider should position the casters on the edge of the curb, leaving some space between the wheels and the curb before forcefully pushing the wheels up and over the curb.

FIGURE 8.10 Ascending curbs: The rider pops a wheelie up the curb on the go (while moving). (A) The rider must carefully time when she pops the wheelie when ascending curbs with forward momentum. If the rider pops the wheelie too soon, it will be difficult to maintain the wheelie and the casters will drop down and hit the curb. If the rider pops the wheelie too late, the casters won't clear the curb. (B) The rider needs to give only a slight push forward after the casters clear the curb. (C) Momentum carries the back wheels up and over the curb.

Descent

The backward or forward approaches are the two basic methods of descending a curb. Using the backward approach, the rider backs up to the edge of the curb so the wheels are on the edge of the curb. The rider then leans forward and places his or her hands far back on the handrims and controls descent of the wheelchair as the back wheels roll off the curb. When the back wheels are off the curb the rider lifts into a slight wheelie and turns 90 degrees to the right or left to prevent the footplate(s) from hitting the top of the curb (Fig. 8.11). An alternative backward approach is to roll off with momentum. In this technique the rider squares the rear wheels to the curb and pulls back on the handrims while immediately leaning forward and grabbing the front frame of the wheelchair. The wheelchair will roll off with casters coming down solidly. This method takes less skill but requires some space for roll out. It is critical that the user not grab the wheels after beginning the roll off because the momentum will pull the wheelchair over. Once all four wheels are on the level, the rider can reach the handrims and brake the wheelchair.

To descend a curb using the forward approach, the rider pushes the wheelchair forward, and just as the casters approach the edge of the curb the patient lifts into a wheelie. The wheelie is maintained as momentum carries the wheels off the curb. The rider maintains the sliding grip (as used during incline descent) to maintain the wheelie so the wheels land first, then the casters (Fig. 8.12). If the casters

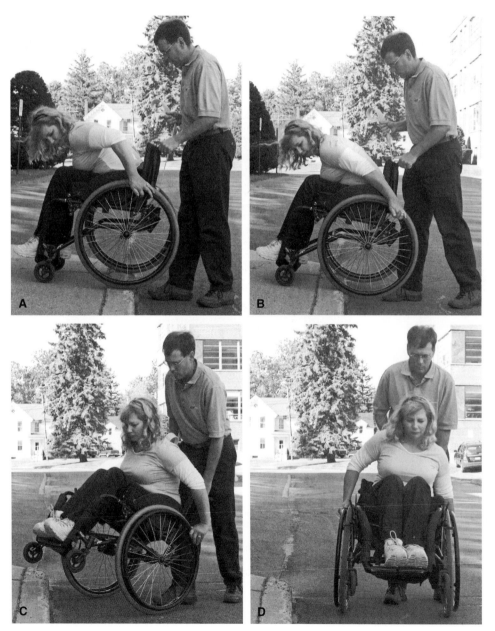

FIGURE 8.11 Backward approach to descending a curb. (A) The rider gradually approaches the edge of the curb and leans forward. (B) The back wheels are slowly lowered over the edge of the curb. Once the back wheels are safely on the ground, the rider (C) pops a wheelie and (D) rotates 90 degrees to prevent the footplate from getting stuck on or hitting the edge of the curb.

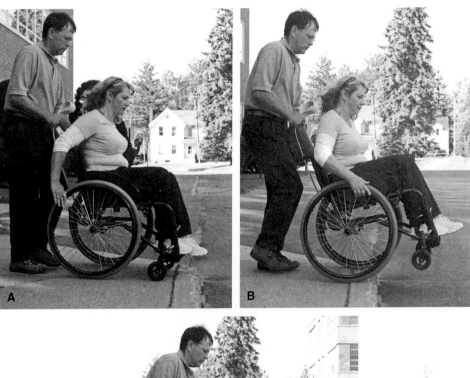

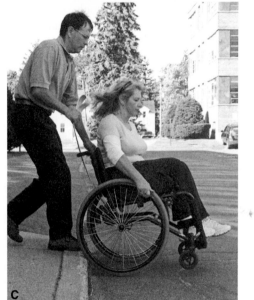

FIGURE 8.12 Forward approach to descending a curb. (A) The rider approaches the curb while moving forward. (B) The rider pops a wheelie as the front casters approach the edge of the curb. (C) The rider maintains the wheelie until the back wheels contact the ground. This prevents the wheelchair from tipping over forward.

land first, the wheelchair will most likely tip over forward. This technique is analogous to an airplane landing, with the back wheels underneath the wings touching the ground before the front wheels underneath the cockpit do. Similar to ascending a curb on the go as described above, skill and timing with popping a wheelie are essential for mastering this task.

Safety is again essential when teaching riders to ascend and descend curbs. If something goes wrong when practicing these skills, the rider is most likely to lose balance in a forward direction and may fall out of the wheelchair. For example, if descending a curb in a wheelie in a forward direction the casters contact the ground before the wheels, the wheelchair will tip over forward. The therapist must have one hand on the anterior trunk/shoulder and one hand on the gait belt or push handle that is posterior to the rider, allowing the

therapist to help the rider recover safely when necessary. Figures 8.11A–D and 8.12A–C illustrate appropriate positioning of the therapist. Also, when initially teaching the rider to ascend or descend curbs, the therapist can set up practice on small curbs (1 to 2 in. high) and progress to higher curbs (6 to 8 in. high) as the rider's skill improves.

Hopping

Hopping a wheelchair is a unique skill that is very empowering to the rider. Mastery of hopping provides the ability to move laterally in either direction or hop and rotate in either direction. Hopping is a very useful skill in tight spaces, allowing the rider to "move over" just a bit. This is frequently needed to clear the arc of a door or in public transit situations.

To teach how to hop a chair, instruct the rider to attempt and practice the maneuver. The only other key instruction is that the rider must hold onto the rear wheels to hop. If the rider does not "get it" with this much instruction, move on to the similar but easier maneuver of walking the wheelchair forward. This is essentially tilting the wheelchair onto one wheel and then the other with a slight forward pull before the wheel lands using weight shifting. It still requires hand contact maintained on the rear wheels. This maneuver is less useful but as a teaching tool allows the rider to begin to intuit how the wheelchair can hop.

Escalators

Riders should learn escalators after they have mastered emergency stair egress. The position on the escalator will be the same as in the two-railing descent of a stairway. Instruction using live escalators should begin with going up. Before attempting to board an escalator the rider should have wheelie skills. Ideally, prerequisite skills include a 30-second static wheelie balance, the ability to move into a wheelie independently, and the ability to lift casters to move over obstacles while moving forward. The main reason for the wheelie skills is the transition at the top of the escalator. The moving tread of the escalator disappears under a fairly aggressive lip that, if the rider is not attentive to lifting the casters over, can cause a dangerous forward fall from the wheelchair, which stays behind and causes a pileup of the people coming up behind the wheelchair rider.

The rider wheels onto the flat aspect of the escalator at the bottom, grabs both sides of the moving handrails, and leans forward. The stairs will position themselves under the rider. As the stairs establish themselves, the rider will usually sit up more to achieve a comfortable balanced position.

Red Flag: Caution—sometimes the handrails are not moving in precise synchrony with the stairs, so the wheelchair rider may need to regrip the handrails soon after boarding. This is particularly important when handrails are moving faster than stairs.

When arriving at the top, the rider sits more upright as the stairs give way to a flat platform. Keeping the hands on the hand rails, the rider can push down slightly or lean the trunk back slightly, to lift the casters over the lip. Alternatively, once the flat platform is established, the rider can return hands to the rear wheels, lift into a small wheelie, and then propel off the escalator.

When teaching this skill, the therapist can lean into the back of the wheelchair to stabilize it on the escalator stairs to lessen the rider's effort and reduce the risk of falling backward out of the wheelchair. The therapist can also assist with the small wheelie to exit the escalator. Note that if the therapist helps push the wheelchair but is not assisting in the wheelie, it might cause the chair to get stuck on the lip.

Red Flag: In older buildings escalators may narrow at the top. It is essential that the rider know that the escalator is wide enough for the wheelchair at both the top and bottom. Any escalator where two people can stand side by side is of sufficient width for most wheelchairs.

Going down the escalator is done in the exact same position as going up. This means that the rider approaches the escalator and turns around just before the top of the escalator so that the rear wheels are on the down side. The rider then puts both hands on the handrails and leans forward during the transition onto the escalator. The therapist should precede the rider onto the escalator and continue to step up to maintain position at the top of escalator until the rider is prepared to move. The therapist can assist by leaning into the backrest to stabilize the wheelchair and inform the rider that the bottom is approaching. When the bottom approaches, the rider should lean forward and push back off the handrails to get the rear wheels over the lip of the escalator. The rider should not turn around to a forward position until well clear of the escalator platform and handrails.

Some facilities do not approve of wheelchairs on escalators and have taken steps (e.g., upright barriers) to block wheelchair access. If you are new to the escalator in question, it is important to know that both the top and bottom have clear wheelchair access. In most private facilities with escalators, polite education of the security personnel will ensure unchallenged ability to ride the escalator.

Outcome Measures

It is important to use standardized outcome measures to assess a patient's wheelchair mobility skills and to document outcomes. The *Wheelchair Skills Test* tests a rider's ability to perform 32 different wheelchair skills including forward propulsion, turns, wheelies, ramps, curbs, and descending stairs.[9,10] The *Wheelchair Circuit* assesses three aspects of wheelchair mobility: tempo, technical skill, and physical capacity during nine different tasks.[11,12] The results of these tests can also be used to provide feedback on performance and motivation to patients.

SUMMARY

Wheelchair skills are important for community living and full social participation for an individual who will use a manual wheelchair for full-time mobility.[1] These skills should not be considered components of advanced rehabilitation or relegated to skills to be learned from peers. Wheelchair skills can and should be integrated throughout the rehabilitation process. Basic skills such as propulsion through a door that opens away from the rider can be taught early, while more demanding skills such as curbs and emergency egress should be incorporated later into the plan of care as the patient's rehabilitation progresses. The principles of motor learning apply to teaching wheelchair skills. It is important to structure the practice and feedback schedule to ensure success and safety so that motor learning is achieved.

REFERENCES

1. Hosseini, SM, et al. Manual wheelchair skills capacity predicts quality of life and community integration in persons with spinal cord injury. Arch Phys Med Rehabil, 2012; 93:2237–2243.
2. Hastings, J, et al. The differences in self-esteem, function, and participation between adults with low cervical motor tetraplegia who use power or manual wheelchairs. Arch Phys Med Rehabil, 2011; 92:1785–1788.
3. Hastings, JD. Seating assessment and planning. Phys Med Rehabil Clin N Am, 2000; 11:183.
4. Hastings, JD, Fanucchi, ER, and Burns, SP. Wheelchair configuration and postural alignment in persons with spinal cord injury. Arch Phys Med Rehabil, 2003; 84:528–534.
5. Hastings, JD, and Betz, KL. Seating and wheelchair prescription. In Field-Fote, EC (ed): Spinal Cord Injury Rehabilitation. Philadelphia: F.A. Davis, 2009.
6. Kwarciak, AM, et al. Redefining the manual wheelchair stroke cycle: identification and impact of nonpropulsive pushrim contact. Arch Phys Med Rehabil, 2009; 90:20–26.
7. Richter, WM, et al. Stroke pattern and handrim biomechanics for level and uphill wheelchair propulsion at self-selected speeds. Arch Phys Med Rehabil, 2007; 88:81–87.
8. Collinger, JL, et al. Shoulder biomechanics during the push phase of wheelchair propulsion: a multisite study of persons with paraplegia. Arch Phys Med Rehabil, 2008; 89:667–676.
9. Kirby, RL, et al. The wheelchair skills test (version 2.4): measurement properties. Arch Phys Med Rehabil, 2004; 85:794–804.
10. Kirby, RL, et al. The Wheelchair Skills Test: a pilot study of a new outcome measure. Arch Phys Med Rehabil, 2002; 83:10–18.
11. Kilkens, OJ, et al. The Wheelchair Circuit: Construct validity and responsiveness of a test to assess manual wheelchair mobility in persons with spinal cord injury. Arch Phys Med Rehabil, 2004; 85:424–431.
12. Kilkens, OJ, et al. The wheelchair circuit: reliability of a test to assess mobility in persons with spinal cord injuries. Arch Phys Med Rehabil, 2002; 83:1783–1788.

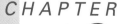

Interventions to Improve Standing and Standing Balance Skills

JoAnn Moriarty-Baron, PT, DPT, and Susan B. O'Sullivan, PT, EdD

This chapter focuses on standing control and interventions that can be used to improve standing and standing balance skills. Careful examination of the patient's overall status in terms of impairments and activity limitations that affect standing control is necessary and should include musculoskeletal alignment, range of motion (ROM), and muscle performance (strength, power, endurance). Examination of motor function (motor control and motor learning) focuses on determining the patient's weightbearing status, postural control, and intactness of neuromuscular synergies required for static and dynamic control. Examination of sensory function includes utilization of sensory (somatosensory, visual, and vestibular) cues for standing balance control and central nervous system (CNS) sensory integration mechanisms. Finally, the patient must be able to safely perform functional movements (activities of daily living [ADL]) in standing in various environments (clinic, home, work [job/school/play], and community).

Standing

General Characteristics

Standing is a relatively stable posture with a high center of mass (COM) and a small base of support (BOS) that includes contact of the feet with the support surface. During normal symmetrical standing, weight is equally distributed over both feet (Fig. 9.1). From a lateral view, the line of gravity (LoG) falls close to most joint axes: slightly anterior to the ankle and knee joints, slightly posterior to the hip joint and posterior to the cervical and lumbar vertebrae, and anterior to the thoracic vertebrae and atlanto-occipital joint (Fig. 9.2). Natural spinal curves (i.e., normal lumbar and cervical lordosis and normal thoracic kyphosis) are present but flattened in upright stance depending on the level of postural tone. The pelvis is in neutral position, with no anterior or posterior tilt. Normal alignment minimizes the need for muscle activity during erect stance.

Postural stability in standing is maintained by muscle activity that includes (1) postural tone in the antigravity muscles throughout the trunk and lower extremities (LEs) and (2) contraction of antigravity muscles. The gluteus maximus and hamstrings contract to maintain pelvic

alignment, the abdominals contract to flatten the lumbar curve, the paravertebral muscles contract to extend the spine, the quadriceps muscles contract to maintain knee extension, and the hip abductors contract to maintain pelvic alignment during midstance and during lateral displacements.

Limit of stability (LOS) is the amount of maximum excursion possible in any one direction without losing balance; it is determined by the distance between the feet and the length of the feet as well as the person's height and weight. The normal adult anterior/posterior LOS is approximately 12 degrees; the normal medial/lateral LOS is approximately 16 degrees. Together they make up the *sway envelope,* the path of the body's movement during normal standing. In an intact person, sway cycles intermittently from side to side and from heel to toe, with the midpoint of sway being *centered alignment.*[1]

Static postural control, also referred to as *stability,* is required to maintain the standing position. *Dynamic postural control,* also referred to as *controlled mobility,* is necessary to control movements within the posture (e.g., weight shifting or upper extremity [UE] reaching or LE stepping movements). In addition, the term *dynamic balance* is used to describe the ability to maintain postural control while in motion or while moving through space and can be thought of as the postural control required for active movements such as walking or running.

Anticipatory postural control refers to adjustments that occur in advance of the execution of voluntary movements. The postural system is pretuned to stabilize the body; for example, a person readies his or her posture before lifting a heavy weight or catching a weighted ball. *Reactive balance control* refers to adjustments that occur spontaneously in response to unexpected changes in the COM (e.g., perturbations) or changes in the support surface. *Postural fixation reactions* stabilize the body against an external force (e.g., a thrust). *Tilting reactions* reposition the COM within the BOS in response to changes in the support surface (e.g., standing on an equilibrium board). *Adaptive balance control* refers to the ability to adapt or modify postural responses relative to changing task and environmental demands. Prior experience (learning) influences a person's adaptability and shapes his or her strategy selection.[1,2]

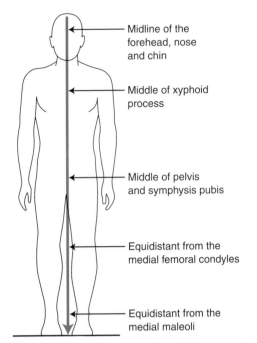

FIGURE 9.1 Normal postural alignment—frontal plane In optimal alignment, the LoG passes through the identified anatomical structures, dividing the body into two symmetrical parts.

Modified Standing

Often those who sustain significant neurological insult lack the prerequisite intersegmental coordination and postural control required for standing. Modified standing activities allow the patient to develop these skills in a position that closely approximates the desired standing posture but with increased limb support and reduced strength demands on the trunk and LE antigravity muscles.

Modified standing, also referred to as **modified plantigrade,** is an early standing posture that involves four-limb weightbearing (UEs and LEs). The patient stands next to a treatment table with both shoulders flexed (45 to 70 degrees), elbows extended, hands flat on the treatment table and weightbearing, and feet in symmetrical stance position (Fig. 9.3). The hips are flexed and the knees extended; the ankles are dorsiflexed. This creates a stable posture with a wide BOS and a high COM. The BOS and the degree of UE weightbearing can be increased or decreased by varying the distance the patient is standing from the table. The patient need not demonstrate complete knee extensor control required for upright standing in modified standing as the position of the COM is in front of the weightbearing line. This creates an extension moment at the knee, aiding weak extensors. As control develops, the patient can progress from flat hand to fingertip support and from bilateral to unilateral UE support to free standing. The LEs can be progressed from a symmetrical stance to a step position (Fig. 9.4). An alternative arm position is placing both hands on a large ball (less stable surface) to increase the challenge (Fig. 9.5). This position

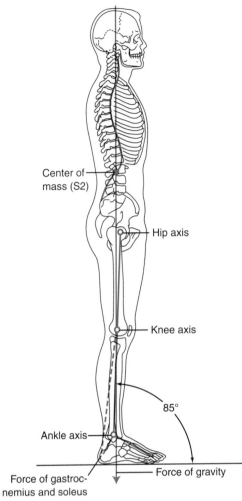

FIGURE 9.2 Normal postural alignment—sagittal plane In optimal alignment, the LoG passes through the identified anatomical structures.

increases the required shoulder flexion ROM and weight borne on the LEs. Unilateral UE weightbearing can also be accomplished by positioning the patient sideways next to a treatment table or a wall with the shoulder in abduction.

Clinical Note: For patients who demonstrate UE flexor hypertonicity (e.g., the patient with traumatic brain injury [TBI] or stroke), modified standing is a better choice for early standing compared with standing in the parallel bars and pulling on the bars. Pulling encourages increased flexor tone, whereas modified plantigrade promotes UE extension and weightbearing. The modified position combines LE muscles in an out-of-synergy pattern (the hips are flexed with the knees extended). Thus it is a useful treatment activity for the patient with stroke who demonstrates strong abnormal LE synergies. In addition, this position is relatively familiar, so it can be used for patients who have cognitive impairments, and it is fairly easy to attain with the assistance of the therapist. Patients who are motivated to stand are likely to find this task highly rewarding.

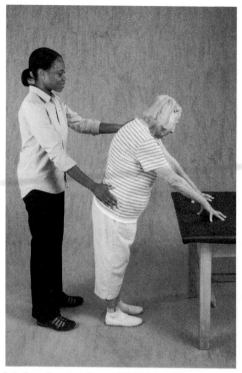

FIGURE 9.3 Standing, holding in modified plantigrade Patient is holding with the LEs in a symmetrical position and the UEs using tabletop fingertip support. The therapist is applying resistance to the upper trunk and pelvis using the technique of stabilizing reversals.

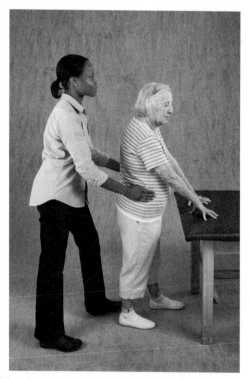

FIGURE 9.4 Standing, holding in modified plantigrade, step position Patient is holding with the LEs in a step position and the UEs using tabletop fingertip support. The therapist is applying resistance to the pelvis using the technique of stabilizing reversals.

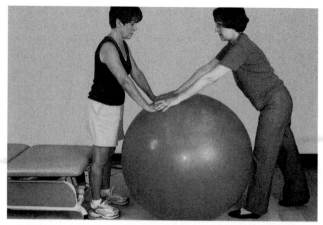

FIGURE 9.5 Standing, holding in modified plantigrade, hands on ball Patient is holding with the LEs, both hands resting lightly on a large ball.

Modified Standing, Holding

The patient can practice active holding or resisted holding. During active holding, important factors to consider when examining stability control include the ability to maintain correct alignment with minimal postural sway (maintained center of alignment) and the ability to maintain the posture for prolonged times.

During resistive holding, the patient is asked to hold steady while the therapist applies resistance in alternating directions. The proprioceptive neuromuscular facilitation (PNF) technique of *stabilizing reversals* can be used. The therapist's manual contacts are placed on the pelvis (see Fig. 9.4), on the pelvis and contralateral upper trunk (see Fig. 9.3), or on the upper trunk bilaterally. Resistance is applied first in one direction and then the other (anterior/posterior, medial/lateral, or diagonally with the LEs in step position). Light approximation can be given to the top of the shoulders or the pelvis to increase stabilizing responses. Verbal cues (VCs) include *"Hold, don't let me pull you backward, hold."* The therapist must then give a transitional command, *"Now, don't let me push you forward,"* before sliding the hands to resist the opposite muscles and again instructing the patient to *"hold"*; this allows the patient the opportunity to make appropriate anticipatory postural adjustments.

The PNF technique of *rhythmic stabilization* can also be used. One hand is placed on the posterior pelvis on one side, pushing forward, while the other hand is on the anterior contralateral upper trunk, pulling backward, providing resistance to isometric contractions of trunk flexors, extensors, and rotators. Verbal cues include *"Don't let me move you, hold, hold; now don't let me move you the other way."*

Outcomes

Motor control goal: stability (static postural control)
Functional skill achieved: patient is able to maintain upright standing with UE support independently with minimal sway and no loss of balance, a lead-up activity to standing with no UE support

Modified Standing, Weight Shifts

Dynamic postural control is necessary for moving in a posture (e.g., weight shifting) or moving the limbs while maintaining postural stability. These movements disturb the COM and require ongoing postural adjustments to maintain upright standing. Initially, the patient's attention is directed to the key task elements required for successful postural adjustments and movement. With increased practice, the postural adjustments become more automatic.

Weight-shifting activities forward and backward in modified standing can be used to increase ROM; these activities may be ideal for patients who are anxious about ROM exercises. Improved ROM in shoulder flexion can be achieved by shifting the weight backward (hands remain fixed on the table) by positioning the feet farther away from the treatment table. Improved ROM in ankle dorsiflexion can be achieved by weight shifts forward. Weight shifts with the patient facing a corner, each hand on adjacent walls, can be used to improve ROM of upper trunk and shoulder flexors (e.g., in the patient with a functional dorsal kyphosis and forward shoulders). The patient actively shifts weight first forward (increasing loading on the UEs) and then backward (increasing loading on the LEs). Weight shifts can also be performed from side to side (medial/lateral shifts) with the LEs in a symmetrical stance position or diagonally forward and backward with the LEs in a step position. Unilateral active reaching activities can be used to promote weight shifting in all directions or in the direction of instability (e.g., the patient with stroke). The therapist provides a target (*"Reach out and touch my hand"*) or uses a functional task like removing a tissue from the box to promote reaching. The patient can also put both hands on a ball placed on top of a flat treatment table (Fig. 9.6). The patient moves the ball from side to side, forward and backward, or diagonally forward and backward.

The PNF technique of *dynamic reversals* can be used to provide resistance during weight shifts. The therapist stands at the patient's side for medial/lateral shifts and behind the patient for anterior/posterior shifts. Manual contacts may be placed on the pelvis, the pelvis and contralateral upper trunk, or bilaterally on the upper trunk. The movements are guided for a few repetitions to ensure that the patient knows the movements are expected. Movements are then lightly resisted. The therapist alternates hand placement, resisting the movements first in one direction and then the other. Smooth reversals of antagonists are facilitated by well-timed VCs, such as *"Pull away from me; now, push back toward me."*

Variations in weight shifting include diagonal weight shifts with feet in step position (one foot forward of the other). Resistance is applied to the pelvis as the patient weight-shifts diagonally onto the forward LE and then diagonally backward onto the other LE (Fig. 9.7). Verbal cues include *"Shift forward and away from me; now shift back and toward me."*

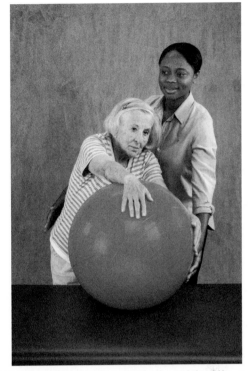

FIGURE 9.6 Standing, modified plantigrade, weight shifts Patient is performing weight shifts with the LEs in a symmetrical position and the UEs supported by a ball placed on the treatment table. The patient moves the ball (forward and backward, side to side) while the therapist provides VCs and guarding.

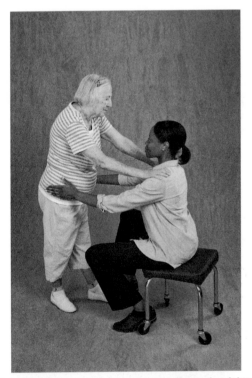

FIGURE 9.7 Standing, modified plantigrade, diagonal weight shifts Patient is performing diagonal weight shifts with pelvic rotation, LEs in step position, and the UEs using light touch-down support on the therapist's shoulders. The patient moves diagonally forward over the more advanced left foot while rotating the pelvis forward on the right. The therapist provides resistance to the pelvis using the technique of dynamic reversals.

Once control is achieved in diagonal shifts, focus may be directed toward pelvic rotation for those who lack it, for example those with Parkinson's disease and stroke. The patient is instructed to shift weight diagonally onto the forward LE while rotating the pelvis forward on the opposite side, then to shift weight diagonally backward while the pelvis is rotated backward. The therapist resists the motion at the pelvis (Fig. 9.8). This activity is a lead-up to stepping. Verbal cues include *"Shift forward and twist; now shift backward and twist."*

If the elbows flex, the upper trunk may also move forward as the pelvis rotates forward, producing an undesirable ipsilateral trunk rotation pattern. The therapist can isolate the pelvic motion by instructing the patient to keep both elbows fully extended.

Clinical Note: People who have difficulty initiating weight shifts from the pelvis often compensate by flexing the knee to bring the COM forward. This substitution should be discouraged because it does not simulate the normal weight shift used in gait.

Modified Standing, Stepping

While in modified standing, the patient can progress to taking a step forward with the dynamic limb while weight shifting diagonally forward. Movements can be active or

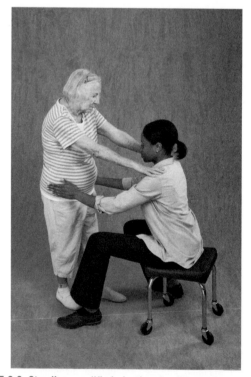

FIGURE 9.8 Standing, modified plantigrade, diagonal weight shifts in step position Patient is performing diagonal weight shifts with the LEs in step position and the UEs using light touch-down support on the therapist's shoulders. The patient moves diagonally forward and over the more advanced left foot. The therapist provides resistance to the pelvis using the technique of dynamic reversals.

resisted. If resisted using dynamic reversals, the therapist maintains manual contacts on the pelvis to facilitate the accompanying pelvic rotation. Verbal cues include *"Shift forward and step; now shift backward and step."*

Flexibility and Strengthening Exercises

Adequate core (trunk) stability and extremity flexibility and strength are required for normal posture and balance. Table 9.1 includes standing activities that can be done in the clinic or at home to achieve these goals. The patient should be positioned next to a treatment table and instructed to use light touch-down fingertip support as needed for balance during these activities. The patient is cautioned not to "hold on tight" and to use the minimal amount of touch-down support necessary, progressing from bilateral support to unilateral support as soon as possible. When these activities are part of a home exercise program (HEP), the patient can stand at the kitchen counter for support (sometimes called "kitchen sink exercises").

Before exercises are performed, it is important to ensure that there is an adequate warm-up to elevate muscle temperature and improve flexibility. Flexibility exercises (stretching) should be performed slowly, with gradual progression to the point of tightness (end range). Ballistic or dynamic stretching (repetitive bouncing) is contraindicated. Patients should be cautioned to maintain a normal breathing pattern and to avoid breath holding. Patients should also be cautioned to stop exercising if they feel unsafe or if unusual pain develops.

Exercises to improve muscular strength and endurance can be performed as active exercises or against resistance using weight cuffs (see Figs. 9.9 and 9.10) or elastic resistive bands (see Figs. 9.11, 9.12, and 9.13). Key muscles (major muscles of the trunk and extremities) important for posture and balance are targeted. The patient performs a set of exercises (8 to 12 repetitions), working to the point of volitional fatigue while maintaining good form. The importance of adequate rest to ensure good form should be stressed. The patient should practice under close supervision at first and then progress to independent practice. An activity diary can be used to document practice sessions at home.

Clinical Note: The Biomechanical Ankle Platform System, or BAPS, board is a dome board commonly used clinically to promote proprioceptive information and increase ankle strength required for postural ankle strategies. In addition to providing various dome heights, this device also includes pegs and weights for selective ankle muscle strengthening.

The therapist should incorporate appropriate exercises for specific muscle groups as indicated and include exercises that address holding (isometric exercise), lifting (concentric exercises), and lowering (eccentric exercises). An ideal exercise to address concentric and eccentric control of the major LE muscles is a partial squat.

TABLE 9.1 Activities to Improve Flexibility and Strength Needed for Normal Posture and Balance

Activity	Purpose
Flexibility Exercises	
Standing, full-body stretches, arms overhead reaching toward ceiling	Improves ROM of trunk flexors and anterior shoulder muscles
Standing, PNF bilateral, symmetrical UE flexion-abduction-external rotation patterns using resistive bands (Fig. 9.12)	Improves ROM of anterior chest and shoulder muscles
Standing, side stretches leaning over to one side	Improves ROM of trunk lateral flexors
Standing, trunk twists, shoulders abducted; twisting around to one side, then the other; head turns, eyes follow the movement	Improves ROM of trunk and head rotators, stimulates lateral semicircular canals of vestibular system
Standing upright on bottom stair or step, hand(s) on railing, feet pointed straight ahead, one foot remains in middle of stair while the other foot is shifted back, and the heel is lowered toward the floor until a stretch is felt in the calf.	Improves ROM in the gastrocnemius muscle
Sitting in bed so that back is straight against headboard or wall, one leg is placed out straight with knee in extension while the other foot is placed on the floor. Flex the ankle that is on the bed so that the toes move toward the head. Stretch will be felt in the back of the thigh, knee, and calf.	Improves ROM in the hamstrings and gastrocnemius muscles
Kneeling beside bed (use bed for support if needed), place one foot on floor in front of body while other leg remains kneeling, then lean forward onto front foot until a stretch is felt in the hip.	Improves ROM in the hip flexors
Strengthening Exercises	
Standing, heel rises	Improves gastrocnemius-soleus muscle strength
Standing, toe-offs	Improves anterior tibialis muscle strength
Sitting in chair, feet in front of body, weight on heels, ankle is rotated outward so that toes move up and away from other foot. If using resistive band, tie the band to chair leg and loop other end around toe of shoe.	Improves posterior tibialis and peroneal muscle strength
Sitting in chair, feet in front of body, weight on heels, ankle is rotated inward so that toes move toward other foot. If using resistive band, tie the band to chair leg and loop other end around toe of shoe.	Improves anterior tibialis muscle strength
Standing, side kicks: lateral leg lifts with or without resistive band at ankle (Fig. 9.11)	Improves gluteus medius strength
Standing, backward kicks with knee straight: backward leg lifts with or without resistive band at ankle	Improves gluteus maximus strength
Standing, front kicks with knee straight: leg lifts forward in front of body with knee straight, with or without resistance at ankle (see Fig. 9.10).	Improves hip flexor and quadriceps strength
Standing, hands lightly resting on table, partial squats, or with body leaning against a wall, wall squats (Fig. 9.13 without a ball and Fig. 9.14 with a ball)	Improves quadriceps and hip extensor strength
Standing, marching in place	Improves hip flexor strength and hamstring strength

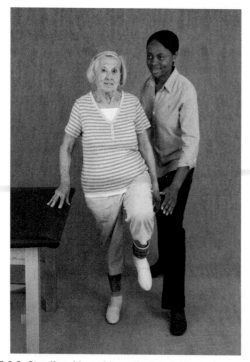

FIGURE 9.9 Standing, hip and knee flexion Patient is performing lifts using a 2-lb (0.9-kg) weight cuff and light fingertip support with one hand.

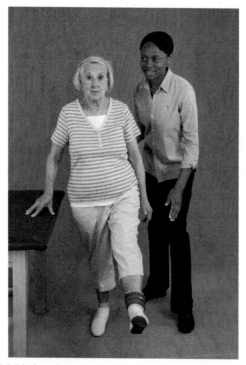

FIGURE 9.10 Standing, hip flexion with knee extension Patient is performing lifts using a 2-lb (0.9-kg) weight cuff and light fingertip support with one hand.

Standing, Partial Wall Squats

The patient stands with the back against a wall, with feet about 4 in. (10 cm) from the wall. The patient is instructed to bend both knees while sliding the back down the wall (Fig. 9.13).

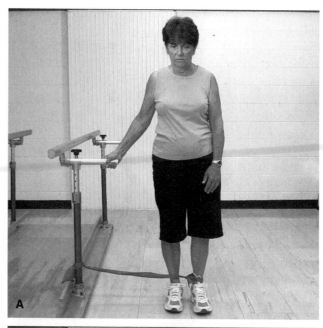

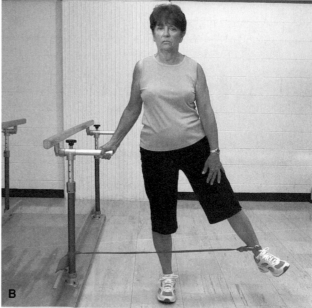

FIGURE 9.11 Standing (A) and hip abduction (B) using an elastic resistance band and support of one hand.

Movement is restricted to partial range; the patient is instructed to stop when no longer able to see the tips of the toes (knees are not allowed to move forward in advance of the toes). The hips are maintained in neutral rotation to ensure proper patellar tracking. The pelvis is also maintained in neutral.

Partial wall squats are an important activity for the patient with quadriceps weakness. The patient is required to maintain control during both eccentric (lowering) contraction and concentric (raising) contractions. The patient is instructed not to move the knee into hyperextension. A small towel roll or ball can be placed between the knees. The patient is instructed to hold the towel roll in position by

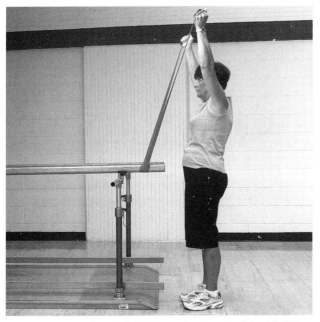

FIGURE 9.12 Standing, PNF UE bilateral symmetrical flex/abd/ER patterns with resistive bands In standing, the patient moves both UEs into flex/abd/ER patterns using resistive bands, stretching the anterior chest muscles and strengthening the upper back, scapular girdle, and shoulder muscles.

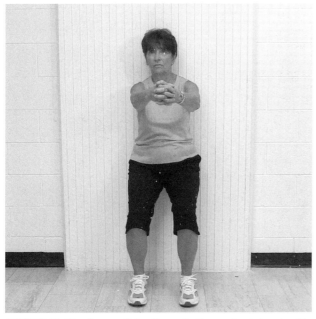

FIGURE 9.13 Standing, partial wall squats The patient stands with both feet about 2 ft (0.6 m) from the wall, hip-width apart. The patient leans back against the wall and slowly lowers, bending both knees. The patient is cautioned not to allow the knees to advance in front of the toes. The patient holds the position for 2 to 3 seconds and then slowly returns to standing. The therapist provides verbal instructions and guarding.

squeezing both knees together during the squat. This enhances contraction of the vastus medialis and improves patellar tracking. An elastic resistive band placed around the thighs can be used to increase the stabilizing activity of the hip abductors during partial wall squats. Partial wall squats

are an important lead-up activity for independent sit-to-stand transfers and stair climbing. Bilateral partial squats can be progressed to unilateral (single-limb) partial squats.

Clinical Note: Partial squats should be performed with a slight posterior pelvic tilt in the presence of low back pain. The patient can also stand with the back supported by a medium-sized ball placed in the lumbar region (Fig. 9.14). The feet are positioned directly underneath the body, with the trunk upright. The ball is resting on the wall. As the patient moves down into the partial squat position, the ball rolls upward, facilitating the movement. The correct size ball also helps to maintain a normal lumbar curve.

Postural Control in Standing

Sensory Components

Independent standing (unassisted vertical postural orientation) is maintained by multiple and overlapping sensory inputs; the CNS organizes and integrates sensory information and generates motor responses for controlling body position.

The *somatosensory (tactile and proprioceptive) system* responds to support-surface inputs about the relative orientation of body position and movement. The somatosensory systems influence postural responses through the stretch reflexes, postural tone, and automatic postural reactions.

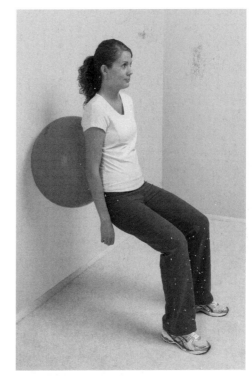

FIGURE 9.14 Standing, partial wall squats with a ball A ball is placed between the wall and the patient's low back to assist during the partial wall squat.

The *visual system* responds to visual cues about the environment and the relationship of the body to objects in the environment. It provides input for optical righting reactions of the head, trunk, and limbs and contributes to upright head position and normal alignment of the head and body. It assists in regulating postural tone and guides safe movement trajectories.

The *vestibular system* responds to gravity acting on the head. It stabilizes gaze during movements of the head by using the vestibulo-ocular reflex (VOR). This reflex allows objects to remain stable in the visual field while the head moves in space. The vestibular system provides input to labyrinthine righting reactions of the head, trunk, and limbs and contributes to upright head position and normal alignment of the head and body. This facet of the system allows one to remain upright in relation to gravity without the use of visual cues, for instance, walking in the dark. It helps to regulate postural tone through the action of vestibulospinal pathways. In addition, the vestibular system acts to mediate conflicting information from the somatosensory and visual systems to accurately perceive movement in space. See Chapter 13: Interventions for Vestibular Rehabilitation for additional information regarding the vestibular system.

Normal Postural Synergies

Synergies are functionally linked muscles that are constrained by the CNS to act cooperatively to produce an intended movement.[3–6] The following normal postural strategies used to maintain upright stability and balance are examples of these synergies.

- *Ankle strategy* involves small shifts of the COM by rotating the body about the ankle joints; there is minimal movement of the hip and knee joints. Movements are well within the LOS (Fig. 9.15A).

- *Hip strategy* involves larger shifts of the COM by flexing or extending at the hips. Movements approach the LOS (Fig. 9.15B).
- *Change of support strategies* are activated when the COM exceeds the BOS and strategies must be initiated that reestablishes the COM within the LOS. These include the *stepping strategy,* which involves realignment of the BOS under the COM achieved by stepping in the direction of the instability (Fig. 9.15C), and UE *grasp strategies,* which involve attempts to stabilize movement of the upper trunk, keeping the COM over the BOS.

Clinical Note: To evaluate a person's ability to effectively utilize and integrate sensory inputs in the clinic without sophisticated equipment, the Modified Clinical Test for Sensory Interaction in Balance (mCTSIB) is recommended. The mCTSIB utilizes four different sensory test conditions:

- Condition 1: eyes open, stable surface (EOSS)
- Condition 2: eyes closed, stable surface (ECSS)
- Condition 3: eyes open, foam surface (EOFS)
- Condition 4: eyes closed, foam surface (ECFS)

Three 30-second trials are used to assess and document the postural strategies utilized, loss of balance, or amount of increased postural sway. Subjective complaints of nausea or dizziness are also recorded. The test is stopped if the person alters the starting posture (feet shoulder-width apart, arms crossed at the chest), utilizes a stepping strategy, or requires assistance to prevent loss of balance.[1,2]

Red Flag: Patients recovering from stroke have a tendency to fall posteriorly and toward the hemiparetic side under eyes-closed conditions, so the therapist should be ready to protect the patient from a fall.

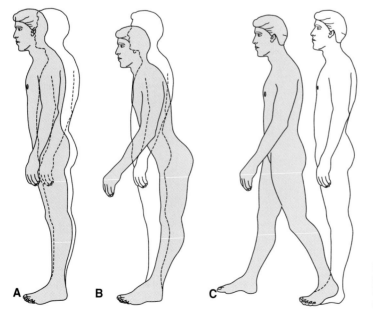

FIGURE 9.15 Normal postural strategies Three automatic postural strategies used by adults to maintain balance (COM over BOS) are the (A) ankle strategy, (B) hip strategy, and (C) stepping strategy.

Clinical Notes:

· **Ankle Strategies:** Although ankle-foot orthoses have many benefits, such as providing ankle stability and preventing foot drop, they prevent the use of normal ankle strategies.
· **Hip Strategies:** People with a history of low back pain may be reluctant to utilize normal hip strategies due to fear of increasing pain.
· **Stepping Strategies:** A "staggering gait" pattern is an example of the overuse of the stepping strategies to help maintain postural control (e.g., the patient with cerebellar dysfunction).

Clinical Note: The patient with bilateral LE paralysis (e.g., paraplegia) can obtain foot/ankle and knee stability through bilateral knee-ankle-foot orthoses; the hips can be stabilized by leaning forward on the iliofemoral (Y) ligament.

Common Impairments in Standing

Although not all-inclusive, impairments in standing can be broadly grouped into those involving alignment, weightbearing, and specific muscle weakness. Changes in normal alignment result in corresponding changes in other body segments; malalignment or poor posture results in increased muscle activity, energy expenditure, and postural stress. Box 9.1 presents common impairments in standing posture and weightbearing. Figures 9.16 and 9.17 demonstrate the postural changes seen in many older adults. Loss of spinal flexibility and strength results in a flexed, stooped posture with a forward head, dorsal kyphosis, and increased hip and knee flexion.

General Considerations in Improving Standing Control

Patients with impairments in static postural control benefit from activities that challenge standing control. Progression is obtained by varying the level of difficulty. For example, greater challenges can be incorporated into standing activities by modifying the BOS, the support surface, the use of UEs, and sensory inputs. During initial practice, the patient should be encouraged to focus full attention on the standing task and its key elements. With practice, the level of cognitive monitoring will decrease as motor learning progresses. Once an autonomous level of learning is achieved, postural responses are largely automatic, with little conscious thought for routine postural adjustments.[1,2]

Strategies to Ensure Safety

Patients who are unstable in standing are likely to have heightened anxiety and a fear of falling. It is important for the therapist to demonstrate the ability to control for instability and falls to instill patient confidence. General safety tips are presented in Box 9.2.

BOX 9.1 Common Impairments in Standing Postural Alignment and Weightbearing

· **Asymmetrical standing** with weight borne primarily on one LE with little weight on the other LE results in increased ligament and bone stress on the weightbearing side; the knee is usually fully extended on the stance limb (e.g., the patient with stroke who stands with weight borne more on the less affected side).
· **Trunk extensor weakness** is typically associated with a *forward head position,* rounded thoracic spine *(kyphosis)* with a flattened lumbar curve, creating a forward displacement of the COM near or at the anterior LOS. The hips and knees are typically flexed (Fig. 9.4). This flexed, stooped posture is seen in many elderly people (Fig. 9.5).
· A **flexed-knee posture** increases the need for quadriceps activity; it also requires increased hip extensor and soleus activity for accompanying increases in hip flexion and dorsiflexion.
· **Excessive anterior tilt of the pelvis** increases lumbar lordosis and produces a compensatory increase in thoracic kyphosis; lumbar interdiscal pressures are increased. The abdominals are stretched, and the iliopsoas becomes shortened. Excessive lumbar lordosis produces shortening of the lumbar extensors.
· **Excessive dorsal kyphosis** produces stretching of the thoracic trunk extensors and shortening of the anterior shoulder muscles.
· **Excessive cervical lordosis** produces shortening of the neck extensors.
· **Genu valgum** produces medial knee joint stresses and pronation of the foot with increased stress on the medial longitudinal arch of the foot.
· **Pes planus** (flat foot) results in depression of the navicular bone and compressive forces laterally; increased weight is borne on the metatarsal heads.
· **Pes cavus** (high-arched foot) results in increased height of the longitudinal arch with a depressed anterior arch and plantarflexion of the forefoot; toe deformity (claw toes) may also be present.
· **Gastrocnemius-soleus weakness** results in limited sway and a wide BOS. **Quadriceps weakness** results in unstable sway; the knees are hyperextended (genu recurvatum) and the trunk may be inclined forward to increase stability. The patient without active knee control compensates by keeping the hips slightly flexed, with increased lordosis.
· **LE spasticity** results in decreased function; the actions of the LE muscles and balance reactions are compromised. The LEs are typically adducted and internally rotated (scissoring position) with feet plantar flexed and inverted.

Floor-to-standing transfers should be practiced by all patients and their caregivers in preparation for recovery should a fall occur. Functional skills acquired during earlier movement transitions (supine to side-sit, side-sit to quadruped, quadruped to kneeling, kneeling to half-kneeling, and half-kneeling to standing) provide the building blocks (lead-up skills) for a successful floor-to-standing transfer. This movement transition can be accomplished by having

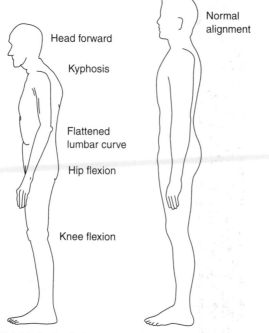

FIGURE 9.16 **Postural changes seen in many older adults** Loss of spinal flexibility and strength can lead to a flexed, stooped posture with a forward head, dorsal kyphosis, and increased hip and knee flexion.

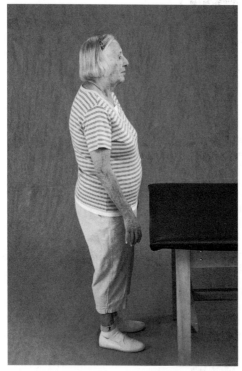

FIGURE 9.17 **Postural changes associated with aging** This patient demonstrates a slight forward head and dorsal kyphosis.

the patient practice moving into quadruped, then kneeling, half-kneeling, and finally standing. The patient uses both UEs for support and the forward LE to push up into standing (Fig. 9.18). As an alternative to manual assistance, the patient can be instructed in how to use a solid

---

BOX 9.2 General Safety Considerations

- Initial early standing may require support devices, such as a standing frame or a frame with a body weight support (BWS) harness. A predetermined percentage of body weight is supported by the BWS device. As control is achieved, the percentage of weight support is decreased (e.g., 30 % support to 20% support to 10% support to no support).
- Activities can progress to modified standing with the use of parallel bars or by standing next to a treatment table using *light fingertip, touch-down support*. The patient can also stand with his or her back to the wall or positioned in a corner (corner standing).
- Gait (guarding) belts should be used as necessary for the patient who is at risk for falls. Lower extremity splints or orthoses may be necessary to stabilize the position of a limb.
- Collaborative treatments (co-treat sessions) with two or more professionals may be necessary for very involved patients (e.g., the patient with TBI and poor standing control).
- The patient should be instructed in safely getting on and off any equipment to be used during balance activities (e.g., wobble board, foam, inflated disc, or ball).

---

piece of furniture (e.g., chair) to assist with a weight shift forward from half-kneeling to sitting, then transition to standing.

Clinical Note: Light touch-down (fingertip) support may be used initially. However, interventions designed to improve independent standing are best addressed without the use of UEs because this puts greater demands on the postural support system (i.e., trunk and LEs). Standing hands free is important for use of the hands in various different functional tasks. In contrast, grasping and pulling on objects (e.g., parallel bars) decrease the demands on the postural support system and provide compensatory control using the UEs. If progression is planned to walking using an assistive device such as a walker or cane, practice in pulling will not transfer well to the control needed for using the devices.

Red Flag: Training with mirrors may be contraindicated for patients with visual-perceptual spatial deficits (e.g., some patients with stroke or TBI).

Strategies to Improve Motor Learning

The therapist should instruct the patient in the correct standing posture and demonstrate the position and activity to provide an accurate *reference of correctness*. It is important to focus the patient's attention on key task elements and improve overall sensory awareness of the correct standing posture and position in space (intrinsic feedback). Using externally focused VCs such as *"bring your pants pockets over your shoe laces"* can be more effective than internally

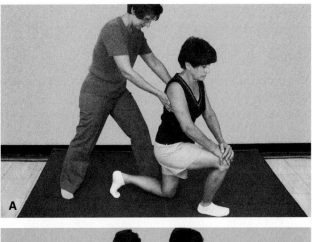

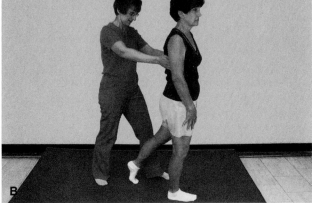

FIGURE 9.18 Floor-to-standing transfer The patient moves into half-kneeling and places both hands on the front knee. From there the patient shifts forward and over the foot, pushes off with both hands, and stands up. (A) The therapist can assist by holding onto the patient's upper trunk (the therapist stands behind the patient). (B) The patient moves into the standing position.

based ones such as *"bring your hips over your feet."*[7] Suggested verbal instructions and cueing are presented in Box 9.3.

Augmented feedback (e.g., tapping, light resistance, and verbal cueing) should focus attention on *key errors* (those errors that, when corrected, result in considerable improvement in performance, allowing other task elements to then be performed correctly). Slowed responses of some muscles may result in inadequate responses or falls. Tactile and proprioceptive cues can be used to call attention to missing elements. For example, tapping on a weak quadriceps can be used to assist the patient in generating an effective contraction to stabilize the knee during standing. Augmented feedback should also emphasize positive aspects of performance, providing reinforcement and enhancing motivation. As soon as appropriate, augmented feedback should be reduced and finally withdrawn to ensure optimal motor learning.[7,8]

Dual-task control—the ability to perform a secondary task (motor or cognitive) while maintaining standing control—can be used to assess the patient's postural control without the use of active cognitive monitoring (having to think about standing posture). Thus, it can be used to evaluate the shift from the cognitive to the associative stage of motor learning.

BOX 9.3 General Verbal Instructions and Cues

- *"Stand tall, hold your head up, and keep your chin tucked with your ears over your shoulders."*
- *"Look up and focus on the target directly in front of you."*
- *"Keep your back straight with shoulders over your hips and hips over your feet."* Alternatively, *"Keep your shirt buttons pointed straight ahead and bring your pants pockets over your shoelaces."*
- *"Keep the bottom of your chest bone directly over your belly button."*
- *"Keep your weight equally distributed over both feet."*
- *"Breathe normally and hold this posture as steady as you can."*
- *"Imagine you are a soldier standing guard at the Tomb of the Unknown Soldier; stand tall and on guard."*

The patient is asked to perform a secondary motor task (pouring water from a pitcher into a glass) or a secondary cognitive task (count backward from 100 by 7s). Any decrement in postural control is noted.

Clinical Note: To capitalize on the motor learning principles of attention, practice, motivation, feedback, and positive reinforcement, virtual reality and gaming devices are being employed as therapeutic interventions to improve dynamic balance. However, the best use of these devices for rehabilitation has yet to be determined with extensive evidence-based research.[9]

Interventions to Improve Static Control in Standing

The patient is standing, with equal weight on both LEs. The feet are positioned parallel and slightly apart (a symmetrical stance position); knees should be extended or in slight flexion, not hyperextended. The pelvis is in neutral position. An alternative standing position is with one foot slightly advanced of the other in a step position. An elastic resistive band can be placed around the thighs (the LEs in a symmetrical stance position) to increase the proprioceptive input and promote pelvic stabilization by the lateral hip muscles (gluteus medius and minimus).

Clinical Note: Knee instability in which the knee buckles due to quadriceps weakness can be managed initially by having the patient wear a knee immobilizer splint. The patient can also practice standing on an inclined surface facing forward. The forward tilt of the body and anterior displacement of the COM provide a posteriorly directed moment (force) at the knee, helping to stabilize it in extension.

Standing, Holding

The patient can practice active holding or resisted holding. Resistance is used to recruit and facilitate contraction of postural muscles in patients who lack active control. The PNF techniques of stabilizing reversals and rhythmic stabilization can be performed (previously described in the modified standing position). In stabilizing reversals, the therapist's hands may be placed on the pelvis, the pelvis and contralateral upper trunk (Fig. 9.19), or the upper trunk bilaterally. Verbal cues include *"Don't let me push you backward, now don't let me pull you forward."* In rhythmic stabilization, one hand is placed on the posterior pelvis on one side, pulling forward, while the other hand is on the anterior contralateral upper trunk, pushing backward. Verbal cues include *"Don't let me move you* [twist you]—*hold, hold; now don't let me move you* [twist you] *the other way, hold."*

Outcomes

Motor control goal: stability (static postural control)
Functional skill achieved: patient able to maintain standing independently with minimal sway and no loss of balance for all ADL

Interventions to Improve Dynamic Control in Standing

Interventions to promote dynamic stability or weight shifting in standing are important lead-up skills for many ADL (both basic and instrumental) typically performed in the standing position, such as showering, cooking, and cleaning, for example. The ability to shift body weight from one LE

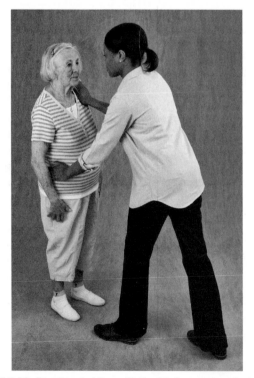

FIGURE 9.19 Standing, holding with the LEs in a symmetrical position The therapist is applying resistance to the upper trunk and pelvis using the technique of stabilizing reversals (both hands pushing back).

to another in standing is also an important lead-up activity for unilateral stance, stepping, and bipedal gait.

Standing, Weight Shifts

The patient is encouraged to actively weight-shift forward and backward (anterior/posterior shifts) and from side to side (medial/lateral shifts) with the LEs in a symmetrical stance position. In a step position, the patient can perform forward and backward diagonal weight shifts, simulating normal weight transfer during gait. Reeducation of LOS is one of the first goals in treatment. The patient is encouraged to shift weight as far as possible in any one direction without losing balance and then to return to the midline position. Initially, weight shifts are small range. but gradually the range is increased (moving through *increments of range*).

Clinical Note: Patients with ataxia (e.g., primary cerebellar pathology) exhibit too much movement and have difficulty holding steady in a posture (maintaining stability). Initially, weight shifts are large and then are progressed during treatment to smaller and smaller ranges (moving through *decrements of range*) to finally holding steady.

Resisted weight shifts (e.g., dynamic reversals) can be used to recruit and facilitate postural muscles. The therapist stands at the patient's side for medial/lateral shifts and either in front of or behind the patient for anterior/posterior shifts. Manual contacts are placed on the pelvis or on the pelvis and contralateral upper trunk. The movement is guided for a few repetitions to ensure that the patient knows the movements expected. Movements are then lightly resisted. The therapist alternates hand placement, resisting the movements first in one direction and then the other. Smooth reversals of antagonists are facilitated by well-timed VCs, such as *"Pull away from me; now push back toward me."*

Clinical Note: A hold may be added in one direction if the patient demonstrates difficulty moving in that direction. For example, the patient with stroke is hesitant to weight-shift onto the hemiplegic LE. Adding the hold increases the stabilizing responses on that side and is a momentary pause (held for one count). The VCs include *"Pull away from me, and hold; now push back toward me."*

The patient can also perform diagonal weight shifts with the LEs in step position (one foot forward of the other) (Fig. 9.20). The therapist is diagonally in front of the patient, either sitting on a stool or standing. Manual contacts are on the anterior or posterior pelvis. Resistance is applied to the pelvis as the patient shifts weight diagonally forward over the limb in front and then diagonally backward over the opposite limb. The VCs include *"Shift forward and toward me; now shift backward and away from me."*

Once control is achieved in diagonal shifts, the patient can be instructed to shift weight diagonally forward onto the forward limb (step position) while rotating the pelvis forward on the opposite side. Weight is then shifted diagonally

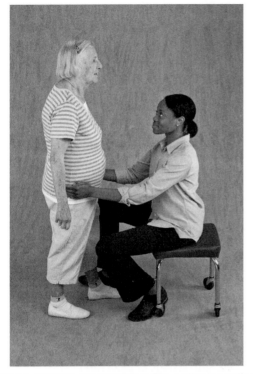

FIGURE 9.20 Standing, weight shifting The patient practices weight shifting forward and backward with the LEs in step position. The therapist provides resistance with both hands at the pelvis using the technique of dynamic reversals. Sitting on a rolling stool allows the therapist to be positioned at pelvic height.

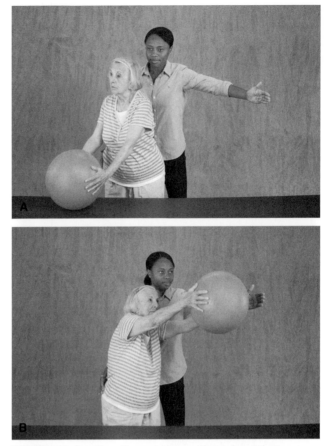

FIGURE 9.21 Standing, diagonal lifting with head and trunk rotation (A) The patient picks up the small ball with both hands and (B) lifts the ball up and across to the left. The therapist provides the target and VCs to maximize head and trunk rotation.

backward while the pelvis is rotated backward. The therapist resists the motion at the pelvis. Verbal cues include *"Shift forward and twist; now shift backward and twist."* The upper trunk may move forward on the same side that the pelvis rotates forward, producing an undesirable ipsilateral trunk rotation pattern. The therapist can isolate the pelvic motion by providing verbal or manual cues. The patient is instructed to hold the UEs in front with the shoulders flexed, elbows extended, and the hands clasped, or the hands can be lightly supported on the therapist's shoulders to stabilize the upper trunk motion. Verbal cues include *"Clasp your hands and hold your arms directly in front of you. Keep them forward; don't let them move from side to side. Now shift forward and twist. Now shift back and twist."*

Standing, Limb Movements

Active movements of the UEs or LEs can be used to challenge dynamic stability control and balance (Fig. 9.21). Postural adjustments are required during every single limb movement. Limb movements can be performed individually or in combination (bilateral symmetrical or reciprocal UE movements). Progression is to increased range and increased time on task. For example, the patient folds laundry (Fig. 9.22), picks an object up off a low stool (Fig. 9.23) or off the floor, or sweeps with a broom (Fig. 9.24). One of the major benefits of these UE activities is that the patient focuses full attention on the UE movements and the task challenges imposed; postural control to maintain standing is largely automatic.

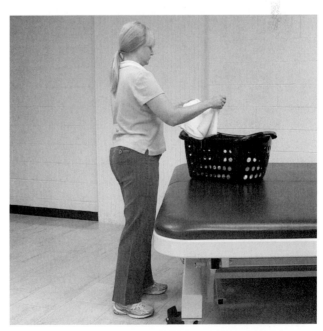

FIGURE 9.22 Standing, folding laundry The patient performs the task of folding laundry, which challenges dynamic standing balance. This functional activity incorporates weight shifting and trunk rotation while completing a bilateral manual task.

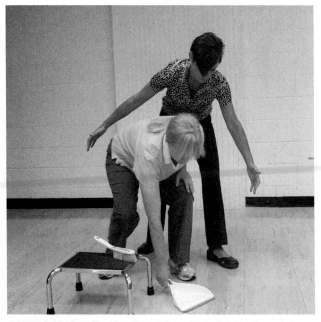

FIGURE 9.23 Standing, bending and reaching The patient lowers the COM from standing by reaching to a low stool and progresses the activity as she retrieves an object from the floor. The therapist provides guarding to ensure safe practice.

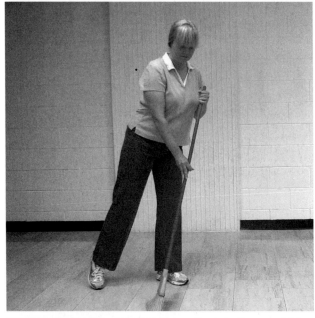

FIGURE 9.24 Standing, sweeping The patient performs weight shifting with the feet in step position while sweeping.

Box 9.4 provides examples of functional task training activities that improve dynamic standing balance.

Standing, Stepping

This activity is initiated with the LEs in step position. The patient shifts weight diagonally forward over the anterior support limb (stance limb) and takes a step forward with the dynamic (swing) limb. The movements are then reversed;

BOX 9.4 Activities That Promote Weight Shifting in Standing

Reaches and Lifts
- Reaching to place items forward, backward, and on a diagonal, such as reaching in or out of a refrigerator or oven
- Placing items on and off a shelf overhead (cupboard) and below waist height (dishwasher)
- Lifting a ball up with both hands, turning, and moving the ball diagonally up and across the body (Fig. 9.21) (The size and weight of the ball can be varied.)
- Reaching forward or sideways to a target (*"Reach out and touch my hand."*)
- Playing bean bag toss
- Folding laundry and placing it in a basket placed off to the side or on a chair next to the person (Fig. 9.22)
- Drying dishes and placing them in a dish drainer
- Reaching down to touch the floor or to pick an object up off the floor (Fig. 9.23)
- Sweeping using a broom (Fig. 9.24)

LE Activities
- Marching in place (This activity can be combined with reciprocal arm swings or head turns.)
- Toe-offs and heel-offs; moving the weight backward onto both heels, lifting the toes, then moving the weight forward onto the toes and balls of the feet, lifting the heels)
- Placing the foot on a stool or low stair (Fig. 9.27)
- Placing the foot on a small ball and rolling the ball in all directions (The size of the ball can be varied.)
- Stopping a rolling ball and kicking it

the patient takes a step backward using the same dynamic limb. Footprint or other markers on the floor can be used to increase the step length and improve the accuracy of stepping movements (Fig. 9.25). Lateral side steps and crossed steps can also be practiced (Fig. 9.26). Verbal cues include *"Shift your weight over onto your right* [or left] *foot. Now step forward with your left foot"* and *"Now shift back over your right foot and step back."*

The patient can also be instructed to place one foot up on a step positioned directly in front (Fig. 9.27). This variation requires increased hip and knee flexion of the dynamic limb. Lateral or side step-ups can also be practiced (Fig. 9.28). The height of the step can be varied from a low of 4 in. (10 cm) to a normal step height of 7 in. (18 cm). Verbal cues include *"Shift your weight over onto your right (or left) foot. Now place your left foot up on the step. Now bring it down."*

To progress dynamic balance and prepare for gait, stepping can be resisted with the therapist sitting on a rolling stool or standing in front of the patient. Manual contacts are on the pelvis. The therapist applies light stretch and resistance to facilitate forward pelvic rotation as the swing limb

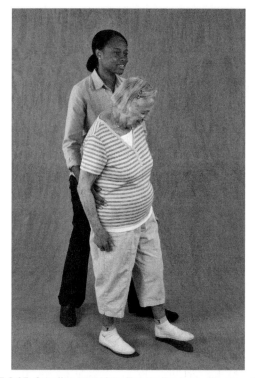

FIGURE 9.25 Standing, stepping The patient practices active stepping using footprint floor markers.

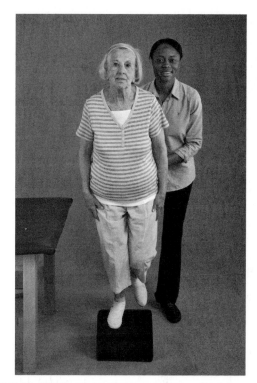

FIGURE 9.27 Standing, forward step-ups The patient steps up onto a 4-in. (10-cm) step positioned in front; the foot is then returned to the start position (symmetrical stance position). The therapist provides verbal cueing and guarding.

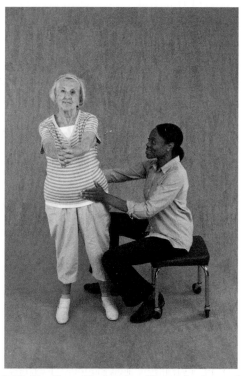

FIGURE 9.26 Standing, sidestepping The patient practices stepping out to the side and back with the dynamic limb; the static (support) limb does not change position. The therapist provides resistance with both hands on the pelvis.

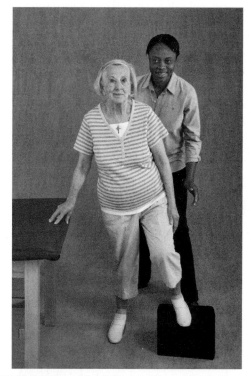

FIGURE 9.28 Standing, lateral step-ups The patient steps up onto a 4-in. (10-cm) step positioned to her left side; the foot is then returned to the start position (symmetrical stance position). Light touch-down support of one hand may be necessary. The therapist provides verbal cueing and guarding.

moves forward and backward. This is a useful activity to promote improved rotation of the pelvis during stepping. Verbal cues include *"Shift forward and step; now shift backward and step."* A resistive band may be used in place of manual contacts from the therapist (Figs. 9.29 and 9.30).

Clinical Note: If the patient is unable to maintain postural control during voluntary limb movements, it may be an indication that conscious control (cognitive monitoring) is still required. This is a characteristic finding in the patient with primary cerebellar damage who must compensate by "paying attention" to every movement. With increased dependence on cognitive monitoring, automatic (nonconscious) control of posture is very difficult to impossible.

Examining Postural Instability

For patients with postural instability, effective use of therapeutic interventions depends on the identification of the areas of deficit and the underlying causative factors of imbalance. The therapist must analyze and synthesize information obtained from specific tests and measures (e.g., ROM, strength, balance assessment tools) in combination with observational analysis to design a plan of care that reduces underlying impairments and improves functional mobility and safety. Initial task selection for therapeutic interventions should be aimed at the remediation of the contributing factors to instability.

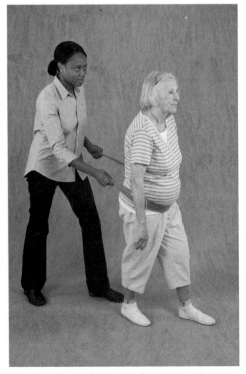

FIGURE 9.29 Standing, resisted stepping The patient steps forward against resistance and then steps back. The therapist provides resistance using an elastic resistive band positioned around the patient's pelvis.

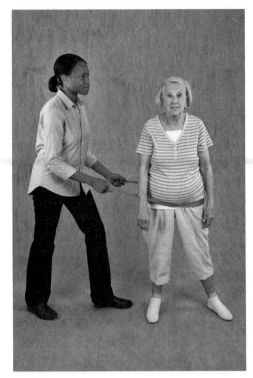

FIGURE 9.30 Standing, resisted sidestepping The patient steps out to the side against resistance and then steps back. The therapist provides resistance using an elastic resistance band positioned around the patient's pelvis.

During the examination, the therapist can glean important clues regarding the underlying causes of unsteadiness by the patient's description of activity limitations and participation restrictions. Many times the patient's subjective report provides key information regarding the source of the unsteadiness. For example, complaints of spinning dizziness or vertigo indicate a vestibular dysfunction, whereas complaints of feeling unsteady or "off balance" implicate postural instability. Critical questions for the examiner to ask include:

- Have you experienced any feelings of unsteadiness or dizziness?
- Have you fallen or lost your balance?
- How many times did you fall in the past week (or month)?
- When was your last fall, and what were you doing when it occurred?
- In general, how safe do you feel?
- Are you able to complete all of your usual everyday activities without losing your balance?

Often the circumstances of a fall will illuminate ineffectual or inefficient balance strategies.

ROM and strength measurements assist in determining the patient's capability to utilize normal postural synergies for balance since deficits in joint motion or weakness impede the ability to maintain the COM over the BOS. Findings from balance assessment tools not only identify those at risk for falls but also often reveal areas of functional deficit and may implicate errors in sensory organization and/or impaired postural synergies (Table 9.2). When assessing a patient with

TABLE 9.2 Examination of Postural Instability

Examination Domain	Factors in Postural Instability
Impairments	Postural malalignment • Scoliosis or leg-length discrepancy • Congenital or acquired deformities leading to alterations in COM over BOS ROM deficits in the • Head and neck • Ankles (especially in dorsiflexion) • Hips (especially in extension) Impaired somatosensory inputs • Decreased cutaneous information in LEs • Decreased proprioception /kinesthesia in the LEs • Visual deficits • Vestibular deficits: complaints of dizziness Muscle weakness • Anterior and posterior tibialis • Peroneals • Gluteus maximus and medius • Trunk
Limitations and Restrictions	Difficulty walking with reduced vision • Poor lighting or at night • When feet cannot be seen Loss of balance while standing and doing tasks at sink or counter Loss of balance when reaching overhead or toward floor Loss of balance while walking • When turning • In small or enclosed spaces • With distractions • On uneven surfaces: carpet, grass, hills, gravel • In busy environments • With rapid head movements Difficulty going up or down stairs
Test and Measures; Identification of Fall Risk	***Sensory Organization Test (SOT)***[6] or ***Modified Clinical Test of Sensory Interaction in Balance (m-CTSIB)*** [10–16] • Identifies sensory condition(s) where LOB occurs • Provides indication of a sensory dependency or a sensory selection problem • Identifies presence of a directional preponderance to the LOB ***Functional Reach (FR) or Multidirectional Reach Test (mFR)***[17–19] • Examines maximal distance a patient can reach forward while maintaining a fixed BOS • Presence of a directional preponderance to the LOB • Utilization of abnormal ankle strategies or hip strategies when reaching ***Berg Balance Test (BBT)***[28–30] • Examines 14 items of functional balance (sitting and standing) • Score indicative of fall risk • Maximum score is 56; patients who score <45 are at high risk for falls.

(table continues on page 204)

TABLE 9.2 Examination of Postural Instability *(continued)*

Examination Domain	Factors in Postural Instability
	Performance-Oriented Assessment of Mobility (POMA)[25–27] • Examines nine items of balance (sitting and standing) and eight items of walking • Score indicative of fall risk • Maximum score is 28; patients who score <19 are at high risk for falls. **Timed Up and Go (TUG)[26,27]** • Examines functional balance during rise from chair, walk 3 m, turn, and return to chair • Timed performance • Normal test ≤10 sec • Patients who score greater than 20 sec are at increased risk for falls. • TUG (cognitive): Patient performs a cognitive task while walking. **Dynamic Gait Index (DGI)[28–32]** • Examines eight items of dynamic gait • Score indicative of fall risk • Patients with a history of falls have a mean score of 11+ or –4. **Activities-Specific Balance Confidence (ABC) Scale[33]** • Identifies conditions where person is confident • Identifies conditions where person is less confident • Identifies a pattern when the person is less confident **Community Balance and Mobility Scale (CB&M)[34]** • Designed to evaluate high-level balance and mobility deficits in patients with balance impairments and reduced community living • Examines 13 challenging tasks • Scored on a 5-point scale: specific criteria for each item • Maximum possible score 96 • Patients with TBI (day hospital setting), mean score of 62

Observational Gait Analysis	Identification of characteristics that indicate dynamic postural instability:
	• Increased BOS throughout gait cycle
	• Use of grasp strategies (touching wall or furniture)
	• Inadequate foot clearance during swing phase
	• Ankle instability during stance phase
	• Stepping strategies used while walking (staggering gait)
	  • With a decreased BOS
	  • While turning
	  • With head turns side to side or up and down

high-level deficits, the therapist must select appropriate tests and measures that capture the patient's limitations.[30,31] For example, the *Community Balance and Mobility Scale* measures high-level balance skills needed for community interaction (see Table 9.2. Examination of Postural Instability).[31]

Interventions to Improve Balance Control

Therapeutic interventions selected must remediate musculoskeletal impairments that hinder use of the hip, ankle, and stepping strategies while practicing the synergies themselves and reintegrating them into functional movement. Reliance on visual or somatosensory input can be retrained by exposing the patient to conditions that require involvement of the underutilized modality while improving patient confidence under these conditions. For instance, a person who relies on visual information for orientation should practice standing on a variety of surfaces with the eyes closed or with vision distorted (e.g., wearing dark sunglasses). A person who relies on somatosensory information should practice standing on compliant or uneven surfaces with and without visual information. Vestibular inputs can be stimulated by situations that limit use of visual and somatosensory information such as standing on foam with head turning side to side.

The therapist focuses on the primary components of postural control, including the neuromuscular synergies and sensory integration. Progression is from voluntary movements (anticipatory control) to automatic movements (reactive control). Box 9.5 presents Examples of Interventions to Improve Standing Control.

Promoting Ankle Strategies

Small shifts in COM alignment or slow sway movements result in activation of an ankle strategy. The patient is instructed to sway gently forward and backward and then return to centered alignment using ankle motions (dorsiflexion and plantar flexion). The trunk and hips move as one unit, with the axis of motion at the ankles; thus, flexion and extension movements at the hips are not permitted. Slow VCs can be used initially to pace the movements. Gentle perturbations applied at the hips or shoulders, either with manual contacts or using a resistive band, can also be used to activate ankle strategies (Fig. 9.31). A small displacement backward activates dorsiflexors and a forward weight shift, whereas a small displacement forward activates plantarflexors and a backward weight shift. Standing on a tipper board (bidirectional board) (Fig. 9.32) or rocker board (Fig. 9.33; multidirectional dome board) and gently rocking the board stimulates ankle actions. Small weight shifts performed while standing on a split foam roller (flat side up) can also be used to activate ankle synergies (Fig. 9.34).

Promoting Hip Strategies

Larger shifts in COM alignment or faster sway movements result in activation of a hip strategy and frequently occur in conditions where the use of ankle strategies is limited, such as standing on a small BOS (standing on a ladder) or on a compliant surface (standing in the sand). The patient is instructed to sway farther into the range and increase the speed of sway. Hip flexors or extensors serve to realign the COM within the BOS. Thus the upper trunk is moving opposite the direction of the lower body, with the axis of motion occurring at the hips. Stepping is discouraged. For example, the patient can be instructed to stand with back toward the wall approximately 12 inches away. The patient then brings his or her buttocks to rest on the wall, then the shoulders to the wall, and finally returns to standing (Fig. 9.35).

Moderate perturbations applied at the hips while standing on flat floor surface or larger, faster tilts on a rocker board can also be used to stimulate anterior-posterior hip strategies. Standing on a split foam roller (flat side up) can be used to produce larger weight shifts and hip strategies, as can standing on a foam cushion, especially with eyes closed (Fig. 9.36).

Medial/lateral adjustments in the COM are accomplished mainly by hip strategies. Tandem standing (heel-toe position) on the floor, or standing tandem lengthwise on a foam roller can be used to promote medial/lateral hip strategies (see Fig. 9.34).

Promoting Stepping Strategies

Larger shifts in which the COM exceeds the LOS result in activation of *stepping strategies*. The patient practices leaning

---

BOX 9.5 Examples of Interventions to Improve Standing Control

Base of Support
A wide-based stance is a common compensatory change in patients with decreased control. Postural control can be challenged by altering the BOS as follows:

- Progress from feet apart to feet close together to *in step* (one foot in front of the other) to *tandem stance* (heel-toe position).
- Progress from bilateral UE support (e.g., parallel bars) to unilateral UE support (e.g., next to the treatment table) to no UE support.

    Note: Light touch-down support (fingertip support) is preferred to holding on (e.g., grabbing onto parallel bars). Progress to no UE support.

Support Surface
The type of support surface can influence postural alignment and control.

- A fixed support surface (e.g., tile floor) provides a stable initial base.
- Progress from standing on a fixed support surface to standing on a carpet, dense foam pad, or mobile surface (e.g., inflated disc, foam roller, wobble board).

Sensory Inputs
Sensory support and modification can influence postural alignment and control.

- Somatosensory cues are maximized by having the patient barefoot or wearing flexible-sole shoes.
- Somatosensory inputs can be varied to increase difficulty: Progress from both feet in contact with a fixed support surface (tile floor) to feet positioned on a soft compliant surface (e.g., dense foam, inflatable dome disc) to standing on a moving platform.
- Visual inputs can be varied to increase difficulty in maintaining standing: Progress from EO to EC.
- Visual cues and perceptual awareness of proper alignment can be assisted by using a mirror; a vertical line can be placed on the mirror; the patient can wear a shirt with a vertical line drawn or taped on the front to align with line on the mirror.
- The role of vestibular inputs can be increased by standing on foam with EC or adding head movements in any stance position.

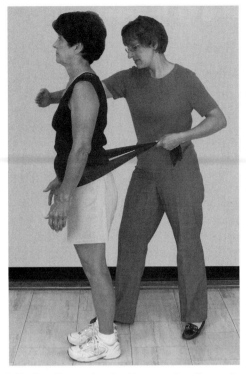

FIGURE 9.31 Standing, resisted ankle strategies The patient leans forward against the resistive band and returns to upright standing, practicing ankle strategies. The band provides both resistance and increased kinesthetic awareness of the movement.

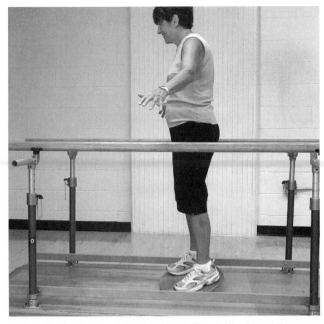

FIGURE 9.33 Standing on rocker board The patient practices ankle strategies using bilateral plantar flexion to maintain standing on the multidirectional dome board. Although the patient is placed in the parallel bars for safety, she is not to use the UEs for support.

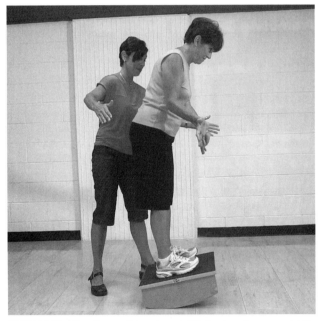

FIGURE 9.32 Standing on tipper board While standing on a bidirectional board, the patient practices ankle strategies used to recover from a posterior displacement of the COM. In this case, the patient demonstrates the transition from an ankle strategy to a hip strategy.

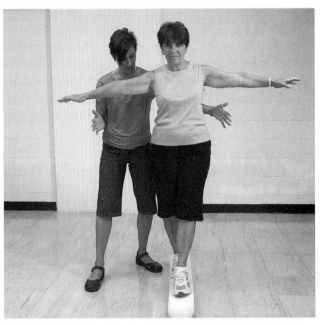

FIGURE 9.34 Tandem standing on a foam roller with flat side up The patient practices maintaining stability with a decreased BOS on a compliant surface using ankle strategies and lateral hip strategies. The therapist readies for a potential for a loss of balance in the medial/lateral direction.

forward until the COM exceeds the BOS. This requires the patient to step forward to prevent a fall. Increased backward lean will result in a backward step, while increased sideward lean will result in a side step or crossed step. The patient then takes a return step to centered alignment. Stepping should be practiced in all directions, progressing from small steps to wider and wider steps. A circle can be drawn on the floor around the patient to encourage symmetry of stepping responses in all directions. The patient is instructed to lean forward (or backward or sideward) against resistance provided by the therapist and to take a step to maintain balance. The therapist suddenly releases the resistance while guarding the patient to protect against a fall. As an alternative, an elastic

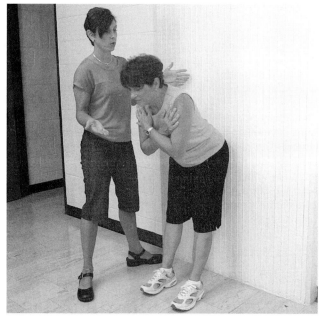

FIGURE 9.35 Standing, bottom to wall exercise The patient practices hip strategies by bringing her bottom to the wall, her shoulders to the wall, and then returns to standing away from the wall. The therapist provides instruction and guarding as needed.

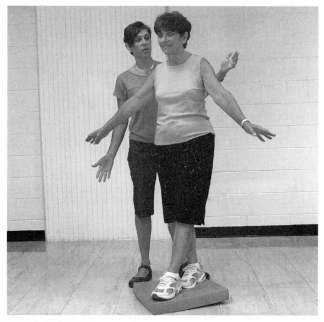

FIGURE 9.36 Tandem standing on foam with EC The patient stands with a reduced BOS on a compliant surface with eyes closed to practice lateral hip strategies.

resistive band may be applied around the hips to provide the perturbation challenge (Fig. 9.37). Sample exercises to improve postural synergies are presented in Table 9.3.

Promoting Balance Control Using Force-Platform Biofeedback

Force-platform biofeedback is an effective training device for patients who demonstrate asymmetrical weightbearing or

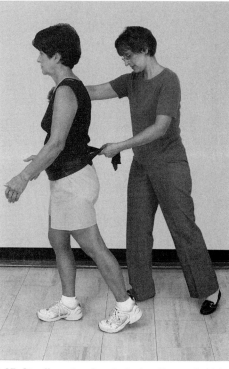

FIGURE 9.37 Standing, stepping strategies The patient leans forward as far as possible against a resistive band. The therapist suddenly releases the tension on the band causing the patient to perform a stepping strategy in the forward direction. The therapist utilizes appropriate guarding techniques for safety.

for those with problems in force generation, producing either too much force (hypermetria) or too little force (hypometria) when weight shifting. Force-platform biofeedback training devices (e.g., Biodex Balance System SD [Fig. 9.38] or NeuroCom Balance Master) can be used to provide center-of-pressure (COP) biofeedback. The weight on each foot is computed and converted into visual feedback regarding the locus and movement of the patient's COP. A computer provides data analysis and training modes using an interactive format. These devices can be used to improve postural symmetry (percent weightbearing and weight-shift training), postural stability (steadiness), LOS (total excursion), and postural sway movements (shaped and modified to enhance symmetry and steadiness).

 Clinical Notes

- The patient recovering from stroke typically stands with more weight on the less affected limb and needs to be instructed to shift weight toward the more affected side to assume a symmetrical stance position. Center-of-pressure biofeedback can be effective in improving symmetrical alignment.
- The patient with Parkinson's disease who demonstrates hypometric responses can be encouraged to achieve larger and faster sway movements using COP biofeedback. The patient with cerebellar pathology who demonstrates hypermetric responses can be encouraged to achieve smaller and smaller sway movements.

TABLE 9.3 Sample Exercises to Improve Postural Synergies

Goal	Primary-Level Exercise	Intermediate-Level Exercise	High-Level Exercise
Improve Ankle Strategies	Gastrocnemius/soleus stretching BAPS board sitting, all directions Ankle exercises using resistance band, all directions Dynamic reversals weight shifting in anterior/posterior direction Standing 6 in. away from a countertop or sink, swaying forward so hip pockets move toward the surface, then sway back to start position Standing on foam: low density to high, EO to EC	BAPS board standing in single-leg stance with UE support Practice swaying toward/away support surface against resistance (Fig. 9.31) Transition from standing on heels to standing on toes without UE support Single-leg stance on solid surface	Performing ankle dorsiflexion and plantarflexion while standing on rocker board (Fig. 9.33) Heel-to-toe standing on a foam roller, flat side up (Fig. 9.34) Marching on foam pad or compliant surface (Fig. 9.40) Single-leg stance on compliant surface Standing on foam throwing/catching a weighted ball Mini-squats on inflated dome (Fig. 9.42) Jogging on mini-trampoline or inflated dome (Fig. 9.43)
Improve Hip Strategies	Dynamic reversals kneeling-to-heel sitting Standing 8–12 in. away from wall, bring bottom to wall then return to stand (Fig. 9.35) Sit-to-stand movement but using a raised surface to promote hip movement rather than full sitting Heel-to-toe standing on a solid surface for medial/lateral stability, EO to EC (Fig. 9.36)	Standing across foam roller with round side down, with or without perturbations at hips or foam roller Bilateral shoulder flexion/extension with resistance band held in hands and tied on doorknob Walking on heels, and walking on toes for short distances	Standing in tandem on foam Throwing/catching weighted ball from the side (Fig. 13.23) Walking with resistance at hips Practice hula-hoop
Improve Stepping Strategies	Multidirectional hip strengthening using resistive band (Fig. 9.11) Unexpected release of resistance applied to trunk with vision (Fig. 9.37)	Sidestepping and braiding Walking with quick head turns side to side	Walking forward or sidestepping with changes to treadmill speed Walking while surface is perturbed (moving carpet) External nudges while walking Walking while catching and throwing a weighted ball

BAPS, Biomechanical Ankle Platform System.

Red Flag: Learning that occurs as a result of practice on these devices is task specific and should not be expected to transfer automatically to functional balance tasks (e.g., improved performance in sit-to-stand transfers, walking, or stair climbing). The *specificity of training rule* applies here. Practice of the specific functional balance tasks is required if balance performance is to be improved.[3]

Interventions to Improve Sensory Control of Balance

A complete sensory examination (somatosensory, visual, and vestibular) is necessary to determine which sensory systems are intact, which are disordered, and which are absent. Central nervous system sensory integration mechanisms should also be examined (e.g., CTSIB or mCTSIB).

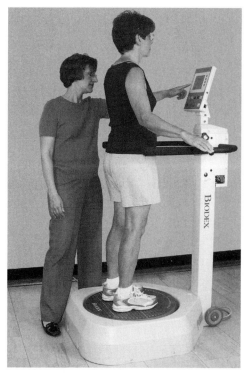

FIGURE 9.38 Standing, balancing on a force platform The patient stands on a Biodex Balance Machine. The therapist can select from two testing/training protocols: postural stability and dynamic limits of stability. During *postural stability,* the patient attempts to keep the board steady with centered alignment using varying levels of difficulty of board tilt (platform perturbation). The machine calibrates the time in balance and provides a stability index. During *limits of stability,* the patient maintains centered balance and, on signal, tilts the board (moving the cursor) to a predetermined box (range); the patient then moves the cursor back to centered alignment. Information is provided about patient excursion and accuracy in varied directions (limits of stability). The therapist provides VCs to direct the patient's attention to the biofeedback information provided.

Intervention focuses on improving the function of individual systems and the interaction among systems.

Strategies to Improve Utilization of Surface Information

The goal is to increase reliance on somatosensory inputs while simultaneously reducing reliance on visual information. The patient stands on a firm, or flat support surface while vision is altered or imprecise.

This can be accomplished with the following activities and strategies:

- Standing, eyes open (EO) to eyes closed (EC)
- Standing, full lighting to reduced lighting to a dark room
- Standing with lenses that reduce visual input (dark or petroleum-coated goggles)
- Standing, dual tasking with eyes engaged with a reading activity (a printed card held in front)
- Standing, with eyes reading a card held against a busy checkerboard pattern
- Marching in place, EC

Strategies to Improve Utilization of Vision

The goal is to increase reliance on visual inputs while simultaneously reducing reliance on somatosensory information. The patient should initially be instructed to keep the eyes focused on a stationary target directly in front of his or her eyes then progress to varied ocular inputs.

This can be accomplished with the following activities and strategies:

- Standing on a compliant surface; progressing from carpet (low pile to high pile) to foam cushion (firm density) of varying height (2 to 5 in. [5 to 12 cm]), EO
- Standing on a moving surface (wobble board or foam roller), EO
- Marching in place on foam, EO

Strategies to Improve Utilization of Vestibular Inputs

The patient with reduced or compromised visual and somatosensory inputs needs to increase reliance on vestibular inputs. This is sometimes referred to as a *sensory conflict situation,* requiring resolution of the conflict (misinformation) by the vestibular system. This can be accomplished with the following activities and strategies:

- Standing on foam, EC
- Standing on foam with eyes engaged in reading task
- Standing on foam catching and throwing a ball vertically and/or from hand to hand
- Standing on foam with vision distorted (dark or petroleum-coated goggles)
- Tandem standing, head turning side to side and or up and down
- Tandem standing on foam, EC
- Marching in place on foam, EC

Progression to Intermediate-Level Interventions to Improve Balance Control

Progression of therapeutic interventions is unique to the individual patient, his or her goals, and potential for improvement. Therapists must creatively design treatment sessions that address all facets of the system in aggregate without compromising safety. Frequently used progressions include reducing the BOS from standing in stride to single-leg stance, transitioning from a stable support surface to a compliant or moving one, reducing or altering visual inputs, adding vestibular stimulation through head turning, adding a secondary motor or cognitive task, external perturbations, and adapting the task by altering the speed and direction of movement or the surrounding environment. Appropriate interventions overlap and are not mutually exclusive (Figs. 9.39 and 9.40).

Standing, Single-Limb Stance

The patient stands on one LE and lifts the other off the ground, maintaining the standing position using single-limb

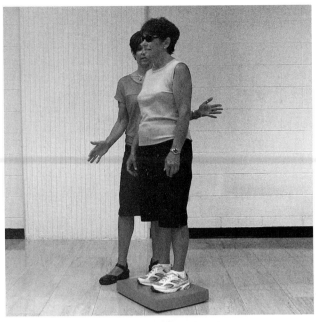

FIGURE 9.39 Standing on foam wearing dark glasses To promote the use of vestibular inputs, the patient practices standing on a compliant surface wearing dark glasses that alter vision.

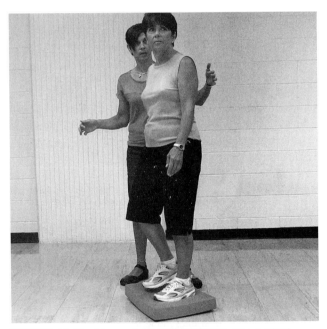

FIGURE 9.40 Marching on foam with head turns The patient practices marching in place (limb movements) while standing on foam as vestibular inputs change with head rotation.

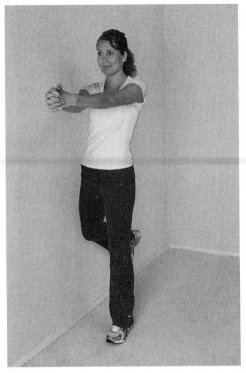

FIGURE 9.41 Standing, single-limb stance, limb abduction The patient stands sideways next to a wall on one limb and lifts the other limb into hip extension with knee flexion. The dynamic limb is abducted with the knee pushing against the wall. The UEs are held with shoulders flexed, elbows extended, and hands clasped together (hands-clasped position). The therapist instructs the patient to push as hard as possible into the wall. The patient is not allowed to lean on the wall (no contact of the wall with the shoulder or hip is allowed).

Manual Perturbations

The therapist applies small, quick perturbations forward or backward (sternal nudge), displacing the patient's COM in relation to the BOS. The patient responds with a counter movement to maintain balance. The challenges should be appropriate for the patient's range and speed of control. Progression is to varying the direction of the displacements (e.g., lateral, diagonal). Excessive perturbations such as vigorous pushes or shoves are not appropriate. Initially with patients who lack stability control, the patient can be informed of the direction of the perturbation (*"Don't let me push you backward"*). This assists the patient in readiness, engaging anticipatory postural control mechanisms. As control improves, the therapist progresses to using unexpected perturbations, emphasizing reactive, involuntary postural strategies. The patient is instructed to *"maintain your standing balance at all times."* The BOS can also be varied to increase or decrease the difficulty (wide BOS to narrow BOS). Altering the support surface to foam can also increase the likelihood of a stepping strategy, especially with EC.

Manual perturbations prepare the patient for unexpected challenges to balance (force displacements) that may occur in everyday life (e.g., standing and walking in crowded situations). To practice being nudged while stepping, small, quick displacements can be provided by the

stance. The patient is instructed to maintain the pelvis level. A pelvis that drops on the side of the dynamic limb indicates hip abductor weakness on the opposite (static limb) side (positive Trendelenburg sign). For the patient with adequate trunk control, single-limb stance with resisted hip abduction with knee flexed (knee pressed laterally to the wall) can be used to promote hip stabilizing responses in the abductors. This technique can be helpful for the person with a positive Trendelenburg sign (Fig. 9.41).

therapist standing behind the patient using an elastic resistive band to provide resistance to the forward step. The therapist should use appropriate safety precautions, carefully guarding to prevent falls in patients with delayed stepping responses.

Mobile and Compliant Surfaces

Rocker Board

The patient stands on a rocker board (also known as a wobble board or tipper board) that allows movement in one or more planes. A limited-motion board (Fig. 9.32) provides bidirectional challenges, and a dome board provides multidirectional challenges (Fig. 9.33). The profile of a domed-bottom rocker board can be varied from low dome to high dome to increase the excursion and difficulty. The subject stands on the device and practices maintaining a centered balanced position; the board is not allowed to touch down on any side. The patient then practices self-initiated tilts (e.g., toe to heel, side to side, and rotations—clockwise and then counterclockwise), first with touch-down contact of the board with the ground and then with no touch-down. Initially the patient can use light touch-down support with fingertips on a wall or table or poles but should progress rapidly to no UE support. The foot position (BOS) or type of board can be varied to increase or decrease the level of difficulty. The therapist should use appropriate safety precautions, guarding to prevent falls. See Appendix 9A for equipment sources.

Ø **Red Flag:** These devices are inherently unstable. Gradual progression is indicated (e.g., from bidirectional board to low-dome board to high-dome board). The patient should be instructed to use caution when getting on and off the board and utilize support as needed. The feet should be positioned on the board using a wide stance, centrally located over the board. The area surrounding the board should be kept free of obstacles in case the patient needs to step off quickly. Placing the dome on a carpeted surface rather than a tile surface reduces the tendency of the board to move. Finally, the patient should be instructed to keep his or her eyes focused directly in front on a target.

📝 **Clinical Note:** Patients with profound somatosensory impairments may need to look at their feet during these activities to augment feedback and improve task performance and learning.

Foam Rollers

The patient can practice standing in neutral position on split foam rollers. For greatest stability, initially the flat sides are face down. As standing control improves, the flat side can be positioned face up to provide a mobile surface (see Fig. 9.34). Progression can include arm raises, head and trunk rotations, catching and throwing a ball, and mini-squats. The therapist should use appropriate safety precautions, guarding to prevent falls.

Inflated Disc or Foam Pad

The patient can practice standing on a compliant surface such as a closed-cell foam pad (Airex Balance Pad) or inflated disc (BOSU Balance Trainer). The soft, compliant surface requires continual adjustments by postural muscles (primarily foot and ankle muscles) to achieve stability on the device. Various activities can be performed while standing on the compliant surface: head turns, mini-squats (Fig. 9.42), bouncing compressions, single-leg stance marching, jogging (Fig. 9.43), and throwing and catching a ball. Standing with EC significantly increases the level of difficulty and postural instability. Standing with EC eliminates visual support for balance; when EC is combined with already reduced somatosensory supports, the patient is left dependent on vestibular inputs for balance.

Therapy Ball Activities

The patient stands with one foot flat on the floor and the other placed on a small ball. The patient actively rolls the ball (forward, backward, in circles) while maintaining upright balance using a single-limb stance. The therapist stands in front of the patient and guards as needed. The therapist can also stand in a mirror-image position with one foot placed on the same small ball. The therapist's foot is used to move the ball and stimulate reactive balance challenges for the patient. Both the therapist and the patient can hold onto a wand for added stabilization (Fig. 9.44).

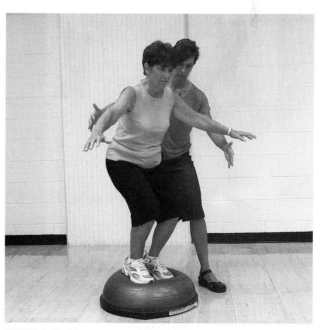

FIGURE 9.42 Mini-squats on BOSU Balance Trainer The patient practices lowering and raising the COM through a limited ROM while adjusting to the continuously shifting surface of the dome. Because of the difficulty of the task, the therapist must be vigilant to protect the patient from a fall.

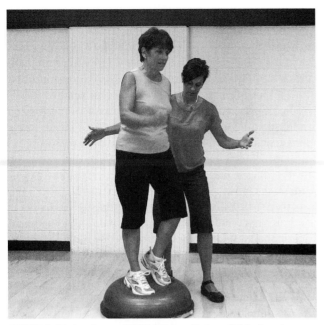

FIGURE 9.43 Jogging on BOSU Balance Trainer While jogging on the dome, the patient uses anticipatory adjustments to increase the speed of movement and reactive postural control to adapt to rapid changes in the support surface. The therapist guards the patient for safety.

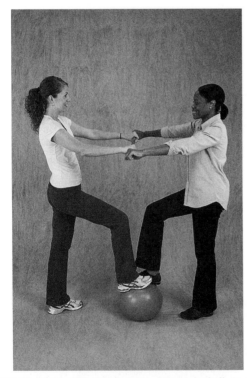

FIGURE 9.44 Single-limb standing: one foot on the ball The patient stands with one foot resting on a small ball positioned in front. The patient moves the ball (forward and back, side to side, and in circles) while balancing on the static limb. The therapist can also put one foot on the same ball (mirror-image position as shown) and move the ball, thereby requiring reactive balance strategies. Stability in single-limb stance can be improved by having both the patient and therapist hold on to a dowel.

Progression to High-Level Interventions to Improve Balance Control

Activities and Strategies for Improving Adaptive Balance Control

Adaptive balance control refers to the ability to modify or change balance responses based on changing conditions (e.g., either task or environmental demands). Such responses are sometimes referred to as *complex balance skills.* Interventions to promote adaptive balance control should therefore include a variety of challenges to balance, including task variations and environmental changes.

Task modifications should be gradual at the start, progressing to more significant challenges as control develops. The therapist can increase the challenge to balance control by manipulating the speed and range of the activity and by external pacing of the activity (using VCs [counting], manual cues [clapping], a metronome, or music with a consistent tempo [marching music]). Based on the principles of neuroplasticity, treatment interventions should focus on tasks that challenge the patient.[1,2]

Environmental modifications should be gradual at the start, progressing from a closed (fixed) environment with minimal distractions to a more open, variable (changing) environment. The patient practices first in the clinic environment (e.g., a quiet room or hallway, progressing to practice in a busy clinic gym). The patient then practices in simulated home, community, and work environments, and finally in real-life environments. One real-life community-based program that promotes adaptive postural control is tai chi.

Clinical Note: Tai chi is an ancient Chinese martial art form of slow mindful movements and postures that emphasize body awareness, flexibility, strength, and balance (see discussion in Chapter 5: Interventions to Improve Sitting and Sitting Balance Skills). Tai chi bridges therapeutic interventions in the clinic with community integration. Appendix 9B presents a tai chi standing routine.

Clinical Note: Current advances in technology and virtual reality enable researchers and clinicians to simulate advanced balance challenges in a clinical environment. The Wii Fit Virtual Reality Gaming System[35] can be used to improve balance, postural stability, and confidence with functional activities.[36] Highly advanced systems such as STABLE (Stability and Balance Learning Environment) and CAREN Computer Assisted Rehabilitation Environment) from Motek Medical[37] provide cutting-edge interactive learning activities to assess and train static and dynamic postural control and high-level gait. Surround screens provide visual stimulation that is synchronized with support platform perturbations to simulate real-world activities such as crossing the street and walking on winding paths. The high expense of this system currently limits its application to major research facilities.

In addition to the demands for postural control previously discussed, tasks that involve vertical displacement or acceleration of the COM require that the system manage the movement of the body in space at changing speeds and with a reduced BOS. To accomplish high-level tasks such as jumping, plyometric forces must be generated and stabilized while counteracting ground reaction forces. At this stage of balance training, the role of the therapist is to design practice activities to approximate the desired level of performance while maintaining patient safety.

Standing, Lunges

The patient stands with feet hip-width apart and steps forward about 2 ft (0.6 m) with the dynamic limb, allowing the heel of the static limb to lift off the ground. The patient lowers into a lunge position by partially flexing the knee and keeping the knee directly over the foot (*partial lunge;* Fig. 9.45). The position is held for 2 or 3 seconds, and then the patient pushes back up into standing. The trunk is maintained upright with the hips in neutral position. If the patient bends forward during the activity (flexes the trunk), he or she can be instructed to hold a dowel behind the back or in front as a reminder to keep the trunk upright. Partial lunges with the foot of the dynamic limb placed on a foam pad or inflated dome cushion increase the difficulty of the activity. Lunges are another activity in which the patient is required to maintain control during both eccentric (lowering) contraction and concentric (raising) contractions.

Partial lunges can progress to *full lunges,* in which the patient comes down onto one knee and then pushes back up into standing (Fig. 9.46). Lunges can also be progressed by varying the direction of the dynamic limb. Wide-stance, sideways lunges can be performed. The patient steps out to the side, bending the knee on the dynamic limb and lowering the body down. The patient then pushes back up and moves the dynamic foot back into symmetrical standing. Backward lunges involve a step backward and lowering of the body.

Jumping, Hopping, and Bounding

During *jumping,* the patient is instructed to stand with feet hips-width apart, hips and knees flexed in a partial squat position, and told to "push off" through the feet. Early attempts at jumping usually result in inadequate propulsion upward and poor coordination of the limb and trunk segments. Using compliant surfaces such as a small trampoline or BOSU Balance Trainer can help with early-stage plyometric training and improve muscle strength, power, and timing. The

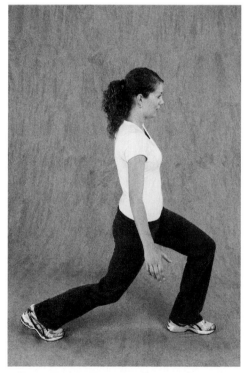

FIGURE 9.45 Standing, partial lunge The patient stands with feet hip-width apart. The patient steps forward about 2 ft (0.6 m) with the left leg, allowing the right heel to lift off the ground and the left LE to slowly lower the body into a partial lunge position. The position is held for 2 to 3 seconds; then the patient slowly pushes back with the left LE and returns to standing. The therapist provides verbal instructions and guarding.

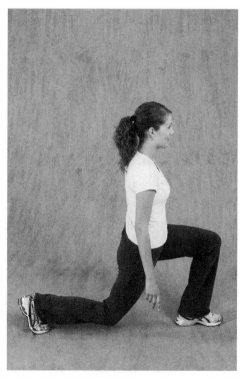

FIGURE 9.46 Standing, full lunge The patient stands with feet hip-width apart. The patient steps forward about 2 ft (0.6 m) with the left LE, allowing the right heel to lift off the ground as the right knee is slowly lowered to the floor (half-kneeling position). The position is held for 2–3 seconds, then the patient slowly pushes back to standing with the left LE. The therapist provides verbal instructions and guarding.

compliant surface offers the patient the opportunity to practice close-chain plantar flexion and synergistic timing without the instability of the feet leaving the support surface. Directional changes, such as jumping forward and backward and side to side (slalom) increase the difficulty of the task, and targets can be placed on the floor to increase the amplitude of the jump (Fig. 9.47).

Hopping on one foot adds the increased postural demands of single-leg support to jumping. Playing the game of "hopscotch" combines coordination of jumping from bilateral LE stance, to hopping on one foot, and incorporates reaching to the floor to retrieve the marker from the grid (Fig. 9.48) *Bounding* is a jump forward from single-leg stance on one side to single-leg stance on the opposite side and is a combination of the activities described above.[28] For training purposes, the patient may stand on either leg to start. The length of each bound can be increased and the surface altered as the patient progresses (Fig. 9.49).

🚫 **Red Flag:** Plyometric training places substantial demands on the cardiovascular system, and all patients should be cleared for high-intensity activity before beginning such activities. Special care should be taken with people who have neurological conditions that impact autonomic nervous system regulation.

Outcomes

Motor control goal: improvement in all aspects of balance performance (anticipatory, reactive, adaptive, and propulsive)

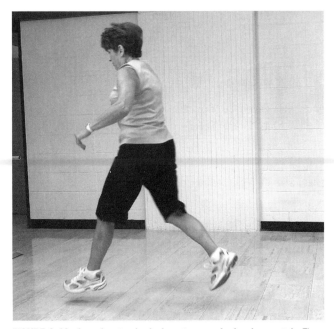

FIGURE 9.48 Jumping to single-leg stance, playing hopscotch The patient begins by standing on one leg, then jumps to land in single-limb stance on the opposite foot.

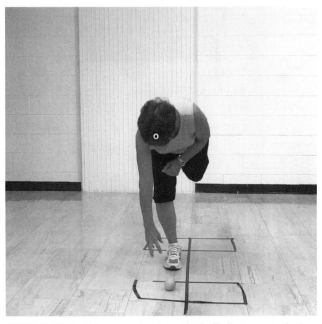

FIGURE 9.49 Bounding: jumping from single-limb stance to single-limb stance The patient plays a variation of the childhood game of hopscotch using a grid outlined on the floor. The patient begins in standing with one foot in each of the boxes at the far end of the grid; she then hops to one foot. She maintains the single-limb position as she lowers her COM to retrieve a ball off of the floor, and then raises her COM to return to single-limb stance. To complete the game, she jumps to place each foot in the boxes at the end of the grid.

Functional skills achieved: patient demonstrates appropriate functional balance during high-level and advanced tasks

See Table 9.4: Therapeutic Interventions to Improve Postural Control.

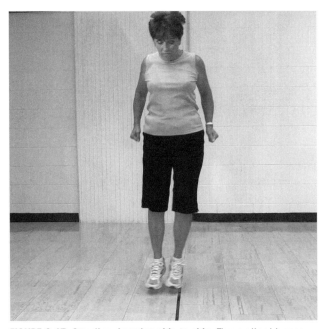

FIGURE 9.47 Standing, jumping side to side The patient jumps laterally from one side of a line marked on the floor to the other side of the line to practice changing the direction of propulsion.

TABLE 9.4 Therapeutic Interventions to Improve Postural Control

Basic-Level Exercise	Indications
Modified standing, feet symmetrical, rolling ball in all directions (Fig. 9.6) Modified standing (toe rises and heel-offs) Standing with partial body weight in an overhead harness Standing, feet symmetrical on solid surface or foam with EO to EC for 30 sec Standing on solid surface or foam playing balloon volleyball or catch Standing, feet in heel-to-toe (tandem) position on solid surface EO or EC for 30 sec (Fig. 9.36) Standing, feet symmetrical 8 in. away from wall, bring bottom to touch wall, return to standing (Fig. 9.35) Standing, feet symmetrical/in step position with head turns side to side and up/down Standing, resisted ankle strategies (Fig. 9.31) and stepping strategies using resistive band (Fig. 9.29)	Those who present with impairments that constrain the use of normal postural strategies including those with: • History of falling • Peripheral neuropathy • LE radiculopathy • Stroke: early recovery or with considerable impairments • Traumatic Brain Injury (TBI) early recovery or with considerable impairments • Advanced multiple sclerosis (MS) • Advance Parkinson's disease (PD) • Cancer survivors • Incomplete spinal cord injury

Intermediate-Level Exercise	Indications
Standing on wobble board Standing, single-leg stance on solid surface Standing, feet in step, on a foam roller with round side down (Fig. 9.34) Single-leg stance, with foot on a ball; standing on a solid surface and catching and throwing a weighted ball Walking with head turning side to side and up/down Walking over different-height objects placed in an obstacle course Reaching to retrieve an object from the floor, return to stand (Fig. 9.23) Modified tai chi or yoga	Those who wish to be independent in the community: • Various stages of recovery from stroke • TBI • Early MS • Early PD • Cancer survivors • Concussion or mild TBI • Vestibulopathy

High-Level Exercise	Indications
Partial lunges Walking against a heavy resistance band with quick stops and starts Standing on foam roller, with round side down, against quick manual perturbations; standing, heel to toe, on compliant surface, and catching and throwing a weighted ball against a plyometric surface, head on and from the side Standing on a compliant surface, kicking a ball against a wall or plyometric surface Lifting weighted objects from floor or overhead Squats on inflated disc (BOSU trainer) (Fig. 9.42) Tai chi (see Appendix 9B) Yoga	Those who wish to return to an active lifestyle and low-intensity sports (golf, bowling) • Moderate to mild impairments from stroke, TBI, MS, PD • Concussion or mild TBI • Vestibulopathy

Advanced-Level Exercise	Indications
Full lunges, forward/backward, side to side (Fig. 9.47) Jumping up/down, forward/backward, side to side Playing hopscotch (Fig. 9.48) Bounding; standing in single-leg stance, then hop to other foot and land in single-leg stance (Fig. 9.49) Jogging on a trampoline	Those who wish to return to running or sports: • Multitrauma • Concussion • High-functioning TBI • Cancer survivors • Young stroke

EO, eyes open; EC, eyes closed

Compensatory Training

When significant postural and balance activity limitations persist, compensatory strategies are necessary to ensure patient safety. Cognitive strategies can be taught to substitute for missing automatic postural control. Sensory substitution strategies emphasize the use of more stable, reliable sensory inputs for balance. Assistive devices may be indicated to ensure patient safety and to prevent a fall. Additionally, footwear designed to improve ankle stability may be beneficial. Two types of commercially available athletic shoes serve this purpose; stability and motion control shoes. Both limit pronation and supination of the foot, with motion control shoes providing maximum support. Compensatory balance strategies are presented in Box 9.6.

Clinical Note: If more than one sensory system is impaired, as in the patient with diabetes who has peripheral neuropathies as well as retinopathy, or vestibular loss, sensory compensatory strategies are generally inadequate. Some balance activity limitations will be evident.

Student Practice Activities

Student practice activities provide an opportunity to share knowledge and skills as well as to confirm or clarify understanding of the treatment interventions. Each student in a group will contribute his or her understanding of, or questions about, the strategy, technique, or activity being discussed and demonstrated. Dialogue should continue until a consensus of understanding is reached. The student practice activities in Box 9.7 focus on improving task analysis in standing. Activities in Box 9.8 focus on the application and assessment of interventions to improve standing balance control, and those in Box 9.9 focus on selecting appropriate interventions.

BOX 9.6 Compensatory Balance Strategies

The patient is taught to do the following:

- Widen the BOS when turning or sitting down
- Widen the BOS in the direction of an expected force (e.g., step position)
- Lower the COM when greater stability is needed (e.g., crouching when a threat to balance is imminent)
- Wear comfortable, well-fitting shoes with rubber soles for better friction and gripping (e.g., athletic shoes)
- Stability- and motion control–type athletic shoes are designed to enhance ankle stability. Use light touch-down support as needed to increase somatosensory inputs and stability
- Use an assistive device as needed (e.g., a cane or walker) to provide support for standing

- Use a vertical or slant cane to increase somatosensory inputs from the hand
- Rely on intact senses, heightening patient awareness of available senses
- Use an augmented feedback device (e.g., auditory signals from a limb-load monitor or biofeedback cane) to provide additional sensory feedback information
- Recognize potentially dangerous environmental factors (e.g., low light or high glare for the patient who relies heavily on vision)
- Focus vision on a stationary visual target rather than a moving target
- Minimize head movements during more difficult balance tasks requiring vestibular inputs (sensory conflict situations)

BOX 9.7 STUDENT PRACTICE ACTIVITY: TASK ANALYSIS IN STANDING

OBJECTIVE: To analyze the standing posture of healthy people

EQUIPMENT NEEDS: Foam cushions and wobble boards (bidirectional and multidirectional [dome])

PROCEDURE: Work in groups of two or three. Begin by having each person in the group stand in a symmetrical stance position, with feet apart and shoes and socks off. Then have each person stand with feet together in tandem (heel-toe position) and repeat on dense foam. In each condition, have the person begin with EO and progress to EC. Then have each person practice weight shifts to the LOS in all positions and conditions (feet apart, feet together, feet in tandem position while standing on the floor and on foam). Finally, have each person stand on a wobble board, using both bidirectional and multidirectional (dome) boards. Have each person practice standing centered on the board (no tilts), then have each person practice slow tilts to each side.

OBSERVE AND DOCUMENT: Using the following questions to guide your analysis, observe and record the variations and similarities among the different standing patterns represented in your group.

▲ What is the person's normal standing alignment?
▲ Does the person complain of instability, dizziness, vertigo, or nausea when performing any of these activities?

BOX 9.7 STUDENT PRACTICE ACTIVITY: TASK ANALYSIS IN STANDING (continued)

▲ What changes are noted between normal, feet together, tandem, on foam positions? Change from EO to EC? Position of UEs?

▲ Which postural strategies are observed and which are absent? In what order do they occur (ankle→hip →stepping or other variation)?

▲ Are postural strategies symmetrical? (Is one LE more active than the other?)

▲ During weight shifts exploring the LOS, are the shifts symmetrical in each direction?

▲ If loss of balance occurs, which direction does the person fall or lean toward?

▲ During standing on a wobble board, how successful is the person at maintaining centered alignment on the board (no touch down)? What are the positions of the UEs?

▲ What types of pathology/impairments might affect a patient's ability to achieve or maintain standing?

▲ What compensatory strategies might be necessary?

▲ What environmental factors might constrain or impair standing?

▲ What modifications are needed?

BOX 9.8 STUDENT PRACTICE ACTIVITY: INTERVENTIONS TO IMPROVE STANDING AND STANDING BALANCE CONTROL

OBJECTIVE: To practice administering balance tests and activities and assess patient performance

EQUIPMENT NEEDS: Tipper board (wobble board), bidirectional and multidirectional dome, BAPS board, split foam rollers, inflated domes, small balls (inflated and weighted), and force-platform training device

DIRECTIONS: Working in groups of three to four students, perform the balance activities listed below. Members of the group will assume different roles (described below) and will rotate roles each time the group progresses to a new activity.

▲ One person assumes the role of therapist (for demonstrations) and participates in discussion.

▲ One person serves as the patient (for demonstrations) and participates in discussion.

▲ The remaining members participate in task analysis of the activity and discussion of the questions. One member of this group should be designated as a "fact checker" to return to the text content to confirm elements of the discussion (if needed) or if agreement cannot be reached.

Thinking aloud, brainstorming, and sharing thoughts should be continuous throughout this activity! Carry out the following activities for each activity performed.

1. Discuss the *activity,* including patient and therapist positioning, indication(s) for use, and appropriate VCs and manual contacts.

2. Perform the *exercise* using the designated therapist and patient. Follow up with an assessment of the demonstration, including:
   • Proper safety precautions
   • Recommendations and suggestions for improvement
   • Strategies to make the activity either *more* or *less* challenging for the patient.

3. Discuss the answers to the *questions* presented at the end of each activity.

If any member of the group feels he or she requires additional practice with the activity and technique, time should be allocated to accommodate the request. All group members providing input (recommendations, suggestions, and supportive feedback) should also accompany this practice.

A. Standing on Solid Surface, Manual Perturbations to Balance

Goal: To displace the patient's COM outside of BOS for assessment of LOS and responsiveness of postural balance strategies.

Activity 1: Patient stands on a stationary surface (floor) while therapist provides a nudge to tap patient out of stance position. Displacing nudges should be given from all directions (anterior, posterior, left and right). Violent perturbations (pushes or shoves) are not necessary!

▲ Therapist uses asymmetrical manual contacts, unpredictable challenges.

▲ Challenges should be appropriate for patients range and speed of control.

▲ Narrow or expand patient's BOS as indicated.

▲ EO to EC

The therapist should note:

▲ Amount of force required to displace COM

▲ Available sway envelope before patient experiences loss of balance (LOB)

▲ Whether vision impacts performance

Questions
1. Which balance strategies does the person use? Which are not used (e.g., hip, ankle, stepping)?

2. Identify possible impairments that might impact a patient's ability to maintain postural control.

3. Identify possible activity limitations and participation restrictions if occluding vision substantially impacts a patient's performance on this task.

(box continues on page 218)

BOX 9.8 STUDENT PRACTICE ACTIVITY: INTERVENTIONS TO IMPROVE STANDING AND STANDING BALANCE CONTROL (continued)

B. Standing, Static Balance Using Rocker Board

Goal: To assess and enhance the patient's ability to maintain postural control on a solid, movable surface.

Activity 1: Instruct the patient to stand on the center of the board in a stable position. Provide UE touch-down support as needed and unilateral UE support progressing to no support. The therapist directs the patient to start with self-initiated postural tilts in varying directions.

Question: What type of postural control does this activity require (e.g., anticipatory, reactive)?

Activity 2: Next, have the therapist tilt the board in varying directions.

Question: Which type of postural control is this (e.g., anticipatory, reactive)?

Activity 3: The therapist then varies the task by:
▲ Varying the speed, range, direction of displacement
▲ Varying BOS
▲ Varying type of board to increase or decrease difficulty limited motion
  • Bidirectional to dome board
  • Multidirectional to low dome to high dome (increased range of excursion)

Question: Which balance strategies do these activities enhance?

C. Practice Standing on Foam Rollers

Goal: To assess and enhance the patient's ability to maintain postural control on a compliant and movable surface.

Activity 1: The therapist instructs the patient to stand across half foam roller (perpendicular to the long axis of the roller) with flat side up maintaining static control.

Question: Which balance strategies does this activity enhance?

Activity 2: The therapist then directs patient to assume tandem stance (heel to toe) along the foam roller with flat side up maintaining static control.

Question: Which balance strategies does this activity enhance?

Activity 3: The therapist then varies the task (tandem stance on foam roller with flat side up) by:
▲ Progressing to dual-task training: singing a song, throwing a ball
▲ Double limb support progressing to single-limb support
▲ Practicing step-ups onto the foam roller: one foot at a time or alternate feet

D. Activities on BOSU Balance Trainer

Goal: To assess and enhance the patient's ability to maintain high-level dynamic balance on a movable surface

Activity1: The therapist instructs the patient to stand on BOSU, feet close together in the center of the dome, knees bent slightly, to perform the following tasks:
▲ Side-to-side weight shifts from foot to foot
▲ Partial squats with arms extending forward
▲ Partial squat with hands reaching to touch outside of knees
▲ Bouncing (compressions)
▲ Jump up and stick landing (jump up and land in a fixed position)
▲ Mogul jumps: side-to-side jumps
▲ Step down and up with knee lift, flex arms forward with knee lift
▲ Single-leg stance
▲ Single-leg squats

Activity 2: Reverse orientation of the BOSU so that the flat side is up and perform the following tasks:
▲ Practice lunges, forward and from side
▲ Practice slowly stepping on and off the BOSU in all directions:
  • Walk up and step down forward
  • Walk up forward and step down backward
  • Walk up and step down from side

Question: How does changing the surface of the BOSU (flat side up) alter the demands of the balance task?

E. Standing in Single-Leg Stance and Manipulating BAPS

Activity 1: The subject is allowed light fingertip support for stability and safety with this activity. The therapist instructs the patient to stand with one foot aligned to match the footprint on the BAPS board, with knee relaxed (not hyperextended), and perform the following tasks:

▲ Ankle dorsiflexion, plantar flexion, inversion and eversion
▲ Clocks: The patient is instructed to rotate and tip the board so that its edge contacts the floor in a clockwise fashion. Repeat in the opposite or counterclockwise direction.

  The therapist then:
▲ Increases the size of the ball underneath the BAPS board
▲ Adds weight with pegs and/or plates

Questions
1. What is the goal of this task?
2. Which balance strategy does this activity enhance?

BOX 9.9 STUDENT PRACTICE ACTIVITY: PRACTICE SELECTING APPROPRIATE INTERVENTIONS

OBJECTIVE: Based on selected clinical problems and patient data, practice clinical decision-making skills by selecting appropriate therapeutic interventions for improving postural instability. The significant findings from a physical therapy examination are presented for each clinical case.

DIRECTIONS: Based on the clinical information provided, select and list three appropriate therapeutic interventions for that patient. Interventions chosen should be those that would be employed during the first three therapy sessions.

Case 1

ROM: lacks 10 degrees of ankle DF on right and left
Strength: right and left anterior tibialis 2+/5
Sensation: intact throughout BLEs
Balance: LOB in posterior direction standing with EO and closed on a solid surface
Gait/Locomotion: lack of toe clearance on right and left
Fall Risk Assessment: DGI score = 18/24
Activity Restriction/Participation Limitations: difficulty walking on carpet; trips frequently but does not fall

INTERVENTIONS:
1.
2.
3.

Case 2

ROM: WNL throughout BLEs
Strength: ankle strength 3+/5 in all muscle groups, right gluteus medius 3–/5, left gluteus medius 2+/5
Sensation: minimally diminished sensation to light touch and pinprick in both lower legs and feet
Balance: able to stand on solid surface and foam with EO and closed for 30 seconds; unable to stand in tandem (heel to toe)
Gait/Locomotion: takes many quick steps to right and left when attempting to walk a straight line
Fall Risk Assessment: on BBT: unable to place foot on a stool without LOB: criteria score = 0/4; requires close supervision when turns 360 degrees: criteria score = 1/4
Activity Restriction/Participation Limitations: LOB when turning right or left while walking; must use railing on stairs

INTERVENTIONS:
1.
2.
3.

Case 3

ROM: lacks 5 degrees of ankle DF on right and lacks 8 degrees on left
Strength: BLE strength grossly 3/5
Sensation: severely diminished to absent sensation to light touch and pinprick in both lower legs and feet
Balance: able to stand on solid surface and foam with eyes open for 30 seconds; unable to stand with EC on solid or compliant surface without LOB
Gait/Locomotion: walks with decreased gait speed and tends to look down
Fall Risk Assessment: on ABC: 20 percent confident that unsteadiness will not occur when walking in a crowded mall where people walk rapidly past
Activity Restriction/Participation Limitations: reports two falls in past month walking outdoors at night

INTERVENTIONS:
1.
2.
3.

ABC scale, Activities-Specific Balance Confidence Scale; BBT, Berg Balance Test; BLEs, both lower extremities; DF, dorsiflexion; DGI, Dynamic Gait Index; LOB, loss of balance; ROM, range of motion; WNL, within normal limits

SUMMARY

This chapter presented the foundational requirements for standing and for static and dynamic balance control. The importance of accurate utilization and interpretation of examination findings and the identification and evaluation of sensory and motor impairments has been stressed. Interventions to remediate these factors, activity restrictions, and participation limitations were presented, and sample pathways for progression were highlighted. The level of challenge during standing may be modified by manipulating both the activity (task) and the environment. Finally, compensatory and safety strategies were discussed.

This chapter has emphasized the importance of tailoring the balance training program to the individual patient. Sound clinical decision-making will guide identification of the most appropriate activities and techniques for an individual patient. Many of these interventions will provide the foundation for developing home management strategies to improve function. Although some of the interventions described clearly require the skilled intervention of a physical therapist, many can be modified or adapted for inclusion in a HEP for use by the patient (self-management strategies), family members, or others who are participating in the patient's care.

REFERENCES

1. Shumway-Cook, A, and Woollacott, M. Motor Control–Translating Research into Clinical Practice, ed 4. Baltimore, Lippincott Williams & Wilkins, 2012.
2. OSullivan, S, Schmitz, T, and Fulk, G. Physical Rehabilitation, ed 6. Philadelphia, F.A. Davis, 2014.
3. Nashner, L. Adaptive reflexes controlling human posture. Exp Brain Res, 1976; 26:59.
4. Nashner, L. Fixed patterns of rapid postural responses among leg muscles during stance. Exp Brain Res, 1977; 30:13.
5. Nashner, L, and McCollum, G. The organization of human postural movements: a formal basis and experimental synthesis. Behav Brain Sci, 1985; 9:135.
6. Peterka, R. Sensorimotor integration in human postural control. J Neurophysiol, 2002; 88:1097.
7. Magill, RA. Motor Learning and Control; Concepts and Application, ed 9. New York, McGraw-Hill, 2011.
8. Schmidt, RA, and Lee, TD. Motor Control and Learning: A Behavioral Emphasis, ed 5. Champaign IL, Human Kinetics, 2011.
9. Lohse, K, et al. Video games and rehabilitation: using design principles to enhance engagement in physical therapy. J Neurol Phys Ther, 2013; 37:166–174.
10. Shumway-Cook, A, and Horak, F. Assessing the influence of sensory interaction on balance: suggestion from the field. Phys Ther, 1986; 66:1548.
11. Wrisley, D, and Whitney, S. The effect of foot position on the modified clinical test of sensory interaction and balance. Arch Phys Med Rehabil, 2004; 85:335–338.
12. Anacker, S, and Di Fabio, R. Influence of sensory inputs on standing balance in community-dwelling elders with a recent history of falling. Phys Ther, 1992; 72:575–581; discussion 581–584.
13. Cohen, H, et al. A study of the clinical test of sensory interaction and balance. Phys Ther, 1993; 73:346–351; discussion 351–354.
14. Di Fabio, R, and Anacker, S. Identifying fallers in community living elders using a clinical test of sensory interaction for balance. Eur J Phys Med Rehabil, 1996; 6:61–66.
15. Di Fabio, RP, and Badke, MB. Relationship of sensory organization to balance function in patients with hemiplegia. Phys Ther, 1990; 70:542–548.
16. Ricci, NA, et al. Sensory interaction on static balance: a comparison concerning the history of falls of community-dwelling elderly. Geriatr Gerontol Int, 2009; 9:165–171.
17. Duncan, P, et al. Functional reach: a new clinical measure of balance. J Gerontol, 1990; 45:M192.
18. Duncan, P, et al. Functional reach: predictive validity in a sample of elderly male veterans. J Gerontol, 1992; 47:M93.
19. Newton, R. Validity of the multi-directional reach test: a practical measure for limits of stability in older adults. J Gerontol Med Sci, 2001; 56A:M248.
20. Berg, K, et al. Measuring balance in the elderly: preliminary development of an instrument. Physiother Can, 1989; 41:304.
21. Berg, K, et al. Measuring balance in the elderly: validation of an instrument. Can J Public Health, 1992; 83(suppl. 2):S7.
22. Donoghue, D, and Stokes, E. How much change is true change? The minimum detectable change of the Berg Balance Scale in elderly people. J Rehabil Med, 2009; 41:343.
23. Tinetti, M, et al. A fall risk index for elderly patients based on number of chronic disabilities. Am J Med, 1986; 80:429.
24. Tinetti, M, and Ginter, S. Identifying mobility dysfunctions in elderly patients: standard neuromuscular examination or direct assessment? JAMA, 1988; 259:1190.
25. Faber, MJ, Bosscher, RJ, and van Wieringen, PC. Clinimetric properties of the Performance-Oriented Mobility Assessment. Phys Ther, 2006; 86:944.
26. Podsiadlo, D, and Richardson, S. The timed "Up and Go": a test of basic mobility for the frail elderly persons. J Am Geriatr Soc, 1991; 39:142.
27. Pondal, M, and delSer, T. Normative data and determinants for the timed "Up and Go" test in a population-based sample of elderly individuals without gait disturbances. J Geriatr Phys Ther, 2008; 31:7.
28. Shumway-Cook, A, et al. Predicting the probability of falls in community dwelling older adults. Phys Ther, 1997; 7:812–819.
29. Romero, S, et al. Minimum detectable change of the Berg Balance Scale and Dynamic Gait Index in older persons at risk for falling. J Geriatr Phys Ther, 2011; 34:131.
30. Jonsdottir, J, and Cattaneo, D. Reliability and validity of the Dynamic Gait Index in persons with chronic stroke. Arch Phys Med Rehabil, 2007; 88:1410.
31. McConvey, J, and Bennett, SE. Reliability of the Dynamic Gait Index in individuals with multiple sclerosis. Arch Phys Med Rehabil, 2005; 86:130.
32. Marchetti, GF, et al. Temporal and spatial characteristics of gait during performance of the Dynamic Gait Index in people with and people without balance or vestibular disorders. Phys Ther, 2008; 88:640.
33. Powell, LE, and Myers, AM. The Activities Specific Balance Confidence Scale. J Gerontol Med Sci, 1995; 50:M28–M34.
34. Howe, J, et al. The Community Balance and Mobility Scale: a balance measure for individuals with traumatic brain injury. Clin Rehabil, 2006; 20:885–895.
35. Wii Fit Virtual Reality Gaming System. Nintendo of America. Retrieved January 20, 2014, from www.nintendo.com.
36. Rendon, A, et al. The effect of virtual reality gaming on dynamic balance in older adults. Age Ageing, 2012; 41:549.
37. Motek Medical. Rehabilitation. Amsterdam, Netherlands. Motek Medical. Retrieved January 20, 2014, from www.motekmedical.com/

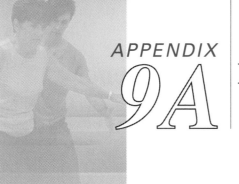

Equipment Resources

Balls, Rocker Boards, Inflatable Discs, Foam Pads, and Rollers

Orthopedic Physical Therapy Products (OPTP)
3800 Annapolis Lane
Minneapolis, MN 55447
www.optp.com
800-367-7393

BOSU Balance Trainer

BOSU Fitness, LLC
3434 Midway Drive
San Diego, CA 92110
www.BOSU.com

Ball Dynamics International, LLC

14215 Mead Street
Longmont, CO 80504
www.fitball.com
800-752-2255

Balance Platform Training Systems

Balance Master
NeuroCom International, Inc.
9570 SE Lawnfield Road
Clackamas, OR 97015
www.onbalance.com
800-767-6744

Biodex Balance System SD

Biodex Medical Systems, Inc.
20 Ramsay Road
Shirley, NY 11967-4704
www.biodex.com
800-224-6339

Elastic Resistance Bands

Thera-Band/Hygenic Performance Health
1245 Home Avenue
Akron, OH 44310-2575
www.thera-band.com
800-321-2135

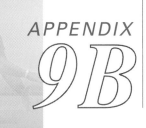

9B Standing Tai Chi Sequence

Preparation

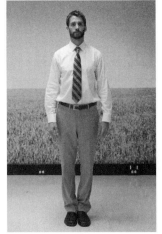

Stand tall and relaxed with feet together.

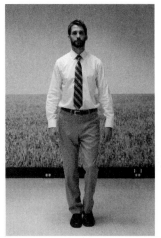

Unweight left leg by bending knee.

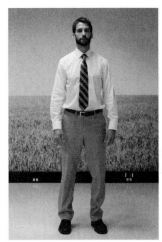

Step left. Feet shoulder-width apart. Slight bend in knees.

Raise Hands

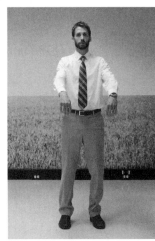

With soft arms leading with wrists, arms float up.

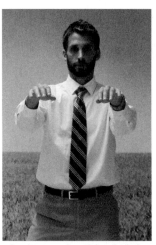

Hands rise to shoulder height.

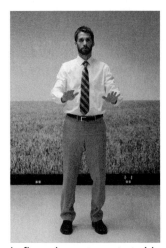

Hands float down to rest at sides.

Hold Ball

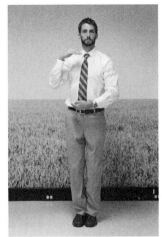

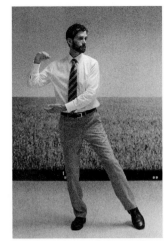

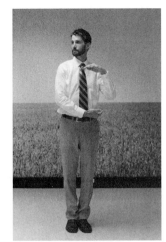

Hold ball on right with slight trunk rotation to right.

Look left and step left, leading with toe.

Step right foot in. Hold ball on left.

Repeat Hold Ball Sequence to Opposite Side

Part the Wild Horse's Mane

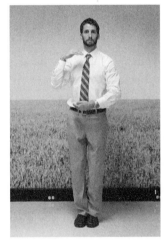

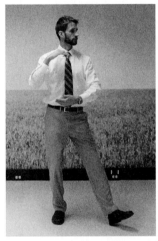

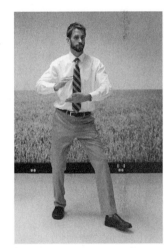

Hold ball on right with slight trunk rotation to right.

Look left. Step left, leading with heel.

Hands pass over one another as if parting a horse's mane.

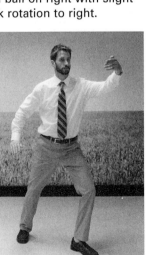

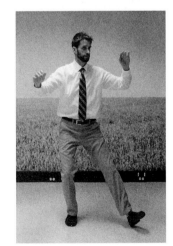

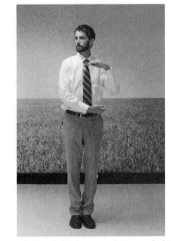

Continue to extend arms apart and shift weight left.

Unweight left toes and pivot, left foot straight ahead.

Unweight right leg and step right foot in. Hold ball on left.

Repeat Part the Wild Horse's Mane Sequence to Opposite Side

(continues on page 224)

Single Whip

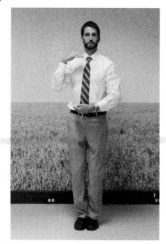

Hold ball on right with slight trunk rotation to right.

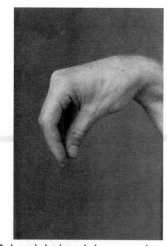

Relax right hand downward, fingertips touching thumb.

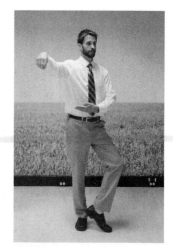

Unweight left heel and pivot on ball of foot while extending right arm out to side.

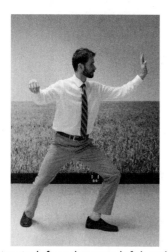

Step to left and sweep left hand palm across face, rotate palm away from face and extend left arm.

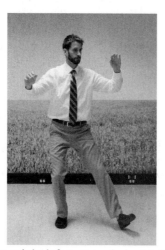

Unweight left toes and pivot left foot straight ahead.

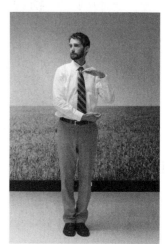

Step right foot in. Hold ball on left.

Repeat Single Whip Sequence to Opposite Side

Closing Position

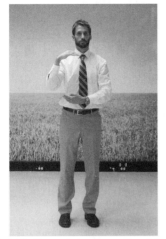

Hold ball on right. Feet shoulder-width apart.

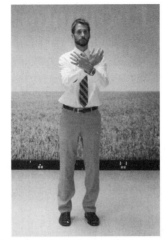

Cross wrists in front of heart, palms facing in.

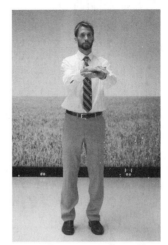

Uncross wrists, extending elbows.

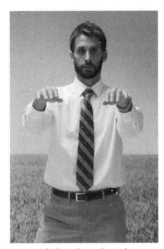

Arms straight ahead, palms facing down.

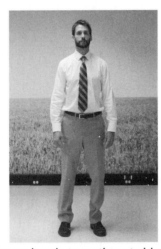

Return hands to resting at side, palms facing back.

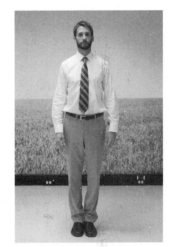

Unweight left leg and step left leg in, feet together.

Developed by Edward W Bezkor, DPT, OCS, MTC. Adapted from Li, F. Transforming traditional Tai Ji Quan techniques into integrative movement therapy—tai ji quan: moving for better balance. J Sport Health Sci, 2014; 3(1):9–15.

CHAPTER 10

Interventions to Improve Locomotor Skills

CRISTIANA K. COLLINS, PT, PhD, CFMT, NCS, AND
THOMAS J. SCHMITZ, PT, PhD

Human locomotion is a foundational component of independent function; it represents the final and highest level of motor control (skill). It involves consistent, highly coordinated and precisely timed movements that allow for economy of effort and adaptability to changes in both task demands and the environment. It is also a skill commonly affected by impairments and activity limitations resulting in participation restrictions. Recovery or improvement in ability to walk is a high priority for many people seeking physical therapy because it enhances participation in domestic, education, work, and social life and is associated with an overall improvement in quality of life.[1-3]

The continuum of locomotor training strategies involves multiple environments (e.g., parallel bars, indoor, community). An overview of locomotor training strategies is presented in Box 10.1. Interventions complimentary to locomotor training include cardiovascular and strength training and interventions to improve transfer skills (see Chapter 7: Interventions to Improve Transfer Skills) and standing control and standing balance (see Chapter 9: Interventions to Improve Standing and Standing Balance Skills).

This chapter focuses on interventions to address locomotor dysfunction. In combination with data obtained from the gait analysis, consideration of the requirements and foundational elements of bipedal locomotion provides a broad perspective on the multiple factors contributing to walking dysfunction. Hedman and colleagues[4] conducted a Delphi survey to determine whether a panel of 58 experts could achieve consensus on the requirements of bipedal locomotion. Full consensus was reached on five locomotor task requirements: *initiation, termination, anticipatory dynamic balance, multitask capacity,* and *walking confidence.* The authors suggest that, with validation, these requirements may provide a framework to categorize locomotor problems and standardize interventions for gait dysfunction.

The foundational elements of bipedal locomotion include (1) the appropriate alignment, strength, and control of the lower extremities (LEs) and trunk to support body mass; (2) the ability to generate locomotor rhythm; (3) dynamic balance control (the ability to maintain stability and orientation with the center of mass [COM] over the base of support [BOS] while parts of the body are in motion); (4) the propulsion of the body in the intended direction; and (5) the adaptability of locomotor responses to changing task and environmental demands.

Developing a plan of care (POC) to enhance gait and locomotor skills requires knowledge of the presenting pathology, the patient's weightbearing status, and impairments and activity limitations that affect movement. Although identification of specific tests and measures is based on the history and systems review, several examination areas are of consistent importance to gait and locomotion: postural alignment and balance control, joint integrity and mobility, motor function (motor control and motor learning), muscle performance (strength, power, endurance), and range of motion (ROM). Examination of sensory function includes the visual and vestibular systems, central sensory integration (the capacity of the brain to organize, interpret, and use sensory information), and the patient's ability to use sensory input from the skin and musculoskeletal system to assist in locomotor control. Other key aspects of examination include perceptual integrity, cognition, attention, and the patient's ability to safely adapt or modify locomotor responses relative to changing task and environmental demands.

Gait: Cycle and Terminology

Gait Cycle

The *gait cycle* is the largest element used to describe human gait. It is divided into two phases, swing and stance, with two periods of double support (Fig. 10.1). The *swing phase* is the portion of the cycle when the limb is off the ground and moving forward (or backward) to take a step (40% of the cycle). The *stance phase* is the portion of the cycle when the foot is in contact with the ground (60% of the cycle). The term *double support time* refers to the period when both feet are simultaneously in contact with the ground as weight is transferred from one foot to the other.

Gait Terminology

The Los Amigos Research and Education Institute, Inc. (LAREI) of Rancho Los Amigos National Rehabilitation Center has developed terminology that subdivides the phases of the gait cycle as follows: Stance includes *initial contact, loading response, midstance, terminal stance,* and *preswing,* and swing includes *initial swing, midswing,* and *terminal swing.*[5] Traditional terminology subdivides the phases of the gait cycle as follows: (1) Stance components

BOX 10.1 Overview of Locomotor Training Strategies

A. Parallel Bars
Instruction and training in:

- Sit-to-stand and reverse with and/or without assistive device
- Static and dynamic standing balance with and/or without assistive device
- Use of appropriate gait pattern with and/or without assistive device while progressing forward and turning (because of limited space, it may not be possible to use an assistive device in standard parallel bars)
- Weight shifting and weight acceptance
- High-stepping
- Stepping forward, backward, sideward, and turning

B. Overground Indoors
Instruction and training in:

- Appropriate gait pattern and assistive device use
- Weight shifting and weight acceptance
- Stepping forward, backward, and sideward
- Crossed-stepping and braiding
- Walking over and around objects (i.e., obstacle course)
- Crossing thresholds and entering/exiting through doorways
- Variations in locomotor task demands (e.g., altering speed, scanning for objects, dual-task activity)
- Stairs
- Falling and transitioning from the floor to standing
- Running

C. Overground Community
Instruction and training in:

- Curb climbing, negotiating ramps, stairs, and sloped surfaces
- Walking over even and uneven terrain
- Walking within imposed timing requirements (e.g., crossing at a stoplight, on/off elevators, escalators)
- Walking for long distances
- Walking at varying speeds, walk using a rhythmic timing device (e.g. metronome)
- Walking while scanning for objects in the environment
- Dual-task training while walking (cognitive and/or motor dual tasks)
- Walking in open environment with distracters
- Entering/exiting transportation vehicles
- Running

D. Body Weight Support/Treadmill
Instruction and training in:

- Stepping on treadmill using BWS with maximally tolerated lower extremity load bearing progressing to no BWS
- Reciprocal stepping pattern with manual assistance at LEs and/or trunk with normal or near normal lower extremity and trunk/pelvis kinematics progressing to no manual assistance
- Production of rhythmical stepping pattern with arm swing and minimal to no weightbearing through the upper extremities
- Progress stepping speeds to normative values based on age
- Walking forward, sideward, and backward
- Strategies to minimize abnormal/compensatory movement patterns
- Strategies to improve aerobic capacity

E. Body Weight Support/Overground
Instruction and training in:

- Walking overground with maximally tolerated lower extremity load bearing progressing to no BWS
- Use of assistive device (if indicated) for walking on level surfaces
- Reciprocal stepping pattern with manual assistance at pelvis with normal or near normal lower extremity and trunk/pelvis kinematics progressing to no manual assistance
- Production of rhythmical, coordinated stepping pattern with arm swing and minimal weightbearing through the upper extremities
- Strategies to minimize abnormal/compensatory movement patterns
- Strategies to maintain/regain balance when perturbed

F. Assistive Devices
Instruction and training in:

- Function and purpose of assistive device
- Sit-to-stand and reverse with assistive device
- Static and dynamic standing balance with assistive device
- Gait pattern
- Use of assistive device and appropriate gait pattern indoor overground and overground in community

Adapted from Fulk, GD, and Schmitz, TJ. Locomotor training. In O'Sullivan, SB, Schmitz, TJ, and Fulk, GD (eds): Physical Rehabilitation, ed 6. F.A. Davis, Philadelphia, 2014, 445–446, with permission.

include *heel strike, footflat, midstance, heel-off,* and *toe-off,* and (2) swing components include *acceleration, midswing,* and *deceleration.* A comparison of the two sets of terminology is presented in Table 10.1 together with a description of key elements that occur within each phase of gait. Table 10.2 presents common terminology used to describe the various parameters of gait.

Task Analysis

Task analysis is a method of determining the nature of underlying abilities required to perform a complex motor task.[6] Applied to gait and locomotion, task analysis involves first breaking down normal performance of the motor

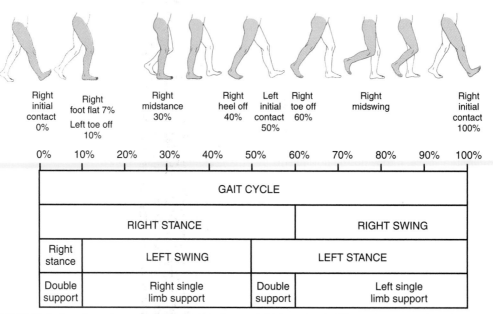

FIGURE 10.1 A gait cycle spans the period between initial contact of the reference extremity (right) and the successive contact of the same extremity. This figure shows the gait cycle with major events: stance and swing phases for each limb and periods of single and double support. The stance phase constitutes 60% of the gait cycle, and the swing phase constitutes 40% of the cycle at normal walking speeds. Increases or decreases in walking speeds alter the percentages of time spent in each phase. From Olney, SJ, and Eng, J. Gait. In Levangie, PK, and Norkin, CC: Joint Structure and Function, ed 5, Philadelphia, F.A. Davis, 2011, 526, with permission.

TABLE 10.1 Gait Terminology Comparison and Related Key Movements

Stance Phase		
Rancho Los Amigos	**Traditional**	**Key Movements**
Initial contact: beginning of stance when the heel or another part of the foot contacts the ground (component of initial double-limb support)	**Heel strike:** beginning of stance when the heel contacts the ground	Quadriceps are active at heel strike through early stance to control small amount of knee flexion for shock absorption; pretibial group acts eccentrically to oppose plantarflexion moment and prevent foot slap.
Loading response: from initial contact until the contralateral extremity leaves the ground for swing (final component of initial double-limb support)	**Foot flat:** occurs immediately following heel strike, when the sole of the foot contacts the floor	As body weight is transferred to lead limb, hip is stable, knee flexes to absorb shock, forefoot lowers to ground, plantarflexors are active from loading response through midstance to eccentrically control forward tibial advancement.
Midstance: begins when contralateral foot leaves the ground and ends when the body is directly over the supporting limb (first half of single-limb support)	**Midstance:** the point at which the body passes directly over the reference extremity	Trunk moves from behind to in front of ankle; the hip, knee, and ankle extensors are active to oppose antigravity forces and stabilize the limb; hip extensors control forward motion of the trunk; hip abductors over the supporting limb stabilize the pelvis during unilateral stance; plantarflexors propel the body forward.

TABLE 10.1 Gait Terminology Comparison and Related Key Movements *(continued)*

Stance Phase		
Rancho Los Amigos	**Traditional**	**Key Movements**
Terminal stance: Begins with heel rise and ends with contralateral initial contact (second half of single-limb support)	**Heel-off:** the point following midstance when the heel of the reference extremity leaves the ground	Trunk continues to move forward relative to foot; peak activity of the plantarflexors occurs just after heel rise to generate forward propulsion of the body.
Preswing: Second double support period from initial contact of contralateral extremity to lift off of the reference extremity	**Toe-off:** the point following heel-off when only the toe of the reference extremity is in contact with the ground	Body weight unloads from reference limb as it prepares for swing. Hip and knee extensors (hamstrings and quadriceps) contribute to forward propulsion.
Swing Phase		
Rancho Los Amigos	**Traditional**	**Key Movements**
Initial swing: the point when the reference extremity leaves the ground to maximum knee flexion of the same extremity (first third of swing)	**Acceleration:** from reference extremity toe-off to point when reference extremity is directly under the body	Hip, knee, and ankle flex for clearance and forward advancement; quadriceps provide forward acceleration of limb with reduced activity by midswing as pendular motion takes effect; hip flexors assist forward limb propulsion.
Midswing: from maximum knee flexion of reference extremity to a relatively vertical tibial position (middle third of swing)	**Midswing:** the reference extremity passes directly below the body; extends from the end of acceleration to the beginning of deceleration	Continued advancement of limb with knee extension and neutral ankle; contraction of hip and knee flexors and ankle dorsiflexors facilitate foot clearance.
Terminal swing: from a relatively vertical position of the tibia of the reference extremity to just prior to initial contact (final third of swing)	**Deceleration:** the portion of the swing phase when the reference extremity is decelerating in preparation for heel strike	Knee achieves maximal extension and ankle is in neutral position; hamstrings act to decelerate the limb, and the quadriceps and ankle dorsiflexors activate to prepare for initial contact.

Adapted from Burnfield, JM, and Norkin, CC. Examination of gait. In O'Sullivan, SB, Schmitz, TJ, and Fulk, GD (eds): Physical Rehabilitation, ed 6. Philadelphia, F.A. Davis, 2014, 255, with permission.

TABLE 10.2 Common Gait Terminology

Acceleration	The rate of change of velocity with respect to time
Cadence	Normal cadence is the number of steps taken per unit of time; the normal range for cadence is 91 to 138 steps per minute. Increased cadence is accompanied by a shorter step length and decreased duration of the period of double support. Running occurs when the period of double support disappears, typically at a cadence of 180 steps per minute.
Double Support Time	The time period of the gait cycle when both LEs are in contact with the supporting surface (double support); measured in seconds
Foot Angle	Degree of toe-out or toe-in; the angle of foot placement with respect to the line of progression; measured in degrees. *Note*: Increased foot angle (turning the foot outward) is often associated with decreased postural stability.

(table continues on page 230)

TABLE 10.2 Common Gait Terminology *(continued)*	
Rhythm	Consistency of gait cycle duration (stride time) from one stride to the next
Stance Time	The duration of the stance phase of one extremity in the gait cycle
Single-Limb Time	The time period of the gait cycle when only one limb is in contact with the floor or other support surface
Step Length	The linear distance between the point of heel strike of one extremity and the point of heel strike of the opposite extremity (in centimeters or meters)
Step Time	The number of seconds that elapse during a single (one) step
Step Width	The distance between feet (BOS), measured from one heel to the same point on the opposite heel; normal step width ranges between 1 and 5 inches (2.5–12.5 cm). Step width increases as stability demands rise (for example, in older adults or very young children).
Stride Length	The linear distance between two consecutive points of foot contact (preferably heel strike) of the same extremity (in centimeters or meters)
Stride Time	The number of seconds that elapse during one stride (one complete gait cycle)
Stride Width	The side-to-side distance between the two feet; step width is increased with instability.
Swing Time	The duration of the swing phase of one extremity in the gait cycle
Velocity (speed)	Also called walking speed, the distance covered per unit of time (meters/second). Average walking speed is 2.2 to 2.8 mph (0.98–1.3 m/s).[a] Velocity is increased by lengthening stride. Velocity is affected by physical characteristics such as height, weight, and gender; it decreases with age and physical disability.

[a]Some estimates of average walking speed are higher (3.5–4 mph [1.6–1.8 m/s]).

skill (i.e., walking) into its component parts to identify the key motor task requirements and underlying abilities needed for efficient performance. This breakdown provides a normative reference on which to base task analysis of gait and locomotor dysfunction. In examining a patient's walking abilities, task analysis allows the therapist to identify missing or compromised components (impairments in body functions and structures) causing or contributing to abnormal gait. As such, task analysis informs the therapist about the link between abnormal movement (patient-selected gait and locomotor strategies) and underlying impairments (e.g., diminished strength, motor function, sensation, ROM). Knowledge of the underlying abilities needed to accomplish motor task requirements allows the therapist to select interventions to address the missing or impaired components. Task analysis may also direct attention to the need for additional tests and measures.

An understanding of normal motor development informs task analysis as well as selection and sequencing of interventions based on motor control task requirements: *transitional mobility, stability* (static postural control), *controlled mobility* (dynamic postural control, mobility on stability), and *skill*. Recall that motor skills develop in a sequential manner (termed *developmental skills* or *developmental sequence skills*). Each stage is a prerequisite for the subsequent stage with eventual progression to controlled movement, as infants and children transition from dependent postures with a low COM and large BOS to postures with a high COM and small BOS. This developmental process also promotes balance and equilibrium reactions and the successful accomplishment of more challenging functional mobility skills such as crawling, cruising, and eventually walking. It also provides insight into the importance of dynamic proximal stability of the trunk for efficient distal mobility of the extremities. Although the rehabilitation process does not require a patient to repeat the developmental sequence, knowledge of normal motor control development provides the basis for analysis of movement and guides selection and sequencing of interventions.

Task analysis involving gait (e.g., observational gait analysis [OGA]) is among the most common forms of task analysis conducted by physical therapists, and a variety of approaches are used. A common method used to organize and structure the OGA is the Rancho Los Amigos Observational Gait Analysis system.[5]

In addition to understanding motor task requirements, knowledge of the normal kinematics and kinetics of human gait is central to performing a gait analysis. This further supports the ability to deconstruct gait into its component parts to establish a normative reference for movement patterns and joint positions. Therapists typically acquire this skill by performing repeated OGA of normal subjects using a segmental approach beginning with the foot/ankle and moving up to the knee, hip, pelvis, and trunk, making sure that each side is considered separately and as a whole.

Models of "normal" movement (e.g., gait characteristics) are important guides to inform the task analysis. However, great variation in normal performance of functional mobility skills can be observed across the life span. An example is the great variation in gait characteristics observed within a population of "normal" people. This has been referred to as the *challenge of normal,* suggesting that movement analysis also be considered from the perspective of efficiency. *Efficient movement* is defined as having adequate mechanical freedom, appropriate neuromuscular function, and effective motor control while engaged in a functional activity with changing task demands.[7,8]

Although the following list is not all-inclusive, data from the gait analysis assist the therapist with the following[5,9]:

• Identifying patient gait characteristics that deviate from a normative reference and their possible causes. Box 10.2 presents some of the more common gait deviations together with their potential causes.

• Establishing the physical therapy diagnosis and prognosis (the predicted level of improvement).

• Developing an appropriate POC to address gait impairments and locomotor dysfunction.

• Sequencing and progressing interventions based on locomotor task requirements.

• Determining the need for assistive, adaptive, or protective equipment and orthotic or prosthetic devices.

• Examining the effectiveness and fit of the devices or equipment selected.

• Promoting improved functional outcomes.

For a comprehensive handling of gait analysis including gait variables and common gait deviations, the reader is referred to the work of Burnfield and Norkin.[10]

Intervention Selection, Sequencing, and Progression

In developing the POC, intervention selection is based on examination data, evaluation, diagnosis and prognosis, and

---

BOX 10.2 Common Gait Deviations and Potential Causes

Stance

Trunk
• *Lateral trunk bending*—result of gluteus medius weakness; bending occurs to same side as weakness
• *Trendelenburg gait*—pelvis drops on contralateral side of a weak gluteus medius; compensatory strategy is lateral trunk bending
• *Backward trunk lean*—result of a weak gluteus maximus; difficulty going up stairs or ramps
• *Forward trunk lean*—result of weak quadriceps (the forward trunk lean decreases the flexor moment at the knee); may also be associated with hip and knee flexion contractures

Pelvis
• *Inefficient/insufficient pelvis posterior depression*—inefficient terminal stance and push-off leading to a decreased stance time on the ipsilateral side and a shortened step length on the contralateral side

Hip
• *Excessive hip flexion*—result of weak hip extensors or tight hip and/or knee flexors
• *Limited hip extension*—result of tight or spastic hip flexors or weak hip extensors
• *Antalgic gait* (painful gait)—stance time abbreviated on the painful limb, resulting in an uneven gait pattern (limping); uninvolved limb has shortened step length, since it must bear weight sooner than normal

Knee
• *Excessive knee flexion*—result of weak quadriceps (the knee wobbles or buckles) or knee flexor contractures; causes difficulty going down stairs or ramps; forward

trunk bending occurs to compensate for weak quadriceps
• *Hyperextension*—result of weak quadriceps, plantarflexion contracture, or extensor spasticity (quadriceps and/or plantarflexors)

Foot/Ankle
• *Toes first*—at initial contact, toes touch floor first—result of weak dorsiflexors, spastic or tight plantarflexors; toes first may also be due to shortened LE (leg-length discrepancy), a painful heel, or a positive support reflex
• *Foot slap*—foot makes floor contact with audible slap following initial contact, result of weak dorsiflexors or hypotonia; slap compensated for with a *steppage gait*
• *Foot flat*—entire foot contacts ground at initial contact—result of weak dorsiflexors, limited ROM, or an immature gait pattern
• *Excessive dorsiflexion with uncontrolled forward motion of the tibia*—result of weak plantarflexors
• *Excessive plantarflexion* (equinus gait)—heel does not touch the ground, result of spasticity or contracture of the plantarflexors; eccentric contraction poor, as in tibia advancement
• *Varus foot*—at initial contact, the lateral side of the foot touches first; foot may remain in varus throughout the stance phase—the result of spastic anterior tibialis or weak peroneals
• *Claw toes*—result of spastic toe flexors, possibly a plantar grasp reflex
• *Inadequate push-off*—the result of weak plantarflexors, decreased ROM, or pain in the forefoot

(box continues on page 232)

BOX 10.2 Common Gait Deviations and Potential Causes (continued)

Swing

Trunk and Pelvis
- *Decreased amplitude in trunk and pelvic rotation*—seen in the elderly and characteristic of several known neurological disorders (e.g., the patient with stroke or Parkinson's disease)
- *Insufficient forward pelvic rotation* (pelvic retraction)—result of weak abdominal muscles and/or weak hip flexor muscles (for example, in the patient with stroke)

Pelvis
- *Inefficient/insufficient pelvis anterior elevation*—inefficient pelvic anterior elevation leading to pelvic anterior or posterior rotation on the transverse plane, pelvic retraction, pelvic hiking, or a combination of the above

Hip and Knee
- *Insufficient hip and knee flexion*—result of weak hip and knee flexors or strong extensor spasticity, resulting in an inability to lift the LE and move it forward
- *Circumducted gait*—LE swings out to side (abduction/external rotation followed by adduction/internal rotation)—the result of weak hip and knee flexors and/or ankle plantarflexors
- *Hip hiking* (quadratus lumborum action)—compensatory response for weak hip and knee flexors and/or ankle plantarflexors or extensor spasticity

- *Excessive hip and knee flexion* (steppage gait)—compensatory response to a shortened contralateral lower limb or the result of same-side dorsiflexor weakness (e.g., resulting from neuritis of the peroneal nerve in the patient with diabetes)
- *Abnormal synergistic activity or spasticity* (e.g., the patient with stroke):
  - Use of a strong flexor synergy pattern—excessive abduction with hip and knee flexion
  - Use of a strong extension synergy pattern—excessive adduction with hip and knee extension and ankle plantarflexion (scissoring)
- *Insufficient knee flexion*—result of extensor spasticity, pain, decreased ROM, or weak hamstrings
- *Excessive knee flexion*—result of flexor spasticity; flexor withdrawal reflex

Foot/Ankle
- *Foot-drop*—result of weak or delayed contraction of the dorsiflexors or spastic plantarflexors
- *Varus or inverted foot*—result of spastic invertors (anterior tibialis), weak peroneals, or an abnormal synergistic pattern (e.g., in the patient with stroke)
- *Equinovarus*—result of spasticity of the posterior tibialis and/or gastrocnemius/soleus; or structural deformity (club foot)

---

goals established for the individual patient.[9] Knowledge of motor control task requirements and the progression of developmental skills can guide and inform clinical reasoning for selecting, sequencing, and progressing interventions applicable to multiple pathologies and health conditions (e.g., cardiovascular, musculoskeletal, neuromuscular, integumentary, multisystem).

For example, upon examination of a patient's gait, the therapist notes difficulty achieving weight acceptance with inadequate hip extension from midstance to heel-off on the left LE. Causes may include decreased ROM in ankle dorsiflexion and hip extension (mobility impairments), or decreased strength in posterior pelvic depression and hip extension (controlled mobility impairments), or a combination of both. Knowledge of motor task requirements guides selection of appropriate interventions, as mobility impairments require significantly different interventions than controlled mobility impairments.

The POC should not only outline the potential treatment activities appropriate for the individual patient but must also address the sequence in which these activities should be performed. As such, an understanding of the motor task requirements (mobility, stability, controlled mobility, skill) and the progression of motor skills (e.g., order of activities selected, proximal to distal progression, modifying BOS and COM) provide the clinician with a basis for appropriately sequencing and progressing the interventions for each patient. This information informs clinical reasoning

and allows novice clinicians (who may spend more time on reflection-on-action) to determine how or why an intervention did or did not work and how to progress the POC. It also allows expert clinicians (who may spend more time reflecting-in-action) to modify the treatment plan in real treatment time as they determine which component of the motor task requirement is the primary barrier to functional progression as interventions are applied.[11] Appendix 10A is an example of selection, sequencing, and progression of interventions within the context of two subsequent treatment sessions for the patient with traumatic brain injury (TBI) who is presented in Case Study 2 (see Part II: Case Studies).

Role of the Pelvis

The work of Perry and Burnfield[12] clearly describes both the phases and kinematics of gait.

In addition to the well-understood kinematics of the hip, knee, and ankle, it has been shown that during the gait cycle the pelvis moves 4 degrees in the sagittal plane, 4 degrees in the frontal plane, and 10 degrees in the transverse plane. Combined with the kinetics and kinematics of the LEs and the trunk, these pelvic motions allow for the least disruption in the body's COM during walking. From a clinical and functional perspective, it is evident that these three-dimensional pelvic motions do not occur in isolation of one another but are present as combined pelvic motions that occur throughout the gait cycle (Table 10.3). An understanding

TABLE 10.3 Three-Dimensional Motion of the Pelvis During Swing and Stance

	Phase Segment	Motion of the Pelvis
Swing	Initial swing (acceleration) to midswing	The pelvis moves into anterior elevation.
	Terminal swing (deceleration)	The pelvis moves eccentrically into anterior depression to allow for heel strike.
Stance	Initial contact (heel strike)	The pelvis continues to move into anterior depression eccentrically to achieve heel strike.
	Loading response (foot flat) to midstance	From loading response to midstance, the pelvis moves into posterior depression to allow for weight shift and weight acceptance onto the stance limb.
	Terminal stance (heel-off)	From midstance toward terminal stance, the pelvis continues to move into posterior depression to allow for efficient push-off; at heel-off, the pelvis moves into relative posterior elevation with combined anterior and posterior elevation as the opposite limb moves toward heel strike.
	Preswing (toe-off)	The pelvis begins to move into anterior elevation engaging a dynamically stable core for the limb to move into swing.

of these three-dimensional motions is important when considering the normal gait cycle and when examining a patient's gait pattern.

The pelvis functions as a "connector" between the LEs and the trunk and, as such, plays an important role in dynamic trunk stability necessary for efficient locomotion. Knowledge of LE position relative to the pelvis during swing and stance further informs the gait analysis (Table 10.4).

Recall that the reciprocal nature of the gait cycle contributes to minimizing displacement of the COM during gait and optimizing energy expenditure. As the LEs progress forward in a reciprocal manner, the trunk responds with reciprocal counterrotation, which in turn promotes reciprocal arm swing. Similar to the pelvis, the scapula also functions as a "connector" linking the upper extremity (UE) and the trunk during locomotion. The scapula and pelvis demonstrate both ipsilateral and contralateral reciprocal movements throughout the gait cycle allowing for efficient trunk counterrotation during gait. (Table 10.5).

Training Principles

Although locomotor training strategies vary based on specific patient presentation (e.g., impairments, diagnosis and prognosis, patient goals), they share common principles. Interventions are selected that are[13]:

- Impairment based
- Task oriented to the specific task of walking
- Goal directed and meaningful to the patient
- Shaped and progressed to maximally challenge the patient's capabilities
- Performed multiple times (high number of repetitions)

Clinical Note: Feedback and practice directly influence motor learning. When a functional skill is practiced inefficiently, the motor learning of that ineffective practice is reinforced. Conversely, when components of efficient movement are repeated and practiced, motor learning of these components is appropriately reinforced, can be transferred to other functional tasks, and leads to permanent changes in performance.

TABLE 10.4 Position of the Lower Extremity Relative to the Pelvis During Swing and Stance

Phase	Lower Extremity Motion	Pelvis Motion
Swing	Flexion, adduction, external rotation	Anterior elevation - Flexion (posterior rotation), slight adduction, and external rotation
Stance	Extension, abduction, internal rotation	Posterior depression - Extension (anterior rotation), slight abduction, and internal rotation

TABLE 10.5 Ipsilateral and Contralateral Reciprocal Movements of the Pelvis and Scapula During Swing and Stance[a]

Phase	Phase Segment	Right Pelvis	Left Pelvis	Right Scapula	Left Scapula
Swing	(R) Initial swing through midswing	Anterior elevation (AE)	Posterior depression (PD)	PD	AE
	(R) Terminal swing	Anterior depression (AD)	Posterior elevation (PE)	PE	AD
Stance	(R) Initial contact	AD	PE	PE	AD
	(R) Loading response to midstance	PD	AE	AE	PD
	(R) Terminal stance (heel-off)	Combined AE and PE	AD	AD	PE
	(R) Preswing (toe-off)	AE	PD	PD	AE

[a]The right (R) lower extremity is used as the reference limb.

Prerequisite Requirements

The foundational prerequisite requirements to initiate interventions to improve locomotor skills include appropriate weightbearing status, musculoskeletal (postural) alignment, ROM, muscle performance (strength, power, and endurance), motor function, balance, and static and dynamic standing control. Many of these prerequisites are dependent on intact neuromuscular synergies (necessary for static and dynamic control), intact sensory (somatosensory, visual, and vestibular) systems, and intact central nervous system sensory integration mechanisms. Also required is the ability to safely stand while engaged in UE functional movements (e.g., reaching) under varying environmental demands (e.g., dual-task activity). Locomotor training is initiated once the patient has achieved adequate mobility and stability, with the ability to initiate and control the pelvis and LE in appropriate sequence for swing and stance.

Clinical Note: A common difficulty that people with locomotor control deficits encounter is the inability to use dissociated movements during gait. Scooting in the seated position provides a safe initial opportunity for learning and practicing dissociated movements of the pelvis and trunk (see Chapter 5: Interventions to Improve Sitting and Sitting Balance Skills).

Interventions to Improve Locomotor Skills

HIGH-STEPPING

High-stepping is used to reinforce the components of swing and stance and to assist the patient in developing an improved kinesthetic sense of the components of gait. When the hip is brought higher than 90 degrees of flexion, the influence of the cross-extension reflex is recruited, facilitating motor output in extension of the stance LE and flexion of the swing LE. This activity is highly effective in facilitating components of both swing (pelvis anterior elevation with hip flexion, adduction, and external rotation; knee flexion; and ankle dorsiflexion) and stance (pelvis posterior depression with hip extension, abduction, and internal rotation; knee extension; and ankle plantarflexion).

The patient stands in a stride position with one foot forward and one foot back. Given the potential challenges to balance during this activity it is safest when initially performed next to a treatment table (for support) or inside parallel bars. The patient is assisted (guided) or resisted (facilitatory) through weight shifting anteriorly onto the forward limb with a high step taken by the posterior limb. Attention must be directed to proper alignment and control of the stance LE. Appropriate resistance[7,8] can be used on the dynamic (swing) limb as it moves into a high-step position with the hip moving beyond 90 degrees of flexion for facilitation of a cross-extension response. Emphasis is placed on pelvis posterior depression on the stance limb and pelvis anterior elevation on the dynamic limb (Fig. 10.2). Appropriate resistance to the pelvis and the LE is used on the swing side while approximation is applied through the pelvis and LE on the stance side. A static high-step position can be used to emphasize each component of gait as it challenges strength, endurance, and balance while providing the patient with increased kinesthetic and proprioceptive input.

Light facilitatory resistance can be applied to pelvis on the stance limb during forward weight shift from midstance to terminal stance to further emphasize weight shifting and

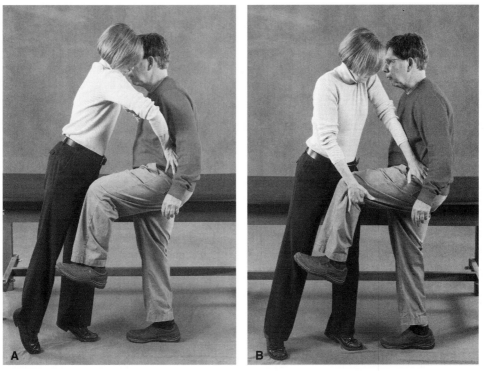

FIGURE 10.2 High-stepping can be used to facilitate components of both stance and swing phases of gait. (A) Facilitation of pelvic posterior depression on stance limb and anterior pelvic elevation on swing side. (B) Manual assistance provided to increase hip flexion with facilitation (light resistance) of pelvic anterior elevation on swing side.

weight acceptance together with pelvic posterior depression, hip extension, and knee control. Variations in location of manual contacts (MCs) and the amount and direction of resistance can be used to provide increased focus on a particular component of gait.

Manual contacts include application of resistance to pelvis anterior elevation and LE flexion on the dynamic side and approximation through pelvis posterior depression and LE extension on the stance side. Hand placements for the stance side are on the superior and slightly anterior iliac crest with the therapist's forearms in line with the pelvic diagonal (i.e., in line with the patient's heel). Verbal cues (VCs) include *"Shift forward onto your front leg, and step high with your opposite leg."*

FORWARD AND BACKWARD WALKING

The patient practices walking forward and backward as a progression from high-stepping. The therapist focuses on appropriate timing and sequencing, beginning with the weight shift forward and diagonally or backward and diagonally with weight acceptance onto the stance limb. The movements are repeated to allow for a continuous movement sequence.

Clinical Note: The BOS created by an efficient gait cycle is relatively narrow, allowing for minimal lateral shifts in the COM as the body moves in a forward progression. When a wider BOS is used owing to decreased balance, the therapist must be aware of the increased lateral weight shift necessary during locomotor training. As balance improves, attention must be placed on facilitating a return to a narrower BOS to improve gait efficiency. Additionally, initial locomotor training is most often performed at a speed less than normal, diminishing the beneficial effects of momentum occurring in normal gait and increasing movement and balance demands. This must also be taken into consideration when manual facilitation is being used during locomotor training.

Manual contacts can be used to guide movements and facilitate missing elements. For example, in the presence of a retracted and elevated pelvis (a problem that exists for many patients with stroke and LE spasticity), the therapist can facilitate anterior pelvic elevation during swing by placing the hands on the lateral, superior, and slightly anterior aspect of the pelvis. For backward progression, the therapist's hand can be placed over the gluteal muscles and posterior thigh to facilitate hip extension. Approximation through the pelvis can be used to facilitate weight acceptance on the stance limb. This also helps to prevent the knee on the stance limb from hyperextending. For forward progression VCs include *"Shift forward, and step"* and for backward progression, *"Shift backward, and step."*

To progress the activity of walking forward and backward, the therapist can do the following:

• Decrease the amount of manual facilitation, placing increasing demands on active control

- Alter the environment by progressing from walking in parallel bars, to next to parallel bars or a wall, to overground walking (i.e., decrease level of assistance)
- Increase the step length from initially reduced to normal
- Change the speed of walking from initially reduced, to normal, to an increased pace
- Modify the BOS from feet apart (wide base), to normal, to feet close together (narrow base), to tandem walking (heel-to-toe pattern). Keep in mind that although a wider BOS will provide increased stability, a wider base will also lead to increased weight-shift demands.
- Vary the acceleration or deceleration by having the patient practice stopping and starting or turning on cue
- Include dual-task walking, such as walking and talking, walking and turning the head (right or left and up or down), walking holding a tray with a glass of water, and walking while bouncing a ball
- Alter the environment by (1) varying the walking surface from flat to carpeted to irregular (outdoors), (2) including anticipatory timing demands, such as the time required to cross a street at a stoplight, and (3) including goal-directed leisure or occupational requirements (return-to-work skills)

> **Clinical Notes:** In the presence of UE flexor spasticity, tone may be reduced by muscle elongation and sustained stretch using an inhibitory pattern. Initially, the therapist slowly moves the limb into the lengthened range while gently rotating the limb (rhythmic rotation). Once full range is gained, the therapist maintains the elongated position using an inhibitory pattern in which the shoulder is extended, slightly abducted, and externally rotated with the elbow, wrist, and fingers extended.

Upright or vertical alignment with adequate control of head/trunk is important for postural alignment and balance during walking. If present, shortening of hip and knee flexors and hip extensor weakness should be addressed within the POC. The patient who demonstrates a kyphotic posture and looks continually down at the feet should be instructed to *"Look up"* at a target (placed directly in front of the patient). Vertical walking poles can also be used to assist upright posture while walking.

RESISTED PROGRESSION

Resisted progression is an ideal technique to facilitate trunk, pelvic, and LE motion. The therapist is positioned standing either in front of (Fig. 10.3) or behind the patient. As the patient moves forward, the therapist positioned in front moves in a reverse or mirror image of the patient's movements. The therapist provides maintained and appropriate resistance to the forward progression by placing both hands on the lateral, superior, and slightly anterior aspect of the pelvis bilaterally. The therapist's forearms should be aligned with the anterior elevation motion diagonal of the pelvis so that resistance is applied correctly to facilitate pelvis anterior elevation together with hip flexion (Fig. 10.3A). If the forearms drop,

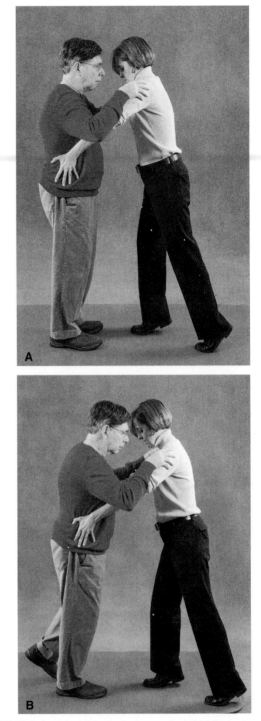

FIGURE 10.3 Resisted forward progression (A) begins in a comfortable stance position. (B) Weight is shifted over right stance LE as patient steps forward with the left. The MCs are on the pelvis for application of appropriate resistance and approximation.

becoming more parallel to the ground, the resistance will promote an unwanted trunk flexion response not conducive to efficient walking. The same MCs should be used if resisting the patient's forward progression from behind. Resistance should be appropriate (facilitatory) to encourage proper timing of the pelvic movements. Approximation can be applied down through the top of the pelvis to promote stabilizing responses as weight is accepted on the stance limb (Fig. 10.3B). A quick stretch to the pelvic anterior elevators can be added as needed to facilitate the initiation of the pelvic motion on the swing limb. An alternative position for MCs is on the pelvis and contralateral shoulder for adding facilitation of the trunk. Overall timing can be facilitated with appropriate VCs. Verbal cues for forward progression include *"Step forward, beginning with your right leg and step,"* and for backward progression, *"Step backward, beginning with your left leg and step."*

Red Flag: Problems can arise if the therapist's movements are not synchronized with the patient's. The pacing of the activity depends on the timing of the therapist's VCs. Movements can become uncoordinated or out of synchronization if the manual resistance on the pelvis is too great. The patient will feel as if he or she is "walking uphill" and may respond with exaggerated movements of the trunk (e.g., forward head and trunk flexion). This defeats the overall purposes of facilitated walking—that is, to improve timing and sequencing of gait and to decrease effort.

Comments

- Alternatively, resisted progression during forward and backward walking can be achieved using an elastic resistive band wrapped around the patient's pelvis. The therapist holds the resistive band in line with the desired pelvic motion of anterior elevation either from behind as the patient moves forward (Fig. 10.4A) or from the front as the patient moves backward (Fig. 10.4B).
- A wooden dowel can also be used to accomplish a forward resisted progression (Fig. 10.5).
- Two wooden dowels can also be used to promote reciprocal arm swing and trunk counterrotation. The therapist is positioned either behind as the patient walks forward (Fig. 10.6A) or in front as the patient walks backward (Fig. 10.6B). Both patient and therapist hold on to the dowels. The therapist is then able to assist in sequencing the arm swings and guide trunk counterrotation during forward and backward progressions. Similarly, reciprocal arm swing and trunk counterrotation can be promoted using elastic resistive bands and applying light resistance. (Note that this activity requires two resistive bands of approximately the same length.) The ends of the bands are held bilaterally by patient and therapist, allowing the therapist to assist and guide movement and to apply light facilitatory resistance. This is a particularly useful activity for patients with Parkinson's disease who frequently demonstrate reduced trunk rotation and arm swing.

Outcomes

Motor control goal: skill

Functional skill achieved: patient is able to ambulate independently with appropriate timing and sequencing of movement components

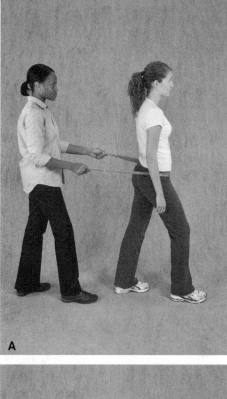

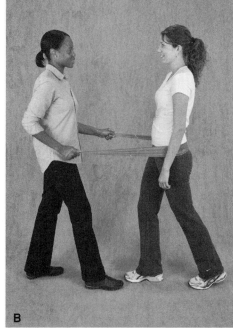

FIGURE 10.4 During (A) forward and (B) backward walking progressions, resistance may be applied using an elastic resistive band wrapped around the patient's pelvis.

Indications: impaired timing and sequencing of locomotor movement components

Side-Stepping

Walking sideways is not only valuable for its functional benefits of training side-stepping, it is also an excellent activity for both hip strengthening and stance stability. A side step involves open kinetic chain abduction and placement of the

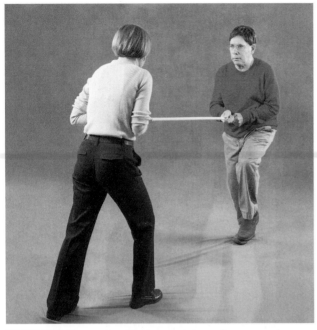

FIGURE 10.5 Forward resisted progression using a wooden dowel that is held by both the patient and therapist.

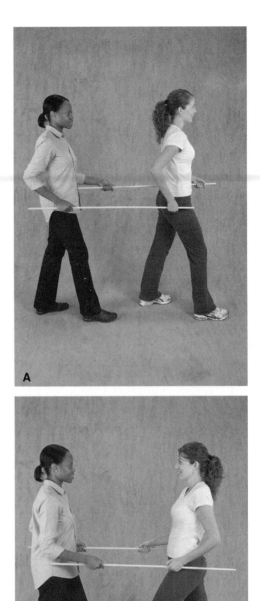

FIGURE 10.6 Wooden dowels held by both the patient and the therapist can be used to promote reciprocal arm swing and trunk counterrotation in either a (A) forward or (B) backward progression. This allows the therapist to assist in sequencing and guiding arm swing and trunk counterrotation.

dynamic limb to the side and closed kinetic chain abduction (stability) on the stance limb. Once the dynamic limb is placed on the ground with appropriate weight shifting and weight acceptance, the remaining limb is then moved parallel to the first *("Step together")*. Abductors are active on both the dynamic limb (to move the limb) and the static limb (to keep the pelvis level). Side-stepping has important functional implications for movement in confined or crowded areas or working at an elevated surface (e.g., kitchen countertop). However, the energy requirements are comparatively high and should be considered in treatment planning.

Resisted Progression

To apply resisted progression in side-stepping, the therapist is positioned (with a wide BOS) at the side of the patient's abducting limb (Fig. 10.7A) as the patient shifts weight toward the stance limb (to unweight abducting limb). Manual resistance is applied to the pelvis on the side of the abducting limb. The patient sidesteps by moving the dynamic limb into abduction (Fig. 10.7B) and then transfers weight onto this limb (Fig. 10.7C). This movement is followed by adduction of the opposite limb (Fig. 10.7D). Side-stepping can also be practiced with the patient and therapist facing each other holding a dowel (Fig. 10.8). Verbal cues include *"Step out to the side, beginning with your left leg, and then step together with the opposite leg. And again, step out to the side; then step together."*

Clinical Note: The therapist may also apply resistance during side-stepping by standing on the stance side and holding an elastic resistive band wrapped around the lateral aspect of the pelvis on the abducting side.

CROSSED-STEPPING

Crossed-stepping is abducting the leading dynamic limb with foot placement followed by moving the opposite leg up, across, and in front of the original side step leg. Emphasis should be placed on keeping the pelvis level. The movements

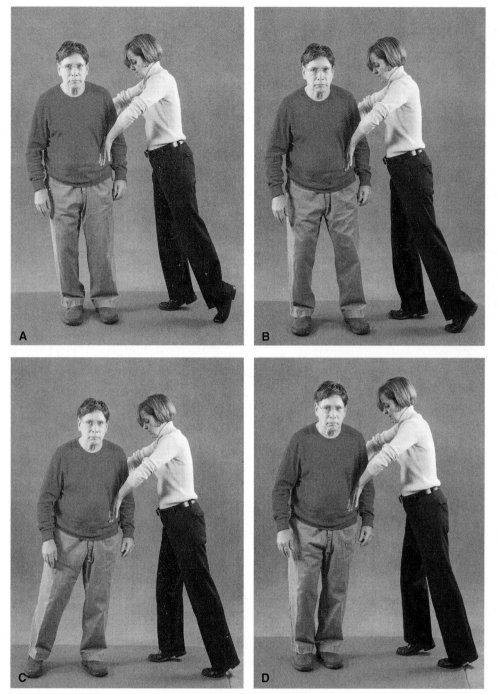

FIGURE 10.7 Walking, side-stepping, resisted progression (A) The patient shifts weight to the right LE for the initiation of side-stepping. (B) The patient side steps by moving the left LE into abduction. (C) Weight is then shifted onto the left LE. (D) The patient then moves the right LE parallel to the left (step together).

are then repeated to allow for a continuous movement sequence. The therapist is positioned behind the patient. Movements can be guided and facilitated using MCs on the pelvis. A progression can then be made to the application of resistance (resisted progression) with MCs on the pelvis, the thigh, or the distal LE. Verbal cues include *"Step out to the side, beginning with your left leg; then step up and across with*

the right leg. And again, step out to the side and up and across."

Braiding

The patient begins in a comfortable stance position (Fig. 10.9A) with the therapist positioned at the side of direction of movement. Approximation is applied through

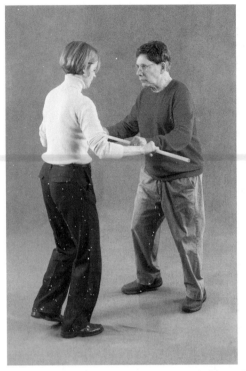

FIGURE 10.8 Side-stepping toward the right with the patient and therapist facing each other holding a wooden dowel.

the stance LE. The patient takes a side step (Fig. 10.9B) and shifts weight onto this limb (Fig. 10.9C). The opposite limb then cross-steps up and across in front (Fig. 10.9D) (LE moves in a flexion, adduction, external rotation [FLEX/ADD/ER] proprioceptive neuromuscular facilitation [PNF] pattern). This sequence is followed by another side step, then a crossed-step backward and behind the first limb (the LE moves in a PNF extension, adduction, external rotation [EXT/ADD/ER] pattern). The movements are repeated to allow for a continuous movement sequence.

Braiding is a highly coordinated sequence that is difficult for many patients to learn. The therapist can facilitate learning by standing in front of the patient and modeling the desired steps. Initially, the patient may require light touch support of both hands in a modified plantigrade position (supported standing). A treatment table, the outside of the parallel bars (or oval parallel bars), or a wall can be used as the support surface.

Alternatively, light touch support can be provided by having the therapist place both hands directly in front, with the elbows flexed and forearms supinated, and having the patient lightly place his or her hands on top of the therapist's hands. A wooden dowel held horizontally by both the therapist and patient can also provide support (Fig. 10.10). For these activities, the patient and therapist face each other and move in unison. Verbal cues should be well timed to ensure a continuous movement sequence and include *"Step out to the side; now step up and across; step out to the side; now step back and behind."*

Resisted Progression

The therapist is behind the patient, standing slightly to the side in the direction of the movement. As the patient moves sideward in braiding, the therapist moves in the same sequence and timing with the patient. The therapist provides maintained resistance to the sideward progression by placing one hand on the side of the pelvis. Alternatively, the therapist can alternate resistance between the anterior pelvis resisting the forward pelvic motion and crossed-step in front and the posterior pelvis to resist the backward pelvic motion and crossed-step behind. Resistance should be appropriate (facilitatory) to encourage proper timing of the pelvic movements. If needed, a quick stretch to the pelvis can be added to facilitate the initiation of the pelvic motion.

Outcomes

Motor control goal: skill

Functional skill achieved: patient ambulates independently using complex stepping patterns (side-stepping, crossed-stepping, braiding)

Indications: used to facilitate lower trunk rotation, pelvic and LE patterns in combination with upright postural control and to promote protective stepping strategies for balance

Clinical Note: Although decreased walking speeds are used in lower (initial) levels of locomotor training, the reduction in speed removes the normal element of momentum present in gait resulting in demands for larger lateral weight shifts, which increase the challenge to balance. As the speed of walking increases, so do the requirements for timing and control. In general, older adults will demonstrate reduced walking speed compared with younger adults.[14,15] However, the level of speed reduction varies considerably across individuals.[16] This slower walking velocity has been associated with multiple factors. Some examples include changes in interjoint coordination (reduced adaptability of neuromuscular control),[17] information processing,[18] and body composition.[19] It is also associated with muscle atrophy and weakness,[20,21] decreased sensory acuity,[22-24] underlying disease (e.g., cardiovascular, degenerative joint disease), and secondary lifestyle factors such as nutrition, fitness level, and body weight.

ASCENDING/DESCENDING STAIRS

Ascending stairs involves a step-over-step pattern. The patient transfers weight onto the stance limb and lifts the dynamic limb up and onto the step. Weight is then transferred onto this limb as it extends and moves the body up and onto the step. Quadriceps and gluteal activity powers the elevation of the body. A combination of the reciprocal motion of pelvis anterior elevation on the dynamic side and pelvic posterior depression on the stance side is instrumental in lifting the LE up onto the step. Upper extremity support using a handrail is typically needed during early stair-climbing training to steady the body. The patient should not be

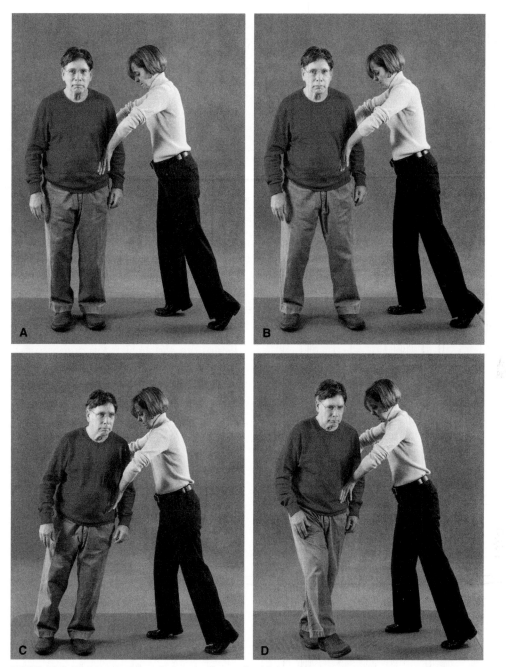

FIGURE 10.9 Walking, braiding To begin, the patient is in a (A) comfortable stance position and (B) sidesteps to the left. (C) Weight is shifted onto the left LE and (D) the right LE is then moved up and over the opposite limb (crossed-step). Approximation force is applied through the stance LE.

allowed to use the handrail to pull the body up the stairs. Progression should be from light touch support to no UE support. Assistance and/or resistance may be used with the therapist's hands placed on the lateral, superior, and slightly anterior aspect of the pelvis as done during resisted progression. Verbal cues include *"Alternate shifting weight over one leg and stepping up with the other. Now, shift and step up, shift and step up again."*

Descending stairs involves a similar weight transfer onto the stance limb with an accompanying eccentric contraction of hip and knee extensors to lower the body to the next step. Note that efficient mobility and controlled mobility of pelvis anterior depression on the descending side are key elements to safely and efficiently lowering the extremity without compensations such as dropping of the pelvis, excessive knee flexion on the stance LE, or decreased control of the descending LE. Weight is then transferred onto this limb as it extends and accepts weight. The patient then shifts weight forward over the stepping limb. The therapist should observe for, and prevent, excessive trunk flexion or extension. The sequence is repeated to allow for completion of a set of steps. Early training in

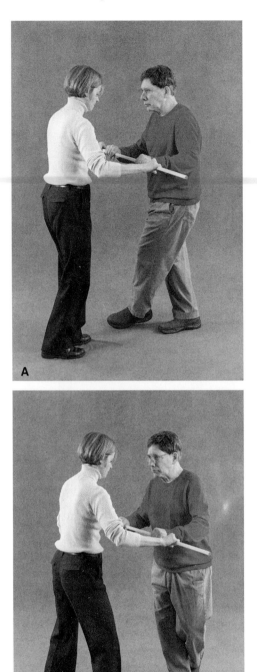

descending stairs also may involve using a handrail, with a progression from light touch support to no UE support. Verbal cues include *"Alternate shifting weight over one leg and stepping down with the other. Now, shift and step down, shift and step down again."*

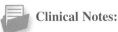 **Clinical Notes:**

- Ensure patient and therapist safety during stair-climbing activities. Proper guarding techniques must be implemented during both facilitation and practice of the activity.
- Important preparatory activities for stair climbing include bridging, sit-to-stand transfers, transitions between kneeling and heel-sitting, partial squats, high-stepping, and stepping activities.
- Step-ups and step-downs can be initially practiced using a low-rise step (4 in. [10 cm]) placed in front of the patient with progression to higher steps and finally to a normal-rise step (7 in. [17.5 cm]) (Fig. 10.11). Commercially available small interlocking aerobic steps are effective for this purpose. This activity requires weight shifts toward the support limb to free the dynamic limb for placement on the step. The therapist provides assistance as needed. Assistance with the weight shifts and LE lifting may be required and can be accomplished by MCs placed on the patient's pelvis or LE, respectively.
- During practice of step-ups and step-downs, having the patient clasp both hands together with shoulder flexion and elbow extension (reaching forward) may be helpful in initially facilitating forward weight transfer (this positioning is also effective for inhibiting UE spasticity). The patient may require assistance during forward weight shift onto the step. The therapist can guide forward weight shift and assist knee extension using a manual contact directly over the lower thigh and pressing downward over the quadriceps. During descent, the therapist can guide the correct foot placement and again provide stimulation over the quadriceps.

Outcomes

Motor control goal: skill

Functional skills achieved: patient climbs up and down stairs independently and negotiates curbs in the community

Indications: impaired ability to transfer weight onto the stance limb and simultaneously lift the opposite dynamic limb up and onto a step; inability to ascend/descend stairs

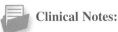 **Clinical Note:** Marked weakness of hip and knee extensors and ankle plantarflexors may preclude stair climbing until adequate gains in strength are achieved. Decreased pelvic mobility and controlled mobility can significantly limit the ability to efficiently ascend or descend stairs.

FIGURE 10.10 Walking, braiding Support can be provided using a wooden dowel held horizontally by both the patient and the therapist. The patient and therapist face each other and move sideward together. *Not shown:* The activity begins in a comfortable stance position. The patient alternates between stepping (A) anteriorly over opposite foot and (B) stepping posteriorly behind opposite foot.

Strategies for Varying Locomotor Task Demands

Locomotion is an automatic postural activity. Neural control originates from subcortical and spinal centers (spinal pattern generators). The cerebellum and cortex adapt locomotion to specific task demands, environmental changes, and correct motor patterns. Later-stage locomotor intervention strategies using distracters such as ongoing conversation or dual-task activities can provide confirmation of a developing level of autonomous control.

Varying locomotor task demands is also critical to establishing adaptability and *resistance to contextual change.* This refers to the patient's ability to maintain the same quality of locomotor skills with task variations or in new or altered environments. For example, a patient who has learned a new locomotor skill in one environment (e.g., walking on indoor level surfaces with a cane) can apply the skill in different environmental contexts (e.g., walking in a shopping mall or on outdoor surfaces). Because learning is task- and environment-specific, practice should include high levels of variation in both task demands and the environments in which they are practiced. Examples of strategies to vary locomotor task demands follow; additional examples are presented in Box 10.3. Box 10.4 offers sample strategies for varying environmental demands. Ideally, the patient will demonstrate adequate control of the components of gait and adequate locomotor skill before progressing to these activities. However, a patient may need to be progressed to varied task and environmental demands despite residual limitations in gait because these activities are critical to daily living and safety during locomotion. Proper guarding techniques should be used when introducing the challenges outlined below because these may initially result in a loss of balance.

- Practice walking with cues for head turns, such as *"Look right," "Look left," "Look up,"* and *"Look down"* (Fig. 10.12).
- Practice walking with cues for speed changes, such as *"Walk slow"* and *"Walk fast."*
- Practice walking with cues for directional changes and abrupt starts and stops, such as *"Turn right," "Turn left," "Pivot 360 degrees," "Stop,"* and *"Start."*
- Practice walking with an external pacing device such as a metronome or personal listening device using marching music to increase speed and improve rhythm.
- Practice walking on varied indoor surfaces, such as tile, wood flooring, and carpeting; difficulty can be increased by having the patient step on and off inflatable discs or foam pads placed strategically on the floor (Fig. 10.13).
- Practice walking through an obstacle course, over and around obstacles (Fig. 10.14), or over a floor grid to improve foot placement.
- Practice dual-task activities such as walking:
  - while engaged in a conversation (Walkie-Talkie test) or a cognitive task (e.g., counting backward by 7s from 100)
  - while holding a ball and moving it side to side with outstretched arms (Fig. 10.15)

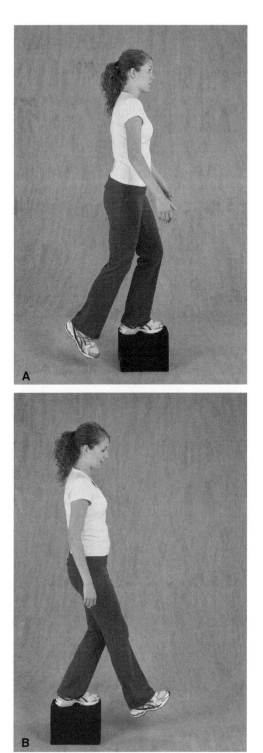

FIGURE 10.11 Step-ups and step-downs Initial practice in preparation for stair climbing can be accomplished using a step placed directly in front of the patient. *Not shown:* To begin, the patient is in a comfortable stance position. (A) The patient then weight-shifts laterally toward the support limb and places the dynamic left limb on the step. The right limb moving up to the step follows this. *Not shown:* Both feet are now positioned on the step. (B) The patient again weight-shifts toward the support limb and steps down, leading with the right limb. A progression is to stepping up and down without the interval of double support (i.e., both feet on the step).

BOX 10.3 Strategies for Varying Locomotor Task Demands

Upright Postural Alignment
- Practice walking upright; the therapist assists the patient in vertical trunk posture using manual and verbal cues, such as *"Look up and stand tall."*
- Use long poles or a body weight support harness to promote upright alignment and reduce UE support, forward head, and flexed trunk position (common with the use of an assistive device such as a walker).
- Progress UE support provided by assistive device to light touch support, then to use of a pole or wall for support as needed, and finally to no support.

Foot Placement/Toe Clearance
- Practice heel-toe initial contact using VCs such as *"Step with heels first."*
- Practice high-step marching in place and then high-step walking accompanied by marching music.
- Practice walking with even steps using footprints attached to the floor.
- Practice increasing step length and/or step width using footprints or a floor grid.
- Practice walking with altered BOS; progressing from wide base (8 to 12 in. [20 to 30 cm] apart) to narrow base (2 in. [5 cm] apart) to tandem (heel-to-toe).
- Practice step-to-walking (i.e., take a long step with one limb and then bring the opposite limb even with the first on the next step).
- Practice walking on a 3-inch (8-cm) wide line taped to the floor, on a split half-foam roller, or low balance beam.

Single- and Double-Limb Support
- Practice controlled lateral and diagonal weight shifts.
- Combine diagonal weight shifts with pelvic movements for stepping forward and backward.

Forward Progression and Push-off
- Practice toe rises in stance; progress to heel-walking.
- Practice heel-rises in stance; progress to toe-walking.
- Practice forceful push-off on cue during walking.
- Practice alternating between heel-walking and toe-walking (i.e., walk a certain number of steps on heels and then the same number on toes).

Walking Against Resistance
- Practice walking against manual resistance using resisted progression.
- Practice walking against resistance from an elastic resistive band around the pelvis.
- Practice pool walking (ideal initial supportive environment for patients with ataxia).

Trunk Counterrotation and Arm Swing
- Practice walking with exaggerated arm swings.
- Practice walking with wooden dowels held horizontally and grasped by both therapist and patient.

Walking Sideward
- Practice walking using lateral side steps, with resisted progression (manual and elastic resistive bands).
- Practice walking using crossed-steps and side steps.
- Practice walking using braiding.

Walking Backward
- Practice walking backward (retro-walking).
- Practice large backward steps (exaggerated knee flexion in combination with hip extension).

Step-Ups/Step-Downs
- Practice stepping up and stepping down; vary the step height, progressing from low (4 in. [10 cm]) to high (8 in. [20 cm]).
- Practice lateral step-ups.
- Practice forward step-ups.
- Practice stepping onto and off of varied surfaces (e.g., foam pad, half-foam roller, inflatable disc, BOSU Balance Trainer).

Stopping, Starting, and Turning on Cue
- Practice abrupt stops and starts on verbal cue.
- Practice turns on verbal cue, progressing from a quarter turn to half turn to full turn; progress from wide-base to narrow-base turns.
- Practice figure eight turns.

Visual Input
- Practice walking alternating between eyes open (EO) and eyes closed (EC); three steps with EO and then three steps with EC.

Head Movements
- Practice walking with alternating head movements; alternate between taking three steps with head to the right and then three steps with head to the left.
- Practice walking with varying head movements on VCs, such as *"Look right,"* *"Look left,"* *"Look down,"* and *"Look up."*
- Practice walking with diagonal head movements on VCs, such as *"Look over your right shoulder"* and *"Look down toward your left hip."*

Timed Walking, Increasing Speed, and Locomotor Rhythm
- Practice walking at a self-selected comfortable speed and then increasing speed to fast walking.
- Use pacing cues to vary speed, such as *"Walk slow"* and *"Walk fast."*
- Use a metronome or brisk marching music to increase speed and improve locomotor rhythm.
- Practice alternating short bursts of fast walking (on verbal cue) with walking at a comfortable speed.

Duration of Walking
- Progress to longer distances with fewer rest intervals.

Dual-Task Walking
- Walk and talk.
- Walk and count by threes.
- Walk and bounce or toss a ball or carry a tray.

Compensatory Responses to Unexpected Perturbations
- Change the speed of the treadmill, or stop and start the treadmill while the patient is walking on it.
- Practice resisted forward progression using an elastic resistive band with unexpected release of resistance.
- Practice walking while recovering from small external perturbations given manually.

BOX 10.4 Strategies for Varying Environmental Demands

Walking Surfaces
- Practice walking on a variety of indoor and outdoor surfaces.
  - Indoor surfaces: tile, linoleum, low- and high-pile carpet, and hardwood and laminate flooring
  - Outdoor surfaces: sidewalks, concrete, gravel, asphalt, and grassy terrains

Stair Climbing
- Practice stair climbing using a handrail; progress to stair climbing without the use of a handrail.
- Practice stair climbing one step at a time; progress to step over step; alter requirements for step height and number of steps.

Obstacles
- Practice walking while avoiding or contending with obstacles in the environment such as the following:
  - Walking over and around a static obstacle course created with objects of varying heights and widths (e.g., step stool, chair, cans, yardstick, stacking cones, books, and so forth); altering requirements for foot clearance, step length, step time, and walking speed
  - Walking with dynamic (moving) obstacles in the path (e.g., revolving door, elevator, or escalator)
  - Walking on varying paths (e.g., changing environment)
  - Walking with two individuals navigating the same obstacle course (collision avoidance)

Slopes or Ramps
- Practice walking on ramps and slopes of varying heights.
  - Gradual incline: using smaller steps
  - Steep incline: smaller steps using a diagonal, zigzag pattern (step length decreases with increasing slope)
- Requirements for navigating slopes or ramps include the following:
  - Descent is associated with increased knee flexion (stance) and increased ankle and hip motions (swing); during descent, peak moments and powers are higher at the knees.

- Ascent is associated with decreased speed, cadence, and step length.

Open Environments
- Practice walking in busy, open community environments (e.g., a busy hallway, hospital lobby, shopping mall, or grocery store).
- Practice finding solutions to real-life functional problems, such as the following:
  - Pushing or pulling open doors
  - Pushing a grocery cart
  - Car transfers: getting into and out of a car
  - Getting on and off a bus or other public transportation vehicle
  - Carrying a bag of groceries
- Practice walking and traversing unfamiliar routes and unfamiliar places.
- Practice stepping up and down curbs.

Time Requirements
- Practice walking with anticipatory timing requirements, such as the following:
  - Crossing at a stoplight
  - Moving on and off moving walkways
  - Moving on and off an escalator
  - Walking through automatic revolving doors

Visual Conditions
- Practice walking in varying visual conditions, such as the following:
  - Full lighting with progression to reduced and low lighting
  - With dark glasses to alter visual conditions
  - Varied lighting conditions (e.g., outside to inside lighting)

- while holding a tray or carrying a grocery bag or laundry basket
- while catching and throwing a lightly weighted ball or tapping a balloon
- while bouncing a ball
- while pushing and pulling loads (e.g., a grocery cart)
- through doorways and opening and closing doors
- stopping to pick an object up off the floor
- increased distances that simulate community distances (e.g., 1,200 ft [366 m]) or increased times that simulate the times needed for crosswalks (e.g., approximately 2.62 ft/sec [0.8 m/s] for a 40-ft [12-m] crosswalk)
- outdoors under different conditions (e.g., terrain, illumination, and weather) or in busy, noisy environments (e.g., busy hallways or clinic entrances and shopping malls)
- while practicing recovery strategies, such as stops or starts on a treadmill

Clinical Notes: The level of task difficulty is increased considerably by adding a second task *(dual-task activity)*. Initially, such activities require constant cognitive monitoring and may be mentally fatiguing and prone to errors when the patient becomes distracted. To begin, a closed environment is most effective. The patient should be guarded cautiously during the introduction of new or novel dynamic locomotor tasks; a gait (guarding) belt or an overhead harness may be warranted to ensure

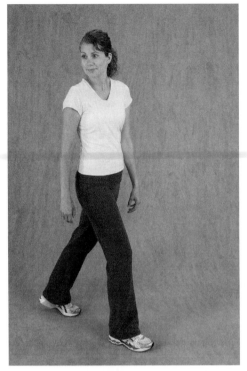

FIGURE 10.12 Walking with head turns to the left and right on VCs (in this example, the head is turned toward the right). A variation is to have the patient look up and down while walking.

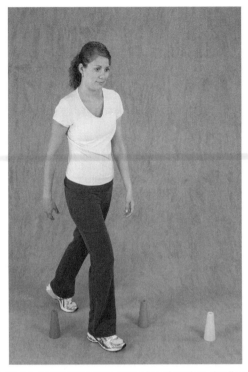

FIGURE 10.14 Walking through obstacles placed on the floor An obstacle course can be created using a variety of common objects. In this example, the course was created using stacking cones.

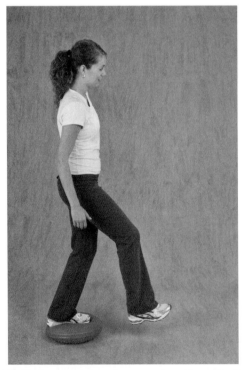

FIGURE 10.13 The walking surface can be altered by the tactical placement of inflatable discs on the floor. The patient steps up onto the disc with one limb and uses the opposite limb to step beyond the disc and make contact with the floor surface.

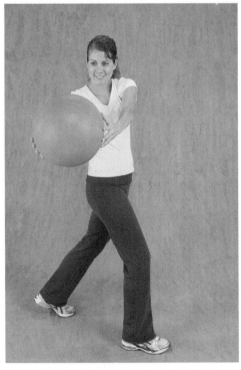

FIGURE 10.15 Dual-task locomotor activity With the shoulders flexed to approximately 90 degrees and the elbows extended, the patient moves the ball from side to side while walking.

patient safety. Most important, careful observance of safety precautions will improve patient confidence and trust in the therapist's ability to provide safe treatment.

Body Weight Support and Treadmill Training

The use of a body weight support (BWS) system and a treadmill (TM) combined with verbal and manual guidance from the therapist is an important intervention for improving locomotor skills. The desired amount of body weight is supported through a trunk harness donned by the patient that attaches to an overhead suspension system; the system's wheeled base (locking casters) allows positioning of the unit over a TM (Fig. 10.16). The unit can then be moved away from the TM for progression to overground locomotion. As a safety strategy, the suspension system may also be used without actually supporting body weight (the patient supports full body weight). This provides a safe and effective environment for the patient and therapist to focus on improving locomotor skills and its components without undue attention devoted to preventing falls.

Unique to the combined use of BWS and a TM is the ability to facilitate automatic locomotion using intensive task-oriented practice. Neural control of locomotion arises from subcortical and spinal centers (spinal pattern generators). As such, reciprocal locomotor patterns can be produced at the spinal cord level in the absence of supraspinal input.[25] This is a central tenet supporting the use of this approach. The constant speed of the TM (speed of walking is controlled) provides rhythmic input that helps to reestablish or reinforce coordinated reciprocal LE locomotor patterns.

Of critical importance to successful outcomes early on is the *hands-on* role of physical therapists and physical therapist assistants (trainers). The BWS system and TM allow access to the patient's hips, pelvis, and LEs to manually assist, provide sensory input, guide, or adjust locomotor rhythm, limb placement, weight shifts, and symmetry. Guided movements are coordinated to simulate a normal gait, and ensure that upright posture and balance are maintained. The sensory input (e.g., joint proprioceptors of hip, knee, and ankle; pressure receptors of foot) from appropriately timed manually assisted limb movements promotes function-induced recovery.[25,26] This sensory input provides spinal level *facilitation* and *inhibition* of flexor-extensor motor neuron pools at the appropriate time in the gait cycle.[27]

BWS and TM Training: Management Strategies

A significant body of literature has provided the following general guidelines for using BWS and TM locomotor training.[25,27–38]

- The adjustable straps are attached to an overhead BWS suspension system (see Fig. 10.16). The BWS unit is positioned over a TM, providing trainer access to the trunk/pelvis, hips, knees, and ankle/foot. If patient

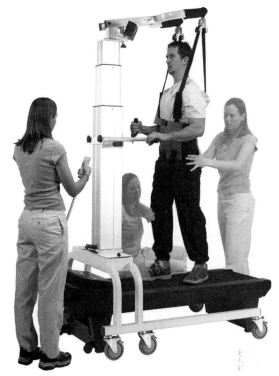

FIGURE 10.16 Body weight support system positioned over a treadmill base As the patient progresses, the support system is moved away from the platform base for overground locomotor training. (Courtesy of Mobility Research, Tempe, AZ 85281)

involvement is bilateral, trainers will need to be positioned on both sides of the TM.

- The BWS system supports a portion of the patient's body weight (e.g., starting at 40% with progressions to 30%, 20%, 10%, and then no BWS). Decreasing the amount of body weight supported is an important measure of progression.

- Increasing the TM *speed* is another important measure of progression. Initially, slow TM speeds are used (e.g., 0.52 mph [0.23 m/s]); then the speed is gradually increased as the patient's locomotor skills improve (e.g., to 0.95 mph [0.42 m/s]).

- Total locomotor training time recommendations range from 30 to 60 minutes with intervening rest intervals. Duration is increased gradually. On average, the patient training is intense (e.g., 5 days per week for 6 to 12 weeks). With severe involvement, however, initial training bouts may be as short as 3 minutes with 5-minute rest intervals.[35]

- After initiating locomotor training, trainers provide manual assistance to normalize gait. With unilateral involvement, for example, one trainer may provide assistance with foot placement while another trainer assists at the trunk and pelvis to promote upright posture and pelvic rotation. In the presence of muscle weakness, poor balance, or other impairments, the physical therapist must determine whether the patient's walking strategies are effective, what elements are consistent with the task of walking and should be promoted, and what elements are inconsistent that need to be modified or eliminated. Decreasing the amount of *manual assistance* provided is another important measure of progression.

- Parameters are established for the percentage of body weight supported, the TM speed, the duration of training bouts and rest intervals, and the amount and location of manual assistance. In the planning of treatment parameters, the following guidelines are considered:
  - LE weightbearing should be maximized, whereas UE support is minimized.
  - Sensory cues and input via appropriate handling techniques should be optimized to ensure the desired or most favorable stepping pattern (assisted by trainers).
  - Normal walking kinematics should be promoted, with emphasis on trunk, pelvis, and limb movements.
  - Recovery of function should be maximized and compensatory movements minimized or eliminated.
  - Manual assistance is limited to only that which is essential for accomplishing the desired movement.
  - As reciprocal patterns of movement begin to develop, locomotor training is progressed by reducing the amount of body weight supported, increasing the TM speed, and reducing the amount of manual guidance. Progression continues until the patient is walking, independently supporting full body weight at a speed of 1.0 mph (0.44 m/s).[35]
- Locomotor training using BWS is continued by progressing to overground walking. When the casters are unlocked, the BWS unit becomes mobile and can be moved away from the TM for use on overground surfaces. Elimination of the rhythmic steady-state input from the TM causes the overground walking speed to be initially reduced. The unit is manually moved by the trainers to keep pace with the patient's forward progression. The use of an assistive device may be introduced during BWS overground walking. The same parameters continue to be used to monitor progress: amount of body weight support, speed, and manual assistance.
- The patient progresses to overground walking without BWS and without an assistive device. The desired walking speed will vary based on the demands of the environment the patient will be negotiating. For example, functional speeds required for community ambulation average 2.8 mph (1.3 m/s) in a normal healthy population.[39]

Appendix 10B presents an overview of locomotor training appropriate for patients with spinal cord injury (SCI); the information provides the framework for Case Study 3.

Conventional Gait Training Versus Weight Support and Treadmill

While intervention strategies differ, conventional gait training and BWS using a TM share common principles. They are both task oriented (to the specific task of locomotion), goal directed, shaped and progressed maximally within the patient's capabilities, and require repeated practice.[13] They share the common goal of achieving optimum locomotor function for the individual patient.

Developing an appropriate POC to address locomotor dysfunction requires consideration of multiple environments (e.g., parallel bars, assistive devices, BWS and TM, overground progressions, negotiating the community). The selection of the optimal environment together with complementary interventions (e.g., strengthening, balance activities, transfer training) is based on patient diagnosis and health status, cognitive status, impairments, and the patient's weightbearing status.[13]

Robotics

An area of research that holds potential for reducing the personnel requirements of BWS and TM training is robotic-assisted BWS TM training (Fig. 10.17). This approach incorporates a computer-controlled, driven (motorized) gait orthosis that provides passive control of individual joints and stabilization during TM stepping. These exoskeletal devices are secured to the patient's LEs and provide controlled reciprocal stepping movements to approximate normal gait kinematics.[40–45]

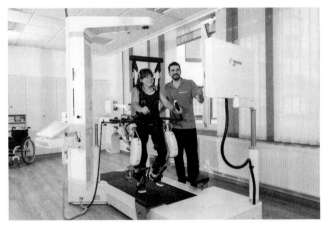

FIGURE 10.17 The Lokomat is a driven gait orthosis that provides passive movement and stabilization of the LEs during BWS TM training. (Courtesy of Hocoma AG, Inc., Zurich, Switzerland.)

Outcome Measures

Outcome measures provide important evidence about the efficacy of interventions designed to improve gait and locomotor skills. Two categories of commonly used measures include timed and distance-based tests. Timed walk tests such as the *2-, 6-,* and *12-Minute Walk Test* (12MWT) require the patient to walk for a specified number of minutes, and the total distance walked is recorded.[46–52] Distance-based measures such as the *10-Meter Walk Test* (10MWT) and *50-Foot Walk Test* (50FTWT), require the subject walk a specified number of meters while being timed so that velocity may be calculated.[53–55]

The *Timed Up and Go* (TUG) test measures the time required to rise from a chair, walk 3 meters, turn, walk back to the chair, and sit down. During the test, the subject wears regular footwear and uses any assistive device normally required.[56–59]

The *Functional Independence Measure-Locomotor* (FIM-L) is a subscale of the Functional Independence Measure (FIM) that uses a 7-point scale based on level of assistance required to ambulate (e.g., 1 = total assistance, 7 = independent without equipment). The FIM-L includes two distinct subscales, walking and wheelchair use, allowing application to a continuum of locomotor abilities.[55,60]

The *Dynamic Gait Index* (DGI) is a performance-based tool used to quantify gait dysfunction in older adults during level walking and in response to challenges to balance and postural control (e.g., altering walking speed, turning head, walking with a pivot turn). It includes eight tasks with a 4-level ordinal scale (e.g., 3 = no gait dysfunction, 0 = severe impairment) and a maximum score of 24. A score of 19 or less indicates risk of falling.[24,61–64]

The *Functional Gait Assessment* (FGA) is a modified version of the DGI. It is a 10-item assessment that includes seven tasks from the original DGI and three new items (walking with a narrow BOS, backward, and with eyes closed [EC]). It also uses a 4-point ordinal scale with a maximum score of 30. Lower scores indicate greater impairment.[65–68]

Observational gait analysis (OGA) involves visual observation of the kinematic patterns of movement implemented during walking.[24] This is an approach commonly used by physical therapists to examine and document gait dysfunction. Examples of outcomes measures used to organize and structure the OGA include the *Rancho Los Amigos Observational Gait Analysis* system,[5] the *Rivermead Visual Gait Examination* (RVGA),[69,70] and the *Gait Assessment Rating Scale* (GARS).[71]

The *Modified Emory Functional Ambulation Profile* (mEFAP) measures the time to walk over five common terrain variations (including a hard floor and carpeted floor), an "up and go" task (rising from chair, 3-meter walk, and return to seated position), navigating an obstacle course, and stair climbing. Scoring involves time to complete each task multiplied by a factor assigned to the level of assistive or orthotic device used.[73,74]

Box 10.5 presents Student Practice Activities that focus on interventions and management strategies to improve locomotor skills.

BOX 10.5 STUDENT PRACTICE ACTIVITY: INTERVENTIONS AND MANAGEMENT STRATEGIES TO IMPROVE LOCOMOTION

OBJECTIVE: Sharing skill in the application and knowledge of treatment interventions to enhance locomotion.

EQUIPMENT NEEDS: Step stool, ball, inflated disc, two poles, two elastic resistive bands, a treadmill, and several common objects to create an obstacle course (e.g., staking cones, plastic cups, books, soup cans, and so forth).

STUDENT GROUP SIZE: Four to six students.

DIRECTIONS: Divide into pairs, with one person serving as the patient/subject and the other functioning as the therapist (reverse roles prior to addressing the guiding questions).

1. **Practice walking forward and backward.** Direct the patient/subject to practice walking forward and backward as the therapist guards and directs the activities. Complete the following activities:
   - Increase the step length from initially reduced to normal.
   - Change the speed of walking from slow to normal to fast; progress to treadmill walking (if available).

- Modify the BOS from feet apart (wide base) to normal to feet close together (narrow base) to tandem walking (heel-to-toe pattern).
- Vary the acceleration or deceleration by having the patient/subject practice stopping and starting or turning on cue.
- Practice dual-task walking, such as walking and counting backward by 7s from 100, walking and turning the head left or right and up or down on cue, and walking and bouncing a ball.
- Vary the walking surface from flat to on and off foam to irregular (outdoors).
- Using an elastic resistive band, practice both forward and backward resisted progressions. Depending on the direction of movement, the therapist stands either in front of or behind the patient holding the ends of the band.
- Practice walking forward and backward on a treadmill, and practice walking with stops and starts of the treadmill.
- Practice walking through an obstacle course.

(box continues on page 250)

BOX 10.5 STUDENT PRACTICE ACTIVITY: INTERVENTIONS AND MANAGEMENT STRATEGIES TO IMPROVE LOCOMOTION (continued)

Guiding Questions

Considering the variations in locomotor tasks just practiced:

▲ What did you learn about changes in postural stability demands with each activity?

▲ What activities provided the *greatest* and *least* challenges to postural stability?

▲ Compare and contrast the rhythmic stepping patterns used during forward versus backward walking. What differences did you notice?

▲ As the speed of walking was reduced and increased, what changes occurred in the requirements for timing and control?

▲ Multiple muscle groups are active in alternating between forward and backward walking. Differentiate between the muscles that contribute to dynamic limb advancement (swing phase) during forward versus backward progressions.

▲ What insights did the activities provide that can be applied clinically?

▲ Describe the importance of synchronizing the therapist's movements with those of the patient's during resisted progression. How is pacing of the activity maintained?

▲ What strategies can be used to assist in sequencing arm swings and promoting trunk counterrotation during forward and backward progressions?

▲ How did walking on a TM affect locomotor rhythm?

▲ Did the level of task difficulty change by adding a second task *(dual-task activity)*? What impact did the dual task have on cognitive monitoring? Was the quality of performance affected by the addition of a second task?

2. **Practice walking, side-stepping.** Direct the patient/subject to sidestep by abduction and placement of the dynamic limb to the side; the remaining limb is then moved parallel to the first. Complete the following activities:
   • Practice active side-stepping in each direction.
   • Apply resisted progression in side-stepping using an elastic resistive band (around the lateral aspect of the pelvis on the abducting side).
   • Change the speed of side-stepping from reduced to normal to increased.
   • Practice side-stepping on a treadmill.

Guiding Questions

▲ What are the functional implications of side-stepping?

▲ During side-stepping, what action is provided by the hip abductors on the dynamic limb? On the static limb?

▲ As the speed of walking was reduced and increased, what changes occurred in the requirements for timing and control?

▲ What changes in timing and rhythm occurred during side-stepping on the TM?

3. **Practice walking, side-stepping, and crossed-stepping.** Instruct the patient/subject to abduct the leading dynamic limb with foot placement followed by movement of the remaining limb to a parallel position with the first (a symmetrical stance) and then crossed-stepping by moving the leg up, across, and in front of the original side step limb. Complete the following activities:
   • Practice active side-stepping and crossed-stepping in each direction.
   • Apply resisted progression in side-stepping and crossed-stepping using manual resistance.
   • Alter the speed of side-stepping and crossed-stepping from reduced to normal to increased.

Guiding Questions

▲ What are the clinical indications for the use of side-stepping and crossed-stepping?

▲ As the speed of side-stepping and crossed-stepping was altered, what changes occurred?

4. **Practice walking, braiding.** Direct the patient to begin with a side step and follow with a crossed-step up and over in front (PNF LE FLEX/ADD/ER pattern), then a side step, and then a crossed-step backward and behind the first limb (PNF LE EXT/ADD/ER pattern). Complete the following activities:
   • Practice active braiding in each direction.
   • Apply resisted progression in braiding using manual resistance.

Guiding Questions

▲ Braiding is a challenging sequence to learn for many patients. How can the therapist help the patient learn this new skill?

▲ What therapeutic goal(s) can be addressed using braiding?

5. **Directions:** Working in a small group, respond to the following:
   • Describe strategies for varying locomotor task demands during training.
   • Describe strategies for varying environmental demands during training.
   • What are the prerequisite requirements for the initiation of stair climbing?
   • Describe the rationale for locomotor training using BWS and a TM. What benefits are associated with this approach?

SUMMARY

Improving or reestablishing locomotor skills is often the highest priority for patients seeking skilled physical therapy intervention. Locomotion is an essential function that supports and enhances effective interaction with the environment. It represents the highest level of motor control (skill) and requires the integrated function of many interacting systems. The foundational requirements of walking include dynamic stability of the trunk, support of body weight, locomotor rhythm, dynamic balance, propulsion of the body in the desired direction, and the ability to adapt to changing task and environmental demands. Establishing an effective POC to improve locomotor skills requires a comprehensive gait analysis and knowledge of the impairments and activity limitations that affect movement. An important focus of intervention is promoting adaptation skills through variations in both locomotor task and environmental demands. Finally, the therapist must consider the demands of the patient's home, community, and work environment to achieve successful outcomes.

REFERENCES

1. Soh, S, et al. Determinants of health-related quality of life in people with Parkinson's disease: a path analysis. Qual Life Res, 2013; 22:1543.
2. Steptoe, A, et al. Enjoyment of life and declining physical function at older ages: a longitudinal cohort study. CMAJ, 2014; 186:E150.
3. Duncan, RP, and Earhart, GM. Measuring participation in individuals with Parkinson disease: relationships with disease severity, quality of life, and mobility. Disabil Rehabil, 2011; 33:1440–1446.
4. Hedman, LD, et al. Locomotor requirements for bipedal locomotion: a Delphi survey. Phys Ther, 2014; 94:52.
5. Pathokinesiology Service and Physical Therapy Department. Observational Gait Analysis Handbook. Downey, CA, Los Amigos Research and Education Institute, 2001.
6. Schmidt, RA, and Lee, TD. Motor Control and Learning, ed 5. Champaign, IL, Human Kinetics, 2011.
7. Saliba, VL, Johnson, GS, and Wardlaw, C. Proprioceptive Neuromuscular facilitation. In Basmajian, JV, and Nyberg, R, (eds). Rational Manual Therapies. Baltimore, Williams & Wilkins, 1993, p 243.
8. Johnson, G, and Saliba Johnson, V. PNF 1: The Functional Application of Proprioceptive Neuromuscular Facilitation, Course Syllabus, Version 7.9, Steamboat, CO, Institute of Physical Art, 2014.
9. American Physical Therapy Association. Guide to Physical Therapist Practice, Version 3.0. Alexandria, VA, American Physical Therapy Association, 2014. Retrieved on March 16, 2015 from http://guidetoptpractice.apta.org.
10. Burnfield, JM, and Norkin, CC. Examination of gait. In O'Sullivan, SB, Schmitz, TJ, and Fulk, GD, eds. Physical Rehabilitation, ed 6. Philadelphia, F.A. Davis, 2014, 255.
11. Wainwright, SF, et al. Novice and experienced physical therapist clinicians: a comparison of how reflection is used to inform the clinical decision-making process. Phys Ther, 2009; 90:75.
12. Perry, J, and Burnfield, J. Gait Analysis: Normal and Pathological Function, ed 2. Thorofare, NJ, Slack, 2010.
13. Fulk, GD, and Schmitz, TJ. Locomotor Training. In O'Sullivan, SB, Schmitz, TJ, and Fulk, GD (eds). Physical Rehabilitation, ed 6. Philadelphia, F.A. Davis, 2014, 444.
14. Himann, JE, et al. Age-related changes in speed of walking. Med Sci Sports Exerc, 1988; 20:161.
15. Forrest, KY, Zmuda, JM, and Cauley, JA. Correlates of decline in lower extremity performance in older women: a 10-year follow-up study. J Gerontol A Biol Sci Med Sci, 2006; 61:1194.
16. White, DK, et al. Trajectories of gait speed predict mortality in well-functioning older adults: the health, aging and body composition study. J Gerontol A Biol Sci Med Sci, 2013; 68:456.
17. Chiu, S, and Chou, L. Effect of walking speed on inter-joint coordination differs between young and elderly adults. J Biomech, 2012; 45:275.
18. Light, K. Information processing for motor performance in aging adults. Phys Ther, 1990; 70:821.
19. Beavers, KM, et al. Associations between body composition and gait-speed decline: results from the Health, Aging, and Body Composition Study. Am J Clin Nutr, 2013; 97:552.
20. Ikezoe, T, et al. Atrophy of the lower limbs in elderly women: is it related to walking ability? Eur J Appl Physiol, 2011; 111:989.
21. Gibbs, J. Predictors of change in walking velocity in older adults. J Am Geriatr Soc, 1996; 44:126.
22. Schulte, OJ, Stephens, J, and Joyce, A. Brain Function, Aging, and Dementia. In Umphred, DA (ed). Neurological Rehabilitation, ed 5. St. Louis, Mosby/Elsevier, 2007, 902.
23. Hooper, CD, and Dal Bello-Haas, V. Sensory Function. In Bonder, BR, and Dal Bello-Haas, V. Functional Performance in Older Adults, ed 3. Philadelphia, F.A. Davis, 2009, 101.
24. Shumway-Cook, A, and Woollacott, MH. Motor Control Translating Research into Clinical Practice, ed 4. Philadelphia, Wolters Kluwer/Lippincott Williams & Wilkins, 2012.
25. Field-Fote, EC. Spinal cord control of movement: implications for locomotor rehabilitation following spinal cord injury. Phys Ther, 2000; 80:477.
26. Visintin, M, and Barbeau, H. The effects of body weight support on the locomotor pattern of spastic paretic patients. Can J Neurol Sci, 1999; 16:315.
27. Kosak, MC, and Reding, MJ. Comparison of partial body weight-supported treadmill gait training versus aggressive bracing assisted walking post stroke. Neurorehabil Neural Repair, 2000; 14:13.
28. Brown, TH, et al. Body weight-supported treadmill training versus conventional gait training for people with chronic traumatic brain injury. J Head Trauma Rehabil, 2005; 20:402.
29. Behrman, A, and Harkema, S. Locomotor training after human spinal cord injury: a series of case studies. Phys Ther, 2000; 80:688.
30. Behrman, A, et al. Locomotor training progression and outcomes after incomplete spinal cord injury. Phys Ther, 2005; 85:1356.
31. Hesse, S, et al. Treadmill training with partial body weight support compared with physiotherapy in nonambulatory hemiparetic patients. Stroke, 1995; 26:976.
32. Macko, RF, et al. Treadmill exercise rehabilitation improves ambulatory function and cardiovascular fitness in patients with chronic stroke: a randomized, controlled trial. Stroke, 2005; 36:2206.
33. Mehrholz, J, Pohl, M, and Elsner, B. Treadmill training and body weight support for walking after stroke. Cochrane Database Syst Rev, 2014; CD002840.pub3.
34. Salbach, NM, et al. A task-oriented intervention enhances walking distance and speed in the first year post stroke: a randomized controlled trial. Clin Rehabil, 2004; 18:509.
35. Seif-Naraghi, AH, and Herman, RM. A novel method for locomotion training. J Head Trauma Rehabil, 1999; 14:146.
36. Sullivan, K, Knowlton, BJ, and Dobkin, BH. Step training with body weight support: effect of treadmill speed and practice paradigms on poststroke locomotor recovery. Arch Phys Med Rehabil, 2002; 83:683.
37. Lucareli, PR, et al. Gait analysis following treadmill training with body weight support versus conventional physical therapy: a prospective randomized controlled single blind study. Spinal Cord, 2011; 49:1001–1007.
38. Sullivan, K, et al. Effects of task-specific locomotor and strength training in adults who were ambulatory after stroke: results of the STEPS randomized clinical trial. Phys Ther, 2007; 87:1580.
39. Perry, J, et al. Classification of walking handicap in the stroke population. Stroke, 1995; 26:982.
40. Hornby, TG, et al. Kinematic, muscular, and metabolic responses during exoskeletal-, elliptical-, or therapist-assisted stepping in people with incomplete spinal cord injury. Phys Ther, 2012; 92:1278.
41. Israel, JF, et al. Metabolic costs and muscle activity patterns during robotic- and therapist-assisted treadmill walking in individuals with incomplete spinal cord injury. Phys Ther, 2006; 86:1466.
42. Lewek, MD, et al. Allowing intralimb kinematic variability during locomotor training poststroke improves kinematic consistency: a subgroup analysis from a randomized clinical trial. Phys Ther, 2009; 89:829.

43. Colombo, G, et al. Treadmill training of paraplegic patients using a robotic orthosis. J Rehabil Res Dev, 2000; 37:693.

44. Colombo, G, Wirz, M, and Dietz, V. Driven gait orthosis for improvement of locomotor training in paraplegic patients. Spinal Cord, 2001; 39:252.

45. Hesse, S, et al. A mechanized gait trainer for restoring gait in nonambulatory subjects. Arch Phys Med Rehabil, 2000; 81:1158.

46. Oliver, R, et al. The Six-Minute-Walk Test in assessing respiratory function after tumor surgery of the lung: a cohort study. J Thorac Dis, 2014; 6:421.

47. Bohannon, RW, et al. Comparison of walking performance over the first 2 minutes and the full 6 minutes of the Six-Minute Walk Test. BMC Res Notes, 2014; 7:269.

48. Southard, V, and Gallagher, R. The 6MWT: will different methods of instruction and measurement affect performance of healthy aging and older adults? J Geriatr Phys Ther, 2013; 36:68.

49. Hanson, LC, McBurney, H, and Taylor, N. The retest reliability of the six-minute walk test in patients referred to a cardiac rehabilitation programme. Physiother Res Int, 2012; 17:55.

50. Fulk, G, et al. Clinometric properties of the six-minute walk test in individuals undergoing rehabilitation post stroke. Physiother Theory Pract, 2008; 24:195.

51. Kosak, M, and Smith T. Comparison of the 2-, 6-, and 12-minute walk tests in patients with stroke. J Rehabil Res Dev, 2005; 42:103.

52. Butland R, et al. Two-, six-, and 12-minute walking tests in respiratory disease. Br Med J (Clin Res Ed), 1982; 284:1607.

53. Peters, DM, Fritz, SL, and Krotish, DE. Assessing the reliability and validity of a shorter walk test compared with the 10-Meter Walk Test for measurements of gait speed in healthy, older adults. J Geriatr Phys Ther, 2013; 36:24.

54. Lin, JH, et al. Psychometric comparisons of 3 functional ambulation measures for patients with stroke. Stroke, 2010; 41:2021.

55. Jackson, AB, et al. Outcome measures for gait and ambulation in the spinal cord injury population. J Spinal Cord Med, 2008; 31:487.

56. Podsiadlo, D, and Richardson, S. The Timed "Up & Go": a test of basic functional mobility for frail elderly persons. J Am Geriatr Soc, 1991; 39:142.

57. Ng, SS, and Hui-Chan, CW. The Timed Up & Go Test: its reliability and association with lower-limb impairments and locomotor capacities in people with chronic stroke. Arch Phys Med Rehabil, 2005; 86:1641.

58. Shumway-Cook, A, Brauer, S, and Woollacott, M. Predicting the probability for falls in community-dwelling older adults using the Timed Up & Go Test. Phys Ther, 2000; 80:896.

59. Ayan, C, et al. Influence of the cognitive impairment level on the performance of the Timed "Up & Go" Test (TUG) in elderly institutionalized people. Arch Gerontol Geriatr, 2013; 56:44.

60. Poncumhak, P, et al. Reliability and validity of three functional tests in ambulatory patients with spinal cord injury. Spinal Cord, 2013; 51:214.

61. Forsberg, A, Andreasson, M, and Nilsagård, Y. Validity of the Dynamic Gait Index in people with multiple sclerosis. Phys Ther, 2013; 93:1369.

62. Dye, D, Eakman, AM, and Bolton, KM. Assessing the validity of the Dynamic Gait Index in a balance disorders clinic: an application of Rasch analysis. Phys Ther, 2013; 93:809.

63. Herman, T, et al. The Dynamic Gait Index in healthy older adults: the role of stair climbing, fear of falling and gender. Gait Posture, 2009; 29:237.

64. Lubetzky-Vilnai, A, Jirikowic, TL, and McCoy, SW. Investigation of the Dynamic Gait Index in children: a pilot study. Pediatr Phys Ther, 2011; 23:268.

65. Wrisley, DM, et al. Reliability, internal consistency, and validity of data obtained with the functional gait assessment. Phys Ther, 2004; 84:906.

66. Wrisley, DM, and Kumar, NA. Functional gait assessment: concurrent, discriminative, and predictive validity in community-dwelling older adults. Phys Ther, 2010; 90:761.

67. Leddy, AL, Crowner, BE, and Earhart, GM. Functional gait assessment and balance evaluation system test: reliability, validity, sensitivity, and specificity for identifying individuals with Parkinson disease who fall. Phys Ther, 2001; 91:102.

68. Yang, Y, et al. Validity of the functional gait assessment in patients with Parkinson disease: construct, concurrent, and predictive validity. Phys Ther, 2014; 94:392.

69. Lord, SE, Halligan, PW, and Wade, DT. Visual gait analysis: the development of a clinical assessment and scale. Clin Rehabil, 1998; 12:107.

70. Lord, S, et al. Visual gait analysis: the development of a clinical examination and scale. Clin Rehabil, 1998; 12:107.

71. Wolfson, L, et al. Gait assessment in the elderly: a gait abnormality rating scale and its relation to falls. J Gerontol, 1990; 45:M12, 199.

72. Baer, HR, and Wolf, SL. Modified Emory Functional Ambulation Profile: an outcome measure for the rehabilitation of poststroke gait dysfunction. Stroke, 2001; 32:973.

73. Liaw, LJ, et al. Psychometric properties of the modified Emory Functional Ambulation Profile in stroke patients. Clin Rehabil, 2006; 20:429.

74. Wolf, SL, et al. Establishing the reliability and validity of measurements of walking time using the Emory Functional Ambulation Profile. Phys Ther, 1999; 79:1122.

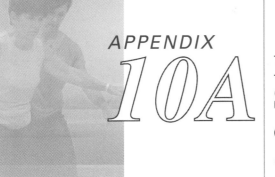

Example of Selection, Sequencing, and Progression of Interventions Within the Context of Two Subsequent Treatment Sessions for a Patient with Traumatic Brain Injury (Case Study 2)

Case Study 2 is presented in Part II on p. 332.

Patient Information	
Patient	Case Study 2: Traumatic Brain Injury: Balance and Locomotor Training
Medical Diagnosis	Traumatic brain injury (TBI)
Medical History	2 years post-TBI sustained during a motor vehicle accident
Precautions/Contraindications	• Patient requires repetition of instructions and demonstrations • Patient demonstrates decreased safety awareness
Systems Review and Tests and Measures	Refer to Case Study 2 (p. 332)
Outcomes of Episode of Care (Long-Term Goals)	1. The patient will ambulate independently without an assistive device, demonstrating symmetrical stance time and step length with efficient weight shifting and weight acceptance during bilateral stance with good dynamic balance in 6–8 weeks. 2. The patient will transition sit-to-stand independently from a standard chair without an assistive device, demonstrating symmetrical weightbearing and appropriate trunk alignment with adequate hip and knee extension bilaterally upon completion of standing in 6–8 weeks. 3. The patient will ascend and descend five steps using a step-over-step approach with contact guard demonstrating proper weight acceptance and LE control for balance and safety at each step in 6–8 weeks. 4. The Berg Balance Test score will improve to 50/56 in 6–8 weeks.
Short-Term Goals	1. The patient will ambulate with contact guard without an assistive device, demonstrating symmetrical weight shifting and efficient weight acceptance on the left LE with adequate hip and knee extension during stance and symmetrical right step length for 3/5 steps in 2 weeks. 2. The patient will be able to maintain single-limb stance on the left LE with a high step on the right LE and adequate control of the left LE for 30 seconds in 2 weeks. 3. The Berg Balance Test score will improve to 45/56 in 2 weeks. 4. The patient will be able to maintain static standing with feet together for 45 seconds without assistance in 2 weeks.

Plan for Treatment Session 1	
Activity Limitations Being Addressed in This Treatment Session	Although the patient demonstrates impairments in UEs and LEs bilaterally leading to gait dysfunction, this treatment session will focus on improving the left LE stance phase of gait. Patient ambulates with straight cane and demonstrates: • Decreased weight shift to left • Decreased left stance time • Decreased right step length • Inadequate weight acceptance on left for midstance • Absent left pelvic posterior depression with inadequate hip and knee extension throughout stance • Absent dynamic trunk control for efficient upper and LE function. • The lack of weight acceptance and the absent engagement between the trunk and the left LE leads to absent left push-off, as would be expected. • Left swing phase is dominated by hip flexion with absent dynamic engagement of the trunk. • Although the left UE appears to have a larger arm swing than the right UE, there is no active engagement of the left scapula with absent dynamic engagement/control of the trunk. • Left arm swing is excessive at the glenohumeral and the elbow joints but lacks scapula control and engagement with the trunk and the left LE. The patient's BOS is widened in an attempt to decrease the challenge to balance and make gait possible and safe. While safer, the wider BOS is also contributing to decreased activation of the trunk, left pelvis, and left LE. The patient does not have an appropriate BOS with efficient alignment up the chain for appropriate weight shifting and weight acceptance onto the left LE.
The Focus of This Treatment Session	Appropriate weight shift and weight acceptance onto the left LE for left stance and right swing.
Functional Pre- and Posttest(s) for This Treatment Session to Be Performed at the Beginning and End of the Treatment Session	• Single-limb stance time on the left LE • Numbers of steps in 3 or 5 meters • Sit-to-stand time and symmetry of weightbearing • Observational gait analysis

Treatment Session 1 Interventions

Intervention 1

Patient Position: left sidelying

Activity: right pelvis anterior elevation and posterior depression

Technique: rhythmic initiation (RI) and combination of isotonics (COI)[7,8]

Manual Contact/Facilitation/Input: MCs for both pelvic patterns will initially be aimed at passive motion to assure that the patient demonstrates mobility of all components. The focus will then shift to assessment and facilitation of the patient's ability to initiate a contraction of both patterns with a dynamically stable trunk in preparation for LE activity. Facilitation may be done through a quick stretch at the beginning of the ROM or through stretches through the range, as deemed appropriate during the intervention. A maintained hold or another quick stretch may be used when the patient begins to lose control of the contraction to facilitate increased motor unit output, to reeducate the pattern, to provide the patient with increased kinesthetic awareness of the motion being facilitated, and to assist in reintegrating that motion into the patient's movement repertoire by providing increased firing of the homunculus.

Rationale: The treatment session begins on the less-involved side to allow examination of the patient's ability to respond to verbal and manual input, determine spinal and pelvic mobility, teach the patient the activities and patterns that will be applied on the more involved side, and set the patient up for a successful response to facilitate rapport and motivate the patient for the remainder of the treatment session. The session begins with the pelvis to assess and facilitate appropriate trunk activation for dynamic stability (proximal stability for distal mobility).

INTERVENTION 2

Patient Position: right sidelying

Activity: left pelvis anterior elevation and posterior depression—focus on posterior depression

Technique: rhythmic initiation and combination of isotonics (COI)[7,8]

Manual Contact/Facilitation/Input: same as for Intervention 1

Rationale: The treatment session progresses using the same activity and techniques on the more involved (left) side for the same purposes. Pelvis anterior elevation and posterior depression is the appropriate PNF diagonal to promote improved weight acceptance for stance. Greater emphasis should be placed on the posterior depression pattern since the focus of this treatment session is the stance phase of gait. Initial activities concentrate on the pelvis since the patient lacks dynamic trunk activation and control and demonstrates an absent engagement of the pelvis during gait. Facilitation of the proper pelvic patterns with dynamic trunk activation is crucial prior to working on the LE components of stance.

INTERVENTION 3

Patient Position: right sidelying

Activity: left pelvis posterior depression with left LE EXT/ABD/IR pattern.

Technique: prolonged holds at the end of pelvis posterior depression with LE EXT/ABD/IR progressing to COI[7,8]

Manual Contact/Facilitation/Input: facilitation of the left LE EXT/ABD/IR pattern with pelvic posterior depression is initiated with approximation that is maintained based on the patient's response. Once the patient demonstrates a proper response, the therapist will continue the approximation together with building resistance to facilitate increased motor unit recruitment and kinesthetic awareness of weightbearing in proper alignment with pelvis posterior depression. When an efficient activation is recruited, the manual input will change to resist an eccentric contraction away from EXT/ABD/IR and posterior depression with a concentric return and approximation again applied at end range (COI). The therapist will perform several repetitions; increasing the demand on the ROM excursion until the patient is able to perform pelvic posterior depression with left LE EXT/ABD/IR from the beginning of the range.

Rationale: This activity mimics stance in a sidelying position. It allows the therapist to facilitate the proper positioning of the pelvis and LE at the end range of the EXT/ABD/IR pattern without challenging the patient's balance. It allows the patient to experience the proper components required for improved stance in a stable

and safe position. Approximation and end range holds prepare the patient for weightbearing with improved weight acceptance and stability.

INTERVENTION 4

Patient Position: standing in stride position with left foot forward and right foot back in parallel bars

Activity: weight shifting from the back right LE to the front left LE with a focus on proper movement and alignment of the pelvis bilaterally without excessive pelvic rotation in the transverse plane and without a drop of the pelvis in the frontal plane. Attention is directed to proper alignment and control of the LEs as the patient weight-shifts from the back LE (right) onto the front LE (left).

Technique: rhythmic initiation for weight shifting with MCs focusing on pelvis anterior elevation on the right (quick stretch and appropriate resistance as needed) and posterior depression on the left (approximation)

Manual Contact/Facilitation/Input: The therapist will initially assist the patient in this weight shift by providing MCs on bilateral pelvis to facilitate and assure that the patient is able to maintain both sides level while weight shifting forward. Care must be taken to assure that proper guarding and blocking of the left knee is provided to facilitate control of knee extension and prevent buckling or hyperextension as the patient shifts weight onto the left LE. As the patient demonstrates increased control of the weight shift, the therapist's manual input transitions from assistive to resistive, reinforcing the efficient coordination of all segments while promoting strengthening across the LEs, pelvis, and trunk.

Rationale: This activity brings the patient to upright standing where he will be required to integrate the components facilitated and practiced in a non-weight bearing and safe position into a functional and more challenging position. The activity begins with RI for simple weight shifting over several repetitions to allow the patient to experience the proper sequencing required for efficient weight shifting. The activity progresses to include resistance only when, and if, the therapist determines that the patient is demonstrating an effective motor strategy that includes appropriate sequencing and quality of activation in all segments with the ability to control the forward transition of the pelvis without excessive rotation or frontal plane motion.

INTERVENTION 5

Patient Position: standing in stride position with left foot forward and right foot back in parallel bars

Activity: weight shifting forward to the left LE with a high step taken by the right LE. Attention is directed to proper alignment and control of the left LE in stance. Appropriate resistance is applied to the swing LE (right) while it is taken into a high step position with the hip moving beyond 90 degrees of flexion. Emphasis is placed on proper pelvic anterior elevation of the swing right LE with proper pelvic posterior depression of the stance left LE.

Technique: appropriate resistance to the right pelvis and right LE (step up leg) with approximation through the left pelvis and left LE (stance leg)

Manual Contact/Facilitation/Input: Manual input, in the form of appropriate resistance is applied to right pelvis anterior elevation with approximation applied to the left pelvis and LE. This assures that the trunk is active and dynamically stable and that the pelvis moves in appropriate diagonals while the LEs hold their positions in FLEX/ADD/ER (right) and EXT/ABD/IR (left). The therapist's manual contact can shift from the right pelvis to add resistance to the right LE flexion pattern. With the right hip brought above 90 degrees of flexion, the therapist is invoking the influence of the cross-extension reflex, further facilitating motor output in the left LE extension pattern. If the patient is stable, MCs can shift again so that one hand is on the right pelvis facilitating pelvis anterior elevation while the other is on the right LE facilitating the LE flexion pattern. During this activity the therapist must assure that the stance leg is guarded appropriately throughout the duration of the intervention to prevent buckling or hyperextension as the patient fatigues.

Rationale: Once the patient demonstrates appropriate weight shifting from the right to the left LE with appropriate trunk, pelvis, and LE control for stance, the therapist progresses the session to high-stepping where all components of stance on the left LE and swing on the right LE will be exaggerated for increased facilitation and reinforcement with increased neurological output as a result of the influence of the cross-extension reflex. In addition to emphasizing the components of gait, this activity allows for work on hip and knee control, strengthening, and balance in stance.

General Comments (All Treatment Sessions)

• Each activity is practiced several times with the physical therapist's focus on proper initiation of movement appropriately followed by strengthening with constant attention to the quality of movement. Once fatigue begins to affect the patient's ability to respond with appropriate initiation and adequate control of the motion, a different demand is placed on the segment (change type or direction of contraction), or the treatment is progressed to the next activity.

• At the conclusion of Intervention 5, the components of gait (with emphasis on stance of the left LE), have been trained in isolation in both non-weightbearing and weightbearing positions and have been practiced using a therapist-controlled weight shifting and stepping activity. The patient is now ready for all components to be taken back into the whole activity of gait (criterion skill), and the treatment session *must* conclude with gait training emphasizing the integration of all the components worked on throughout the session (*whole task training*). The therapist's role providing MCs, resistance, and VCs decreases in favor of active, independent practice of the functional skill focused on during that treatment session.

• Practice sequences where elements of a task are broken down into component parts (e.g., initiation of movement, weight shifting and weight acceptance, stepping strategies), are always followed by practice of the task in its entirety as an integrated whole to optimize motor learning.

Rationale for the Sequencing of Activities Within This Treatment Session

• Several clinical reasoning frameworks were utilized in this treatment session. From a perspective of principles of therapeutic exercise, the interventions began in positions with a large BOS and low COM and progressed to positions with a smaller BOS and higher COM. Initially, focus was on one movement (pelvis) and progressed to greater degrees of freedom and number of joints involved when the LE was added to the activity. From a task-oriented approach, the session broke the task (gait) into its components, worked on the components, and then put the components back together into the whole task; whole task practice is a crucial component of facilitating improved functional task performance. From the perspective of motor task requirements and a developmental approach, the treatment sessions followed a progression from sidelying to standing and worked on proximal stability for improved distal mobility. It included mobility activities, progressed to stability and controlled mobility, and concluded with a skill level activity.

• Across all activities the physical therapist uses appropriate verbal and manual cues, repetition, and feedback to augment treatment and promote motor learning. Progression is to active, independent practice without verbal and manual cues.

Suggestions for Treatment Progression Within the Episode of Care

Assuming that the patient responded well to this treatment session, the focus of subsequent sessions would be as follows:

1. Combination of pelvis and scapula patterns (mass flexion and elongation patterns and reciprocal scapula/pelvis patterns) for improved trunk control during functional activities and improved unilateral and contralateral reciprocity for all functional tasks

2. Focus on swing phase, similar to this session, now that the patient has improved control of stance and therefore has better dynamic stability and improved balanced to work on swing

3. Similar sessions can be used to improve motor control on the right LE.

Independent of the focus of a specific treatment session, all sessions should have a:

• A focus that connects to the patient's short- and long-term goals

- A specific functional activity the session is aiming to improve, that is, improved walking
- Pre- and posttest that will demonstrate to the patient and therapist that the activities worked on have indeed had an effect on a task that is relevant to the patient and to achievement of identified goals
- A functional training component at the end of each session so that gains in mobility, stability, or controlled mobility are placed back into the context of the criterion functional skill, that is, improved walking
- Home exercise program (HEP) that reinforces, through repetition, the gains made in each session; use of an activity log to document practice times and outcomes

Plan for Treatment Session 2	
Activity Limitations Being Addressed in This Treatment Session.	Assuming that the previous treatment session was successful, the patient's gait will demonstrate improved weight shift and weight acceptance onto the left LE, leading to increased stance time with pelvic posterior depression and hip extension on the left LE. Additional gait deviations include: • Swing phase of left LE is initiated with posterior pelvic retraction demonstrating absent dissociation between the pelvis and the trunk or the pelvis and the hip • Absent trunk counterrotation with decreased reciprocal arm swing • Wide BOS • Decreased dynamic balance
The Focus of This Treatment Session	This treatment session will focus on dynamic trunk control for improved dissociation between left scapula and left pelvis throughout the gait cycle and improved swing of the left LE.
Functional Pre- and Posttest(s) for This Treatment Session to Be Performed at the Beginning and End of the Treatment Session	• Observation of rolling for dissociation of trunk, pelvis, and left LE • Observation of patient's ability to clear the foot when stepping up onto a step • Observational gait analysis focusing on quality of left LE swing phase

Treatment Session 2 Interventions

Intervention 1

Patient Position: right sidelying
Activity: left mass trunk flexion pattern (left scapula anterior depression and left pelvis anterior elevation)
Technique: rhythmic initiation and COI[7,8]
Manual Contact/Facilitation/Input: MCs for anterior depression of the left scapula (midline of the rib cage and inferior to coracoid process) and anterior elevation of the left pelvis (lateral, superior and slightly anterior iliac crest) begin with passive facilitation of the mass flexion pattern from a starting position of mass elongation (scapula posterior elevation and pelvis posterior depression). The patient is instructed to assist with the mass flexion pattern; manual input progresses from passive to active assistive to resisted as the patient increases active control of the activity. To promote increased motor output of the trunk into mass flexion, the activity will progress to COI[7,8] as follows:
- A prolonged hold facilitated at end-range mass flexion
- Followed by a slow eccentric lengthening through part of the range
- Then concentric contraction back into full mass flexion
- Continuing to eccentric lengthening through a larger range
- Again back to a concentric pull toward mass flexion

This activity will continue until the patient is able to control eccentric lengthening into full mass elongation followed by a concentric contraction through the full range of mass flexion.
Rationale: The treatment session begins with a mass trunk pattern to increase motor output to the trunk and to promote irradiation between the left scapula and the left pelvis with an emphasis on assuring that both scapula and pelvis are able to move on a dynamically stable trunk. Rhythmic initiation is used first to teach the proper motion and to assure that the patient can initiate motion of both components efficiently and with proper timing. Once his ability to initiate this pattern is established, the emphasis changes to COI[7,8] for continued strengthening and improved eccentric control.

Intervention 2

Patient Position: right sidelying
Activity: left mass trunk flexion pattern and mass elongation pattern
Technique: dynamic (isotonic) reversals
Manual Contact/Facilitation/Input: MCs for anterior depression of the left scapula (midline of the rib cage and inferior to coracoid process) and anterior elevation of the left pelvis (lateral, superior and slightly anterior iliac crest) will begin by resisting mass flexion from the beginning of the range. MCs will change to resist posterior elevation of the left scapula (superior and slightly posterior to the acromion) and posterior depression of

the left pelvis (inferior ischial tuberosity) into full range of mass elongation. MCs will alternate to facilitate/resist movement into mass trunk flexion followed by mass trunk elongation.

Rationale: The treatment session progresses to a reversal between mass trunk flexion and mass trunk elongation to begin to challenge the patient's ability to reverse directions, to assure that the patient has the ability to initiate movement of the left scapula and left pelvis in both patterns within that diagonal, to promote strength in mass elongation and continue to strengthen mass flexion, and to improve coordination.

INTERVENTION 3

Patient Position: right sidelying

Activity: left scapula posterior depression with reciprocal left pelvis anterior elevation

Technique: COI[7,8] followed by dynamic (isotonic) reversals

Manual Contact/Facilitation/Input: MCs for left scapula posterior depression (inferior and medial border of the inferior angle of the scapula) and left pelvis anterior elevation (lateral, superior and slightly anterior iliac crest) begin by passively positioning the patient at the end range of each pattern (left scapula posterior depression and left pelvis anterior elevation, reciprocal patterns) and facilitating an end-range hold to maximize motor unit output of both components in a reciprocal pattern in preparation for gait. Once an adequate contraction at end range is obtained, the activity progresses to eccentric lengthening followed by concentric shortening allowing increasing ROM with each repetition until the patient is asked to move into scapula posterior depression and pelvis anterior elevation reciprocally from the beginning of the range with proper timing and coordination.

Rationale: The treatment progresses from mass trunk patterns to reciprocal trunk patterns given that functional movements involve reciprocity. This reciprocal combination replicates the swing phase of the left LE with reciprocal arm swing and trunk counterrotation in a stable sidelying position.

INTERVENTION 4

Patient Position: sitting and scooting

Activity: weight shifting side to side with pelvis anterior elevation and anterior weight shift emphasizing dissociated forward scooting in a chair

Technique: rhythmic initiation

Manual Contact/Facilitation/Input: Manual contact should begin bilaterally on pelvis (lateral, superior and slightly anterior iliac crest) facilitating proper weight shift side to side to assure unweighting of one side for proper forward scooting. Once proper weight shifting is facilitated, the manual contact can shift to assist and then resist pelvis anterior elevation of the unweighted side with a lift and anterior glide of the LE. The activity

is repeated side to side and can progress to resistance of pelvis anterior elevation and the LE anterior glide as the patient develops increased control and improved dissociation of the trunk and pelvis.

Rationale: The seated position provides a large BOS on which the patient can begin to experience weight shifting to one side with pelvis anterior elevation on the other side. It is a progression from a dependent sidelying position but not as challenging as a standing position given that it involves less degrees of freedom.

INTERVENTION 5

Patient Position: standing in stride position with right foot forward and left foot back in parallel bars

Activity: weight shifting forward to the right LE with a high step taken by the left LE. The therapist assures that the patient demonstrates adequate alignment and control of the right LE in stance. Appropriate resistance is applied to swing of left LE while it is taken into a high step with the hip moving beyond 90 degrees of flexion. Emphasis is placed on proper anterior elevation of the swing left LE with proper posterior depression of the stance right LE.

Technique: appropriate resistance to left pelvis anterior elevation and left LE flexion/adduction/external rotation (FLEX/ADD/ER) during swing

Manual Contact/Facilitation/Input: Manual input, in the form of appropriate resistance, is applied to left pelvis anterior elevation with approximation applied to the right pelvis and LE assuring dynamic stability through the right LE. The therapist's manual contact applies resistance to left pelvis anterior elevation and left LE flexion for swing. It is important to ensure the left hip is brought higher than 90 degrees of flexion, invoking the influence of the cross-extension reflex further facilitating motor output to both LEs. During this activity the therapist must assure that the stance leg is guarded appropriately to prevent buckling or hyperextension as the patient fatigues.

Rationale: Progressing this treatment session to a standing position now allows all the components practiced in sidelying and in sitting to be combined into the standing position where the patient is required to control stance on the right LE while once again bringing the left pelvis into anterior elevation for forward progression. Focus is on dynamic stability of the trunk with appropriate arm swing, necessary components for improved balance and increased efficiency of gait.

General Comments

• As stated following the initial treatment session, it is crucial that the components of gait addressed throughout the treatment session be integrated back into gait (criterion skill), allowing for practice of the whole task (parts-to-whole training). Physical therapy interventions must focus on improving functional skills; thus all treatment sessions must conclude with the practice of the whole task with less therapist input to promote learning and independent control of the functional task. In addition, a HEP aimed at emphasizing and reinforcing the functional task addressed during treatment is a crucial element of the POC.

Rationale for the Sequencing of Activities Within This Treatment Session

The sequencing of this treatment session allowed for practice of component parts of the task (left scapula posterior depression, left pelvis anterior elevation and left LE FLEX/ADD/ER) before the components were combined for practicing the whole task (gait with emphasis on left LE swing). A developmental progression moving from sidelying to sitting and later to standing and gait was also utilized, with treatment beginning in a more stable position with a larger BOS and lower COM and progressing to the highest functional position of standing and walking. Treatment was initiated with more passive activities and progressed to independent practice with less therapist input and more independent control by the patient.

Suggestions for Treatment Progression Within the Episode of Care

The two initial treatment sessions proposed for this patient addressed (A) the stance phase of gait to promote a stable BOS and improved trunk control and dynamic stability; and (B) the swing phase of gait to improve trunk dissociation and gait efficiency. Assuming that these interventions were successful, future treatment sessions can progress to ambulation on different level surfaces such as stairs and improved endurance. Continued gait training for decreasing BOS and improving balance would be indicated. Once the components of gait have been facilitated, gait training on a treadmill may be indicated for increased automaticity and independent control of gait. Specific focus on UE function would also be indicated.

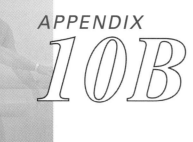

Brief Overview of Locomotor Training Using a Body Weight Support System and a Treadmill for a Patient With Spinal Cord Injury (Case Study 3)

Elizabeth Ardolino, PT, MS; Elizabeth Watson, PT, DPT, NCS; Andrea Behrman, PT, PhD; Susan Harkema, PhD; and Mary Schmidt-Read, PT, DPT, MS

Case Study 3 is presented on p.337.

Conventional gait-training interventions after SCI focus on increasing independence by using compensatory methods to address deficits in strength, motor control, balance, and sensation. Typical gait-training goals for patients with SCI address compensation for paresis or paralysis using braces and assistive devices. Locomotor training (LT) using a BWS system and a treadmill (TM) is an intervention based on the activity-dependent plasticity and motor learning capacity of the spinal cord.[1–4]

A network of spinal interneurons process and integrate both ascending sensory input and descending supraspinal input to generate the motor output of walking.[5] With diminished supraspinal drive after incomplete SCI, LT targets the promotion of locomotor-specific input to the neural axis to promote locomotor output below the level of the lesion.[6] Intense repetitive and task-specific practice of walking (through LT) is aimed at fostering neurological recovery of balance and gait as well as improving the overall health and quality of life for patients with SCI and other neurological disorders.

Locomotor training is based on the following four principles:[1,7]

1. **Maximize LE weightbearing.** Patients are encouraged to bear as much body weight on the LEs as often as possible, while decreasing the amount of weightbearing through their UEs.
2. **Optimize the use of sensory cues.** Locomotor training utilizes appropriate manual facilitation from therapists to optimize the quality of the stepping pattern, while walking at or near preinjury walking speeds.
3. **Optimize kinematics for each motor task.** Locomotor training focuses on upright posture, proper pelvic rotation, and appropriate interlimb coordination for walking. Patients initiate stepping by beginning in a stride

position, with hip extension of the trailing limb. Emphasis is placed on the use of standard kinematics for sit-to-stand transitions, standing, and other tasks.
4. **Maximize recovery and minimize compensation.** Patients are assisted, when needed, to perform movements using typical spatial-temporal components to accomplish a task. Performance of tasks using compensatory strategies (i.e., momentum and leverage) is minimized. Patients attempt to accomplish a task while using the least restrictive assistive devices, without orthoses, and as little physical assistance as possible.

Locomotor training using a BWS system and a TM consists of three main components: *step training, overground examination,* and *community integration.*

Step Training

The *step training* environment includes a BWS system placed over a TM, with physical therapists and physical therapist assistants (trainers) providing hands-on manual assistance. The BWS system and the TM provide an ideal environment for safe practice of the task of walking. Step training consists of four components: *stand retraining, stand adaptability, step retraining,* and *step adaptability.*

- **Stand retraining.** The purpose of stand retraining is to examine how much body weight the patient's LEs can support. The goal is to decrease the body weight support to the lowest amount possible, with the trainers (who have undergone specific training in the techniques of LT) providing as much assistance as needed for the patient to maintain an appropriate upright standing posture.
- **Stand adaptability.** The purpose of stand adaptability is to examine the body weight parameters necessary to maintain independence at different body segments (e.g., trunk, pelvis, right knee, left knee, right ankle, left ankle) during both static and dynamic standing.

- **Step retraining.** The purpose of step retraining is to retrain the nervous system's ability to walk by establishing a kinematically correct stepping pattern at the lowest possible amount of BWS and at normal walking speed (2.2 to 2.8 mph [0.98 to 1.3 m/s]).
- **Step adaptability.** The purpose of step adaptability is to promote independent control of each body segment for the task of walking. Initially, the patient will require more BWS at a slower speed, with gradual progression to less BWS and faster speeds until independence is achieved.

Overground Examination

The purpose of the *overground examination* is to determine the carryover of skills acquired during step training on the TM to the overground progression without BWS. In this component, the therapist examines the patient's ability to perform functional mobility, such as transfers, bed mobility, standing, and ambulation, without the use of assistive devices, braces, or compensations. Goals for the next step training session and for community integration are identified based on the overground performance. The therapist and patient identify the factor(s) limiting successful independent ambulation and then use the information to establish new training goals.

Community Integration

Community integration focuses on the application of LT principles in the patient's home and community environment.

The therapist selects the least restrictive assistive device that allows safe and independent standing and walking. The goal is to increase the amount of weightbearing in more open environments.

Because the ultimate goal of LT is to promote maximal recovery of the nervous system, patients often require an extended course of treatment as compared with more conventional outpatient episodes of care. It is not unusual for patients to need in excess of 40 sessions of LT. Following discharge from acute inpatient rehabilitation, patients typically start by attending LT outpatient sessions five times per week and then, as they advance, progress down to four and then three times per week.

REFERENCES

1. Harkema, S, Behrman, A, and Barbeau, H. Locomotor Training Principles and Practice. New York, Oxford University Press; 2011.
2. Harkema, SJ, Hillyer, J, and Schmidt-Read, M, et al. Locomotor training: as a treatment of spinal cord injury and in the progression of neurologic rehabilitation. Arch Phys Med Rehabil 2012; 93(9):1588–1597.
3. Barbeau, H, and Blunt, R. A novel interactive locomotor approach using body weight support to retrain gait in spastic paretic subjects. In Wernig, A (ed): Plasticity of Motorneuronal Connections. Restorative Neurology, Vol. 5. Amsterdam, Elsevier, 1991, 461.
4. Barbeau, H, Nadeau, S, and Garneau, C. Physical determinants, emerging concepts, and training approaches in gait of individuals with spinal cord injury. J Neurotrauma 2006; 23:571 (review).
5. Harkema, SJ. Plasticity of interneuronal networks of the functionally isolated human spinal cord. Brain Res Rev 2005; 57:255.
6. Edgerton, VR, Niranjala, JK, Tillakaratne, AJ, et al. Plasticity of the spinal neural circuitry after injury. Annu Rev Neurosci 2004; 27:145.
7. Behrman, AL, Lawless-Dixon, AR, Davis, SB, et al. Locomotor training progression and outcomes after incomplete spinal cord injury. Phys Ther 2005; 85:1356.

11 Interventions to Improve Upper Extremity Skills

Sharon A. Gutman, PhD, OTR, FAOTA, and Marianne Mortera, PhD, OTR

This chapter is written from the perspective of the practicing occupational therapist and addresses how impairment of the upper extremity (UE) is treated within the context of daily living skills. The chapter is designed to provide the physical therapist with information to (1) provide effective interventions to improve UE function, (2) understand the unique contributions of the occupational therapist in UE functional skill training, and (3) communicate with occupational therapy colleagues about comprehensive interdisciplinary patient management.

Task Analysis Guidelines

Before planning treatment, the therapist performs a task or activity analysis. Task analysis is the breakdown of activities into their component parts to understand the demands of the activity and identify patient deficits that hinder successful participation in the activity (Box 11.1). Therapists consider three primary components in the activity analysis process: patient body function performance skills, activity demands, and environmental factors. *Patient body function performance skills* refers to the anatomical and physiological components necessary to participate in the activity; the skills are further broken down into the following skill categories: *sensory, perceptual, neurological, musculoskeletal, cognitive,* and *psychosocial*. This chapter focuses on the neurological and musculoskeletal skills needed to perform activities of daily living (ADL).

Activity demands refers to the requirements embedded in each step of the activity. *Environmental factors* are the physical characteristics of the environment that may impede or promote performance and the social and/or cultural values and beliefs that may influence a patient's ability and desire to perform specific ADL. Once an analysis of all three areas is complete, the therapist can modify the activity and/or the environment to enhance the patient's ability to participate. To improve patient performance, therapists can

---

BOX 11.1 The Process of Activity Analysis

Patient Case Sample

The patient is a 72-year-old woman status post cerebrovascular accident (CVA) with a right parietal lobe lesion and resultant underlying impairments in sensation, visual perception, motor functioning, cognition, and psychosocial skills. The following are specific underlying **body function performance skill** impairments.

- **Sensory:** impaired proprioception, kinesthesia, and stereognosis in left UE
- **Perceptual:** left visual and somatosensory neglect noted; exhibits extinction upon double simultaneous stimulation to both UEs
- **Musculoskeletal:** moderate left shoulder weakness; moderate flexor synergy elicited with left UE overhead and side reach; minimal gross grasp and weak trunk control when seated
- **Cognitive:** decreased attention and concentration, able to follow two- to three-step commands, has moderate difficulty with judgment, awareness, and insight; requires frequent prompts to initiate activities
- **Psychosocial:** appears depressed and demonstrates emotional lability; appears to lack motivation to participate in treatment

The therapist considers the following questions:

1. How will the above impairments affect or limit the patient's performance during each ADL task?
2. How will each component of a given ADL task be affected by a combination of impaired performance skill areas?

For example, while engaged in functional activities the patient may have difficulty with the following:

- **Sensory:** During bathing the patient may have difficulty holding a washcloth in the more affected hand without visually compensating for poor tactile sensation and proprioception. Even with the ability to grasp a washcloth as motor function returns, poor tactile sensation and proprioception may make motor function effortful or inefficient during functional hand use in ADL.
- **Perceptual:** Left visual neglect may be demonstrated when the patient ignores the food on the left side of the plate. Extinction may be observed when the patient attempts to cut food bilaterally and the more affected hand starts losing grip on the fork handle as the less affected hand grasps the knife.

BOX 11.1 The Process of Activity Analysis (continued)

- **Musculoskeletal:** The patient may not be able to pull the neck of an overhead nightgown past 90 degrees of shoulder flexion; when attempting this movement, the patient may experience moderately increased hypertonicity at the shoulder and elbow.
- **Cognitive:** The patient may be easily distracted and require frequent VCs to attend to ADL such as brushing teeth. The patient may also present with decreased safety awareness and poor judgment by failing to lock wheelchair brakes during transfers.
- **Psychosocial:** The patient states that she does not want to brush her teeth or get out of bed to participate in ADL training. Frequent encouragement to participate in ADL is often needed to enhance patient motivation.

Activity Demands
The therapist identifies the specific task components or steps of the activity and considers the following questions:

1. What are the specific steps of the activity?
2. How do the underlying impairments affect actual patient performance and what can be done to either

use the activity or the task components of the activity to improve upon the impaired areas?
3. What compensatory strategies can be incorporated to compensate for deficits?

Environmental Considerations
- Physical
- Sociocultural

The therapist considers the following questions:

1. What physical characteristics of the environment may obstruct the patient's performance?
2. What social and/or cultural values and beliefs does the patient hold that may impede her ability to participate in the activity?

Analysis of the above allows the therapist to modify the activity and the environment to improve the patient's performance in specific ADL.

---

also use specific interventions designed to enhance the patient's neurological and/or musculoskeletal function.

Required Body Function Performance (Lead-up) Skills

The following are required body function performance skills, or lead-up skills, for the activities of self-feeding, hygiene, and dressing.

- **Trunk postural stability.** Appropriate upper and lower trunk stability (i.e., upper trunk extension and abdominal stabilization) is essential to maintain an upright-seated position (Fig. 11.1). A neutral pelvis position and hip abduction enhance lower trunk stability. An upright-seated position is necessary for normal UE movement patterns. If the patient is in standing position, proper pelvic and lower extremity (LE) alignment should be encouraged to provide an adequate and stable base of support (BOS). In standing, the pelvis should be properly aligned to encourage a neutral position and upper trunk extension. Standing during performance of ADL may be challenging for the patient, and the therapist may need to provide tactile or verbal cues to help maintain proper standing position.
- **Shoulder stability and mobility.** Cocontraction of the shoulder girdle muscles is needed to support distal UE movement in space during reaching activities, as in reaching for and retrieving utensils for feeding, grooming, or dressing (Fig. 11.2).
- **Elbow stability and mobility.** Cocontraction of the elbow musculature to support distal UE movement in space during reaching is also a required lead-up skill (Fig. 11.3). For example, elbow stability is needed to grasp a drinking glass securely or hold a toothbrush in one's mouth. Elbow

flexion and extension are needed to pull down a shirt over one's pants.
- **Wrist stability and mobility.** The ability to maintain the wrist in a neutral or extended position to allow for grasp and prehension patterns (described below) is required in most ADL (Fig. 11.4). For example, maintenance of the wrist in an extended position

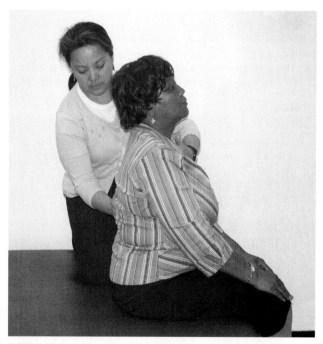

FIGURE 11.1 Postural trunk stability is a necessary lead-up skill for self-feeding. It allows for normal UE movement patterns to occur, and upright posture of head and trunk prevents aspiration of food items.

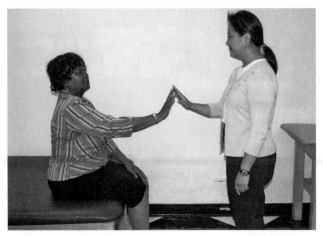

FIGURE 11.2 Shoulder stability and mobility are lead-up skills for self-feeding required for reaching and retrieving utensils and food items. Here the patient practices reaching using the therapist's hand as a target.

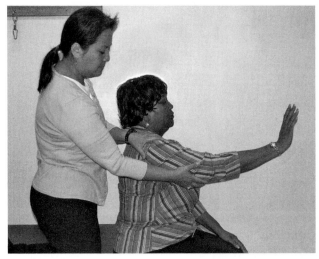

FIGURE 11.3 Elbow stability and mobility are necessary to support distal UE movement in space; they are lead-up skills for self-feeding.

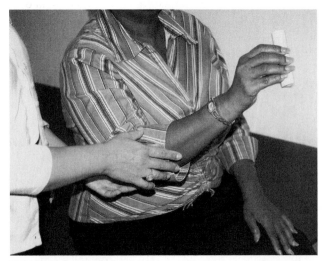

FIGURE 11.4 Wrist stability and mobility allow for grasp and prehension patterns required for self-feeding.

(approximately 20–30 degrees of wrist extension) is required to grasp a milk container and pour the liquid into a glass, manipulate buttons on a shirt, or manage a zipper on a clothing item.

- **Gross grasp.** *Gross grasp* refers to a grip that places an object in contact with the palm and palmar surface of the digits. Gross thumb and finger flexion and extension are needed to grasp and release large food items (such as a sandwich) and drinking glasses (Fig. 11.5), stabilize a bar of soap in one's hand during bathing, or secure a bottle of mouthwash when rinsing after brushing teeth.
- **Prehension patterns.** *Prehension* refers to a hand position that allows for finger and thumb opposition and manipulation of objects. A variety of prehension patterns contribute to hand function and the execution of daily living skills. For example, with *palmar prehension* (also referred to as a three jaw chuck or tripod grasp), the thumb opposes one or more fingers (e.g., the index and long fingers) to retrieve a small object. In *lateral prehension* the thumb and the radial side of the index and long fingers meet, as if holding a key. Prehension patterns are required to hold utensils in feeding—for example, a fork handle (Fig. 11.6), knife, or a mug handle. Prehension patterns are also needed for ADL such as holding a key using lateral prehension (Fig. 11.7). Palmar prehension is used for retrieving small food items such as pretzel nuggets (Fig. 11.8).
- **Thumb and finger manipulation.** The fine motor movements of thumb and finger manipulation are needed for dynamic manipulation of small utensils and food items, such as placing a straw in a glass, tearing open sweetener packets (Fig. 11.9), and opening the plastic wrap on crackers. Thumb and finger fine motor movements are also needed in grooming and dressing tasks, such as tying shoelaces, buttoning a shirt, and flossing teeth.

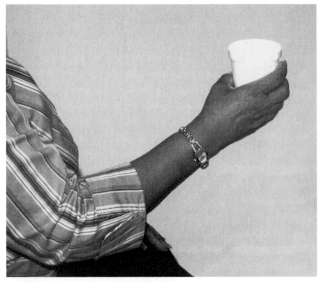

FIGURE 11.5 Gross grasp is required to take hold of and release larger food items and drinking glasses during self-feeding.

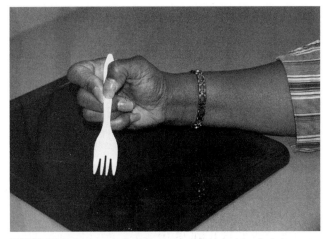

FIGURE 11.6 Prehension pattern is used to hold a fork.

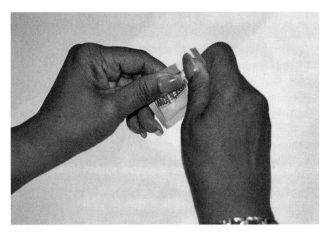

FIGURE 11.9 Thumb and finger manipulation used to open a sweetener packet is a lead-up skill for self-feeding.

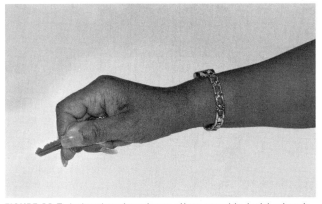

FIGURE 11.7 Lateral prehension pattern used to hold a key is a lead-up skill for self-feeding.

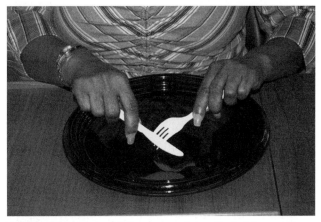

FIGURE 11.10 Bilateral UE movement used to hold an eating utensil in each hand is a lead-up skill for self-feeding.

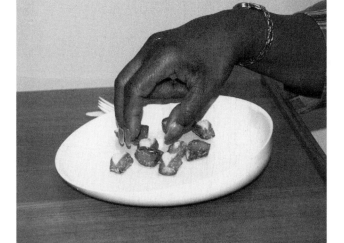

FIGURE 11.8 Palmar prehension pattern used to pick up pretzel nuggets is a lead-up skill for self-feeding.

donning socks, placing toothpaste on a toothbrush, and positioning contact lenses in one's eyes are all examples of bilateral UE movements essential to common ADL performance.

The UE functions needed for ADL tasks depend on a progression of lead-up skills. These skills must be addressed in a specific sequence because each depends on a prerequisite skill in an ordered progression. Adequate trunk stability is a key prerequisite for all UE skills. Once trunk stability has been established, UE skills should be addressed in the following order:

- Shoulder stability and mobility
- Elbow stability and mobility
- Wrist stability and mobility
- Gross grasp and prehension patterns
- Thumb and finger manipulation
- Bilateral UE movements

Bilateral UE integration—the integration of both UEs in coordinated movement to achieve a targeted task—is the highest skill level required for ADL and thus is the final skill addressed in the sequence.

- **Bilateral UE movement.** Two-handed or bilateral UE movement is required for most self-feeding, grooming, and dressing skills. Cutting food with a knife and fork (Fig. 11.10), applying butter to a roll, buttoning a coat,

Activity Analysis of ADL Tasks

Below are three examples of abbreviated activity analysis processes. These examples illustrate how the activities of self-feeding, hygiene, and dressing are analyzed with respect to neurological and musculoskeletal body function performance skills of the UE, activity demands, and environmental factors.

Self-Feeding

Activity Demands and Task Components

1. The patient must be seated upright at a table (or bed with lap tray) with meal, utensils, and drinking glass positioned in front. Adaptive equipment is used as needed. The pelvis and LEs should be properly aligned to encourage a neutral pelvis position with hip abduction when seated because proper pelvic support is necessary for adequate upper-body alignment during self-feeding (Fig. 11.11).

2. The UEs are positioned to encourage shoulder stabilization through cocontraction of the shoulder girdle muscles. Shoulder stabilization is necessary to facilitate the normal movement pattern of forward reach with elbow extension and wrist stabilization so that functional distal hand movements can occur (Fig. 11.12).

3. Food is brought to the mouth via gross grasp (i.e., combined thumb and finger flexion) if finger foods are used (Fig. 11.13). When utensils are used, food is brought to the mouth using prehension patterns to grasp utensil handles (see Fig. 11.6). The normal movement pattern for gross grasp and prehension

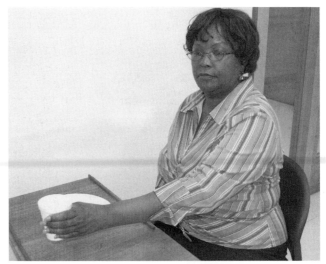

FIGURE 11.12 Shoulder stabilization facilitates the normal movement pattern of forward reach with elbow extension and wrist stabilization so that functional distal hand movements can occur.

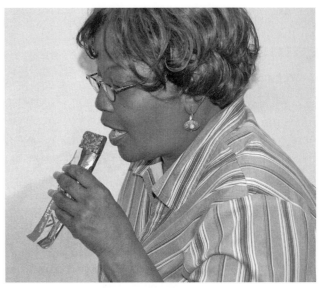

FIGURE 11.13 Food is brought to the mouth via gross grasp for finger feeding (finger foods).

involves finger and thumb flexion/extension patterns to grasp and release items.

4. The hand is brought back and forth from plate to mouth. Owing to the frequency and duration of this movement pattern in self-feeding (i.e., shoulder, elbow, and wrist stabilization against gravity), the patient's endurance and tolerance for this movement pattern must be monitored for fatigue.

5. Liquids are retrieved from the table using a gross grasp for drinking glasses and prehension patterns for mugs with handles and teacups. These patterns allow liquids to be brought to the mouth and returned to the table (Fig. 11.14).

6. Two-handed cutting (Fig. 11.15) and manipulation of food require bilateral UE integration.

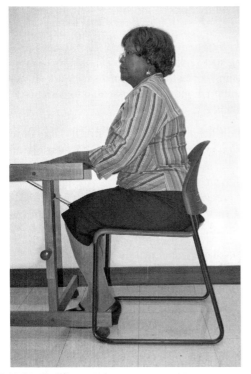

FIGURE 11.11 Upright-seated posture The pelvis and LEs should be properly aligned to encourage a neutral position or slight anterior tilt of pelvis and hip abduction.

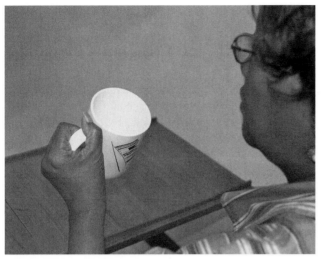

FIGURE 11.14 Liquids are retrieved from the table using gross grasp for glasses and prehension patterns for cups with handles.

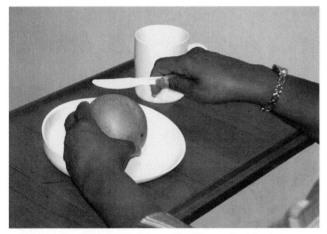

FIGURE 11.15 Bilateral UE integration is required for two-handed cutting and manipulation of foods. The patient holds the knife with one hand and handles the food item in the opposite hand.

Environmental Factors

• The patient must be able to maintain an upright-seated position in a chair or wheelchair.
• The table must be at the patient's midtrunk level.
• The table surface must be large enough and sufficiently stable to accommodate food items, utensils, and the patient's UEs.
• All food items must be consistent with the patient's dietary, nutritional, religious, and social and cultural preferences and restrictions.

Brushing Teeth
Activity Demands and Task Components
1. The patient must be seated upright or standing at a bathroom sink with toothbrush, toothpaste, removable dental prosthetics (e.g., dentures), and cup positioned

in front. Adaptive equipment is used as needed. The pelvis and LEs should be properly aligned to encourage a neutral pelvis position and hip abduction when seated as proper pelvic support is necessary for adequate upper-body alignment while brushing teeth (see Fig. 11.11). In standing, the patient's feet should be shoulder-width apart with weight evenly distributed over both feet, the pelvis should be in neutral alignment, and the upper trunk in slight extension with head in midline.
2. The UEs are positioned to encourage shoulder stabilization through cocontraction of the shoulder girdle muscles. Shoulder stabilization is necessary to facilitate the normal movement pattern of forward reach with elbow extension and wrist stabilization so that functional distal hand movements can occur (see Fig. 11.12).
3. Bilateral hand use is required to remove the toothpaste cap and apply paste to the brush. Gross grasp is used to hold the toothpaste in one hand, and palmar prehension is needed to unscrew the cap with the opposite hand. The dominant hand then grasps the toothpaste and applies it to the brush as the brush is supported in the opposite hand using lateral prehension. Bilateral proximal shoulder and elbow stabilization are also required together with slight wrist extension to support distal grasp and prehension in both hands.
4. To manipulate the toothbrush inside the mouth and brush all tooth surfaces, proximal shoulder and elbow stabilization are required with wrist stabilization and rotation to support distal hand use. Owing to the frequency and duration of this movement pattern when brushing teeth (i.e., shoulder, elbow, and wrist stabilization against gravity), the patient's endurance and tolerance for this movement pattern must be monitored for fatigue.
5. Shoulder forward reach, elbow extension, wrist stabilization, and palmar prehension are required to turn the faucet lever to activate the water flow. Shoulder forward reach, elbow flexion/extension, wrist stabilization, and gross grasp of the cup are required to fill the cup with water, bring it to the mouth, and return it to the sink top (see Fig. 11.14). To release water from the mouth into the sink, slight neck and trunk flexion are needed. Shoulder forward reach, elbow extension, wrist stabilization, and palmar prehension are required to rinse the toothbrush upon completion of brushing. To retrieve a towel from the sink top and wipe the mouth laterally, shoulder forward reach, elbow flexion/extension, wrist stabilization, and gross grasp are required.

Environmental Factors

• The patient must be able to either maintain an upright-seated position in a chair or wheelchair or maintain an upright stance and standing balance at a bathroom sink.
• The sink surface must be sufficiently sized and stable to accommodate items for brushing the teeth. If the sink is unstable, a grab bar must be present to provide UE support and balance if needed in standing.

Donning a Pullover Sweater

Activity Demands and Task Components

1. The patient must be seated in a chair or wheelchair or positioned in unsupported sitting at the edge of a bed or mat. The pelvis and LEs should be properly aligned to encourage a neutral pelvis position and hip abduction with feet flat on the floor because proper pelvic support is necessary for adequate trunk alignment during upper-body dressing (see Fig. 11.11). The upper trunk should be in slight extension with head in midline. Sitting unsupported while performing UE overhead activities will affect the patient's endurance level during dressing, and the patient should be monitored for fatigue.

2. Involvement of the more affected UE in dressing tasks depends on the degree of functional return while the patient uses the less affected limb to perform most task requirements. In this example we describe the use of a more affected UE with initial return of isolated shoulder and elbow movement, weak wrist movement, and limited gross grasp.

3. The patient should attempt to use the more affected UE so that proximal shoulder stabilization is achieved. This can be facilitated by encouraging active shoulder forward reach and gradually progressing to overhead reach against gravity to strengthen the proximal musculature needed to support elbow and hand motions in space. Shoulder stabilization is necessary to facilitate the normal movement pattern of forward reach with elbow extension and wrist stabilization so that functional distal hand movements can occur (see Fig. 11.12). Donning a pullover sweater over one's head requires sufficient strength and endurance of the shoulder musculature to maintain both UEs in an overhead position. Because of this activity's demands, the patient's endurance level must be taken into consideration and monitored. The patient may quickly fatigue if the demand to raise both UEs over the head is too difficult. If the more affected UE presents with significant shoulder weakness, overhead UE use may be too taxing.

4. Bilateral gross grasp, slight wrist extension, elbow flexion, and shoulder overhead reach are needed to grasp the pullover sweater and pull the neck opening over the head. The patient should insert the less affected UE through the corresponding sleeve and then position the more affected UE through the opposing sleeve using shoulder forward reach and elbow extension. If possible, the patient should use bilateral gross grasp and elbow extension to pull the bottom sweater edge over the anterior trunk. Additionally, the patient should be encouraged to use shoulder internal rotation and extension, elbow extension, and gross grasp of the more affected UE to pull the sweater down over the posterior trunk.

Environmental Factors

• As stated above, the patient must be able to maintain an upright-seated position in a chair or wheelchair or edge of bed or mat and maintain good pelvic and trunk control. Both the surface on which the patient is sitting and the amount of trunk or back support will affect how well the patient is able to maintain good pelvic and trunk alignment.

• The seat height of the chair or wheelchair, bed, or mat must allow the patient to sit with both feet flat on the floor to encourage proper LE and pelvic alignment.

• If sitting balance becomes unstable in unsupported sitting, or if the patient experiences progressive trunk fatigue with UE overhead reach, adequate mat or bed space around the patient should be provided in the event that the patient lists toward the more affected side. The therapist should be seated in front of the patient and guard the more affected side to maintain safety.

Clinical Note: Standardized outcome measures to assess UE function have been developed often for specific populations or groups of patients. Examples include the Modified Ashworth Scale, Disability of the Arm, Shoulder and Hand Questionnaire, Motor Assessment Scale, Fugl-Meyer Assessment of Motor Recovery After Stroke, Purdue Pegboard Test, and the Jebsen-Taylor Hand Function Test. A description of these outcome measures together with their indicated use is presented in Table 11.1.

Treatment Strategies and Considerations

The following treatment approaches addressing UE function within the context of the various ADL tasks detailed above are described: *neuromuscular facilitation, proprioceptive neuromuscular facilitation (PNF), compensatory training, motor learning,* and *modified constraint-induced therapy.* The discussion of each approach explains how the therapist can use the intervention to facilitate UE function within the context of ADL. The therapist can also use these approaches to promote UE lead-up skills needed to perform ADL.

Therapists use and sequence the treatment approaches in varying combinations depending on patient needs and UE function. An important consideration when deciding when and how to use these approaches is whether the patient has appropriate UE voluntary movement. Patients who demonstrate sufficient recovery of voluntary movement may not benefit from neuromuscular facilitation or an intensive hands-on approach. Rather, such patients benefit more from direct engagement in ADL retraining. Neuromuscular facilitation and PNF are particularly useful for patients who require development or enhancement of lead-up skills (e.g., patients who demonstrate poor shoulder stabilization; patients with poor reaching, pushing, grasping, and prehension patterns; or patients with poor bilateral UE use owing to movement patterns impaired by increased or decreased tone, weakness, and movement decomposition).

TABLE 11.1 Outcome Measures of UE Function and Performance

Measure: Modified Ashworth Scale (MAS)

Description: The purpose of the MAS is to assess the degree of spasticity in the affected limbs of patients with central nervous system disorders (e.g., stroke, traumatic brain injury, cerebral palsy). The MAS is a six-level ordinal scale ranging from 0 (no increase in muscle tone) to 5 (limb rigid in flexion or extension).

The therapist moves the patient's limb(s) through a ROM and determines degree of spasticity based on observed response. Administering the MAS takes approximately 5 minutes, depending on number of affected limbs.
Indication: The MAS is intended for children (6–12 years) and adults (18–64 years) with muscle tone disorders secondary to central nervous system lesion.
Reference: Bohannon, RW, and Smith, MB. Interrater reliability of a Modified Ashworth Scale of muscle spasticity. 1987; Phys Ther, 67:206.

Measure: Disability of the Arm, Shoulder and Hand Questionnaire (DASH)
Description: The purpose of the DASH is to evaluate upper limb performance and function in patients with musculoskeletal disorders; the DASH may also be used to monitor changes in upper limb function and performance longitudinally over time. The DASH is a 30-item, 5-point ordinal self-report questionnaire designed to assess UE function relative to joint limitation and physical activity in specific tasks. The assessment requires approximately 10 to 30 minutes to complete. An optional component of the measure assesses high-level physical activity during work, sports, or the performing arts. The *Quick*DASH is a short form of the measure consisting of 10 questions and the optional works/sports/performing arts module.
Indication: The DASH is intended for adults (18–64 years) with a range of orthopedic and neurological disorders affecting the UE.
Reference: Beaton, DE, et al. The DASH (Disabilities of the Arm, Shoulder and Hand) Outcome Measure: what do we know about it now? Hand Ther, 2001; 6:109.

Measure: Motor Assessment Scale (MAS)
Description: The purpose of the MAS is to assess the motor function and recovery of patients with stroke during functional ADL (i.e., bed mobility, sitting balance, ambulation, UE performance, and functional hand activities). The MAS is an eight-item performance-based measure with one additional item assessing muscle tone that is not included in the total score (eight items examine motor function and one item assesses general muscle tone). The assessment can be administered in approximately 15 to 30 minutes and scored using a 7-point ordinal scale (from 0 to 6, with 6 indicating optimal performance). Item scores are summed to provide a possible total score of 48 (with the exception of the muscle tone item). Patients are asked to perform each task three times; the best performance of the three trials is recorded.
Indication: The MAS is intended for adults (18–64 years) and elderly (65+) patients with stroke.
Reference: Carr, JH, et al. Investigation of a new motor assessment scale for stroke patients. Phys Ther, 1985; 65:175.

Measure: Fugl-Meyer Assessment of Motor Recovery after Stroke (FMA)
Description: The purpose of the FMA is to measure recovery in sensorimotor function in patients with hemiplegia secondary to stroke. The assessment is performance-based, contains 226-items, and uses a 3-point ordinal scale (0 = cannot perform, 1 = performs partially, 2 = performs fully) that is divided into five domains: *motor function, sensory function, balance, joint range of motion*, and *joint pain*. The patient performs specific movements in daily activities while standing, seated, or in supine, and reports subjective experience of sensation and pain. Administration requires approximately 30 minutes (a shortened version of the FMA requires approximately 10 minutes). The FMA includes a UE subtest that can be used independently. It contains 33 items, uses a 3-point ordinal scale, and has a possible total score of 66. The UE subtest assesses shoulder, elbow, forearm, wrist, and hand movement. Upper extremity function is specifically assessed for reflex activity and voluntary movement within and outside of synergy patterns. Gross and fine motor UE coordination and speed are also assessed.
Indication: The FMA is intended for adolescents (13–17 years), adults (18–64 years), and elderly (65+) patients who have hemiplegia secondary to stroke.
Reference: Fugl-Meyer, AR, et al. (1975). The post-stroke hemiplegic patient. Scand J Rehabil Med, 1975; 7:13.

Measure: Purdue Pegboard Test (PPBT)
Description: The purpose of the PPBT is to measure fingertip dexterity and gross motor function of the fingers, hand, and arm. The measure was originally developed to aid in the selection of employees for industrial and assembly jobs requiring manual dexterity and coordination but has been used extensively in clinical rehabilitation settings. The PPBT consists of a rectangular board with two vertical lines of holes and four cuplike depressions at the top of the board. Tasks require the patient to retrieve small metal pins from the cups and place them into the holes as quickly as possible. Testing trials are in 30- and 60-second periods. Scores can be obtained for right-hand

(table continues on page 270)

TABLE 11.1 Outcome Measures of UE Function and Performance *(continued)*

pin placement, left-hand pin placement, bilateral-hand pin placement, and bilateral assembly of pins and washers. Full administration of the assessment can take approximately 15 to 30 minutes. Scores are interpreted through comparison to standardized normative data.

Indication: The PPBT is intended for children (6–12 years), adolescents (13–17 years), adults (18–64 years), and elderly (65+) with neurological and orthopedic conditions affecting arm, hand, and finger dexterity and coordination.

Reference: Tiffin, J, and Asher, EJ. The Purdue Pegboard: norms and studies of reliability and validity. J Appl Psychol, 1948; 32:234.

Measure: Jebsen-Taylor Hand Function Test (JTHF)

Description: The JTHF is a standardized norm-based performance test used to examine unilateral hand function in a range of daily activities. Hand performance speed in specific tasks is measured rather than quality of movement. Seven tasks are assessed using the nondominant and dominant hands separately (the nondominant hand should be tested before the dominant hand): writing a short 24-character sentence at third-grade reading level (eliminated for children ages 6–7 years), card turning, retrieving and placing small familiar objects in a container (i.e., coins, paper clips, bottle caps), simulated feeding, stacking checkers, lifting and placing light objects (empty cans), and lifting and placing heavy objects (1-pound cans). Each task is timed and requires approximately 10 seconds. Item and total scores are interpreted through comparison to standardized normative data according to age and sex. Reassessment allows intervention progress to be measured over time. The administration of the JTHF requires approximately 15–20 minutes for both hands.

Indication: The JTHF is intended for children (5–12 years), adolescents (13–19 years), and adults (20–94 years) with hand function deficits secondary to orthopedic or neurological injury or disease.

Reference: Jebsen, RH, et al. An objective and standardized test of hand function. Arch Phys Med Rehabil, 1969; 50:311.

Neuromuscular Facilitation

Neuromuscular facilitation is an important intervention for the development of lead-up skills needed to perform feeding, hygiene, and dressing. Selected components of the intervention are described within the context of facilitating the following lead-up skills: *stabilization, reach, grasp,* and *prehension patterns.*

Stabilization

Joint approximation can be used to promote proximal shoulder stabilization via weightbearing activities. The patient is instructed to bear weight on the affected UE, which is positioned in elbow extension and supported by the therapist (Fig. 11.16) or by another support surface (e.g., a platform mat). Approximation can be used to facilitate shoulder/scapular stabilizers and elbow extensors. Sufficient shoulder stability is required before the patient can achieve dynamic distal movement in space against gravity (required for all ADL skills).

Reach

Once shoulder stabilization is established, reaching is addressed. Reaching can be facilitated using active scapular protraction, shoulder flexion, and elbow extension. The patient is initially instructed to slide the UE (gravity minimized) along a tabletop surface in a forward direction as if reaching for a target food item (Fig. 11.17). When this skill is achieved, the patient can begin to practice the higher-level skill of reaching (against gravity) into space to grasp a glass or bread roll (Fig. 11.18). To facilitate agonist contraction of

the anterior deltoid for forward reach, tapping (quick stretch) over the muscle belly can be incorporated. The muscle contraction that is generated, however, is short lasting. Therefore, resistance may be added to maintain muscle contraction. Once these lead-up skills have been performed, the

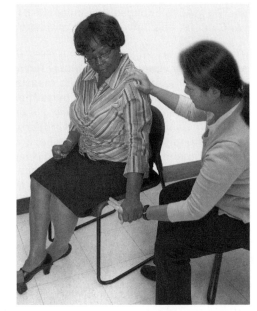

FIGURE 11.16 To enhance UE stabilization, the patient is instructed to bear weight on the more affected UE positioned in elbow extension on a support surface. Support is provided using manual contacts from the therapist. Alternatively, a treatment table or mat surface can be used to support the UE.

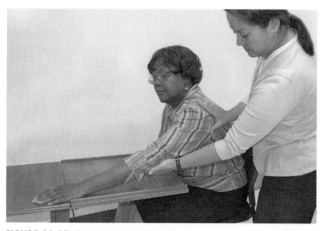

FIGURE 11.17 To facilitate reaching, the patient is instructed to slide the UE (with gravity minimized) along a tabletop as if reaching for a targeted food item.

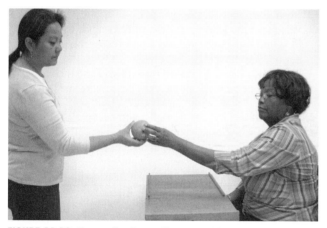

FIGURE 11.18 The patient practices reaching against gravity into space to grasp a food item.

therapist can guide the patient in how to use these skills to perform reaching movements in actual self-feeding, hygiene, and dressing activities.

Grasp and Prehension

An important goal of neuromuscular facilitation is to reduce flexor spasticity and promote extension in patients with UE flexor synergy patterns. For these patients, reduced flexor spasticity in the wrist and fingers is required for grasp and prehension patterns. Functional grasp and prehension patterns involve voluntary active finger and thumb flexion and voluntary active finger, thumb, and wrist extension. Without voluntary grasp and prehension patterns, independence in self-feeding cannot be achieved. Tapping over the respective muscle bellies can facilitate wrist and finger extension; adding resistance to these movements sustains the response. Tapping over the extensor muscles is thought to inhibit the spastic flexor muscles.[1] Once these lead-up skills have been performed, the therapist can guide the patient to practice voluntary wrist and finger extension during a feeding task (e.g., grasp and release of a drinking glass or prehension and

release of small food items, such as a bread roll or cracker). Voluntary wrist and finger extension or gross grasp and release may be practiced when pulling down a pullover sweater.

The Student Practice Activity in Box 11.2 presents a patient example using neuromuscular facilitation.

Clinical Note: When using neuromuscular facilitation techniques, therapists must consistently maintain acute awareness of the patient's quality of UE movement. Compensatory movement patterns should be brought to the patient's attention, and verbal and manual cues should be used to help the patient correct abnormal movement patterns so they do not become learned habits. For example, when attempting forward reach, a patient may compensate with shoulder elevation and abduction rather than appropriate shoulder flexion and scapular protraction. Similarly, patients attempting distal movements may also exhibit excess shoulder movements. Such compensatory movement must be noted immediately and corrected. Correction should begin with verbal and manual cues to offer both auditory and proprioceptive feedback. As the patient begins to demonstrate learning, verbal cues (VCs) should be continued while manual cues are decreased. Eventually, VCs can also be diminished as the patient gains the ability to self-correct inappropriate movement patterns. Practice of desired normal movement patterns should begin with proximal musculature and progress distally as the patient's performance becomes more skilled. Eventually, the practice of both proximal and distal movement patterns can be combined (as they would be in functional activities).

Red Flag: The observation of abnormal movement patterns and the use of compensation strategies in place of appropriate movement may indicate that the patient has been challenged to perform a motor activity that is presently beyond his or her skill level. The range of motion (ROM) or the physical effort required for performing a specific shoulder, elbow, wrist, or hand movement may be too demanding for the patient and could inhibit his or her ability to practice and learn normal movement patterns. In these situations, the therapist should immediately intervene to modify the task to provide a therapeutic challenge that is more appropriate. Increased spasticity in any muscle group also indicates that the patient has been asked to perform an activity that is too demanding. In such cases, facilitating one joint at a time and using gravity-minimized positions may decrease the challenge level of a particular activity.

Proprioceptive Neuromuscular Facilitation

Like neuromuscular facilitation, PNF may also be used to promote the required lead-up skills to feeding, hygiene, and dressing (UE stabilization, reach, grasp, and prehension). Because normal movement patterns are made through a combined use of rotational and diagonal planes, PNF can be

The patient is an 84-year-old man who is 3-weeks status post left CVA resulting in right UE hemiparesis. Minimal active shoulder movement, minimal active elbow and wrist movement, and minimal active finger, thumb, and wrist flexion and extension characterize the quality of right UE movement. There is evidence of a mild flexor synergy pattern against gravity. He also exhibits mild visual-spatial impairment and requires minimal VCs to attend to multiple-step activities.

The patient was initially provided with weightbearing activities for the right UE to facilitate cocontraction of shoulder musculature and active elbow extension. To facilitate active shoulder and elbow movements for forward reaching, he was provided with active-assistive exercises to decrease the effort needed to move against gravity. Once the patient was able to independently support the shoulder and elbow within minimal ROM, he was encouraged to practice grasp and release hand patterns requiring active wrist extension. When he was able to demonstrate UE movement patterns with only a slight flexor synergistic overlay, he was offered a self-feeding task using a plastic fork to prehend and spear lightweight, large food items. He practiced the hand-to-mouth pattern requiring shoulder stabilization with active distal movements several times, incorporating rest breaks as needed. During dressing tasks in which he donned a pullover sweater, he was encouraged to incorporate shoulder forward reach, with shoulder at less than 90 degrees, while incorporating elbow extension to push his more affected UE through the sweater sleeve. When brushing his teeth, the patient used shoulder, elbow, and slight wrist stabilization with bilateral hand use and gross grasp to squeeze the toothpaste tube and apply the paste to the brush.

Guiding Questions

1. How can neuromuscular facilitation techniques be used in conjunction with a therapeutic exercise program? What would a therapeutic exercise program consist of?
2. How would you teach the patient's caregivers to carry out a therapeutic exercise program in his home environment? What contraindications should be noted? What signs or red flags should caregivers be alerted to when working with this patient?
3. What specific lead-up skills would you use to facilitate trunk and postural control to encourage normal UE movement patterns?
4. What specific lead-up skills would you use to facilitate normal UE movement patterns of the shoulder, elbow, wrist, and hand?
5. How can the physical therapist and occupational therapist collaborate to enhance the relearning of normal movement patterns and increase independence in functional ADL?

used to facilitate the normal movement patterns needed for functional activities. Bilateral UE PNF patterns that place demands on trunk control can facilitate the needed lead-up skills in preparation for ADL. PNF guiding principles call for a progression of activities within the stages of motor control: *mobility, stability, controlled mobility,* and *skill.* The following guidelines may be used to promote the lead-up skills needed for self-feeding, hygiene, and dressing.

Trunk Stabilization, Rhythmic Stabilization

Trunk stabilization is critical for adequate UE use. During self-feeding and hygiene activities, patients must be able to use the trunk to lean forward while bringing food or hygiene items to the mouth and to use shoulder stability to facilitate reaching and hand-to-mouth patterns. Trunk stabilization may be enhanced through the PNF technique of *rhythmic stabilization.* Rhythmic stabilization uses isometric contractions against resistance (no motion occurs). To promote initial trunk stabilization using rhythmic stabilization, the patient is positioned sidelying. Appropriate resistance[2,3] is applied simultaneously to the upper trunk flexors with one hand and to the lower trunk extensors with the opposite hand (Fig. 11.19). Repetitions of this technique should be performed in accordance with the patient's tolerance and

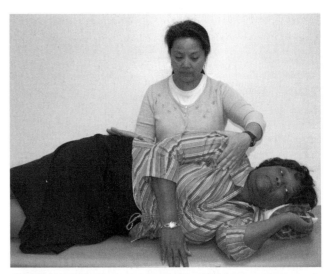

FIGURE 11.19 Rhythmic stabilization in sidelying to promote trunk stability The patient is in sidelying while the therapist applies appropriate resistance to isometric contractions of the upper trunk flexors with one hand and appropriate resistance to the lower trunk extensors with the other hand. Resistance is applied simultaneously to opposing muscle groups (e.g., upper trunk flexors and lower trunk extensors or upper trunk extensors and lower trunk flexors). Although no movement occurs, resistance is applied as if twisting or rotating the upper and lower trunk in opposite directions.

fatigue level. The activity can be progressed to sitting or standing with application of rhythmic stabilization.

Shoulder Stabilization, UE PNF Patterns, Dynamic (Isotonic) Reversals

Shoulder stability is critical to achieving functional reach using hand-to-mouth patterns; forearm and wrist stabilization is necessary for grasp and prehension of eating utensils and grooming items.

Dynamic reversals promote isotonic contractions in one direction followed by isotonic contractions in the reverse direction without relaxation. Verbal cues are used to mark initiation of movement in the opposite direction. The patient may be positioned in supine (which provides good trunk support) or sitting. The patient is instructed to move into the UE flexion/adduction/external rotation (FLEX/ADD/ER) pattern against appropriate resistance, but only to midrange (Fig. 11.20). The shoulder externally rotates and pulls up and across the face, moving into shoulder flexion and adduction. The patient is asked to hold this position for approximately 3 seconds. The patient then moves into the UE extension/abduction/internal rotation (EXT/ABD/IR) pattern against appropriate resistance. The shoulder internally rotates and pushes down and out, moving into abduction and extension (Fig. 11.21). Resistance is gradually increased in both directions before the patient is asked to hold the position. The holding position may be varied at different points in the joint range. Repetitions of dynamic reversals with a hold should be performed in accordance with the patient's tolerance and fatigue level.

Reach with Forearm Stabilization, UE PNF Patterns, Dynamic (Isotonic) Reversals

Once shoulder stabilization has been achieved, forearm stabilization during reaching activities should be addressed. In UE ADL, forearm stabilization is needed to support and maintain the wrist in a position of slight extension

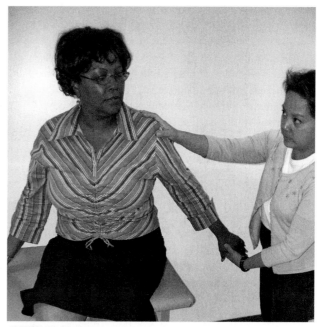

FIGURE 11.21 Sitting, PNF UE pattern, dynamic (isotonic) reversals. The patient moves into the EXT/ABD/IR pattern while the therapist applies continuous resistance to isotonic contractions.

(approximately 20–30 degrees). This prerequisite lead-up skill allows for the appropriate hand manipulation of food, hygiene items, and clothing. The patient is positioned in sitting. Dynamic reversals may be used to promote isotonic contractions of the UE agonists, followed by isotonic contractions of the UE antagonists performed with resistance. The UE FLEX/ADD/ER pattern in which the shoulder flexes, adducts, and externally rotates facilitates reach and hand-to-mouth patterns (this pattern is illustrated in Fig. 11.20 from a supine position). The patient is instructed to close the hand, wrist, and fingers and to pull the limb up and across the face so that the shoulder is adducted and flexed, with the elbow extended. The therapist should apply appropriate resistance (matched to the strength of the patient's contractions) to this UE FLEX/ADD/ER pattern. When the UE is positioned near the end of its range, the patient is instructed to change direction into the UE EXT/ABD/IR pattern. The patient is asked to open the hand and extend the fingers and wrist, with the shoulder internally rotated, pushing down and out (see Fig. 11.21). The shoulder should now be in abduction and extension. The therapist should apply appropriate resistance to this UE EXT/ABD/IR pattern. When these PNF patterns are reversed, movement should be smooth and continuous without relaxation and appropriate resistance maintained from one pattern into the opposite pattern. The Student Practice Activity in Box 11.3 presents a patient example using PNF UE patterns. The reader is referred to Chapter 3: Proprioceptive Neuromuscular Facilitation for further discussion of the principles and techniques presented in this section.

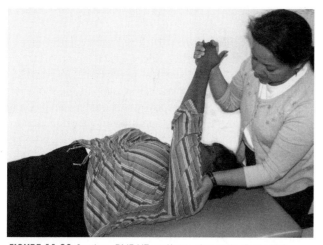

FIGURE 11.20 Supine, PNF UE pattern, dynamic (isotonic) reversals. The patient moves into the FLEX/ADD/ER pattern to midrange while the therapist applies continuous resistance to isotonic contractions.

BOX 11.3 STUDENT PRACTICE ACTIVITY: PATIENT EXAMPLE—APPLYING PNF UE FLEX/ADD/ER AND EXT/ABD/IR PATTERNS

The patient is a 54-year-old woman who is 12-weeks status post right humeral fracture. She is able to demonstrate approximately 0 to 90 degrees of active right shoulder flexion and abduction. Moderate limitations in active internal and external rotation are also noted. Upper extremity PNF patterns and the PNF technique of dynamic (isotonic) reversals were used to promote isotonic contractions of shoulder agonists (i.e., shoulder flexion, adduction, and external rotation), followed by isotonic contractions of shoulder antagonists (i.e., shoulder extension, abduction, and internal rotation) performed with appropriate resistance (dynamic [isotonic] reversals). The therapist guided the patient to move into the UE FLEX/ADD/ER pattern (shoulder adduction and flexion) and applied appropriate resistance. The patient was then instructed to change direction into the UE EXT/ABD/IR pattern, moving the shoulder into abduction and extension against appropriate resistance. Providing resistance with UE PNF patterns can increase joint ROM and muscular strength in shoulder movements while incorporating the rotational and diagonal movements required in hair brushing. Once the patient's shoulder ROM and muscle strength increased, she was given a bathing activity to practice incorporating the combined UE movements needed to perform normal hand-to-body movement patterns.

Guiding Questions

1. How can the above PNF patterns and techniques be used as part of the patient's overall plan of care? Coordinated with what functional activities?
2. How would you instruct the patient's caregivers to carry out a home exercise program?
3. What signs or red flags should caregivers be alerted to when working with this patient?
4. What additional lead-up skills would facilitate UE ROM and strength?
5. How can the physical therapist and occupational therapist collaborate to enhance relearning of normal movement patterns and increase independence in functional ADL tasks?
6. What contraindications should you consider when using PNF patterns and techniques for patients who have sustained a shoulder fracture?

Clinical Note: The therapist should continuously observe the quality of the patient's performance in desired movement patterns and then monitor and adjust the amount of resistance using manual and verbal cueing to correct abnormal postures and positioning. Manual contacts used as cues should be progressively decreased as the patient demonstrates more normal movement patterns. As manual contacts are decreased, verbal cueing continues but is progressively withdrawn as the patient demonstrates self-correction of inappropriate movement patterns, replacing them with normal movements (or with movements approximating normal patterns).

Red Flag: The above PNF techniques are indicated only for patients who possess no less than minimal to moderate active movement and no more than minimal hypertonicity in the UE and trunk. If significant hypertonicity is noted, PNF techniques must be used with caution or may be contraindicated because the application of resistance may increase hypertonicity and reduce the quality of the desired movement patterns. Evidence of pain should also be monitored during the application of gradual increments in resistance and during movement of a joint through its range.

Compensatory Training

A compensatory training approach should be used when UE recovery is limited and prolonged. Activities of daily living function must be promoted through adaptive methods. In the compensatory approach, the less affected UE and all preserved function of the more affected UE are used in the context of direct engagement in ADL retraining. Facilitation techniques are not used because significant return of further function is not expected. Selected adaptive devices can be used to substitute for the absence of foundational UE skills. For example, poor proximal shoulder stability can be addressed using a mobile arm support (described below). Splints designed to enhance wrist support can compensate for the absence of wrist extension, which is a necessary prerequisite skill for gross grasp and prehension. Built-up handles on utensils further aid gross grasp and prehension patterns.

Shoulder Stabilization

A mobile arm support (MAS) can be used to compensate for poor proximal shoulder stability (Fig. 11.22). The MAS attaches to the patient's wheelchair to support the shoulder, elbow, forearm, and wrist. It provides shoulder stabilization so that the distal UE is placed in a position of function to promote movements needed in self-feeding and grooming (i.e., bringing food and hygiene items back and forth from mouth to lap tray).

Reaching

Shoulder stabilization and scapular protraction are prerequisite skills for reaching. Once shoulder stabilization and scapular protraction have been appropriately established through compensatory strategies (e.g., MAS), shoulder forward reach and elbow extension in space can be facilitated

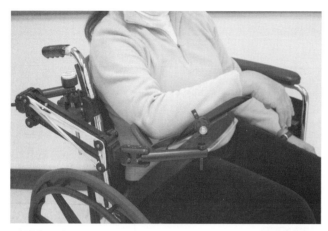

FIGURE 11.22 A mobile arm support can be used to compensate for weak proximal shoulder stability so that distal UE movements can occur.

to promote reaching patterns. The therapist should instruct the patient to practice shoulder forward reach and elbow extension during UE ADL.

Grasp and Prehension

A MAS provides stabilization by compensating for weak proximal shoulder stability, supporting the shoulder in slight abduction and flexion. The MAS forearm trough supports the elbow, forearm, and wrist and facilitates forward reaching, which allows the movements needed for grasping and prehension. For patients who may experience distal return of musculature (e.g., peripheral nerve injury), a dorsal wrist support can be used to provide wrist stabilization (Fig. 11.23) so that thumb and finger flexion can be achieved for gross grasp and prehension of utensils and food items. Once shoulder and wrist stabilization are established, the therapist should instruct the patient to practice gross grasp patterns. For example, the therapist may guide patient practice in grasping a small carton of milk and pouring it into a drinking glass.

Clinical Note: Patients who are not expected to experience distal return (e.g., those with complete spinal cord injury [SCI]) may be candidates for a MAS and dorsal wrist support. Additionally, adaptations to compensate for lost thumb and finger movements are indicated.

Grasp and prehension patterns can also be enhanced using built-up handles on utensils—an adaptive device that compensates for weakness and lack of isolated movement of the finger flexors (Fig. 11.24). A universal cuff—which can hold utensils when isolated finger movements are absent—can be applied to the palmar surface of the hand to compensate for absent finger and thumb movements (Fig. 11.25). Other examples of UE adaptive equipment are presented in Table 11.2.

Bilateral UE Use

After the above prerequisite skills of shoulder stabilization, scapular protraction, shoulder forward reach, elbow extension, and grasp and prehension have been facilitated through

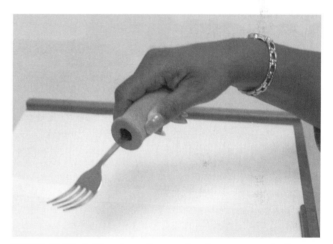

FIGURE 11.24 Built-up handles on utensils compensate for weakness and lack of isolated movement of the finger flexors.

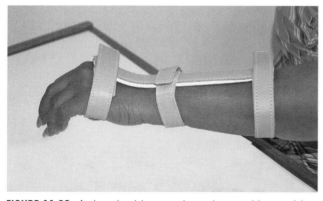

FIGURE 11.23 A dorsal wrist support can be used to provide wrist stabilization so that thumb and finger flexion can be achieved for gross grasp and prehension of utensils and food items.

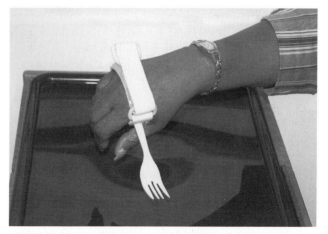

FIGURE 11.25 A universal cuff can compensate for absent finger and thumb movements.

TABLE 11.2 Examples of Upper Extremity Adaptive Equipment

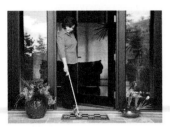

Long-handle reacher (FeatherLite Reacher)

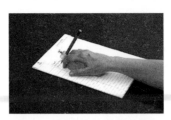

Writing aid (Writing-Bird)

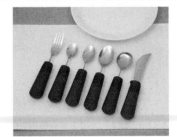

Eating utensils with built-up handles (Good Grips)

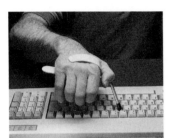

Typing aid

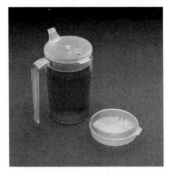

Cup with two lids

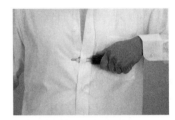

Button hook with built-up handle (Good Grips)

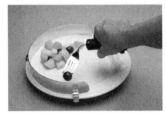

Stainless steel food guard

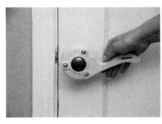

Door knob extender

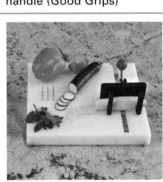

Swedish one-handed cutting board

Images provided courtesy of North Coast Medical, Inc., Gilroy, CA 95020.

compensation, bilateral UE use can be promoted through activities such as washing the face with both hands or picking up a sandwich. The therapist should guide the patient in integrating both UEs within the context of an actual ADL task.

Clinical Note: Many patients perceive adaptive equipment as a sign of disability. Although adaptive devices help patients compensate for lost motor function and can ultimately help them achieve a desired level of independence in ADL tasks, many patients resist using such devices because of fear and stigmatization. For some patients, the use of adaptive devices may represent an admission that little or no further recovery is possible. Because of this perception, the use of adaptive devices must be presented to patients gently and in accordance with their own readiness to accept their injury or illness. The introduction and presentation of adaptive devices must emphasize the patient's ability to achieve independence in desired daily activities. Patients must be allowed to exercise their own freedom to decide whether they are emotionally able or ready to use adaptive devices.

Red Flag: Research regarding the brain's neuroplasticity has demonstrated that motor recovery, in some patients, can occur several years after a neurological insult—long after further motor recovery was thought to be possible.[4] Thus, therapists must understand that the long-term use of adaptive equipment to compensate for poor motor recovery may prevent further potential return.

Patients should be encouraged to use adaptive equipment to increase independence and ADL efficiency, but they should also be provided with a therapeutic exercise program to facilitate the potential return of desired muscle function in involved limbs. The Student Practice Activities in Boxes 11.4 and 11.5 present patient examples using compensatory training strategies.

Motor Learning

Motor learning is used with patients who are able to engage in repeated practice of desired skills and who can cognitively use feedback to modify movement errors. Motor learning relies heavily on actual practice, mental practice, and feedback. Rather than relying on facilitation techniques (e.g., neuromuscular facilitation and PNF) to improve lead-up skills needed for functional skill performance, motor learning is based on the theory that motor skills are best relearned when practice takes place within the context of the actual desired activity (activity- or task-specific training).

Patients who are candidates for active practice should demonstrate some recovery of isolated movement of the shoulder, elbow, wrist, and/or hand. The patient's UE may still present with some weakness or impairment of tone. Motor learning is chiefly used to organize movement patterns (i.e., synergistic movement patterns). Cues, guidance, and feedback are provided to help the patient relearn normal movement patterns as they are practiced in actual activities.

Shoulder Stabilization and Reaching

Selected components of the UE movement pattern during feeding (i.e., shoulder stabilization, scapular protraction, shoulder forward reach, and elbow extension) should initially be addressed in isolation. The patient can be instructed to perform the motor pattern by reaching forward to place the hand on the table surface. *Intrinsic* and *augmented feedback* is used to help the patient understand what normal movement feels like. *Intrinsic feedback* provides proprioceptive and tactile information about the patient's own movement. For example, the patient can be instructed to use the less affected side to reinforce what normal movement feels like when spearing food with a utensil.

Augmented feedback provides information about the patient's movement patterns from external sources (e.g., VCs from the therapist and visual cues from observing one's own movement in a mirror). *Knowledge of performance* is a type of augmented feedback that provides information about the patient's performance of movement patterns. For example, the therapist may offer verbal feedback to the patient about the inappropriate use of shoulder elevation to compensate for impaired shoulder flexion during reaching. The therapist might also use a mirror to show the patient how he or she elevates the shoulder to compensate for impaired shoulder flexion during reaching. *Knowledge of results* is another form of augmented feedback that provides

---

BOX 11.4 STUDENT PRACTICE ACTIVITY: PATIENT EXAMPLE—APPLYING COMPENSATORY TRAINING STRATEGIES

The patient is a 22-year-old male construction worker who is status post C5 incomplete SCI sustained in a work-related accident. An MAS was used to compensate for weak proximal shoulder stability and to facilitate forward reaching during a hygiene activity. It stabilized the shoulder against gravity and provided support to the elbow, forearm, and wrist. The MAS was positioned to facilitate elbow extension and the forearm to move with the assistance of gravity to compensate for poor elbow extension. Because the patient had minimal active elbow flexion, he could engage an eccentric contraction of the biceps to help control the speed of elbow extension. The use of an MAS to compensate for weak proximal stabilization also promoted distal movements (e.g., bringing hygiene items back and forth from sink top to face/head). Additionally, adaptive devices including a dorsal wrist support (Fig. 11.23) and a universal cuff (Fig. 11.25) were used to compensate for poor wrist extension and weak or absent grasp and prehension. Practicing the UE movement pattern of bringing hygiene items back and forth from sink top to face/head during an actual grooming activity also strengthened the musculature that may have been spared following the incomplete SCI. The use of compensatory devices is necessary to promote

independence in grooming when patients do not otherwise have the physical capability needed for basic hygiene skills. However, if there is evidence that motor return is occurring in the shoulder or other musculature, the use of compensatory devices may be diminished as the patient improves and is able to use his own muscle power for self-feeding and other functional activities.

Guiding Questions

1. What shoulder and elbow movements are preserved at the C5 spinal cord level? What movements are lost? How do you think such losses affect specific daily activities?
2. If you were the patient's physical therapist, what type of therapeutic exercise program would you design to enhance UE use? What specific exercises could be used to target the spared musculature at the C5 spinal cord level? How could your therapeutic exercise program support the occupational therapist's effort to help the patient regain independence in hygiene?
3. How can the physical therapist and occupational therapist collaborate to enhance potential return of the UE musculature in patients with incomplete spinal cord injuries?
4. How would you instruct the patient's caregivers to carry out a home exercise program?

BOX 11.5 STUDENT PRACTICE ACTIVITY: PATIENT EXAMPLE—APPLYING COMPENSATORY TRAINING STRATEGIES

The patient is a 52-year-old female schoolteacher with progressive relapsing multiple sclerosis. She presents with incoordination, fatigue, and difficulty maintaining trunk control when sitting unsupported over long periods, such as when getting dressed in the morning while sitting on the edge of her bed. Additionally, she presents with weak bilateral shoulder overhead use and requires frequent rest periods. She enhances her trunk support by performing dressing tasks in a straight-back chair. She was advised to wear hook-and-loop closure cardigan sweaters, rather than pullover sweaters, to minimize overhead reach against gravity and to compensate for lack of fine motor skills needed for buttoning or managing zippers. Practicing the UE movement pattern of overhead reach and donning a sweater in unsupported sitting may be used to maintain existing muscle strength; however, using compensatory strategies may be more prudent to help conserve energy for other ADL or work tasks during the day. The ease of hook-and-loop sweater fasteners that only require lining up sweater front closures will also assist in energy conservation. The use of compensatory strategies during dressing is often necessary to promote independence when patients do not otherwise have the physical capability needed for basic ADL skills. During periods of remission, the patient may be able to engage in dressing tasks with less compensatory strategies, thereby maintaining her current level of independence and UE function.

Guiding Questions

1. What energy conservation strategies can be incorporated into usual ADL tasks during a period of relapse? What signs would indicate difficulty during performance of dressing while seated unsupported?
2. If you were the physical therapist, what type of modifications would you consider to enhance this patient's trunk stability and UE use?
3. What specific precautions would you incorporate in treatment activities during a period of relapse?
4. How can the physical therapist and occupational therapist collaborate to maximize the patient's ability to incorporate energy conservation strategies while engaging in her usual ADL or work tasks?

---

information about the outcome of the movement pattern. For example, after repeated practice and feedback, the patient may be able to spear food with decreased shoulder elevation and increased shoulder flexion. Successfully reaching for and spearing food with a utensil (without excessive shoulder elevation) provides the patient with knowledge that the desired outcome was attained.

Grasp and Prehension

Once normal movement patterns of the shoulder and elbow have been achieved through motor learning principles, wrist stabilization to support grasp and prehension can be addressed using intrinsic feedback. For example, the patient can be instructed to place the less affected wrist in a position of stabilization while bringing a hairbrush to the head. The patient is asked to observe what more normal proprioceptive feedback feels like in response to wrist stabilization. *Knowledge of performance* can provide augmented feedback about wrist stabilization through external sources. For example, a patient who lacks wrist stabilization may overcompensate with shoulder abduction. The therapist can use VCs and a mirror to help the patient understand that he or she is substituting shoulder abduction for wrist stabilization. Through VCs and the visual feedback of a mirror, the patient is guided to practice normal wrist stabilization patterns with increased wrist extension and reduced shoulder abduction. *Knowledge of results* is provided when the patient is able to reach for and grasp a hairbrush with normal shoulder stabilization, scapular protraction, shoulder

forward reach, elbow extension, wrist stabilization, and finger/thumb grasp and prehension patterns.

Bilateral UE Use

Once normal shoulder, elbow, wrist, and finger/thumb movement patterns have been established, the patient can be guided in bilateral UE use. The patient can be instructed to practice bilateral integration by using the less affected UE to pour milk into a cereal bowl while using the more affected UE to stabilize the bowl. Directing the patient's attention to the proprioceptive and tactile information that accompanies bilateral integration can highlight intrinsic feedback. Using an object (e.g., the milk container) with the less involved UE provides proprioceptive information regarding the initial weight of the container, the changing weight of the milk container as the liquid is poured into the bowl, the change in forearm positions from neutral to pronated as the milk is poured from the container, and maintaining shoulder stabilization as the forearm pronates while pouring the milk. *Knowledge of performance* can then be attained when the patient pours the milk with the more affected limb. The therapist may use VCs to help the patient understand that he or she needs to bring the UE closer to midline (through shoulder adduction and elbow flexion) to pour the milk into the bowl instead of onto the table. Auditory cues of the milk as it hits the cereal (instead of the side of the bowl) can also serve as augmented feedback regarding the need to modify motor patterns. Finally, *knowledge of results*—for example, the milk spilling on the tabletop instead of on the cereal—can be used to help the patient correct motor errors until the desired movement pattern is achieved.

Practice

After a patient successfully demonstrates a desired movement pattern, he or she is asked to engage in repeated practice of that movement pattern within the context of a specific activity.

- *Constant practice* rehearses a single motor skill repeatedly until it is mastered. For example, a patient may practice palmar prehension with wrist extension to retrieve similar-sized screws, washers, and bolts presented in a toolbox positioned at midline.
- *Variable practice* involves modifying motor patterns in accordance with the demands of a specific activity. Variable practice involves a higher-level skill than constant practice and should be addressed after constant practice has sufficiently been performed. For example, a patient is given a toolbox of items of varied sizes and weights and is asked to retrieve each item separately. The demands of this activity require the patient to modify grasp and prehension patterns in accordance with each item, as it varies in weight and size.
- *Mental practice* is a form of practice in which the patient uses cognitive rehearsal to improve motor patterns without actually attempting physical movement. For example, as a patient begins to practice desired movement patterns in therapy, the therapist may instruct the patient to spend 15 minutes in the afternoon and before bed mentally rehearsing the performance of reaching to retrieve a pair of eyeglasses using shoulder stabilization without elevation.

When using motor learning, therapists must monitor patients' level of fatigue continuously, which will determine the duration of practice. Augmented feedback that addresses the primary senses (i.e., audition, vision, and sensation) should be provided to best meet patients' unique learning styles. Activities should first be practiced as selected segments. Once mastery of selected segments has been achieved, practice of the activity as a whole is recommended (i.e., parts-to-whole training).

Clinical Note: The type and amount of practice are important considerations for promoting motor learning principles. Research has shown that variable practice (in which the patient is asked to make rapid modifications of the skill to meet the changing demands of the task or environment) is better for retention and generalization of learning compared with constant practice (in which the patient is asked to repeatedly practice a single motor skill that does not change).[5] Therefore, movement patterns should be practiced using varied positions, heights, and ranges. The use of *massed practice* (in which the amount of rest time is less than the total practice time) versus *distributed practice* (in which the amount of rest time is equal to or greater than the total practice time) must also be considered. Massed practice may

lead to decreased movement quality as patients become fatigued. A patient's tolerance and fatigue level must be continuously monitored to determine whether massed practiced can be tolerated or distributed practice must be initiated.

Red Flag: Because practice may easily fatigue a patient with compromised status, therapists must carefully observe for signs of muscular, cardiovascular, and mental fatigue. Fatigue may also lead to an increase in spasticity and a decrease in the quality of the desired movement patterns. The monitoring of heart rate, blood pressure, and oxygen saturation levels is indicated for patients with compromised cardiovascular status. Patients with minimal cognitive impairments may require frequent visual, verbal, and manual cueing to follow prescribed practice protocols. Consequently, generalization of learning may be difficult for such patients, and caregiver training should be initiated in addition to patient instruction. Progression from constant to variable practice is generally contraindicated for patients with severe cognitive impairment. The Student Practice Activity in Box 11.6 presents a patient example using motor learning principles.

Modified Constraint-Induced Movement Therapy

Constraint-induced movement therapy (CIMT or CI therapy) is a treatment approach that improves use of the more affected extremity following a stroke. It includes intense task-specific practice with multiple treatment elements and is discussed fully in Chapter 12: Constraint-Induced Movement Therapy. Modified constraint-induced movement therapy (mCIMT) was developed to provide a less intense movement therapy protocol for patients with chronic stroke.[6] Modified CIMT combines 30-minute structured functional practice sessions with restriction of the less affected UE 5 days a week for 5 hours, during a 10-week period.[7] Several studies found that mCIMT effectively improved the use and function of the more affected UE in patients with neurological disorders.[8–10] Patients who have used mCIMT also reported good adherence with decreased incidence of pain. This therapy is designed as an outpatient intervention and is reimbursable within the parameters of most managed care plans.[7]

mCIMT Protocol

Modified CIMT provides (1) repeated practice attempts that are known to facilitate skill acquisition, (2) purposeful specific practice, (3) a practice schedule that is safe and motivating for participants, and (4) active problem-solving to facilitate learning.

1. Treatment consists of 30 minutes of occupational therapy and 30 minutes of physical therapy, each three times per week for 10 weeks.
2. Occupational therapy focuses on use of the more affected limb in meaningful functional activities that provide opportunity for UE strengthening and control.

BOX 11.6 STUDENT PRACTICE ACTIVITY: PATIENT EXAMPLE—APPLYING MOTOR LEARNING PRINCIPLES

The patient is an 18-year-old male who sustained a traumatic brain injury in a motor vehicle accident. He presents with frontal lobe dysfunction marked by mild attention problems and decreased awareness of disability. He is able to follow two- or three-step directions with minimal verbal and visual cues. He exhibits overall weakness, however, and has moderate active movement in his right UE, including grasp and prehension. The patient currently appears to favor his left UE, although he is right-hand dominant.

Knowledge of performance was used to provide augmented feedback during the use of his right UE in ADL tasks. *Augmented feedback* incorporated visual cues and VCs to provide information about performance of UE movement patterns. Because he was using shoulder elevation to compensate for impaired shoulder flexion during reaching activities, he was provided with VCs to decrease excess shoulder elevation. The therapist initially addressed isolated shoulder movements to minimize the cognitive demands of simultaneously attending to prehension patterns (using a standard-weight fork). The patient was also provided with a mirror to visually cue him to recognize his use of shoulder elevation as a form of compensation for weak shoulder flexion during reaching.

Once the patient was able to perform reaching with appropriate scapular protraction and shoulder forward reach, *variable practice* was used to enhance his hand-to-mouth feeding pattern. He was given a plate of food items that were positioned on different areas of the dish; he was then asked to grasp 1- to 2-in. (2.5–5 cm) foods that required him to vary his reach pattern. The demands of this activity required him to adjust his reach patterns depending on where each food item was positioned on the plate. *Knowledge of results* was attained once he was able to successfully reach for and grasp the different-sized food items while using a normal UE movement pattern.

Guiding Questions

1. What important considerations are required when treating a patient who has both physical and cognitive deficits? What are the cognitive demands required for self-feeding activities?
2. If you were the patient's physical therapist, how would you challenge him to enhance UE control without using therapeutic activities that are too cognitively demanding?
3. What types of cues would best facilitate the patient's performance without causing him to become agitated?
4. How can the physical therapist and occupational therapist collaborate to enhance relearning of normal movement patterns and increase independence in functional tasks such as self-feeding?

---

3. Physical therapy focuses on UE limb strengthening and stretching, dynamic standing balance, and gait activities.
4. Shaping—a principle derived from CIMT—is the use of small steps that progressively increase in difficulty. Shaping is used to slowly but steadily increase motor performance.
5. Shaping techniques, functional activities, and rest periods are alternated for approximately 5 minutes each during therapy.
6. The less affected UE is restrained every weekday for a 5-hour period in which patients must actively attempt to use their more affected UE during daily activities.
7. The less affected UE is restrained using a cotton sling with the hand placed in a meshed, polystyrene-filled mitt with hook-and-loop straps around the wrist.
8. A log is used to record periods of mCIMT in the patient's home; the log is also used to record the specific activities performed during restraint periods of the less affected UE.

Clinical Note: The primary therapeutic factor in both CIMT and mCIMT appears to be the repeated use of the more affected UE, which is theorized to induce cortical reorganization with accompanying functional improvements. Repeated functional practice using the more affected UE (as directed by the protocol) appears to overcome learned nonuse and improves function.

Red Flag: One shortcoming of both CIMT and mCIMT is that patients must demonstrate the minimum active ROM of distal extension in the more affected UE (see Table 12.1 in Chapter 12: Constraint-Induced Movement Therapy). Functional electrical stimulation has been shown to be an effective means to facilitate active wrist and finger extension in patients who fail to meet these criteria but demonstrate traces of motor unit activity in their affected forearms.[11] It is important to identify such patients and attempt to activate distal UE extension through functional electrical stimulation before determining ineligibility for mCIMT. The Student Practice Activity in Box 11.7 presents a patient example using mCIMT.

SUMMARY

This chapter has addressed the basic requirements for UE function within the context of daily living skills. Task analysis guidelines were presented. Activity demands and suggested interventions were discussed for the tasks of self-feeding, hygiene, and dressing, as were the pre-ADL tasks of stabilization, reach, grasp, and prehension. The treatment approaches discussed included *neuromuscular facilitation, proprioceptive neuromuscular facilitation, compensatory training, motor learning,* and modified *constraint-induced therapy.*

BOX 11.7 STUDENT PRACTICE ACTIVITY: PATIENT EXAMPLE—APPLYING MODIFIED CONSTRAINT-INDUCED MOVEMENT THERAPY

The patient is a 62-year-old woman with a history of hypertension and type II diabetes. She is currently 6-weeks status post right CVA with resultant left UE hemiparesis. Moderate active shoulder movement; minimal active elbow and wrist movements; and moderate active finger, thumb, and wrist flexion/extension characterize the quality of left UE movement. On active movement, a moderate flexor synergy pattern emerges. Visual perception and cognition (specifically attention, recall, and basic problem-solving skills) are intact. Although the patient is left-hand dominant, she fails to use her left UE for ADL and requires moderate assistance for most functional self-care activities.

The patient received outpatient occupational therapy three times per week for 30-minute sessions over the course of 10 weeks. She chose two functional activities to address in therapy: self-feeding and donning clothing with moderate assistance. Therapy consisted of practicing feeding techniques for 5 minutes at a time, during which hand-to-mouth patterns were incorporated while using the left hand to prehend a lightweight fork for spearing foods. The hand-to-mouth pattern was repeated three or four times per 30-minute session, leaving time for appropriate rest periods. Shaping was used to decrease compensatory movements (i.e., excess shoulder elevation and abduction) and increase normal movement patterns. In physical therapy, she practiced ambulating with a straight cane (progressing from her current use of a quad cane).

When the patient was at home, her less affected right UE was restrained for 5 hours each day during the performance of routine daily activities (e.g., feeding, dressing, preparing light cold meals, and doing light dusting). The patient's spouse maintained a log of her activities performed while the right UE was restrained. He also assisted with all ADL as needed and secured the UE mCIMT restraint device. After 10 weeks, the patient could independently use a left UE hand-to-mouth pattern to spear large food items with a lightweight fork. She also could independently don upper-body garments, using both UEs and minimal assistance to don lower body garments.

Guiding Questions

1. If you were the patient's physical therapist, what lead-up skills would you select to facilitate normal UE movement patterns in preparation for self-feeding?
2. What type of home exercise program (HEP) would you design for her? How would you instruct the patient's spouse to carry out the HEP? What red flags and contraindications should the spouse be educated about to best facilitate his wife's recovery?
3. How can the physical therapist and occupational therapist collaborate to enhance relearning of normal movement patterns and increase independence in functional tasks such as self-feeding?

REFERENCES

1. Carr, J, and Shepherd, R. Neurological Rehabilitation: Optimizing Motor Performance. New York, Churchill Livingstone, 2011.
2. Saliba, VL, Johnson, GS, and Wardlaw, C. Proprioceptive neuromuscular facilitation. In Basmajian, J, and Nyberg, R (eds): Rational Manual Therapies. Baltimore, Williams & Wilkins, 1993; 243.
3. Johnson, G, and Saliba Johnson, V. PNF 1: The Functional Application of Proprioceptive Neuromuscular Facilitation, Course Syllabus, Version 7.9. Steamboat, CO, Institute of Physical Art, 2014.
4. Bowden, M, Woodbury, M, and Duncan, P. Promoting neuroplasticity and recovery after stroke: future directions for rehabilitation clinical trials. Curr Opin Neurol, 2013; 26:37. DOI: 10.1097/WCO.0b013e32835c5ba0.
5. Shumway-Cook, A, and Woollacott, M. Motor Control: Translating Research Into Clinical Practice, ed 3. Philadelphia, Lippincott Williams & Wilkins, 2007.
6. Shi, Y, et al. Modified constraint-induced movement therapy versus traditional rehabilitation in patients with upper-extremity dysfunction after stroke: a systematic review and meta-analysis. Arch Phys Med Rehabil, 2011; 92:972. DOI: org/10.1016/j.apmr.2010.12.036.
7. Page, S, Boeb, S, and Levinea, P. What are the "ingredients" of modified constraint-induced therapy? An evidence-based review, recipe, and recommendations. Restor Neurol Neurosci, 2013; 31:299. DOI:10.3233/RNN-120264.
8. Page, S, Murray, C, and Hermann, V. Brief report—affected upper-extremity movement ability is retained 3 months after modified constraint-induced therapy. Am J Occup Ther, 2011; 65:589. DOI:10.5014/ajot.2011.000513.
9. Aarts, P, et al. Effectiveness of modified constraint-induced movement therapy in children with unilateral spastic cerebral palsy: a randomized controlled trial. Neurorehabil Neural Repair, 2010; 24:509. DOI: 10.1177/1545968309359767.
10. Smania, N, et al. Reduced-intensity modified constraint-induced movement therapy versus conventional therapy for upper extremity rehabilitation after stroke: a multicenter trial. Neurorehabil Neural Repair, 2012; 26:1035. DOI:10.1177/1545968312446003.
11. Hara, Y, et al. The effects of electromyography-controlled functional electrical stimulation on upper extremity function and cortical perfusion in stroke patients. Clin Neurophysiol, 2013; 124:2008. DOI: org/10.1016/j.clinph.2013.03.030.

Constraint-Induced Movement Therapy

DAVID M. MORRIS, PT, PhD, AND EDWARD TAUB, PhD

Constraint-induced movement therapy, or *CI therapy,* involves a variety of intervention components used to promote increased use of a more-impaired extremity in the clinic setting, the research laboratory, and, most importantly, in the home setting.[1-15] The CI therapy protocol has its origins in basic animal research that led Taub to propose a behavioral mechanism that can interfere with recovery from a neurological insult—*learned nonuse.*[11,16,17] A linked but separate mechanism, *use-dependent brain plasticity,* has also been proposed as partially responsible for producing positive outcomes from CI therapy.[18-25] Substantial evidence has accumulated to support the efficacy of CI therapy for hemiparesis after chronic stroke (i.e., greater than 1-year post injury).[4,26] Evidence for efficacy comes from several studies: an initial small, randomized controlled trial (RCT) of CI therapy in patients with upper extremity (UE) hemiparesis secondary to chronic stroke,[1] a larger placebo controlled trial in patients of the same chronicity and level of impairment,[27] and a number of other studies.[2-9] There has also been a large multisite randomized clinical trial in patients with UE hemiparesis in the subacute phase of recovery (i.e., 3–9 months poststroke).[28-30] Positive findings regarding CI therapy after chronic stroke are also published in several studies from other laboratories employing between-group and within-subjects control procedures and numerous case studies.[31-35] Altogether, several hundred studies on the clinical effects of CI therapy have been published, almost all with positive results. Moreover, the most recent poststroke clinical care guidelines, developed by a working group organized by the *Veteran's Administration and Department of Defense,* describe CI therapy as an intervention that has evidence of benefit for survivors of stroke with mild-to-moderate UE hemiparesis.[35]

Intervention: The CI Therapy Protocol

Constraint-induced movement therapy for the UE consists of four different components. Some of these intervention elements have been employed in neurorehabilitation previously, but usually as individual procedures and at a reduced intensity compared with CI therapy. The main novel features of CI therapy are (1) the introduction of a number of techniques designed to promote transfer of the therapeutic gains achieved in the clinic/laboratory to the home environment,

termed the *transfer package,* and (2) the combination of these treatment components and their application in a prescribed, integrated, and systematic manner. This involves many hours a day for a period of 2 or 3 consecutive weeks (depending on the severity of the initial deficit) to induce a patient to use a more-impaired extremity. In the University of Alabama at Birmingham (UAB) CI Therapy Research Laboratory and Taub Training Clinic, patients are categorized according to their ability to achieve minimal movement criteria with the UE before treatment. To date, six categories, referred to as "grades," have been described (see Table 12.1). The participant in Case Study 5 (see pp. 351–371) exhibits movement that would be categorized as grade 3.

Constraint-induced movement therapy has evolved and undergone modification over the course of its existence. However, most of the original treatment elements remain part of the standard procedure. The present CI therapy protocol, as applied in our research and clinical settings, consists of four main elements with multiple components and subcomponents under each (see Table 12.2).[1,7,9,12,13] These are

1. intensive training of the more-impaired UE for multiple days
2. training with a behavioral technique termed *shaping*
3. applying a "transfer package" of adherence-enhancing behavioral methods designed to transfer gains made in the research laboratory or clinical setting to the patient's real-world environment
4. inducing the patient to use the more-impaired UE during waking hours over the course of treatment, usually by restraining the less-impaired UE (Fig. 12.1).

Each of the elements, component and subcomponent strategies are described in the following sections.

Intensive Training over Multiple Days

Training in the CI therapy protocol occurs over many hours a day for a period of 2 or 3 consecutive weeks, depending on the severity of the initial deficit. In the protocol most commonly used, supervised training occurs on every weekday for 3 hours. Continued use of the more-impaired UE continues while away from therapist supervision and is facilitated by use of behavior management techniques and a restraining device worn on the less-impaired UE. On weekend days, the participant does not come into the clinic for supervised

TABLE 12.1 Grade Criteria—Minimum Active Range of Motion and Motor Activity Log Scores

Impairment[a]	Shoulder	Elbow	Wrist	Fingers	Thumb
Grade 2 (MAL < 2.5 for AOU and HW scale)	Flexion ≥ 45° and abduction ≥ 45°	Extension ≥ 20° from a 90° flexed starting position	Extension ≥ 20° from a fully flexed starting position	Extension of all MCP and IP (either PIP or DIP) joints ≥ 10°[b]	Extension or abduction of thumb ≥ 10°
Grade 3 (MAL < 2.5 for AOU and HW scale)	Flexion ≥ 45° and abduction ≥ 45°	Extension ≥ 20° from a 90° flexed starting position	Extension ≥ 10° from a fully flexed starting position	Extension ≥ 10° MCP and IP (either PIP or DIP) joints of at least two fingers	Extension or abduction of thumb ≥ 10°
Grade 4 (MAL < 2.5 for AOU and HW scale)	Flexion ≥ 45° and abduction ≥ 45°	Extension ≥ 20° from a 90° flexed starting position	Extension ≥ 10° from a fully flexed starting position	Extension of at least two fingers > 0° and < 10°[c]	Extension or abduction of thumb ≥ 10°
Grade 5 (Low MAL < 2.5 for AOU and HW scale)	At least one of the following: flexion ≥ 30° abduction ≥ 30° scaption[d] ≥ 30°	Initiation[c] of both flexion and extension	Must be able to either initiate[e] extension of the wrist or initiate extension of one digit		

Each movement must be repeated three times in 1 minute.

[a]Grade 1 would indicate a patient who has minimal impairment yet is still interested in improving high-level skills (e.g., playing musical instruments, using equipment requiring a high degree of skill). Such patients do not participate in the research but do participate in the clinical programs. Grade 6 patients would fall below the minimum grade 5 criteria.

[b]Informally assessed when picking up and dropping a tennis ball.

[c]Informally assessed when picking up and dropping a washcloth.

[d]Scaption refers to the position between shoulder flexion and abduction. This position is used in many functional skills.

[e]Initiation is defined for the purposes of criteria as minimal movement (i.e., below the level that can be measured reliably by goniometer).

Abbreviations: MAL, Motor Activity Log; AOU, Amount of Use Scale; HW, How Well Scale; MCP, metacarpophalangeal joint; IP, interphalangeal joint; PIP, proximal interphalangeal joint; DIP, distal interphalangeal joint

training but still wears the mitt and uses the more-impaired UE as much as possible. Applying this intense, concentrated practice over consecutive days promotes the confidence needed to overcome learned nonuse and promotes long-lasting neural plastic changes in the brain.

Repetitive, Task-Oriented Training Using Shaping

On each of the weekdays during the intervention period, participants receive training under supervision for several hours each day. The original protocol called for 6 hours/day for this training. More recent studies indicate that a shorter daily training period (i.e., 3 hours/day) is as effective for certain groups of patients (i.e., grades 2 and 3).[33,34] *Shaping* is the training method employed. It is based on the principles of behavioral training.[36–39] In this approach a motor or behavioral objective is approached in small steps by "successive approximations"; for example, the task can be made more difficult

in accordance with a participant's motor capabilities, or the requirement for speed of performance can be progressively increased. Each functional activity is practiced for a set of ten 30-second trials while explicit, immediate feedback is provided regarding the participant's performance after each trial.[39] When increasing the level of difficulty of a shaping task, the progression parameter selected for change should relate to the participant's movement problems. For example, if the participant's most significant movement deficits are with thumb and finger dexterity and an object-flipping task is used, the difficulty of the task would be increased by making the object progressively smaller if the movement problem was in thumb and finger flexion and adduction (i.e., making a pincer grasp), whereas if the movement problem involved thumb and finger extension and abduction (i.e., releasing a pincer grasp), the difficulty of the task would be increased by making the object progressively larger. As another example, if there is a significant deficit in elbow extension (as with the participant in Case Study 5 [see pp. 351–371]) and a

TABLE 12.2 Components and Subcomponents of the CI Therapy Protocol

Repetitive, task-oriented training
- Shaping
- Task practice

Adherence-enhancing behavioral strategies (i.e., transfer package)
- Daily administration of the Motor Activity Log (MAL)
- Home diary
- Problem-solving to overcome apparent barriers to use of the more-affected UE in the real-world situation
- Behavioral contract
- Caregiver contract
- Written home skill assignment with check-off list to determine adherence
- Home practice
- Daily schedule
- Weekly phone calls for the first month after treatment to administer the MAL and problem-solve

Constraining use of the more-affected UE
- Mitt restraint
- Any method to continually remind the participant to use the more-affected UE

pointing or reaching task is used, the shaping progression might involve placing the target object at increasing distances from the participant.

The shaping task is typically made progressively more difficult as the participant improves in performance (Figs. 12.2, 12.3, and 12.4). Generally, only one shaping progression parameter at a time should be varied. However, for higher functioning patients, more than one progression parameter can be changed if the trainer believes that a participant would benefit from varying a second parameter at the same time as the first. The amount of difficulty increase

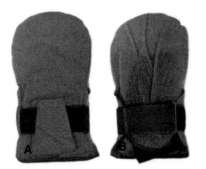

FIGURE 12.1 Protective safety mitt A protective safety mitt is used to restrain the less-impaired UE during CI therapy intervention. (A) palmar view; (B) dorsal view.

should be such that it is likely that the participant will be able to accomplish the task, although with effort. This often makes it possible to achieve a given objective that might not be attainable if several large increments in motor performance were required. Another advantage of this approach is that excessive participant frustration is avoided, assuring continued motivation to engage in the training. The following examples illustrate how a shaping task could be progressed.

A large bank of tasks has been created for each type of training procedure. Therapists are encouraged to provide four forms of interaction during the shaping and task practice activities. Table 12.3 provides a description of these modes of interaction and guidelines for applying them. For each patient, training tasks are selected that consider the following factors:

1. the joint movements that exhibit the most pronounced deficits
2. the joint movements that have the greatest potential for improvement
3. the patient's preference among tasks that have similar potential for producing specific improvement

Frequent rest intervals are provided throughout the training day. The intensity of training (the number of trials per hour [shaping] or the amount of time spent on each training procedure ([task practice]) is recorded.

Adherence-Enhancing Behavioral Methods to Increase Transfer to the Life Situation (Transfer Package)

One of the overriding goals of CI therapy is to transfer gains made in the research or clinical setting into the participant's real-world environment (e.g., home and community settings). To achieve this goal, a set of techniques is employed (the *transfer package*) that has the effect of making the patient accountable for adherence to the requirements of the therapy. In this way the patient becomes responsible for his or her own improvement. The participant must be actively engaged in and adherent to the intervention without constant supervision from a therapist, especially in the life situation where supervision is not available. Attention to adherence is directed toward using the more-impaired UE during functional tasks and obtaining appropriate assistance from caregivers if present (i.e., assistance to prevent excessive struggling but allowing the patient to try as many tasks unaided as is feasible). Attention is also directed to wearing the mitt as much as possible (when it is safe to do so).

Potential solutions to these adherence challenges have been used to increase adherence to exercise in older adults, the population most commonly experiencing stroke and subsequently most likely to receive CI therapy.[40] Two psychological factors, self-efficacy and perceived barriers, have been identified as the strongest and most consistent predictors of adherence to physical activity in older adults.

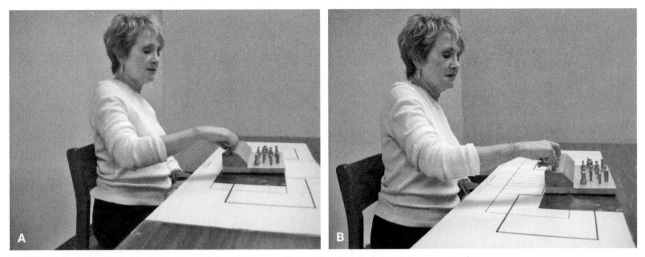

FIGURE 12.2 Task-oriented training A participant is executing a shaping task involving unscrewing a nut from a bolt (A) at a lower level of complexity, with the bolt placed closer to her, and (B) at a higher level of complexity, with the bolt placed farther away.

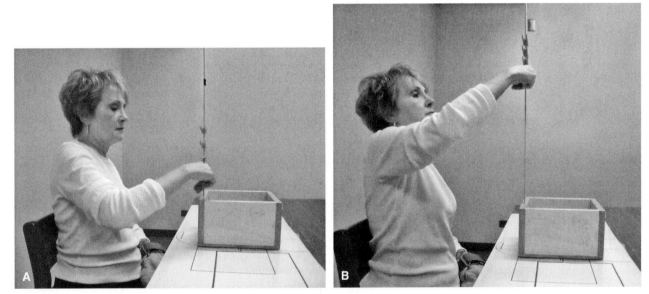

FIGURE 12.3 Task-oriented training A participant is executing a shaping task in which she removes clothespins from a horizontally positioned wooden stick (A) at a lower level of complexity, with the clothespins placed low on the stick, and (B) at a higher level of complexity, with the clothespins placed high on the stick.

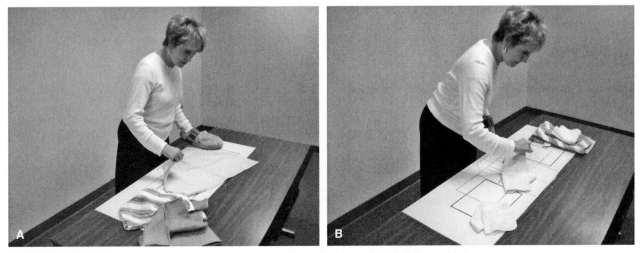

FIGURE 12.4 Task-oriented training A participant is executing a task practice activity in which she folds towels and stacks them during (A) early and (B) later stages of execution.

TABLE 12.3	Forms of Interventionist/Participant Interaction Used During Shaping and Task Practice		
Interaction Type	**Definition**	**Used in Shaping**	**Used in Task Practice**
Feedback	Providing specific knowledge of results about a participant's performance on a shaping trial or task practice session (e.g., the number of repetitions in a set period of time or time required to perform a task or specific number of repetitions)	Provided immediately after each trial	Provided as global knowledge of results at the end of the entire task practice activity
Coaching	Providing specific suggestions to improve movements. Aspects of this procedure are described in the behavioral literature as cuing and prompting.	Provided liberally throughout all shaping trials	Provided throughout entire task practice session, though not as often as in shaping
Modeling	When a trainer physically demonstrates a task	Provided at the beginning of shaping activity; repeated between trials as needed	Provided at the beginning of a task practice activity
Encouragement	Providing enthusiastic verbal reward to participants to increase motivation and promote maximal effort (e.g., *"That's excellent, that's good, keep trying."*)	Provided liberally throughout all shaping trials	Provided throughout entire task practice session though not as often as in shaping

Self-efficacy is defined as a person's confidence in his or her ability to engage in the activity on a regular basis and is related to both the adoption and maintenance of a target behavior.[41–44] Studies demonstrate that self-efficacy can be enhanced through training and feedback.[45–47] *Perceived barriers* may incorporate both objective and subjective components.[48] *Objective obstacles* can be reduced through environmental and task adaptation. *Subjective barriers* may be reduced by such interventions as confidence building, problem-solving, and refuting the beliefs that hinder activity.

A number of individual intervention principles have been successfully applied to enhance adherence to exercise and physical function–oriented behaviors. Four interventions in particular are most relevant to and are utilized in the adherence-enhancing behavioral components of CI therapy: monitoring, problem-solving, behavioral contracting, and social support.

Monitoring is one of the most commonly used strategies and involves asking participants to observe and document performance of target behaviors. The most important type of monitoring carried out in CI therapy is daily administration of the *Motor Activity Log (MAL)*,[1,49,50] a structured, scripted, validated interview that obtains information on how well and how often a participant uses the more-affected arm in 30 common activities of daily living (ADLs). (In addition,

see the Home Diary Section below.[51]) Patients can be asked to record a variety of aspects of these behaviors, including mode of activity, duration, frequency, perceived exertion, and psychological response to the activity. Patients should be asked to submit their monitoring records to therapists to facilitate consistency and completeness of records, but most importantly, to promote adherence to the self-monitoring strategy.

Problem-solving interventions involve partnerships between the therapist and patient that ultimately teach participants to identify obstacles that hinder them, generate potential solutions, select a solution for implementation, evaluate the outcome, and choose another solution if needed.[42]

Behavioral contracting involves asking participants to write out specific activities they normally carry out during the course of a day and then entering into an agreement with the therapist as to which will be carried and how they will be accomplished. Verification of the execution of the contract occurs as part of the diary-keeping aspects of the procedure.

Social support by way of educating and enlisting the caregiver to provide the optimal amount of support (e.g., encouraging the patient's independence with tasks as much as possible but also assisting the patient when absolutely necessary to prevent frustration on the part of the patient) is important to successfully using the mitt restraint and more-involved UE when in the home and community setting.[11] Reviewing the terms of the behavioral contract and administering a caregiver contract with anyone who spends a significant amount of time with the patient will optimize this social support.

Monitoring, problem-solving, contracting, and social support interventions have been used successfully, alone or in combination, to enhance adherence to physical activity in a variety of participant groups with a variety of physical conditions. These are essential aspects of the CI therapy approach. The full range of adherence-enhancing behavioral subcomponents currently employed in CI therapy protocol include daily administration of the MAL, a patient-kept home diary, problem-solving, behavioral contracts with the patient and the caregiver independently, a daily schedule developed by the therapist, home skill assignment, home practice, and a posttreatment contact. Table 12.4 identifies and categorizes each transfer package component according to the adherence-enhancing intervention principle(s) employed. Each transfer package subcomponent is described below, in the order in which they are encountered by the patient during a typical intervention period.

Motor Activity Log (MAL)

In the MAL respondents are asked to rate how much and how well they use their more-affected arm for 30 important ADLs in the home over a specified period on two separate 6-point rating scales (see Tables 12.5 and 12.6).[1,49–51] The MAL is administered independently of the patient and, in the research setting, an informant when available. The MAL provides a standardized, quantified record of patient progress during treatment and can be used as a supplement to a therapist's clinical notes. The tasks include such activities as brushing teeth, buttoning a shirt or blouse, and eating with a fork or spoon (see Table 12.7 and Fig. 12.5) As part of our research, this information is gathered about more-affected UE use in the week and year prior to the participant's enrollment in the project, the day before and after the intervention, on each day of the intervention (i.e., the whole MAL on the first day of each week, alternate halves of the instrument on each of the other weekdays), weekly by phone for the 4 weeks after the end of treatment, and at several times during the 2-year follow-up period. In the clinic, the MAL is administered before training on the first treatment day, on each day during treatment, immediately after treatment, and once a week for the first month after treatment. Several studies concerning the clinimetric properties of the MAL show the measure to be reliable and valid.[49–51] Moreover, the MAL does not produce a treatment effect when administered to persons receiving a placebo treatment at the same treatment schedule as those receiving CI therapy.[27] Preliminary results from an ongoing experiment at UAB suggest that this self-monitoring instrument is an important means of producing a transfer of improved performance from the laboratory/clinic to the life situation when used in conjunction with other aspects of the CI therapy treatment package, particularly concentrated training.[12]

Behavioral Contract

The *behavioral contract (BC)* is a formal, written agreement between the therapist and patient indicating that the patient will use the more-affected extremity for specific agreed-upon activities in the life situation, which are enumerated in the BC. In addition to increasing use of a restraint device (a protective safety mitt) outside of the clinic or laboratory, the BC is helpful in increasing safety in use of the mitt, engaging the participant in active problem-solving

TABLE 12.4 Adherence-Enhancing Intervention Principles Emphasized in Each CI Therapy Transfer Package Component

Transfer Package Component	Monitoring	Problem-solving	Behavioral Contracting	Social Support
Motor Activity Log	X			
Behavioral contract		X	X	X
Caregiver contract			X	
Home diary	X	X		
Home skill assignment		X	X	
Daily schedule	X			X
Home practice	X		X	
Weekly phone calls for first month after treatment	X	X		X

TABLE 12.5 Motor Activity Log Amount of Use Scale

0 Did not use my weaker arm (not used)

1 Occasionally tried to use my weaker arm (very rarely)

2 Sometimes used my weaker arm but did most of the activity with my stronger arm (rarely)

3 Used my weaker arm about half as much as before the stroke (half prestroke)

4 Used my weaker arm almost as much as before the stroke (3/4 prestroke)

5 Used my weaker arm as normal as before the stroke (same as prestroke)

TABLE 12.6 Motor Activity Log How Well Scale

0 The weaker arm was not used at all for that activity (never).

1 The weaker arm was moved during that activity but was not helpful (very poor).

2 The weaker arm was of some use during that activity but needed some help from the stronger arm or moved very slowly or with difficulty (poor).

3 The weaker arm was used for the purpose indicated, but movements were slow or were made only with some effort (fair).

4 The movements made by the weaker arm were almost normal but not quite as fast or accurate as normal (almost normal).

5 The ability to use the weaker arm for that activity was as good as before the injury (normal).

TABLE 12.7 Activities in the 30-Item Motor Activity Log

1. Turn on a light with a light switch
2. Open a drawer
3. Remove an item of clothing from a drawer
4. Pick up a phone
5. Wipe off a kitchen counter or other surface
6. Get out of a car
7. Open a refrigerator
8. Open a door by turning a doorknob
9. Use a TV remote control
10. Wash your hands
11. Turning the water on/off with knob or lever on the faucet
12. Dry your hands
13. Put on your socks
14. Take off your socks
15. Put on your shoes
16. Take off your shoes
17. Get up from a chair
18. Pull a chair away from the table before sitting down
19. Pull a chair toward the table after sitting down
20. Pick up a glass, bottle, drinking cup, or can
21. Brush your teeth
22. Put makeup base, lotion, or shaving cream on face
23. Use a key to unlock a door
24. Write on paper
25. Carry an object in hand
26. Use a fork or spoon for eating
27. Comb hair
28. Pick up a cup by the handle
29. Button a shirt
30. Eat half a sandwich or finger foods

to increase adherence, and emphasizing patient accountability for adherence. The BC is completed at the end of the first day of treatment when the therapist has assessed the patient's functional motor capacity and the participant has experienced using the mitt. The therapist, patient, and a witness sign the BC; this formality stresses the importance of the agreement. Before administering the BC, the therapist emphasizes the following points:

1. Use of the weaker UE outside of the laboratory is just as important as using it in the laboratory, if not more so.
2. The purpose of the BC is to induce the patient to use the more-impaired UE as much as possible.
3. Safety is always the most important consideration, even more than maximal use of the impaired UE.
4. At times, the patient will be asked to perform activities in ways that he or she would not normally carry them out (e.g., using the nondominant UE to brush the teeth). It is not suggested that this approach be adopted permanently. Instead, the patient is asked to perform the activities in this way for the 2- or 3-week treatment period to

encourage use recovery of the more-affected arm. It is usually at this point that the therapist briefly explains use-dependent neural reorganization (i.e., that CI therapy produces an increase in gray matter in motor and motor-associated areas of the brain and increases the integrity of white matter tracts and that this is one of the important mechanisms by which CI therapy achieves its therapeutic effect). It may be helpful to use language that evokes images, such as "every time you use your weaker arm, you send nerve impulses to your brain that help to strengthen it, which will improve your ability to move the arm."

5. The patient will be asked frequently if he or she performed the activities listed in the BC; the BC may be modified (items added or deleted) periodically based on performance.

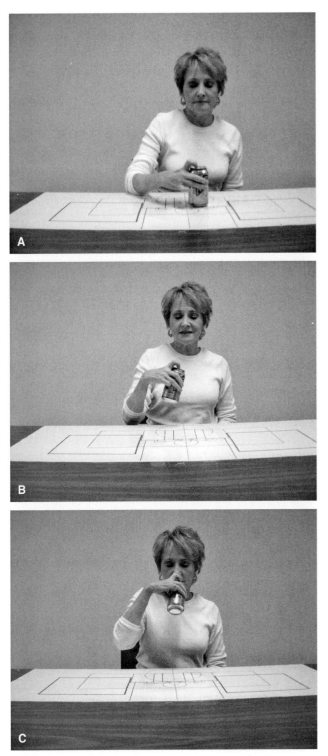

FIGURE 12.5 Wolf Motor Function Test item The patient performs the task by lifting the can using a cylindrical grasp and bringing it close to the lips. The task is timed from starting point to within one inch of the mouth.

6. With some activities on the BC, the participant may need assistance from a caregiver. In many cases, receiving this assistance is preferred to removing the mitt and using the less-impaired arm to complete the task because it maximizes use of the more-affected arm. Activities where it

is acceptable for a caregiver to assist will be discussed, agreed upon by all parties, and identified in the BC by a check in the caregiver assistance column for those tasks.

7. The BC is a formal agreement between the participant and the therapy team, and as such, it should be taken very seriously (as the therapy team does).

The first step in administering the BC involves listing ADLs encountered by the patient on typical weekdays, Saturdays, and Sundays. The times that these activities are usually carried out by the patient and distinguishing activity characteristics (e.g., equipment used, assistance provided) are also listed. Identifying the patient's typical routine is helpful for selecting items for each category of the BC that are important and meaningful to the patient. The ADLs are then categorized in the contract as those to be done with (1) the more-impaired UE with the mitt on, (2) both UEs with the mitt off, and (3) the less-impaired UE only with the mitt off. The specified times agreed upon for "mitt off" activities have mainly to do with safety, the use of water, and sleep; the time interval for when the mitt should be put back on should also be specified.

When formulating the BC, the therapist's goal is to place as many of the patient's activities into the "mitt on, more-impaired UE only" category as is safe and feasible. Sometimes this means that routine activities must be modified; adaptive equipment may be suggested and provided and/or the caregiver enlisted to assist with the task. The caregiver can participate by serving as a "second arm" or by completing components of the task that are not possible for the patient (e.g., cutting meat for the patient during mealtime). When formulating the BC, therapists should consider that patients may need additional time to complete their routine tasks while wearing the mitt and should account for this with an appropriate schedule. For example, a patient may need to wake up 30 minutes earlier than usual to complete routine activities and still arrive at the clinic at the scheduled time. Using an assistive device when walking poses a challenge to mitt use and should be considered when formulating the BC. For example, if the patient must use a straight cane for walking outside the home (e.g., in the yard or community), any outdoor walking should be placed in one of the "mitt off" categories. Also, tasks performed in social situations may pose a particular challenge if the patient is embarrassed to use the mitt in public. This should be discussed frankly with the patient. The therapist should point out that the CI therapy protocol requires full participation and that failure to use the mitt whenever possible will result in a reduced outcome. Patients should be proud of their dedication to improving the use of their UE and be reminded that others will view their efforts in the same way. Still, they may choose to avoid social situations that they anticipate will be uncomfortable for the short 2-week intervention period. That exception is acceptable if it cannot be avoided. When the patient's routine includes long periods of inactivity (e.g., many hours spent watching television), the therapist can add activities to the patient's routine to assure they are moving the more-affected UE as much as possible, thereby maximizing use-dependent plastic brain reorganization.

To promote safety, therapists must point out situations for which the patient should avoid using the mitt. The "mitt off; both hands" category is for activities in which the patient should not use the mitt but could still safely incorporate use of the more-affected UE into the task. Bathing and/or showering are included in this category. Although the mitt should be removed to avoid getting it wet and to allow use of the less-affected UE for maintaining balance, the more-affected UE should still be used as much as possible during the bathing process (e.g., lathering body parts, manipulating a bar of soap). Dressing is also commonly included in this category because it is difficult to place the mitt through a shirt or blouse sleeve. Nevertheless, patients should be encouraged to use their more-affected UE to manipulate buttons, fasten straps, and buckle belts whenever possible. Therapists unfamiliar with the CI therapy protocol may have the tendency to include all bimanual tasks in this category. We believe that many bimanual tasks can be modified for inclusion into the "mitt on; more-affected UE only" category by enlisting the caregiver to serve as a second UE during these tasks. For example, opening a jar cannot usually be effectively executed with one hand. Instead of including this task in the "mitt off; both hands" category, we believe it preferable to ask the caregiver to stabilize the jar while the patient unscrews the lid and to include it in the "mitt on; more-affected UE" category. Activities typically belonging in the "mitt off; less-affected UE" category include those in which it is advisable to use a handrail when ascending or descending stairs, shaving, and cooking. Clumsiness with these tasks could result in injury and should not be risked. Once the mitt is removed, it can be difficult to get the patient to put the mitt back on the less-impaired UE. For that reason, the BC specifies the time the mitt should be removed and then placed back on, reemphasizing the importance of wearing the mitt. The document is often modified during treatment as the patient gains new movement skills. An example of a completed behavioral contract from Case Study 5 is available for review online at Davis*Plus* (www.fadavis.com). The BC, in conjunction with the adherence-enhancing intervention principles of monitoring and problem-solving, is used to transfer treatment into the home and community environment. Since it specifies activities with which caregiver assistance should be provided, it also employs a social support strategy.

Caregiver Contract

The *caregiver contract* is a formal, written agreement between the therapist and the patient's caregiver indicating that the caregiver will be present and available while the patient is wearing the mitt and will aid in the at-home program and more generally in helping to increase more-affected UE use. It is completed after the terms of the BC with the patient are shared with the caregiver. The caregiver contract serves to (1) improve caregivers' understanding of the treatment program, (2) guide caregivers to assist appropriately, and

(3) increase patient safety. An informed caregiver is an important element in the therapeutic process. The caregiver functions as the less-affected arm in assisting the patient when a task would otherwise be impossible when the mitt is being worn. In addition, the caregiver must withhold assistance when the task is within the patient's capacity to complete a task, even if this is done slowly and not well. A tendency to impatience or a counterproductive tendency to help the patient should be avoided. The caregiver contract is signed by the therapist, patient, caregiver, and a witness which, again, formally emphasizes the importance of the agreement. As such, it employs social support to enhance adherence to the treatment protocol.

Home Diary

The *home diary* is maintained daily. Patients list their activities outside the laboratory and report whether they have used their more-affected extremity or not while performing different tasks, especially those listed on the behavioral contract. The home diary and daily review of the MAL constitute the main monitoring aspects of the CI therapy protocol. They heighten patients' awareness of their use of the more-affected UE and emphasize adherence to the BC and the patients' accountability for their own improvement.

Problem-Solving

Discussion of the MAL and home diary also provides a structured opportunity for discussing why the weaker extremity was not used for specific activities and for problem-solving on how to use it more. For example, the patient may state that he or she was unable to pick up a sandwich with one hand and therefore removed the mitt and used the less-impaired UE to assist. The therapist may then suggest that the sandwich be cut into quarters so that it is more easily manipulated with the weaker extremity. As another example, the patient might report an inability to open a door at home because the doorknob is small and difficult to grip. The therapist may provide the participant with a built-up doorknob and suggest using it so the patient can open the door with the more-affected UE.

Home Skill Assignment

Wearing the mitt while away from the clinic or laboratory does not assure that patients will use the more-impaired UE to carry out ADLs that had been accomplished exclusively with the less-impaired UE, or not at all, since the stroke. The *home skill assignment* process encourages patients to try ADLs that they may not otherwise have tried with the more-impaired UE. The therapist first reviews a list of common ADLs carried out in the home. The tasks are categorized according to the rooms in which they are usually performed (e.g., kitchen, bathroom, bedroom, office). Starting on the second day of the intervention period, patients are asked to select 10 ADLs tasks from the list that they agree to try after they leave the clinic or laboratory and before they return for the next day of treatment. Tasks not on the list may be selected if desired by the patient. These tasks are to be carried out while wearing the mitt when possible and it is safe to do so. Therapists guide the patient to select five tasks that the patient believes will be relatively easy to accomplish and five they believe will be more challenging. The 10 items selected are recorded on an assignment sheet and given to patients when they leave the clinic or laboratory for the day. The patients are instructed to check off the ADLs tasks on the assignment sheet as they are performed. Adherence in completion of the assigned tasks is discussed the next morning, and problem-solving is carried out when there is lack of adherence. The goal is for approximately 30 minutes to be devoted to trying the specified ADLs at home each day. Ten additional ADLs are selected for the home skill assignment for that evening. This process is repeated throughout the intervention period with efforts made to encourage use of the more-impaired UE during as many different ADLs in as many different rooms of the patient's home as possible.

Home Practice

During treatment, patients are also asked to spend 15 to 30 minutes at home every day performing specific UE tasks repetitively with their more-affected arm; this is referred to as *home practice-during (HP-D)*. The tasks typically employ materials that are commonly available (e.g., stacking plastic cups). This strategy is particularly helpful for patients who are typically relatively inactive while in their home setting (e.g., spending long periods watching TV) and provides increased structure to using the more-impaired UE. Care must be taken not to overload the patient with too many assignments while away from the clinic or laboratory because this could prove demotivating. Toward the end of treatment, an individualized posttreatment home practice program is drawn up consisting of tasks that are similar to those assigned in HP-D; this is referred to as *home practice-after (HP-A)*. For each patient, toward the end of treatment, a written individualized posttreatment home skill practice program is developed and given to the patient. There are seven separate lists, one for each day of the week, that are to be repeated weekly. Each list contains three repetitive tasks to be carried out for 15 to 30 minutes and 7 ADLs in which the participant is asked to use the more-affected hand selected from a list of approximately 400 ADLs developed by the laboratory. Patients are instructed to carry out these exercises indefinitely.

Daily Schedule

Therapy staff record a detailed schedule of all activities carried out in the clinic on each day of the intervention together with the time devoted to each activity listed. The schedule specifically notes the times when the mitt is taken off and put back on the less-impaired hand. The time and length of rest periods are also included. Specific shaping and task practice activities are listed, including use of only the more-affected UE during lunch whenever patient function is high

enough for this to be feasible. The daily schedule record includes not only the length of time devoted to eating lunch but also what foods were eaten and how this was accomplished. Information recorded on the daily schedule is particularly helpful for demonstrating improvements in daily activities to the patient; this often has a motivating effect to try harder.

Posttreatment Telephone Contacts

Participants are contacted weekly by telephone for the month after treatment. During each contact the "how well" and "how often" scales of the MAL are administered and problem-solving is carried out to address any problems encountered.

Constraining Use of the More-Impaired UE

The most commonly applied UE CI therapy treatment protocol incorporates use of a restraint (either sling or protective safety mitt) worn on the less-impaired UE to prevent patients from succumbing to the strong urge to use that UE during functional activities, even when the therapist is present. Over the last 15 years, the protective safety mitt, which eliminates the ability to use the fingers, has been preferred to restraint of the whole arm by a sling. The advantage of the mitt is that it permits functional use of the less-impaired UE for most purposes while still allowing protective extension of that UE in case of falling, allowing swinging of the limb during ambulation, and to otherwise help maintain balance. Patients are taught to put on and take off the mitt independently, and decisions are made about when its use is feasible and safe. Wearing the mitt for 90% of waking hours is the goal for patients with mild-to-moderate motor deficits. This so-called "forced use" is arguably the most visible element of the intervention to the rehabilitation community and is frequently and mistakenly described as synonymous with CI therapy. However, Taub et al.[2] state "there is . . . nothing talismanic about use of a sling, protective safety mitt or other restraining device on the less-affected UE" as long as the more-impaired UE is exclusively engaged in repeated practice. The term "constraint," as used in the name of the therapy, was not intended to refer only to the application of a physical restraint, such as a mitt, but also to indicate a constraint of opportunity to use the more-impaired UE for functional activities.[2] As such, any strategy that encourages exclusive use of the more-impaired UE is viewed as a "constraining" component of the treatment package. For example, shaping was intended as constituting a very important constraint on behavior; either the participant succeeds at the task or is not rewarded (e.g., by praise or knowledge of improvement).

Preliminary findings by Sterr et al.[33] indicate a significant treatment effect using CI therapy without the physical restraint component. Likewise, our laboratory has obtained similar findings with a group of nine participants when a CI therapy protocol without physical restraint was employed.[2,6,48] However, our study suggested that this group experienced a larger decrement at the 2-year follow-up testing than groups in which physical restraint was employed. If other treatment package elements developed in our laboratory are not used, our clinical experience suggests that just routine reminders alone not to use the less-affected UE, without physical restraint, would not be as effective as using the mitt. Consequently, we use the mitt to minimize the need for the therapist or caregiver to continually remind the patient to remember to limit use of the less-impaired UE during the intervention period.

Unique Aspects of CI Therapy as a Rehabilitation Approach

Three general approaches are commonly employed to improve motor function after stroke.[53] The first, *compensation*, refers to modification of ADLs such that tasks can be performed primarily with the less-affected side of the body. In this way, the more-affected extremities would, at most, be used as a prop or assist. This approach is believed to be particularly useful when spontaneous recovery of function has plateaued and further recovery seems doubtful. In recent years, however, a more optimistic view has been adopted. As a result, emphasis on regaining movement on the more-affected side of the body has been advocated. With one such approach is *true recovery*. A specific function is considered "recovered" if it is performed in the same manner and with the same efficiency and effectiveness as before the stroke. With a *substitution approach*, the more-affected extremities may be used in new way to perform a functional task compared with before the neurological insult. The question regarding which approach to rehabilitation is most effective has been an ongoing debate in the neurorehabilitation field for many years. In a sense, the CI therapy approach cuts through the long-standing discussion noted above. Trends apparent in the content of popular physical rehabilitation textbooks, evaluative criteria for professional educational programs, and topics commonly addressed in continuing education courses suggest that physical rehabilitation still includes a predominance of true recovery, substitution, or compensation approaches to intervention. The CI therapy approach to stroke rehabilitation bypasses compensation entirely and is not concerned with the requirement for the exact replacement of normal or prestroke coordination to produce improved motor function and functional independence. Further, owing mainly to reimbursement policies, most intervention is delivered in shorter treatment periods compared to that required for CI therapy and takes place in a distributed manner. If applied clinically, the CI therapy approach, as used in the UAB research laboratory represents a substantial paradigm shift for conventional physical rehabilitation. The CI therapy approach is inconsistent in a variety of ways with the more conventional compensation and functional recovery approaches, as discussed below.

Using the More-Affected Extremity

Using the protective safety mitt prevents participants from performing ADLs and training activities with the less-affected extremity unless using the less-affected UE is absolutely necessary for safety or to avoid having the restraining device wet with water, even if the less-affected UE would normally be used for that function. For example, if the less-affected UE was the dominant UE before the stroke and the task was typically performed by the dominant UE (e.g., writing), the CI therapy protocol still requires the participant to perform the task with the more-affected, nondominant UE. This remains true for tasks that are bilateral in nature (e.g., folding clothing). Instead of removing the mitt and performing the task with both UEs, the participants perform the task in a modified fashion, with the more-affected UE exclusively or by enlisting the assistance of a caregiver to serve as a "second UE." Many of the CI therapy participants' ADLs are modified during the training period. In this way, the CI therapy protocol does not allow compensation and deviates from a functional recovery approach where all ADLs would be attempted in the "typical" manner they were performed before the stroke. The purpose of the strict adherence to use of the protective safety mitt is not to encourage a permanent change in the way the participant performs ADLs. Rather, use of the protective safety mitt requires the concentrated and repetitive use of the more-affected UE, which leads both to overcoming the strongly learned habit of nonuse and to use-dependent cortical plasticity. Once the treatment period (i.e., 2 or 3 weeks) has ended, participants return the protective safety mitt to the laboratory staff and perform ADLs in the most effective manner possible with enhanced use of the more-affected UE. Interestingly, anecdotal observations suggest that after treatment many participants with more-affected, nondominant UEs begin using the more-affected, nondominant UE for tasks previously performed with the dominant, less-affected UE. Such observations warrant further investigation.

Importance of Concentrated Practice

Although the CI therapy protocol used most often includes some sort of restraint on the less-affected UE, variations in this approach (e.g., shaping only, intensive physical rehabilitation) do not.[2] There is thus nothing talismanic about using a restraining device on the less-affected UE. The common factor in all of the techniques, producing an equivalently large treatment effect, appears to be repeated practice using the more-affected UE. Any technique that induces a patient to use a more-affected UE many hours a day for a period of consecutive weeks should be therapeutically efficacious. This factor is likely to produce the use-dependent cortical plasticity found to result from CI therapy and is presumed to be the basis for the long-term increase in the use of the more-affected limb. Researchers have also shown that repetitive practice is an important factor in stroke rehabilitation interventions.[53,54] Conventional physical rehabilitation, regardless of setting (e.g., inpatient or outpatient) or stage of rehabilitation (e.g., acute, subacute, or chronic), does not provide a sufficient concentration of practice. The conventional schedule falls short not only in the absolute time that using the more-affected UE is required but also in the consecutive nature of the practice periods. Clinical application of CI therapy will likely require a change in the typical scheduling pattern for rehabilitation. Episodes of care will likely need to be modified from short treatment sessions held several times a week for several months to 3.5-hour sessions carried out daily for consecutive days over a 2- or 3-week period. Enhancement of amount of use by means of prescribed home practice exercises, home skill assignments with adherence recorded on a check-off sheet, and monitored home diaries is highly desirable, especially for weekends during treatment. Financial feasibility of this type of approach requires changes in payment structures and policies within reimbursement agencies.

Shaping as a Training Technique

Constraint-induced movement therapy studies predominately use shaping for training activities in the laboratory. Preliminary data suggest that a predominance of shaping in the training procedures is especially effective for lower functioning participants. Use of shaping for higher functioning participants is also beneficial.[12] Thus, shaping would seem to be an effective training procedure for enhancing use of the more-affected UE in the life situation. Although there are many similarities between shaping and the conventional training techniques used by therapists, important differences also exist. Shaping procedures use a highly standardized and systematic approach to progress the difficulty level of motor tasks attempted. Also, feedback provided in shaping is immediate, specific, quantitative, and emphasizes only positive aspects of the participants' performance. In this way, the therapist's input and continuous encouragement motivate the participant to put forth continued and maximal effort. Tasks are used that emphasize movements in need of improvement, but that can be easily accomplished by the participant. Excessive effort is avoided because it may demotivate the participant. The influence of shaping is primarily behavioral and directed at keeping participants motivated along with increasing the use of the UE during training. The main objective is that the patient will use the more-affected UE repeatedly in a concentrated, massed-practice fashion to overcome learned nonuse and induce use-dependent cortical plasticity. Skill acquisition regarding the specific shaping task practiced is not the primary purpose of shaping. Instead, skill attained during practice of a shaping task is a very beneficial byproduct that can generalize into motor performance in the real-world environment. However, the primary objective is to overcome learned nonuse; specific skill acquisition with functional tasks will likely occur during the independent trial and error taking place outside the laboratory using the protective safety mitt during ADLs in the participants' home environments.

Using a Transfer Package

It is our belief that most patients (and therapy professionals) view rehabilitation as occurring primarily under the direct observation and supervision of the rehabilitation professional. We believe that continued use and practice, for many hours daily, away from the rehabilitation facility is critical to achieving permanent changes in plasticity and function. Another unique aspect of the CI therapy approach involves an emphasis on the use of adherence-enhancing behavioral techniques (i.e., the transfer package) to facilitate more-affected UE use. Although the use of similar behavioral techniques has been described in the physical rehabilitation literature, their use in combination and the intensity with which they are used in the CI therapy protocol is different. Using the transfer package provides multiple opportunities for systematically increasing attention to more-affected UE use, promoting participants' accountability for adhering to the CI therapy protocol, and providing structured problem-solving between participants and research personnel. Intensive contact with the therapist establishes an important rapport between therapist and patient that helps the patient take home practice and mitt-wearing requirements of the therapy very seriously. Taken together, the behavioral techniques result in improved adherence to the required CI therapy procedures. Evidence from our research laboratory suggests that this transfer package may be the most important component of the CI therapy protocol.[12,19] Also, studies investigating a CI therapy protocol with a reduced laboratory-training component (e.g., 3.5 hours instead of 6 hours) suggest that the reduced laboratory time produces similar results. A possible explanation for this could be successful carryover of the behavioral techniques used during the treatment period to promote adherence, even when the patient is at home and not in contact with research personnel. These findings highlight the importance of the "out of laboratory" activities and, subsequently, the behavioral techniques needed to assure participants' adherence to them.

Main Effect of CI Therapy: Increased Use

Because a true recovery approach promotes performance of specific functional tasks in a manner similar to that before the stroke, quality of movement would seem to be an important, if not primary, indicator of successful rehabilitation. Results from CI therapy research, as evidenced by the Wolf Motor Function Test,[55] suggest that participants do significantly improve their quality and skill of movement. A more powerful change, however, has been demonstrated with increased use of the more-affected UE in the life situation, as evidenced by the MAL. Participants may well be developing new movement strategies to accomplish functional tasks. If so, this would further distinguish CI therapy from the more true recovery-oriented therapies.

SUMMARY

Much research evidence supports using CI therapy for hemiparesis after chronic stroke (greater than 1 year). Constraint-induced movement therapy is believed to be effective because of two separate but linked mechanisms: *overcoming learned nonuse* and *use-dependent cortical plasticity*. These mechanisms are different from those attributed to more conventional rehabilitation approaches that seek to achieve compensation, true recovery, and/or substitution. As a result, the CI therapy approach represents a significant paradigm shift in physical rehabilitation. With continued investigation, elaboration, and application to clinical settings, CI therapy would appear to hold great promise for the field of physical rehabilitation.

REFERENCES

1. Taub, E, et al. Technique to improve chronic motor deficit after stroke. Arch Phys Med Rehabil, 1993; 74:347.
2. Taub, E, Uswatte, G, and Pidikiti, R. Constraint-Induced Movement therapy: a new family of techniques with broad application to physical rehabilitation–a clinical review. J Rehabil Res Dev, 1999; 36:237.
3. Taub, E, Uswatte, G, and Elbert, T. New treatments in neurorehabilitation founded on basic research. Nat Rev Neurosci, 2002; 3:228.
4. Taub, E. Harnessing brain plasticity through behavioral techniques to produce new treatments in neurorehabilitation. Am Psychol, 2004; 59:692.
5. Morris, DM, and Taub, E. Constraint-induced therapy approach to restoring function after neurological injury. Top Stroke Rehabil, 2001; 8:16.
6. Morris, DM, et al. Constraint-induced (CI) movement therapy for motor recovery after stroke. Neurorehabil, 1997; 9:29.
7. Morris, DM, Taub, E, and Mark, VW. Constraint-induced movement therapy: characterizing the intervention protocol. Europa Medicophysica, 2007; 42:257.
8. Taub, E, and Uswatte, G. Constraint-induced movement therapy: answers and questions after two decades of research. NeuroRehabilitation, 2006; 21:93.
9. Mark, VM, and Taub, E. Constraint-induced movement therapy for chronic stroke hemiparesis and other disabilities. Res Neurol Neurosci, 2004; 22:317.
10. Taub, E. Movement in nonhuman primates deprived of somatosensory feedback. Exerc Sport Sci Rev, 1977; 4:335.
11. Taub, E. The behavior-analytic origins of constraint-induced movement therapy: an example of behavioral neurorehabilitation. Behav Anal, 2012; 35:155.
12. Taub, E, et al. Method for enhancing real-world use of a more-affected arm in chronic stroke: transfer package of constraint-induced movement therapy. Stroke, 2013; 44:1383.
13. Uswatte, G, and Taub, E. Constraint-induced movement therapy: a method for harnessing neuroplasticity to treat motor disorders. Prog Brain Res, 2013; 207:379.
14. Taub, E, Uswatte, G, and Mark, VW. The functional significance of cortical reorganization and the parallel development of CI therapy. Front Hum Neurosci, 2014; 8:396.
15. Taub, E, Mark, VW, and Uswatte, G. Implications of CI therapy for visual deficit training. Front Hum Neurosci, 2014; 8:1.
16. Taub, E. Somatosensory deafferentation research with monkeys: implications for rehabilitation medicine. In Ince, LP (ed): Behavioral Psychology in Rehabilitation Medicine: Clinical Applications. New York, Williams & Wilkins, 1980, 371.
17. Liepert, J, et al. Motor cortex plasticity during constraint-induced movement therapy in stroke patients. Neurosci Lett, 1998; 250:5.
18. Liepert, J, et al. Treatment-induced cortical reorganization after stroke in humans. Stroke, 2000; 31:1210.
19. Kopp, B, et al. Plasticity in the motor system related to therapy-induced improvement of movement after stroke. Neuroreport, 1999; 10:807.
20. Bauder, H, et al. Effect of CI therapy on movement-related brain potentials. Psychophysiology, 1999; 36(abstract):S31.
21. Wittenberg, GF, et al. Constraint-induced therapy in stroke: magnetic-stimulation motor maps and cerebral activation. Neurorehabil Neural Repair, 2003; 17:48.
22. Levy, CE, et al. Functional MRI evidence of cortical reorganization in upper-limb stroke hemiplegia treated with constraint-induced movement therapy. Am J Phys Med Rehabil, 2001; 80:4.
23. Mark, VW, Taub, E, and Morris, DM. Neural plasticity and constraint-induced movement therapy. Eura Medicophys, 2006; 42:269.
24. Gauthier, LV, et al. Remodeling the brain: plastic structural changes produced by different motor therapies after stroke. Stroke, 2008; 39:1520.
25. Uswatte, G, and Taub, E. Implications of the learned nonuse formulation for measuring rehabilitation outcomes: lessons from constraint-induced movement therapy. Rehabil Psychol, 2005; 50:34.
26. Taub, E, Uswatte, G, and Mark, V. Implications of CI therapy for visual deficit training. Front Integr Neurosci, 2014; 8:1.
27. Taub, E, et al. A placebo controlled trial of constraint-induced movement therapy for upper extremity after stroke. Stroke, 2006; 37:1045.
28. Winstein, CJ, et al. Methods for a multi-site randomized trial to investigate the effect of constraint-induced movement therapy in improving upper extremity function among adults recovering from a cerebrovascular stroke. Neurorehabil Neural Repair, 2003; 17:137.
29. Wolf, SL, et al. Effect of constraint-induced movement therapy on upper extremity function 3 to 9 months after stroke: the EXCITE randomized clinical trial. JAMA, 2006; 296:2095.
30. Wolf, SL, et al. Retention of upper limb function in stroke survivors who have received constraint-induced movement therapy: the EXCITE randomized trail. Lancet Neurol, 2007; 7:33.
31. Miltner, WH, et al. Effects of constraint-induced movement therapy on patients with chronic motor deficits after stroke: a replication. Stroke, 1999; 30:586.
32. Kunkel, A, et al. Constraint-induced movement therapy for motor recovery in chronic stroke patients. Arch Phys Med Rehabil, 1999; 80:624.
33. Sterr, A, et al. CI therapy in chronic hemiparesis: the more the better? Arch Phys Med Rehabil, 2002; 83:1374.
34. Dettmers, C, et al. Distributed form of constraint-induced movement therapy improves functional outcome and quality of life after stroke. Arch Phys Med Rehabil, 2005; 86:204.
35. Duncan, PW, et al. Management of adult stroke rehabilitation care: a clinical practice guideline. Stroke, 2005; 36:e100.
36. Skinner, BF. The Behavior of Organisms. New York, Appleton-Century-Crofts, 1938.
37. Skinner, BF. The Technology of Teaching. New York, Appleton-Century-Crofts, 1968.
38. Panyan, MV. How to Use Shaping. Lawrence, KS, HH Enterprises, 1980.
39. Taub, E, et al. An operant approach to rehabilitation medicine: overcoming learned nonuse by shaping. J Exp Anal Behav, 1994; 61:281.
40. Dominick, KL, and Morey, M. Adherence to physical activity. In Bosworth, HB, Oddone, EZ, and Weinberger, M (eds): Patient Treatment Adherence: Concepts, Interventions, and Measurement. Mahwah, NJ, Lawrence Erlbaum Associates, 2006.
41. Trost, SG, et al. Correlates of adults' participation in physical activity: review and update. Med Sci Sports Exer, 2002; 34:1996.
42. Dishman, RK. Determinants of participation in physical activity. In Bourchard, C, Shephard, RJ, Stephens, T, Sutton, JR, and McPherson, BD (eds): Physical Activity, Fitness and Health: International Proceedings and Consensus Statement. Champaign, IL, Human Kinetics, 1994, 214.
43. Sallis, JF, and Owen, N. Physical Activity and Behavioral Medicine. Thousand Oaks, CA, Sage Publications, 1999.
44. King, AC, Blair, SN, and Bild, DE. Determination of physical activity and interventions in adults. Med Sci Sports Exerc, 1992; 24:S221.
45. McAuley, E. The role of efficacy cognitions in the prediction of exercise behavior in middle-aged adults. J Behav Med, 1992; 15:65.
46. Rejeski, WJ, Brawley, LR, and Ambrosius, WT. Older adults with chronic disease: benefits of group-mediated counseling in promotion of physical active lifestyles. Health Psychol, 2003; 22:414.
47. McAuley, E, et al. Exercise self-efficacy in older adults: social, affective, and behavioral influences. Ann Behav Med, 2003; 25:1.

48. DiMatteo, MR. Social support and patient adherence to medical treatment: a meta-analysis. Health Psychol, 2004; 23:207.

49. Uswatte, G, et al. The Motor Activity Log-28: assessing daily use of the hemiparetic arm after stroke. Neurology, 2006; 67:1189.

50. Uswatte, G, et al. Contribution of the shaping and restraint components of constraint-induced movement therapy to treatment outcome. NeuroRehabil, 2006; 21:147.

51. Van der Lee, JH, et al. Clinimetric properties of the Motor Activity Log for the assessment of arm use in hemiparetic patients. Stroke, 2004; 35:1410.

52. Shumway-Cook, A, and Woollacott, M. Motor Control: Theory and Practical Applications, ed 4. Philadelphia, PA, Lippincott, 2012.

53. Butefisch, C, et al. Repetitive training of isolated movements improves the outcome of motor rehabilitation of the centrally paretic hand. J Neurol Sci, 1995; 130:59–68.

54. Hesse, S, et al. Restoration of gait in nonambulatory hemiparetic patients by treadmill training with partial body-weight support. Arch Phys Med Rehabil, 1995; 75:1087–1093.

55. Wolf, SL, et al. Assessing Wolf Motor Function Test as outcome measure for research in patients after stroke. Stroke, 2001; 32:1635–1639.

CHAPTER

13 Interventions for Vestibular Rehabilitation

JOANN MORIARTY-BARON, PT, DPT

The vestibular system is a complex, highly integrated component of the nervous system that usually goes unnoticed until it is disturbed. Consider the person who goes on a ride at an amusement park feeling well but exits experiencing dizziness, unsteadiness, nausea, and difficulty with vision, concentration, and walking. In this instance, we intuitively identify that the person is experiencing "motion sickness" due to excessive stimulation from the ride. However, these are the symptoms that people with vestibular disorders experience. The vestibular system makes up one the seven special senses and is responsible for the awareness of body position in space, maintaining postural control against gravity, and coordinating head and eye movements. Because of the integral role that the vestibular system plays in postural control, the physical therapist must be able to recognize vestibular system involvement to remediate balance impairments. This chapter presents an overview of the vestibular system and introduces entry-level interventions that address limitations and restrictions based on the clinical presentation of the patient.

Overview of the Peripheral Vestibular System

The peripheral vestibular apparatus originates in the inner ear, adjacent to the cochlea, and lies deep within the temporal bone. It comprises the *otoliths* (the utricle and saccule), three *semicircular canals,* and the vestibular portion of the eighth cranial nerve *(vestibulocochlear nerve).* Each ear contains one set of these structures that work as a team to convey information regarding head position to the central nervous system (CNS). A bony outer labyrinth covers a fluid-filled inner membranous labyrinth that contains the five vestibular sensory organs: the *utricle,* which detects lateral head tilt and linear translation of the head in the horizontal plane; the *saccule,* which detects linear translation of the head in the vertical plane; and the three semicircular canals, which detect angular acceleration of the head (rotation).[1] Afferent information from the sensory receptors synapse at *Scarpa's ganglion* then travels to the periphery on the vestibular portion of the vestibulocochlear nerve (Fig. 13.1) .

The distinct arrangement of the hair cells in the utricle and saccule provide the system with precise information regarding the head position in relation to gravity. Both the

utricle and saccule contain a *macula,* a patch of specialized hair cells, on top of which sits a gelatinous cap. The hair cells and macula of the utricle are oriented to detect movement in the horizontal plane, and the hair cells and macula of the saccule are oriented to detect movement in the vertical plane. On top of this gelatinous cap lies a layer of calcium carbonate crystals called *otoconia.* The otoconia serve as a ballast to accentuate the bending of the hair cells. Deflection of the hair cells toward the tallest hair cell (the *kinocilium*) excites the vestibular neurons, whereas deflection of the hair cell away from the kinocilium inhibits the vestibular neurons. The orientations of the hair cells on the macula vary, and this variation informs the central somatosensory system about the head's position in space without visual input (Fig. 13.2).[1]

The three semicircular canals are arranged so that they are at about 90-degree angles to one another, and the horizontal canal is positioned approximately 30 degrees upward from the tip of the nose. The *anterior canal* (also known as the superior canal) detects head rotation with forward motions such as a reaching to the floor or performing a forward roll or somersault. The *posterior canal* detects posterior rotation of the head and is stimulated by movements such as looking up or moving from long-sitting to supine. The *horizontal canal* detects lateral rotation of the head and is

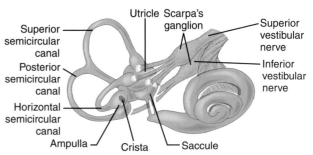

FIGURE 13.1 Anatomy of the vestibular labyrinth Structures include the utricle, sacculus, superior semicircular canal, posterior semicircular canal, and the horizontal semicircular canal. The three semicircular canals (SCCs) are orthogonal with each other. Note the superior vestibular nerve innervating the superior (anterior) and horizontal semicircular canals as well as the utricle. The inferior vestibular nerve innervates the posterior semicircular canal and the saccule. The cell bodies of the vestibular nerves are located in Scarpa's ganglion. Also note that the semicircular canals enlarge at one end to form the ampulla. From Schubert, p. 966,[2] with permission.

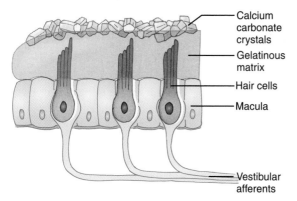

FIGURE 13.2 Otoconia Otoconia are calcium carbonate crystals that are embedded in a gelatinous matrix, which provides an inertial mass. Linear acceleration shifts the gelatinous matrix and excites or inhibits the vestibular afferents, depending on the direction in which the stereocilia are deflected. From Schubert, p. 967,[2] with permission.

stimulated when the head turns to look to the right and left or upon rotation of the body while upright (Fig. 13.3).

As the head undergoes torsional acceleration or rotates through space, endolymph moves within the semicircular canal sharing that plane. Located at the end of each semicircular canal is an enlargement called the *ampulla.* Within each ampulla lies a *cupula,* which is a gelatinous diaphragm that blocks the movement of the fluid in the canal. The cupula houses the *cristae ampullaris* that contains specialized hair cells. When the head rotates in the plane of the canal, the endolymph moves and bends the cupula, thus bending the hair cells located in the cristae. If cupula deflection results in the

hair cells bending toward the kinocilium (the tallest hair cell) the vestibular neurons are excited and movement is detected in the plane of the canal. If the hair cells are deflected away from the cupula, stimulation of the vestibular neurons is inhibited. The anatomical alignment of the semicircular canals in each ear allows them to function in pairs so that the left anterior canal lies in the same plane as the right posterior canal and the right anterior canal lies in the same plane as the left posterior canal. Additionally, rotation of the head to one side increases the firing rate of the vestibular nerve on that side and reduces the firing rate on the opposite side (commonly referred to as a *push-pull mechanism*) (Fig. 13.4).[2]

Overview of Central Vestibular System Connections

The vestibular system is highly integrated with multiple regions within the CNS. The afferent vestibular information primarily interacts with the cerebellum, vestibulospinal tracts, and visual and oculomotor systems. Information leaving the peripheral vestibular apparatus travels via the vestibular nerve to the CNS where it synapses with the *vestibular nuclei* located at the junction of the pons and medulla near the floor of the fourth ventricle.[1,3] There are four main vestibular nuclei on each side of the brainstem: superior, inferior, medial, and lateral. All afferent information received by the vestibular nuclei is shared and sent to the vestibular nuclei on the contralateral side, and together they act as an initial integrator of incoming sensory motor information.[3,4] Projections from the vestibular nuclei may descend with the *medial and lateral vestibulospinal tracts,* project to the *cerebellum,* or ascend to the *oculomotor*

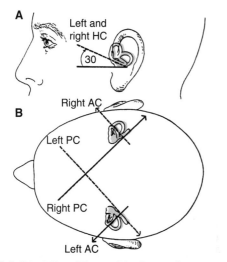

FIGURE 13.3 Orientation of the semicircular canals (A) Orientation of the horizontal semicircular canals (HC) in situ, with the head neutrally aligned. (B) The semicircular canals (ipsilateral anterior and contralateral posterior, and each horizontal) work in pairs. The arrows indicate the angular pitch direction of individual SCC stimulation. The dashed and continuous lines illustrate each SCC has an equally opposing SCC, sensitive to the opposite angular pitch direction of the head; for example, the left anterior canal (left AC) is paired with the right posterior canal (right PC) and collectively recognized as the left anterior right posterior (LARP) plane. From Schubert, p. 969,[2] with permission.

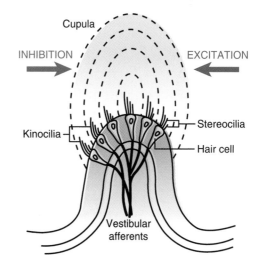

FIGURE 13.4 The cupula of the ampulla The cupula of the ampulla is a flexible, gelatinous barrier that partitions the canal. The crista ampullaris contains the kinocilia and stereocilia sensory hair cells. The hair cells generate action potentials in response to cupular deflection. Deflection of the stereocilia toward the kinocilia causes excitation; deflection in the opposite direction causes inhibition. From Schubert,[2] p. 966, with permission.

nuclei then onto the thalamus and cortex for conscious awareness of body and head position in space. Each of the functions of the vestibular system can be attributed to one or more of these pathways, and although discussed separately, redundancy exists within the system and pathways function cooperatively (Fig. 13.5).

Vestibulospinal Reflex

Afferent information originating from the otoliths and semicircular canal that projects to the *lateral vestibular nucleus* descends ipsilaterally down the spinal cord in the *lateral vestibulospinal tract.* The lateral vestibulospinal tract terminates on the alpha motor neurons (or interneurons that act on the alpha motor neurons) in the anterior horn that excite the postural and limb extensor muscles. This tract ends in the lumbar segments of the cord. The *lateral vestibulospinal reflex* contributes heavily to antigravity postural control and protective extension responses for balance.[4,5] Afferent information originating from the otoliths organs and semicircular canals that projects to the *medial vestibular nucleus* descends down the contralateral spinal cord in the *medial vestibulospinal tract* as part of the *medial longitudinal fasciculus.* The medial vestibulospinal tract facilitates bilateral cervical extensor muscles with fibers terminating at the upper thoracic segments of the cord. The *medial vestibulospinal reflex* allows for head-righting responses and contributes to oculomotor control.[1,2,5] Additionally, both pathways interact with the reticulospinal tract, further influencing postural muscle tone.

Cerebellar Pathways

The cerebellum can be considered the executor of the vestibular system and is responsible for the modulation and adaptation of the system. The cerebellum receives information from the vestibular nuclei and delivers this information to the cerebellar lobes and nuclei for processing. The four cerebellar nuclei are the dentate, the emboliform, the fastigial, and the globus.[3] Each nucleus differs in processing, function, and output. Output from the fastigial nucleus projects directly back to the vestibular nuclei, whereas output from other cerebellar nuclei projects to the thalamus and prefrontal and motor cortices.

The *flocculonodular lobe* (also called the *vestibulocerebellum*) and the *vermis* (midline portion) of the cerebellum receive most of the afferent vestibular inputs. Both structures receive vestibular, visual, auditory, and proprioceptive information from the head, neck, and trunk. Outgoing projections return to the lateral vestibular nucleus then down the lateral vestibulospinal and reticulospinal tracts coordinating the head, neck, trunk, and eyes during movement and the limbs during gait.[1,5]

The flocculonodular lobe plays a principal role in coordinating eye and head movement through its extensive articulations with the visual system. This section of the cerebellum incorporates information regarding head position from the otoliths and semicircular canals via the vestibular nuclei with visual information from the superior colliculus and primary and secondary visual cortices. The flocculonodular lobe interacts with the medial longitudinal fasciculus to control the vestibular ocular reflex through projections to the medial vestibular nucleus (Fig. 13.6).[1]

Vestibulo-ocular Reflex

The *vestibulo-ocular reflex (VOR)* holds special significance when discussing the central vestibular pathways because it is the primary mechanism responsible for *gaze stability* (also called *gaze fixation*). The VOR functions to maintain visual focus on an object despite quick head movements. Consider reading while jogging on a treadmill. Although the head and body are moving, the eyes are kept stable so that the words on the page remain fixed on the fovea of the retina, allowing the reader to see them clearly. To accomplish this task, the vestibular system works in conjunction with the oculomotor system to detect head movement and counteract it using eye movement of equal amplitude in the opposite direction (termed *VOR phase*). The term *VOR gain* describes the relationship of eye velocity to head velocity and normally holds a numerical value of −1. Each semicircular canal excites specific ocular muscles and inhibits the opposing pair, including muscles on both the ipsilateral and contralateral side so that the sum of eye muscle activity enables both eyes to move in the same direction (Table 13.1).

Head movements that occur with normal daily activities rarely take place in a single plane and frequently stimulate the peripheral vestibular sensory apparatus in more than one canal simultaneously. The function of the VOR with head rotation to the left is described in the following example.

Rotation of the head to the left stimulates the left horizontal semicircular canal and simultaneously inhibits the

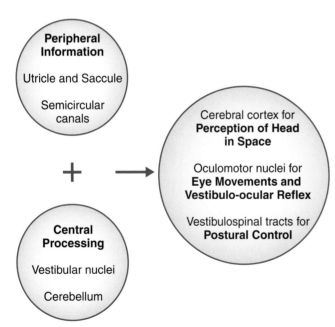

FIGURE 13.5 Fundamental components of the vestibular system

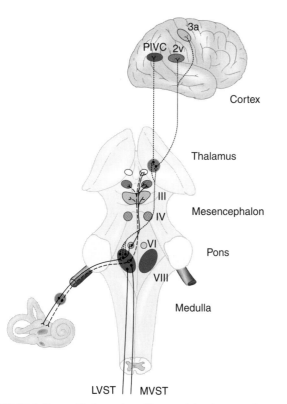

FIGURE 13.6 The vestibular system The semicircular canal (angular) and otolith (linear) input is sent to the vestibular nuclei. From the vestibular nuclei, the input travels to the ocular motor nuclei (III, IV, VI) for mediation of the vestibulo-ocular reflex. For arousal and conscious awareness of the head and body in space, information proceeds further to the thalamus and cortex. For maintenance of postural control, the peripheral vestibular input is sent distally as the medial and lateral vestibulospinal tracts (MVST, LVST). PIVC, parieto-insular vestibular cortex. From Schubert, p. 967,[2] with permission.

right. Afferent information leaving the left ear projects to the ipsilateral vestibular nuclei and ascends to synapse with the oculomotor nuclei within the medial longitudinal fasciculus of the brainstem. This input excites the left oculomotor nucleus and facilitates the left medial rectus muscle, eliciting adduction of the left eye, and simultaneously crosses to the contralateral abducens nucleus, facilitating the right lateral rectus muscle and eliciting abduction of the right eye. Concurrently, the opposing muscles are inhibited. The combined effect is conjugate gaze to the right of equal and opposite amplitude as the head rotates to the left.

Although gaze stability is required for normal function, there are times that the eyes and head must move together, such as when turning the head to scan the visual environment, and in these instances, the cerebellum overrides the VOR (*VOR cancellation*).

Vestibular System Functions

As discussed in Chapter 9: Interventions to Improve Standing and Standing Balance Skills, the sensory components responsible for upright postural control and balance include the somatosensory, visual, and vestibular systems. Owing to its critical role in static and dynamic balance, the pathways of the vestibular system are inextricably linked with all aspects of the postural control system. The otoliths and the semicircular canals detect the direction and rate of movement of the head in space, and the *parieto-insular cortex* processes this information for conscious awareness of body position.[3] Visual information is utilized in conjunction with gaze stability from the VOR to evaluate and interact with the environment. In addition, the vestibulospinal reflexes cooperate with the somatosensory system to regulate postural

TABLE 13.1 Innervation Pattern of Excitatory Input From Semicircular Canals

Semicircular Canal Primary Afferent	Extraocular Motor Neuron	Muscle Activation
(L) Horizontal	(L) oculomotor nucleus (R) abducens nucleus	(L) medial rectus (R) lateral rectus
(R) Horizontal	(R) oculomotor nucleus (L) abducens nucleus	(R) medial rectus (L) lateral rectus
(L) Posterior	(R) trochlear nucleus (R) oculomotor nucleus	(L) superior oblique (R) inferior rectus
(R) Posterior	(L) trochlear nucleus (L) oculomotor nucleus	(R) superior oblique (L) inferior rectus
(L) Anterior (superior)	(R) oculomotor nucleus	(L) superior rectus (R) inferior oblique
(R) Anterior (superior)	(L) oculomotor	(R) superior rectus (L) inferior oblique

L, left; R, right

Adapted from Shubert MC, Table 21.1, p. 968.[2]

tone and automatic postural responses. The unique connections of the vestibular system allow it to regulate postural control under conditions in which somatosensory and visual information conflict or are inaccurate or unavailable. These circumstances are simulated under conditions 5 and 6 of the Clinical Test for Sensory Interaction and Balance Test (CTSIB)[6] (also referred to as the Sensory Organization Test).

Clinical Note: Conditions 5 and 6 of the CTSIB indicate marked vestibular loss or bilateral involvement (Fig. 13.7).

Vestibular Dysfunction

An intact vestibular system provides essential support to normal movement and the ability to accomplish daily activities. Similar to most systems within the human body, the vestibular system can withstand some disruption with limited impact on function. However, the location and extent of the pathological process, as well as the person's response to the disturbance, determine the nature and scope of impairments that the therapist will observe. The term *disequilibrium* describes a balance deficit or the sensation of being "off balance," and can be attributed to an interruption along the vestibulospinal pathways. For example, people with unequal vestibular inputs tend to fall toward the side with diminished input or the weaker side *(lateropulsion)*. The term *vertigo* describes the illusion of movement while the body is at rest and indicates abnormal processing of information regarding head position. Like lateropulsion, vertigo

occurs due to a disparity in strength between the left and right sides of the system. Dysfunction of the vestibulo-ocular pathways results in *oscillopsia,* or the illusion of stable objects moving in the environment owing to a loss of gaze stability. The term *nystagmus* describes involuntary eye movements at rest or with movement. Each of these conditions may occur with disruption of the peripheral or central components of the vestibular system and are not mutually exclusive. Symptoms of vestibular dysfunction frequently overlap due to the multifaceted nature of the system and can include a variety of manifestations. Complaints include dizziness, vertigo, unsteadiness, gait disturbance, frequent loss of balance, and nausea and vomiting. See Box 13.1 for a list of common symptoms of vestibular dysfunction.

Vestibular System Examination and Evaluation

To ascertain a diagnosis, the therapist must navigate the patient through a series of tests and measures designed to determine potential causes of vestibulopathy. In doing so, the therapist must confirm that the pathology lies within the vestibular system and differentiate between a peripheral or central vestibular problem. If it is a peripheral vestibular problem, the therapist must identify the problem as bilateral or unilateral, and if the latter, locate the involved side. Given the complexity of the vestibular system, this problem-solving process requires a comprehensive understanding of each of

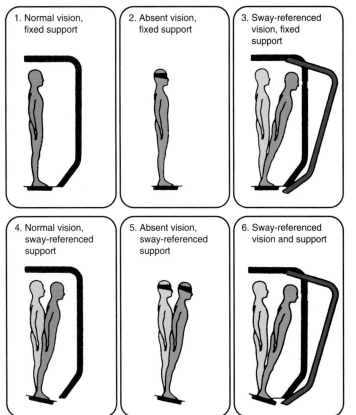

1. Normal vision, fixed support
2. Absent vision, fixed support
3. Sway-referenced vision, fixed support
4. Normal vision, sway-referenced support
5. Absent vision, sway-referenced support
6. Sway-referenced vision and support

FIGURE 13.7 Clinical test for sensory interaction and balance
From Schmitz TJ, and O'Sullivan SB. Examination of coordination and balance. In O'Sullivan SB, Schmitz TJ, Fulk GD (eds): Physical Rehabilitation, 6th ed. Philadelphia, F.A. Davis, 2014.

BOX 13.1 Common Symptoms of Vestibular Dysfunction

- Dizziness
- Vertigo or a spinning feeling or feeling that the world is spinning around the person
- Ringing in the ears (tinnitus) or pressure in the ears
- Difficulty concentrating
- Feeling disoriented
- Difficulty watching a moving object or the television
- Difficulty reading
- Report of a "whooshy" feeling with movement
- Unsteadiness
- Difficulty sitting or standing with drifting to one side (lateropulsion)
- Gait disturbances with difficulty walking a straight path
- Inability to turn head quickly without losing balance
- Frequent falls or near falls
- Losing balance while moving in the dark
- Nausea and vomiting
- Symptoms with riding in a car
- Symptoms with transitional movements such as rolling over in bed, sit-to-stand, or lying down
- Symptoms with head movements, such as looking up overhead or down toward the floor

these factors. This section presents basic tests, measures, and interventions to prepare the novice therapist to establish a preliminary plan of care (POC). As always, the primary goal of rehabilitation is to remediate impairments and return the patient to prior activities. Therapists must always recognize the need to generate a referral when faced with circumstances that lie beyond their scope of expertise. If the patient does not improve with basic interventions within a few weeks after initiating the POC, the therapist should refer the patient to a therapist who has successfully completed the American Physical Therapy Association's competency course in vestibular rehabilitation or to a neurologist. (The American Physical Therapy Association's [www.apta.org] "Find a PT" feature and the Vestibular Disorder Association [www.vestibular.org] are resources to identify local area specialists.)

Ø Red Flag: Contraindications to vestibular rehabilitation include:

- Loss of consciousness
- Acute traumatic brain injury
- Uncontrolled migraine headaches
- Sudden loss of hearing
- Increased pressure in one or both ears to the point of discomfort
- Fluid discharge from ears or nose after trauma or surgery, which may indicate cerebral spinal fluid leak
- Acute neck injuries and resulting pain that would interfere with treatment
- Presence of signs and symptoms associated with stroke

Subjective Report and Patient History

Because a method to directly measure vestibular system function does not exist in the clinical setting, system evaluation relies on subjective reports from the patient and the therapist's ability to accurately administer and interpret appropriate tests and measures. The most effective method to evaluate the vestibular system clinically involves the use of infrared video (Frenzel) goggles. However, fundamental clinical tests and measures often provide adequate information to identify a working diagnosis and to initiate a POC.

Clinical Note: The terms "bedside examination" or "clinical evaluation" refer to tests and measures of vestibular function administered in a physical therapy clinic or hospital room environment. These tests differ from *vestibular function tests* performed in a laboratory environment that require sophisticated instrumentation, including caloric, rotary chair, quantified dynamic visual acuity, and vestibular evoked myogenic potential tests.[4,5]

The word "dizziness" is a highly subjective term whose meaning differs with each person. It may be used to describe a range of sensations from lightheadedness, syncope, imbalance, flu, whirling, and spinning to a general feeling of "funny in the head." The therapist must ascertain the patient's precise meaning of "dizziness" to identify structures implicated in the pathology. Table 13.2 presents a variety of vestibular symptoms with possible sources of dysfunction.

A critical element of the examination entails documenting the severity of the symptoms and the resultant impact on daily life. Often, those recovering from vestibular insult experience noxious symptoms with head and body movement *(motion sensitivity)* and as a result, limit functional activities or deviate from normal movement patterns. A simple but appropriate tool to determine the overall severity of symptoms due to a vestibular disorder is an analog rating scale based on a 10-cm line with anchors at 0 and 10, where 0 indicates no symptoms and 10 represents symptoms of the worst possible severity. The *Motion Sensitivity Quotient (MSQ)* is a clinical test designed to identify provocative movement positions and intensity and duration of symptoms.[2,5] Valid and reliable measures that capture the level of perceived participation restrictions due to vestibular dysfunction include the *Dizziness Handicap Inventory (DHI)* and the *Activities-Specific Balance Confidence Scale (ABC)*[7] (see Table 9.2, p. 203).

Ø Red Flag: Because of the provocative nature of vestibular tests, the therapist should pay close attention to the symptom severity ratings. Vertigo, nausea, and vomiting are symptoms that patients find extremely uncomfortable and anxiety producing. Using the analog rating scale as a guide, the therapist should judiciously select and implement tests that will not overstimulate the patient and cause noxious results. Examination procedures should be administered so that the first tests are least provocative with progression to those likely to be most provocative.

TABLE 13.2 Clinical Presentation of Vestibular Pathology

Clinical Presentation/Symptoms/Complaints	Vestibular System Pathology
Complaints of objects "jumping" in the visual field Unable to see clearly with head movement Symptoms while walking with head movement	Oscillopsia due to loss of vestibular ocular reflex leading to reduced gaze stability
Poor postural trunk control and balance deficits Unsteady gait with wide BOS, unequal step length, and veering side to side while walking	Ataxia due to disturbance in lateral vestibulospinal tract and/or cerebellum
Neck pain, cervical muscle spasm, asymmetrical tightness of neck muscles	Postural misalignment due to disturbance in medial vestibulospinal tract and/or utricular involvement
Consistently drifting toward one side while upright (lateropulsion); can occur with or without visual input Veering to one side while walking	Static postural instability due to disturbance in vestibulospinal tracts and/or cerebellum
Difficulty reading	Reduced saccadic eye control due to dysfunction of the floccular nodular lobe and/or vermis of the cerebellum, medial longitudinal fasciculus
Difficulty watching moving objects such as cars in traffic	Abnormal visual tracking (smooth pursuits) due to dysfunction of the floccular nodular lobe and/or vermis of the cerebellum
Unable to keep eyes still when head is not moving	Spontaneous nystagmus due to disturbance of flocculonodular lobe of cerebellum and/or the vestibular apparatus, vestibular nerve
Complaints of motion sickness with or without vomiting	Nausea due to disruption of reticulospinal pathways

As part of the patient history, the therapist should explore medical history; determine the onset, duration, and severity of symptoms; ask whether there is associated hearing loss, ringing in the ears *(tinnitus)*, or vertigo; and determine whether the patient is experiencing postural imbalance or falls. Each of these factors contributes to the clinical picture of the patient and assists with the evaluation process. For example, the medical history may reveal conditions that indicate CNS involvement such as mild traumatic brain injury (including concussion), transient ischemic attacks, stroke, or multiple sclerosis, whereas manifestations of migraine headaches, anxiety, and panic attacks often mimic vestibular disorders. In contrast, hearing deficits, complaints of pressure in the ear, or tinnitus indicate involvement of the peripheral vestibular apparatus. The presence of vertigo differentiates vestibular system dysfunction from postural imbalance caused by somatosensory and musculoskeletal impairments. Importantly, the nature and mechanism of dysfunction and time since onset of symptoms provide key clues into the origin of the disturbance and underlying pathological process (Table 13.3).

Clinical Note: Oculomotor behavior provides integral clues about the source of vestibular lesions. As tests for oculomotor function tend to be only mildly provocative for the patient, assessing nystagmus (with the exception of the positional tests) and VOR function provides a gentle starting point in the examination process.

Nystagmus

Nystagmus, an involuntary oscillation of the eyes, can occur at rest *(spontaneous nystagmus),* with voluntary eye movement within the orbit *(gaze-evoked nystagmus),* and with changes in head position *(positional nystagmus).*[4] Nystagmus results from central or peripheral vestibular damage and, depending on the site of the lesion, occurs in horizontal, vertical, or torsional directions. The therapist examines spontaneous nystagmus by observing eye movement with the patient at rest; pure vertical or torsional spontaneous nystagmus suggests central vestibular system pathology.[4] In contrast, horizontal spontaneous nystagmus is associated with one-sided peripheral vestibular damage *(unilateral vestibular hypofunction)* and presents with a side-to-side eye motion that contains a quick phase and a slow phase. The quick phase beats toward the intact side (stronger ear). Clinically, nystagmus is named for the quick phase, so eyes that beat quickly to the left are identified as having left-beating nystagmus and indicate right peripheral hypofunction. (This is analogous to the game of tug-of-war where one team is

TABLE 13.3 Common Peripheral Vestibular Diagnoses, Clinical Presentation, and Mechanism of Dysfunction

Diagnosis	Clinical Presentation	Mechanism of Dysfunction
Benign Positional Paroxysmal Vertigo (BPPV)	*Sudden onset* of vertigo or "spinning" dizziness that lasts *seconds* while the person is moving, then subsides. Symptoms reoccur whenever moving in the plane of the involved canal.	Otoconia become dislodged from gelatinous matrix in otoliths and enter semicircular canals, causing a mechanical disruption. Otoconia can be free-floating in canal *(canalithiasis)* or adhere to the cupula *(cupulolithiasis)*
Ménière's Disease *(Endolymphatic hydrops)*	*Episodic bouts* of severe vertigo, tinnitus and pressure in the ear, nausea, vomiting, and disequilibrium that lasts *hours* Symptoms abate or resolve in early stages of disease but residual deficits are seen with repeated bouts over time.[3]	Swelling in inner ear causes increased pressure and damage within the membranous labyrinth. Cause of disease unknown.
Neuronitis/Neuritis	*Sudden onset* of vertigo, nausea and vomiting, disequilibrium and nystagmus that lasts *days* with gradual abatement within a few weeks Hearing remains intact.[3,4]	Inflammation of the vestibular nerve due to a virus
Labyrinthitis	*Sudden onset* of vertigo, nausea and vomiting, disequilibrium, and hearing loss that lasts *days,* with gradually abatement within a few weeks[4]	Inflammation within the labyrinth due to bacterial or viral infection
Acoustic Neuroma/Vestibular Schwannoma	*Gradual or sudden onset* of tinnitus, hearing loss, vertigo or disequilibrium Symptoms depend on the location of tumor.[2,5]	Slow-growing tumors derived from the Schwann cells of the vestibulocochlear nerve Tumor located within the internal auditory canal
Perilymphatic Fistula	*Sudden onset* vertigo and hearing loss[2,3]	An opening between the middle and inner ear Frequently seen with trauma and caused by a rupture in the oval or round window
Semicircular Canal Dehiscence	*Transient* vertigo precipitated by coughing, loud noises, and pressure changes in ear[2,3] *(Tullio phenomena)*	A form of fistula due to lack of temporal bone covering the superior semicircular canal

clearly stronger than the other; the red tie in the middle of the rope goes toward the stronger side.) Gaze-evoked nystagmus is assessed with the eye in all three positions in the orbit: center, right, and left. Normally, the eye remains still in all three positions. Nystagmus that beats in the same direction in one or more positions indicates a peripheral vestibular lesion with the quick phase designating the stronger side. Nystagmus that changes direction in one or more positions in the orbit designates a central vestibular lesion.

Benign Paroxysmal Positional Vertigo

The *Dix-Hallpike* and *roll tests* (Table 13.4) identify positional nystagmus due to benign paroxysmal positional vertigo (BPPV), the most common cause of vertigo in adults.[6] Although BPPV may be precipitated by head trauma or a virus, the precise causative factors remain under investigation. It is postulated that BPPV occurs when the otoconia become dislodged from the macula of the otoliths organs and are displaced into one or more of the semicircular

TABLE 13.4 Examination and Evaluation of Benign Paroxysmal Positional Vertigo

Dix-Hallpike Test for Posterior/Anterior Canal BPPV

Procedure	Positive Findings
• Begin in long-sitting with knees slightly flexed. Head should be close to edge of mat table (Fig. 13.8A). • Rotate subject's head 45 degrees of rotation toward side being tested so chin points toward shoulder. • Gently lay subject into supine position with head extended 30 degrees off table (head can be in evaluator's lap) (Fig. 13.8B). • Maintain position for 1 minute or until spinning sensation stops.[5] • Return subject to long-sitting (Fig. 13.8C).	The subject reports vertigo or spinning sensation that lasts less than 1 minute. The examiner detects a torsional nystagmus that lasts less than 1 minute. Positive findings indicate BPPV on the side that the head is rotated toward. If using Frenzel lenses or infrared goggles: • Up-beating nystagmus indicates involvement of the posterior canal. • Down-beating nystagmus indicates involvement of the anterior canal. • Clockwise rotational nystagmus indicates involvement of the left ear. • Counterclockwise rotational nystagmus indicates involvement of the right ear. These are usually present in combination with a directional (up/down) and torsional component (clockwise/counterclockwise).

Roll Test for Horizontal (lateral) Canal BPPV

Procedure	Positive Findings
• Begin in long-sitting with knees slightly flexed (Fig. 13.9A). • Subject tucks chin to chest (approximately 20–30 degrees of cervical flexion) and lies supine. • With neck flexed, head is fully rotated to side being tested. Position is maintained for 15 seconds (Fig. 13.9B). • The patient's head is returned to midline. The position is maintained for 15 seconds (Fig. 13.9C). • The head is then fully rotated to the opposite side. The position is maintained for 15 seconds (Fig. 13.9D).[5]	Subject reports vertigo that lasts less than a minute but not necessarily "spinning" as the nystagmus is not torsional in nature. While the subject's head is rotated to the left, the examiner detects a horizontal nystagmus toward the left or in the direction of the ground (*geotropic nystagmus*). While the subject's head is rotated to the right, the examiner detects a horizontal nystagmus to the right or toward the ground (*geotropic nystagmus*). ***Note:*** Both conditions must be met to conclude that the subject has canalithiasis.

canals. This displacement disrupts the movement of endolymph on the involved side, resulting in mismatched inputs with the paired intact semicircular canal on the opposite side. The hallmark characteristics of BPPV include vertigo and nystagmus whose onset is direction specific or positional in nature (i.e., only occurs when the head moves in the plane of the involved canal) and occurs within a few seconds after initiation of the movement (once the endolymph begins to move in the canal). The duration of symptoms designates the nature of the BPPV. Nystagmus and complaints of vertigo that last less than 60 seconds indicate BPPV due to *canalithiasis,* where the otoconia are free-floating in the semicircular canal. In contrast, nystagmus and complaints of vertigo that persist as long as the head remains in the provoking position indicates BPPV due to *cupulolithiasis,* where the otoconia adhere to the cupula.[4,5]

Recall that the semicircular canals on each side of the head are stimulated simultaneously, and each elicits a specific pattern of oculomotor excitation and inhibition. In BPPV, the presence of the otoconia in the semicircular canals disrupts endolymph flow, alters the displacement of the cupula, and causes a mismatch in peripheral signals from each ear. This results in uncoordinated patterns of ocular muscle stimulation (nystagmus). Owing to the erratic eye movement, the patient "sees" an unstable visual environment (analogous to a shaky hand with a video camera) and complains of vertigo.

Tests for BPPV require that the head be positioned to maximize the effects of gravity on the canal being tested.

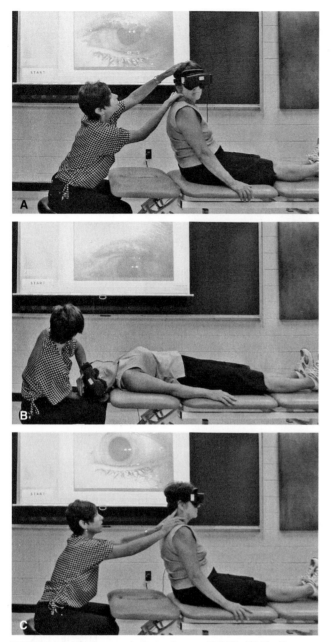

FIGURE 13.8 Test for anterior/posterior canal BPPV (A) Starting position for a right Dix-Hallpike test. The patient is positioned in long-sitting with head rotated toward the side being tested (in this case, to the right). Patient must be positioned so that when fully supine, the head can be extended off the table. The therapist sits on a stool at the end of the table to support the patient during the transition to supine and conduct the test without changing position. The patient is wearing infrared video Frenzel goggles that project the image of the eye to the screen. (B) Second position for a right Dix-Hallpike test. The patient is assisted to supine-lying with head extended 30 degrees and rotated 45 degrees toward side being tested (the right). The therapist sits on a stool at the end of the table to support the patient's head and provide comfort to the patient should vertigo ensue. This positioned is maintained for 30 seconds. The therapist views the image of the eye on the screen to determine the direction, duration, and intensity of nystagmus. If performing this test without goggles, the therapist must look directly at the patient's eyes to obtain this information. (C) Right Dix-Hallpike test, return to sitting. The therapist assists the patient to long-sitting to complete the right Dix-Hallpike test. The test should then be administered to the opposite side.

See Table 13.4 for more information on the administration and interpretation of these tests.

During the Dix-Hallpike test, BPPV that originates on the right side causes the superior pole of the eyes to rotate to the patient's right (counterclockwise as observed by the therapist), whereas BPPV originating on the left side causes the superior pole of the patient's eyes to rotate to the left (clockwise as observed by the therapist). A BPPV that originates in the anterior canal causes the eyeball to jump downward in the orbit, and BPPV in the posterior canal causes the eye to move upward. Typically, BPPV in the posterior and anterior canals includes torsional and vertical components. During the roll test, BPPV that occurs in the horizontal canal results in a lateral movement of the eye with eye movement toward the ground *(geotropic nystagmus)* with the head rotated to the right *and* left, or eye movement away from the ground *(apogeotropic nystagmus)* with the head rotated to the right *and* left.[2–5,7]

BPPV is diagnosed based on the presentation and duration of the nystagmus. For example, during the Dix-Hallpike test, a person who complained of vertigo and demonstrated nystagmus that was up-beating, clockwise, and of short duration would receive a diagnosis of "left posterior canal BPPV due to canalithiasis." A horizontal canal BPPV is named for the side of greatest intensity, direction, and duration of nystagmus. For example, during the roll test a person who complained of short-duration vertigo of greatest severity with the head turned to the right, and demonstrated a geotropic nystagmus with the head rotated to the right and left, would receive a diagnosis of "right horizontal canal BPPV due to canalithiasis." With horizontal canal involvement, an apogeotropic nystagmus signifies cupulolithiasis, whereas geotropic nystagmus signifies canalithiasis. Importantly, the therapist must be cognizant that to establish the presence of BPPV, the specific ocular conditions must be met and that BPPV may occur in more than one canal or bilaterally. The therapist must also recognize that although the direction of nystagmus indicates the involved canal in BPPV, the same ocular pattern may also indicate CNS involvement. For instance, down-beating nystagmus may be a sign of anterior canal BPPV or CNS involvement. The therapist must consider all elements of the examination, including the patient history and findings on tests and measures, to determine a plausible working diagnosis.

Because of the highly provocative nature of these tests, they are best performed toward the end of the examination. It should be noted that patients tend to be alarmed if not cautioned in advance about the potential for provocation of symptoms during testing. It is critical that the therapist explain that the tests are designed to reproduce vertigo and provide instructions to remain in the test position with their eyes open until the vertigo subsides.

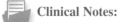 **Clinical Notes:**

• The *sidelying test* may be used as an alternative if the Dix-Hallpike test cannot be tolerated. For this

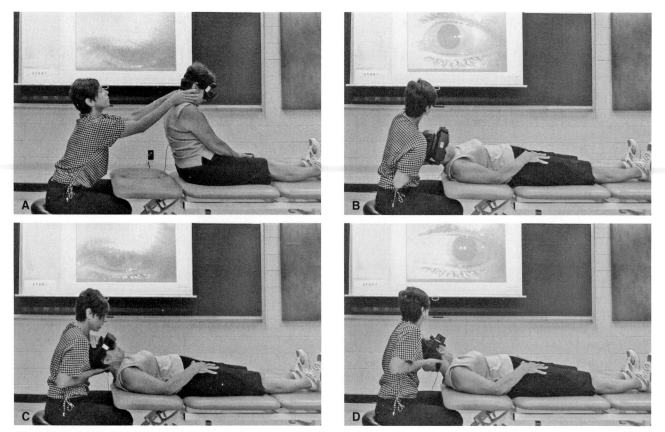

FIGURE 13.9 Test for horizontal canal BPPV (A) Starting position for the roll test. The patient is positioned in long-sitting with the head in neutral and chin tucked toward the chest (between 20 and 30 degrees of cervical flexion). The patient is wearing infrared video Frenzel goggles that project the image of the eye to the screen. (B) Roll test, second position. The patient is assisted to the supine position while maintaining cervical flexion. The therapist rotates the patient's head toward the side being tested (in this case, the right). This position is maintained for 15 to 30 seconds. The therapist determines the direction, duration, and intensity of nystagmus testing using the image of the eye on the screen. Note that the eye has deviated from center and is moving toward the patient's right (to the left of center to the therapist or observer). (C) Roll test, third position. The therapist rotates the patient's head back to midline and allows the patient to recover in this position for 15 to 30 seconds. (D) Roll test, fourth position and return to sitting. The therapist rotates the patient's head to the opposite side (in this case, to the left), testing the other horizontal canal, and maintains this position for 15 to 30 seconds. The therapist views the direction, duration, and intensity of nystagmus using the image of the eye on the screen. Note that the eye has deviated from center and is moving toward the patient's left (to the right of center to the therapist or observer). These finding are consistent with a geotropic nystagmus and horizontal canal BPPV due to canalithiasis. Once the test is concluded, the patient is returned to upright sitting.

test, the patient rotates the head toward one shoulder then lies down on the opposite shoulder. In this case, the downward ear is tested and the therapist identifies the BPPV as described for the Dix-Hallpike test.[5,7]

- Using infrared video Frenzel goggles allows the therapist to perform the oculomotor examination in the absence of light and observe oculomotor behavior uninfluenced by outside sources that could assist with fixation. The therapist views the ocular movement on a monitor that enlarges the eye image for improved clarity, and the examination may be recorded and replayed (Fig. 13.10).
- Spontaneous nystagmus due to peripheral damage usually resolves within 7 days from onset. Therefore, the therapist should suspect a central vestibular problem if spontaneous nystagmus is viewed in room light after 1 week postinjury. Given that the presence of spontaneous nystagmus implicates CNS involvement, the patient's physician should be alerted to this finding.

Smooth pursuit is the ability of the ocular muscles to smoothly follow a slowly moving target, whereas *saccades* (saccadic eye movement) allow the eyes to quickly locate and fix on a near target. Assessing smooth pursuit involves asking the patient to follow the therapist's moving finger as it travels horizontally, vertically, and diagonally approximately 16 in. (40.64 cm) away from the patient's face (Fig. 13.11). (This test is commonly called the "bow tie" test because the evaluator's finger traces the outline of a bow tie when testing.)

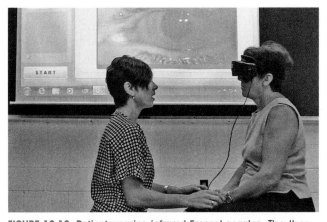

FIGURE 13.10 Patient wearing infrared Frenzel goggles The therapist helps familiarize the patient with the infrared Frenzel goggles before testing. Note the size and clarity of the image of the eye on the screen behind them. In the clinic, a television monitor or computer screen may be used to display the image from the goggles.

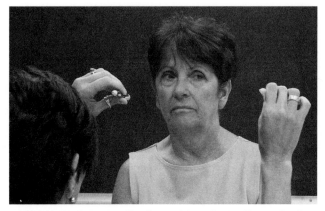

FIGURE 13.12 Saccades The therapist evaluates the patient's ability to locate targets placed in the near visual field (two pens). The patient is instructed to look quickly from the tip of one pen to the tip of the other pen while the therapist observes the patient's ability to hit the targets with appropriate control, speed, and accuracy.

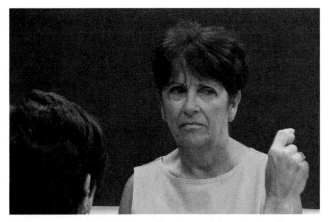

FIGURE 13.11 Smooth pursuits The therapist evaluates the patient's ability to perform smooth pursuits by instructing the patient to follow the moving finger with the eyes, without turning the head. The therapist observes the patient's visual tracking for appropriate control and accuracy.

The therapist tests saccades by providing the patient with two near targets (usually the therapist's nose and finger) and directs the patient to quickly look from one target to another. The therapist moves his or her finger approximately 20 degrees to the left, right, and up and down from the patient's nose so that the patient must locate the therapist's finger in each visual quadrant. The therapist determines the patient's ocular pattern and ability to hit the targets (normally this occurs in one to two eye movements) (Fig. 13.12). Abnormal saccades and smooth pursuits result in multiple, jerky eye movements in an attempt to find or follow the target. Smooth pursuits and saccades rely on normal vestibulocerebellar interaction; therefore, the therapist should suspect a central vestibular lesion if a patient is unable to perform either of these tasks in a normal fashion.

Vestibulo-ocular Reflex

Clinical tests of the VOR include the *Head Impulse Test* (also called the *Head Thrust Test*) and the evaluation of dynamic visual acuity (DVA) using an Early Treatment Diabetic Retinopathy Study (ETDRS) eye chart.[7] Because the VOR functions to fixate the eyes on a target despite head movement, the Head Impulse Test (HIT) reproduces this situation. While seated in front of the patient, the therapist instructs the patient to maintain gaze by looking at a near target (usually the therapist's nose). The therapist rotates the patient's head approximately 20 degrees from side to side until the patient appears comfortable with the rotation. The therapist then performs a small-range, low-amplitude head thrust toward one side while observing the patient's eyes to determine the patient's ability to remain on the focal point. If the patient is unable to maintain fixation, the therapist will observe the patient's eyes perform a quick saccade toward the nose in an attempt to "stay on target." This indicates VOR loss on the side toward which the head was moved (Fig. 13.13). Vestibulo-ocular reflex loss (a positive HIT) may be unilateral or bilateral (in one or both ears). Because the patient usually experiences a startle response with this test, causing him or her to anticipate the abrupt movement to the opposite side, it is best to first test the side suspected of dysfunction. The patient may report mild symptoms of discomfort with this test, so the severity of symptoms should be documented using an analog scale.

Dynamic visual acuity is the ability to see clearly with horizontal head movement. The patient is positioned 4 m (13.12 ft) from the ETDRS eye chart and is asked to identify the lowest line on the chart that can be read clearly. The therapist repeats the test while rotating the patient's head at a rate of 2 Hz (Fig. 13.14). The therapist compares the patient's ability to read with the head still versus moving and a difference of three or more lines on the ETDRS chart indicates VOR loss.

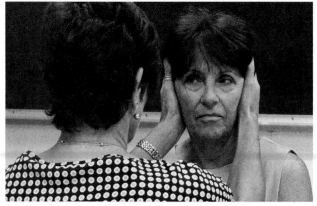

FIGURE 13.13 Clinical test of the VOR, the Head Impulse Test (HIT) While sitting, the therapist evaluates the patient's gaze stability by performing the HIT. The patient is instructed to maintain visual fixation on therapist's nose while the head is rotated to the right and left. The therapist performs a low-amplitude, rotational quick thrust toward the patient's left, requiring that her eyes remain fixed to the right and on target (the therapist's nose). If the patient is unable to maintain gaze stability, the eyes will move with the head during the rotation to the left, and the therapist will observe rapid movement of the eyes to the right to get back on the target.

the therapist must distinguish causative factors. It is critical for the therapist to differentiate between loss of postural control due to musculoskeletal and sensory motor impairments and imbalance due to vestibular dysfunction. Typically with vestibulopathy, there is a temporal association between the onset of vestibular symptoms and postural instability. The *Romberg* and *Sharpened Romberg tests* are useful in identifying lateropulsion, because the patient will tend to lean toward or fall toward the side of vestibular hypofunction. The addition of head rotation and/or neck flexion and extension in positions of reduced base of support (BOS), or on compliant surfaces, further helps to detect vestibular loss (Fig. 13.15). Other static balance tests appropriate for those with vestibular involvement include the *Functional Reach Test (FRT)*, the *Modified Functional Reach Test (mFRT)*, the *Modified Clinical Tests of Sensory Interaction in Balance (mCTSIB)*, and the *Berg Balance Test*[7] (see Table 9.2 on p. 203).

Given that the vestibular system plays an integral role in controlled movement in space, deficits in dynamic balance commonly occur with dysfunction. Tests such as the *Dynamic Gait Index (DGI)* and *Functional Gait Assessment*

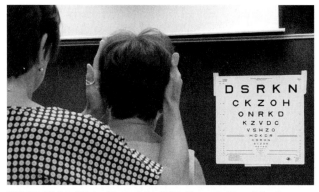

FIGURE 13.14 Clinical test of the VOR, Dynamic Visual Acuity (DVA) The patient is positioned approximately 4 meters away from an ETDRS chart and is instructed to read aloud the lowest line on the chart that can be seen clearly. The therapist then rotates the patient head at a rate of approximately 2 Hz (a metronome can be used to maintain the appropriate speed of head rotation). The patient is asked to read aloud the lowest line that can be seen clearly during head movement. A difference of three or more lines indicates VOR loss. A patient performing this test in standing may find it destabilizing; therefore, the therapist should remain close to insure patient safety.

Clinical Note: If an ETDRS chart is unavailable, the therapist may substitute a Snellen eye chart to assess the clarity of a target with rapid head movement. However, the use of line clarity as a measure of dynamic visual acuity is no longer applicable.

Postural Control

Patients with vestibular dysfunction readily report feelings of postural instability and activity limitations due to imbalance. Often multiple factors contribute to postural instability, and

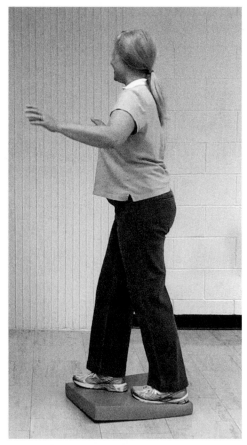

FIGURE 13.15 Static postural control Postural control is examined by having the patient stand in step position on a compliant surface while performing head rotation to the right and left. These conditions increase the demand on the vestibular system for postural control and detect disequilibrium.

(FGA) include items that assess postural control in combination with head movement, with changing gait direction and speed, decreased BOS, and varied visual inputs; therefore, these tests can be used to determine the impact of vestibular system involvement on dynamic balance and gait. Similarly, the *Timed Up and Go (TUG)* and the *TUG (cognitive)* tests include turning while walking and competing mental processing that illuminate potential vestibular involvement[7] (see Table 9.2 on p. 203).

Clinical Note: People who have bilateral vestibular loss exhibit greater impairments in postural control and gaze stability than those with unilateral hypofunction resulting from extensive loss of peripheral input from both sides of the system. On the other hand, those with bilateral vestibular loss tend to have less vertigo than those with unilateral hypofunction because there is less disparity between sides, and although inputs from both sides are diminished, they are more equal. The most common cause of bilateral vestibular loss is ototoxicity secondary to aminoglycoside drugs such as gentamicin and streptomycin.[3,5]

Nonvestibular Dizziness

The process of differential diagnosis requires that the therapist remain vigilant during the examination for those disorders that mimic vestibular dysfunction. Conditions such as high or low blood pressure, migraine headache, anxiety, panic attacks, and drug interactions or side effects can present as episodes of "dizziness."

Orthostatic hypotension may occur immediately following transitional positional movements against gravity such as supine-to-sit and sit-to-stand due to a drop in blood pressure. Similarly, elevated blood pressure can cause complaints of lightheadedness and dizziness. The therapist must carefully monitor blood pressure during the examination to rule out cardiovascular contributions to the patient's complaints.

Antihypertensive, antidepressant, and numerous other medications, may be the source of complaints of dizziness, especially in the elderly population. The therapist should review the patient's medications and note any temporal association between medication and dosing changes and the onset of symptoms. Symptoms that coincide with medications or those that are linked to a particular time of day are likely not vestibular in origin. Because the vestibular examination includes measures of static and dynamic balance, therapists are often the first to detect the impact of medication on postural control, and findings should be reported to the patient's physician.

Migraine headaches frequently simulate BPPV or Ménière's disease in presentation and may occur with or without symptoms of disequilibrium, nausea, vomiting, and headache.[4] Although migraine headaches are usually managed with medication prescribed by the physician, therapists may assist the patient in identifying and managing potential headache triggers, motion sensitivity, and remediating balance disturbances.[5,9] Symptoms related to phobias or specific activities (such as driving over a bridge) also imply that the source of pathology lies outside the vestibular system and may be caused by psychological or emotional conditions. Complaints of "swimming" or "tingling in the head," constant dizziness, and dizziness at rest that occurs in the absence of nystagmus also implicate somatoemotional conditions. Manifestations of anxiety and panic attack that overlap with the symptoms of vestibular disorders include dizziness, unsteadiness, sweating, shortness of breath, nausea, abdominal distress, heart palpitations, hot flashes or chills, and fear. The *Vertigo Symptom Scale* serves as a useful tool in discriminating emotional from vestibular causes of dizziness.[7] In all cases, it is imperative that the therapist communicate findings to the primary care physician and other appropriate members of the health-care team for effective management of the patient (Box 13.2).

Mechanisms of Recovery

With the exception of BPPV, where the otoconia can be removed from the semicircular canals, thus restoring normal function, recovery after vestibular insult occurs through the processes of compensation, adaptation, and habituation. The terms adaptation and compensation overlap in the literature, but the term *compensation* generally refers to the substitution of other structures for lost vestibular function. Compensation includes the use of multiple alternative pathways or strategies for recovery including, but not limited to, the utilization of remaining intact vestibular pathways such as the cervico-ocular reflex and intact oculomotor pathways, the selection of somatosensory pathways such as vision and information from the feet for postural control, increased use of anticipatory balance responses, and general changes in functional movement patterns, such as reduced gait speed to improve dynamic stability.[1,3–5] *Adaptation* may be thought of as a specific mode of compensation that refers to the reestablishment of the gain, phase, or direction of the VOR by the cerebellum.[1,4,5] In the context of learning, *habituation* refers to the decreased response to a noxious stimulus after repeated stimuli.[1,5] Vestibular rehabilitation employs habituation to reduce motion sensitivity by deliberate, repeated practice of movements that provoke symptoms. Regardless of the pathophysiological process involved, recovery of function after vestibular insult may be attributed to the combined effect of these mechanisms (Fig. 13.16).

Early Strategies to Enhance Recovery

Evidence indicates that early mobility and visual stimulation in room light enhance recovery.[4,5] Repeated functional movements reduce symptoms via habituation and promote compensation and adaptation. As stated, provocation of symptoms is an inherent element of the habituation process,

BOX 13.2 *Interpretation of Basic Test Findings*

Findings That Implicate Central Vestibular Involvement
- Constant dizziness
- Purely horizontal or vertical spontaneous gaze-evoked nystagmus
- Direction-changing gaze-evoked nystagmus
- Nystagmus that beats in equal and opposite directions
- Spontaneous nystagmus persisting more than 7 days after onset of symptoms
- Substantial loss of static and dynamic postural control, including posterior loss of balance
- Symptoms consistent with vertebrobasilar artery stroke:
  - Dysphonia
  - Upper- and lower-extremity hemiparesis
  - Facial paralysis
  - Ataxia
  - Vertigo
  - Nausea/vomiting
  - Nystagmus
  - Diplopia
  - Coma
  - Deafness
  - Disconjugate gaze

Findings That Implicate Peripheral Vestibular Involvement
- Vertigo that consistently occurs with head movement in a specific plane or direction
- Positional nystagmus that presents with a torsional and vertical/horizontal component
- Postural instability of varying degrees

- Corresponding tinnitus, pressure in the ears, or hearing loss

Findings That Implicate Unilateral Vestibular Involvement
- Moderate to severe vertigo
- Nystagmus with a quick phase that consistently beats in one direction (right or left)
- Lateropulsion
- Minimal loss of static and dynamic postural control

Findings That Implicate Bilateral Vestibular Involvement
- Mild to no complaints of vertigo
- Oscillopsia with extensive VOR loss
- Substantial loss of static and dynamic postural control
- Nausea with movement

Findings That Implicate Nonvestibular Involvement
- Constant dizziness
- Dizziness that is activity related rather than movement related
- Dizziness that occurs at a certain time of day or has a temporal relationship with medication
- Dizziness that occurs in absence of nystagmus
- No nystagmus with examination in infrared Frenzel goggles
- Fear of falling while seated
- Hyperventilation or shortness of breath related to panic attacks
- Verbalization of unspecified fear or anxiety
- Lightheadedness that occurs with transitions from lying to sitting or sitting to standing

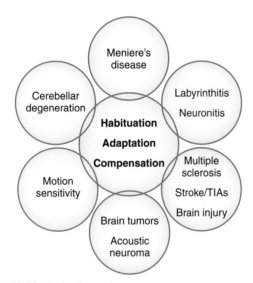

FIGURE 13.16 Mechanisms of recovery

and as a result, patients must practice at intensity levels that elicit symptoms until they resolve. However, it is the therapist's responsibility to establish the patient's tolerance level and modify the selection and intensity of activities to sufficiently promote recovery but not overpower the patient and

jeopardize compliance.[4,5] During the acute stage of a vestibular event, using visual fixation on a stationary target during transitional movements (including gait) mitigates symptoms and improves tolerance to movement. Pausing at points within a transition (resting on one elbow while moving from sidelying-to-sitting) and waiting for the symptoms to subside before continuing the movement is another strategy to enhance tolerance to early movement. In addition, enhancing sensory inputs from the body augments awareness of the body in space through additional proprioceptive and tactile stimulation. Although difficult, patients should be encouraged to walk as soon as possible following an acute event. Early gait characteristics include wide BOS, veering to one side, increased stepping strategies, reduced head and trunk movements, and using furniture or walls for haptic cues. Temporary use of assistive devices may be necessary for postural control and patient safety. After the acute phase, most patients demonstrate decreased gait speed and benefit from a daily walking program to regain previous self-selected speeds for community ambulation. Vestibular suppressant medications such as meclizine that help to alleviate symptoms initially may repress the compensation process and delay recovery with prolonged use and therefore should be discontinued as soon as possible.[4,5]

Clinical Note: Although vertigo and other symptoms range from mild to severe, the magnitude of vestibular symptoms must not be underestimated. During an acute vestibular event, such as labyrinthitis and neuronitis or an acute attack of Ménière's disease, symptoms may be debilitating, rendering the person immobile. It is not uncommon for someone to require hospitalization due to dehydration from vomiting. Many people find the sudden onset and harshness of these symptoms quite distressing but tend to respond positively to reassurances that symptoms generally abate within a few days to weeks. However, those with underlying or preexisting anxiety and/or depression may demonstrate less-effective coping strategies and thus subsequently reduced potential for recovery.

Interventions

Following the patient/client management model, selecting therapeutic interventions is based on examination findings and adheres to the principles of patient-centered care. Regardless of the underlying pathology, the therapist designs specific therapeutic interventions according to impairments revealed during the examination with the goal of resolving the patient's activity limitations and participation restrictions (Fig. 13.17). Successful remediation of vestibular impairments engages the patient as an active participant in the rehabilitation process and requires the patient to comply with the exercise program. The patient must comprehend the value of consistent practice and strictly abide by the therapist's instructions. Establishing clear limits on provocation enhances patient compliance and heightens potential for successful outcomes. As a general rule, vestibular exercises are best performed frequently throughout the day, but for short durations of time. The following methods help to limit overpractice and excessive noxious stimulation while enhancing compliance with vestibular rehabilitation exercises:

- Limit duration and frequency of practice *("Practice three times a day for 5 minutes.")*

- Limit symptom severity during practice *("Don't let your symptoms go above a 6 on the 0–10 scale.")*
- Limit duration of residual symptoms after practice *("Your symptoms shouldn't last more than 20 minutes after you perform your exercises.")*

Interventions to Restore Oculomotor and VOR Function

Consistent with other motor impairments, deficits in smooth pursuits and saccades may be reduced through task-specific practice. Importantly, tasks designed to solely improve oculomotor control must be performed with the head still. Saccades are trained by alternatively looking at two objects in the near visual field and should be practiced in both the horizontal and vertical planes. Almost any object can act as a target as long as the patient can clearly see it. Options include "sticky notes" tacked to the wall or two objects on a desk, such as a coffee mug and a vase. Using common objects like these lets the patient practice saccadic eye control anywhere or at any time during his or her daily routine, thus improving compliance. Reading is another excellent opportunity to practice saccades, because the eyes must jump from one word to the next. Smooth pursuit training requires that the patient focus on a moving target, again without head movement. In this case, the test criteria may be used as an intervention and the patient may follow the therapist's moving finger for task-specific practice. Computer games that require visual tracking of a target across the screen or scrolling "ticker tape" messages on the television offer additional opportunities for practice. Once the therapist ensures that the patient correctly performs each task and does so within established limits of provocation, these tasks may be assigned as part of the home exercise program.

One of the cerebellum's natural functions is to modify the VOR so that a visual image remains stable on the retinal fovea as the person clearly views the object. When visual inputs are altered, such as occurs with normal aging or with the use of corrective lenses, the cerebellum modifies the gain of the VOR to compensate for *retinal slip* (an unstable

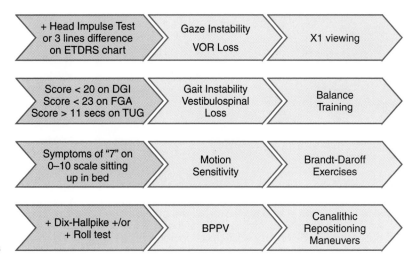

FIGURE 13.17 Framework for interventions

image on the retina).[1,5] Vestibular rehabilitation techniques capitalize on this inherent property of the cerebellum to reduce oscillopsia and restore gaze stability after vestibular insult. During the most common therapeutic intervention, called *times one viewing* (×1 viewing), the patient performs small-amplitude head movement as quickly as possible without losing focus on a visual target. For recalibration to occur, the patient must move the head while maintaining a clear (not blurry) visual focus on the target. Usually, the patient stands or sits approximately 4 feet from a target such as an eye chart, a sticky note (pasted to wall) with a letter boldly printed on it, or the number 12 on a clock. Visual targets that contain a clearly defined outline work best so the patient can easily detect if the object becomes blurred. The direction of the head movement practiced depends on the patient's symptoms. Generally, horizontal head turns (rotation) are more provocative than vertical movement (nodding up and down), and therefore it is more common to practice ×1 viewing while shaking the head in the "no" direction than while shaking the head in the "yes" direction. These activities require head movement within a small range, whereas the speed depends on the intensity of symptoms and can range from slow to rapid. However, the therapist should expect that the patient would find rapid movements more provocative and establish appropriate practice conditions (Fig. 13.18). Below is a sample script the therapist can use when instructing the patient in ×1 viewing exercises:

"Shake your head "no" (or "side to side") as fast, as you can, without the letter "H" on the sticky note getting blurry. Try to maintain this for 1 minute; however, do not let your symptoms go above a 6 on the 0–10 intensity scale. If they do, stop and allow them to return to 0 before attempting the exercise again. Perform this exercise multiple times throughout your day."

If the patient cannot tolerate ×1 viewing exercises while standing, the exercises may be performed while sitting. Should the patient find ×1 viewing exercises in sitting intolerable (as may result from bilateral vestibular loss) *gaze-shifting exercises* offer an alternative compensation training strategy.[5] Gaze shifting addresses eye and head coordination by allowing the patient to first practice saccades, and then head rotation, in sequence. The therapist instructs the patient to alternately look at two targets in the near visual field; the patient begins with the head and eyes aligned with the first target, then moves the eyes to the second target, followed by head movement toward the second target, and repeats the sequence looking back at the first target (eye movement followed by head movement). The patient should practice with targets positioned in both the horizontal and vertical planes with similar guidelines for practice as ×1 viewing exercises (Fig. 13.19).

Progression of ×1 viewing exercises occurs by increasing the speed of the head movement until the patient can shake the head rapidly without symptoms. Once the patient attains this level of proficiency in sitting and standing, the patient performs ×1 viewing while walking forward toward the stationary target and backward away from it. Usually, this results in increased symptoms or disequilibrium. Further progressions include performing ×1 viewing while walking and holding a target (such as a business card or sticky note) at arm's length in front and performing ×1 viewing with the target mounted on a busy visual surface such as a checkered tablecloth, creating a more challenging visual field. See Case Study 9: Peripheral Vestibular Dysfunction video segment for demonstration of ×1 viewing progressions.

Although not utilized as frequently in the clinic as ×1 viewing, a *times two viewing* (×2 viewing) paradigm exists. This exercise requires the patient to maintain a clear visual focus on a target as the head rotates in one direction while the target rotates in the opposite direction. The practice parameters remain the same as those for ×1 viewing exercises.

Red Flag: Note that ×2 viewing exercises are not recommended for patients with bilateral vestibular loss because they may cause excessive retinal slip.

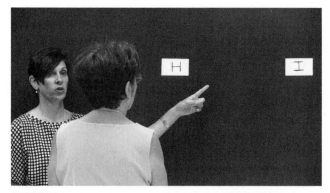

FIGURE 13.19 Gaze-shifting exercises The patient stands aligned with the first visual target (the letter *H*). She is instructed to move her eyes to focus on the second target (the letter *I*), then quickly move her head toward the target. She then duplicates the eye followed by head movements to look back at the first target. The therapist instructs the patient to repeat this procedure multiple times and throughout the day to promote compensation but to limit provocation and prevent overstimulation.

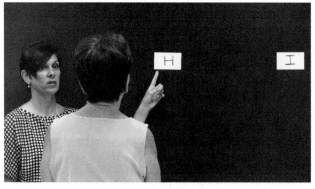

FIGURE 13.18 ×1 Viewing The therapist instructs the patient to shake her head from side to side as fast as she can without the letter *H* moving or becoming blurry. The therapist instructs the patient to repeat the procedure to encourage adaptation but to limit provocation and prevent overstimulation.

Patients with oscillopsia often hold the head still in an attempt to steady their gaze, and eventually this leads to complaints of neck stiffness and pain. The observant therapist notices the lack of normal head movement during activities such as sit-to-stand and during gait. As gaze stability improves, such patients benefit from interventions that reintroduce head movements into daily functional activities. An upper body ergometer may be used to promote upper thoracic trunk and cervical rotation. Initially the patient can be positioned in sitting for increased proprioceptive inputs and stability and then progressed to standing. Note that upper extremity activity creates movement in the visual field that some patients may find distracting or noxious. Once again, the therapist must guard against overstimulation and undesirable consequences (Box 13.3).

Interventions to Resolve Motion Sensitivity

Many people seek therapy because of motion sensitivity: an uncomfortable or noxious transient sensation that occurs during body and head movements after vestibular insult. But these complaints differ from those of vertigo because the patient usually denies a feeling of spinning. Rather, patients tend to described motion sensitivity as a "whooshy" feeling or feeling as if the head has to catch up to the body while moving in space. In response to motion sensitivity, many people alter their normal movement strategies and, in doing so, inadvertently delay or prevent recovery. To remediate motion sensitivity, interventions promote habituation in combination with practice schedules that keep symptoms within a reasonably tolerable level.

Brandt-Daroff exercises, originally used to correct BPPV, are well suited for this purpose because all of the semicircular canals are stimulated in one activity. To perform Brandt-Daroff exercises, the patient begins in short-sitting in the middle of a bed. The patient rotates the head toward one shoulder and lies down onto the side of the opposite shoulder (see Fig. 13.20A and B). This motion usually reproduces symptoms. The patient remains in the sidelying position for 30 seconds or until the symptoms stop. The patient returns to sitting, again waiting for the symptoms to subside before rotating the head to the opposite shoulder and lying down at the other end of the bed (Fig. 13.20C and D). Once again, symptoms may be provoked, and the patient remains in this position for 30 seconds or until symptoms resolve and then returns to sitting. Originally, Brandt-Daroff exercises required that the patient perform the procedure for 5–10 repetitions, three times per day until the symptoms resolved for 2 consecutive days.[2,5] However, many patients find this intensity intolerable, and as an alternative, the

---

BOX 13.3 Compensation, Adaptation, and Habituation Training Strategies for Recovery From Vestibular Insult During Acute and Subacute Phases (Excluding BPPV)

Acute Period Training Strategies (during or immediately after a vestibular event)

- Use visual fixation as *compensation* for lost VOR function; have person fix gaze on a visual target while moving
- Break transitional movements into component parts. Rest between stages and allow disorienting sensation to pass before continuing movement (e.g., when sitting from sidelying, come up part way, then wait for sensation to dissipate before sitting upright)
- When moving head, dissociate head and eye movements; first move eyes toward target, then move head
- Use assistive devices as necessary
- When turning while walking, employ the eye-then-head strategy, then add a quarter-turn of the body using wide steps
- Reduce exposure to busy visual environments

Subacute Period Training Strategies (once movement is tolerated)

- Practice *habituation* exercises. Determine postures, functional tasks, and transitional movements that provoke symptoms. Limit the intensity of symptoms elicited during the practice session to 4 to 6 on 0 to 10 scale.
- Practice Brandt-Daroff exercises
- Break movements down into component parts to improve tolerance. For example, if symptoms are experienced while bending over to feed the dog

from standing, practice reaching to floor from sitting.
- Practice ×1 viewing exercises in sitting and standing: begin adaptation exercises as soon as possible. Use a clear visual target such as the number 12 on a clock, then shake head from side to side (and/or up and down) as fast as possible, keeping the numbers in focus. Limit provocation to 4 to 6 on 0 to 10 scale of symptom intensity. Repeat multiple times throughout day.
- Progress ×1 viewing exercises by performing head shaking as described above under the following conditions:
  - Walking toward and away from target
  - Walking while holding a visual target at arm's length
  - Walking with a visual target mounted on a complex visual background such as a checkered tablecloth
- Practice standing in tandem on floor and foam with eyes open to eyes closed
- Practice walking with head turns starting with head turned to one side looking over one shoulder for a given distance. Then switch to looking to the opposite side. To progress, gradually decrease the number of steps the person takes with the head turned in one direction before rotating head in opposite direction. This increases the speed of head turns from right to left. The subject should not use lateral stepping strategies to maintain a steady gait and should not step outside a 12-inch-wide pathway.

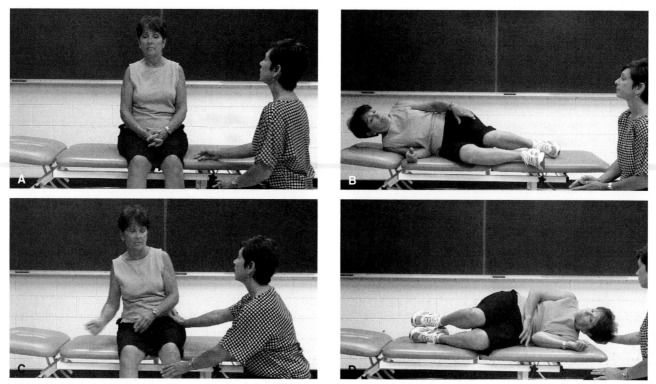

FIGURE 13.20 Brandt-Daroff exercises (A) Starting position. The therapist instructs the patient to sit in the middle of the mat with the head in neutral position. (B) First position, sidelying. The patient rotates the head toward one side (her left) then moves to the sidelying position on the opposite side (her right). In this case, right sidelying is provocative, and the edge of the mat table is elevated to improve patient tolerance to the activity. The patient is instructed to maintain this position until the symptoms subside, plus an additional 30 seconds. (C) Second position, return to sitting. The patient returns to sitting in the middle of the mat. The therapist provides manual contacts for safety and emotional support due to patient complaints of symptoms during this phase of the exercise. The patient is instructed to remain in this position until symptoms subside. (D) Third position, sidelying. The therapist instructs the patient to rotate her head to the opposite side (her right) and to move into left sidelying. The therapist provides support for the patient's head due to the patient's position on the table. The patient remains in this position until symptoms subside plus 30 seconds.

therapist may prescribe Brandt-Daroff exercises for three to five repetitions, three times per day, to improve adherence.

Another method of habituation involves actually practicing those motions that provoke symptoms, but at a slower speed or reduced range of motion. For example, if reaching to the floor from standing produces fairly intense symptoms, then the patient practices standing reaching to the bed or table, followed by sitting on the bed and reaching to the floor. The behavior is shaped until the patient can merge the two components without symptoms. Although most patients readily identify symptomatic movements, the *Motion Sensitivity Quotient* helps to identify and rate provocative positions to prioritize practice.

Motion sensitivity from vertical plane stimulation manifests itself with activities such as riding in an elevator, getting out of the car, and jogging or other fitness activities. Standing on a minitrampoline or BOSU ball offers small-amplitude displacements in the vertical plane and may be progressed by having the patient perform rapid heel raises, then small jumps. Step machines and elliptical

trainers provide advanced stimulation to ready the patient to return to more dynamic activities.

Clinical Note: The following analogy may help patients adopt their habituation exercises: "*If a concert pianist fractures his hand, he does not play skillfully the same the day the cast is removed. He must practice to restore his previous level of proficiency. The same holds true after vestibular disorders: A person must practice for the system to return to its previous level of function.*"

Interventions to Resolve BPPV

Benign paroxysmal positional vertigo is a condition rather than a disease, and unlike other vestibular pathologies, it is a mechanical disruption that can be corrected.[4] The goal in the treatment of BPPV is to remove the otoconia from the canal, thereby reestablishing delivery of synergistic information from the periphery to the central vestibular system. This is accomplished by guiding the patient's head through a series of movements consistent with the plane and shape of the affected canal, utilizing endolymph flow to clear the otoconia (similar to running water to clear a drain pipe). The repositioning maneuver selected depends on the involved canal (anterior, posterior, or horizontal) and type of BPPV (canalithiasis or cupulolithiasis). With cupulolithiasis, the otoconia must first be freed from the cupula, so these techniques tend to be more vigorous. Regardless of the technique used, the patient should sit upright for approximately 20 minutes after repositioning maneuvers.[5]

Several repositioning maneuvers correct both canalithiasis and cupulolithiasis, and these techniques range from simple to complex. The versatile *modified Epley maneuver* is presented in Table 13.5 because it may be used to correct anterior and posterior canal BPPV due to canalithiasis (the most common form of BPPV) (Fig. 13.21).[5] The most commonly used maneuver to correct a horizontal canal

BPPV due to canalithiasis, the *bar-b-que maneuver* (also referred to as the *log roll maneuver*), is also presented in Table 13.5 (Fig. 13.22). The patient may experience symptoms of motion sensitivity for a brief period after repositioning maneuvers, but if the BPPV has cleared, the patient should not complain of positional vertigo. If vertiginous complaints persist, the therapist should retest for BPPV and perform maneuvers as indicated. Repeated maneuvers may be required, but if the BPPV does not clear within a few weeks of treatment, the therapist should refer the patient to a competent vestibular therapist or physician.

Red Flag: Improper execution of the repositioning maneuvers may move the otoconia from the posterior canal to the horizontal canal, converting posterior canal BPPV to horizontal canal BPPV. In this case, the

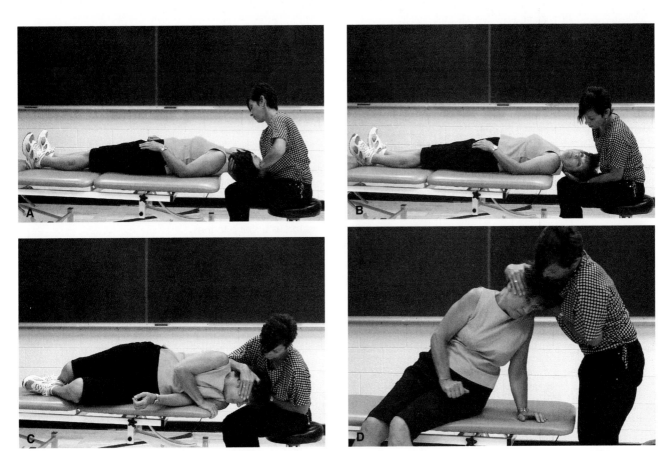

FIGURE 13.21 Right modified Epley maneuver (A) First position. The first position of this canalith repositioning maneuver is the same as the test position for the Dix-Hallpike test (in this case, head extended and rotated to the right). The patient lies supine with the head rotated 45 degrees to the involved side and extended off the table approximately 30 degrees. This position is maintained for 30 seconds. The therapist is seated on a rolling stool at the head of the table to support the patient's head during the procedure. Note that the patient is not wearing the goggles during the repositioning maneuver since the nature of the BPPV has already been determined and the procedure is likely to reproduce vertigo. (B) Second position. While maintaining head and neck extension, the therapist rotates the patient's head 45 degrees to the opposite side (the left) and maintains the position for 30 seconds. (C) Third position. The therapist instructs the patient to roll onto the left shoulder and rotate the head to look at the floor. The therapist supports the patient's head throughout this transition and maintains neck extension. The position is held for 30 seconds. (D) Return to sitting. The patient is assisted to sitting from the left sidelying position. The therapist maintains the patient's head position during the transition to prevent conversion to a horizontal canal BPPV.

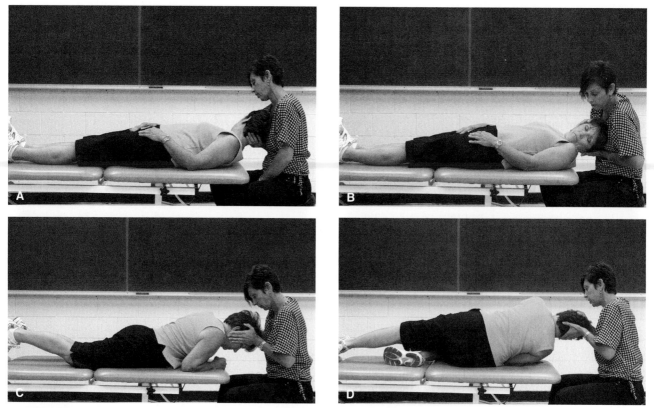

FIGURE 13.22 Bar-b-que maneuver for a horizontal canal canalithiasis (A) Starting position. The first position of this canalith repositioning maneuver is the same as the test position for the roll test (in this case, head flexed approximately 20 to 30 degrees and rotated 45 degrees to the right). The therapist is seated on a rolling stool at the head of the mat table to support the patient's head during the procedure. This position is maintained for 15 seconds or until the symptoms subside. (B) Second position. The therapist maintains head and neck flexion and rotates the patient's head 45 degrees to the left. This position is maintained for 15 seconds or until the symptoms subside. (C and D) Third position. The patient is assisted with rolling to the left side (C) then into prone (D) while the therapist maintains the chin tuck position. The patient should not be allowed to extend the head beyond neutral. This position is maintained for 15 seconds. The patient is assisted from prone to right sidelying then up into sitting. The therapist assists the patient by supporting the head during transitions.

characteristics of the BPPV change, as do the patient's complaints. The therapist must then resolve the horizontal canal BPPV.

Clinical Note: The technique depicted in Table 13.5 is commonly referred to as Epley maneuver in the clinic; however, this is a misnomer as the true Epley maneuver entails vibration at the mastoid process before repositioning and application of a soft cervical collar after repositioning.[5]

Interventions to Restore Postural Control

For many patients recovering from vestibular loss, the inability to walk normally and navigate in the community with confidence is a major concern. The following questions sampled from the DHI are designed to explore activity limitations and participation restrictions imposed by postural instability.[11]

- Because of your problem, is it difficult for you to go for a walk by yourself?
- Does walking down the sidewalk increase your problem?
- Does walking down the aisle of the supermarket increase your problem?
- Because of your problem, is it difficult for you to walk around your house in the dark?
- Does performing more ambitious activities sports, dancing, and household chores, like sweeping or putting the dishes away, increase your problem?
- Because of your problem, are you afraid that people will think that you are intoxicated?
- Because of your problem, are you afraid to leave your home without someone accompanying you?

Responses to these questions in conjunction with findings on tests and measures such as the *Sharpened Romberg* and *Functional Gait Assessment* guide the therapist in choosing interventions to remediate postural instability. Preexisting musculoskeletal and sensory motor impairments that limit the postural control system will impede recovery after vestibular insult; therefore, the therapist should also address these impairments in the POC. Chapter 9: Interventions to Improve Standing and Standing Balance Skills provides

TABLE 13.5 Repositioning Maneuvers to Treat BPPV Due to Canalithiasis

Canalith Repositioning Maneuver for Canalithiasis (modified Epley)	Canalith Repositioning Maneuver for Horizontal Canalithiasis (bar-b-que [log roll] maneuver)
If both sides are positive, **perform repositioning maneuver on side of greatest intensity first. Do not treat both sides in same session.** Procedure:	Perform repositioning maneuver on side of greatest intensity first. Procedure:
• Begin in starting procedure for Dix-Hallpike test with head rotated 45 degrees toward the **involved side.** Lay patient supine with head extended 30 degrees off table (Fig. 13.21A).	• Begin in the starting positioning for the roll test with the patient long-sitting with chin tucked to chest (approximately 20–30 degrees of cervical flexion) and head rotated toward the side with the symptoms of greatest intensity (Fig. 13.22A).
• Keeping head extended, rotate 45 degrees toward **uninvolved** side (Fig.13.21B).	• Wait 15 seconds or until symptoms pass, then rotate head back to midline and wait 15 seconds or until symptoms pass.
• Patient rolls to lie on the uninvolved shoulder and turns head to look at floor (Fig. 13.21C).	• Rotate head fully toward uninvolved side and wait 15 seconds or until symptoms pass (Fig. 13.22B).
• Patient then sits up with head maintained so that chin points at uninvolved shoulder (Fig. 13.21D).	• Roll patient into prone position so that they are looking at floor and wait 15 seconds or until symptoms pass. It is important to maintain the head in flexion as the patient rolls into prone (Fig. 13.22C)
	• Complete the roll so that the patient ends lying on the involved side and return to sitting (Fig. 13.22D).

extensive information regarding postural control and interventions to improve static and dynamic balance. Static stability and weight-shifting techniques will be most beneficial immediately after an acute vestibular event to regain normal postural alignment and correct lateropulsion. Recall that conditions in which somatosensory and visual inputs are unreliable or conflicting maximize vestibular inputs. Therefore, static balance tasks designed to enhance vestibular function should combine a reduced BOS and/or compliant surfaces with head movements and/or oculomotor training. The therapist must tailor practice activities to the specific needs of the patient. For example, during the initial stages of recovery, practice standing with a diminished BOS with eyes open (EO) on a solid surface may offer a substantial challenge. As the patient progresses, a compliant surface and active head movements may be added to increase difficulty, such as standing on foam and tossing a ball from one hand to another. Tandem standing (heel-to-toe) on foam while playing paddle ball is an example of an advanced intervention that involves vestibulo-ocular and vestibulospinal functions while engaging the patient in a dual-tasking activity. Catching and throwing a ball while standing on a compliant surface is another activity that combines visual tracking, eye-head and hand coordination with dynamic postural control and altered somatosensory inputs (Fig. 13.23).

Walking with eyes closed (EC), head turns, and turning are examples of task-specific practice to improve dynamic postural control. The EC condition simulates conditions where vision is removed, such as walking in a dark room. Walking with head turns frequently causes gait disturbance

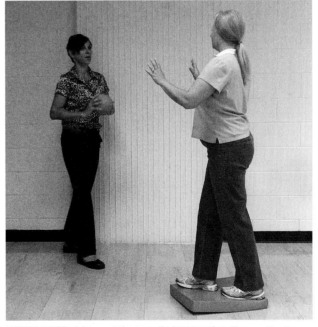

FIGURE 13.23 Advanced therapeutic intervention The patient participates in a game of catch with the therapist while standing in step position on foam with the head turned to the right. These conditions challenge all functions of the vestibular system. The activity can be further progressed by adding a cognitive component such as singing a song.

owing to disruption of the push-pull mechanism. Early practice of this task includes asking the patient to walk 20 ft (6 m) with head turned toward one side, then walking the same path with the head turned toward the opposite side. In the case of unilateral hypofunction, the patient usually deviates from a straight path with the head turned toward the involved side. In this situation, it may be helpful initially for the patient to fixate on a visual target. As always, the therapist must take appropriate measures to ensure patient safety. Progressions include walking the same distance while turning the head every three steps, and finally, every step. An example of a task-specific progression consists of walking with the head turned to speak with someone walking next to the patient. Refer to the Case Study 9: Peripheral Vestibular Dysfunction video (online at Davis*Plus*) for a demonstration of this intervention.

Similarly, walking with quick turns also causes instability for those with vestibular loss. Early strategies to regain postural control with turning involve breaking down components of the task and performing them in sequence. Instead of performing a quick pivot turn, the patient is instructed to perform partial turns, turning 90 degrees twice, rather than 180 degrees at once. When turning, a patient with poor dynamic balance may improve control by first moving the eyes in the direction of the turn, focusing on a visual target, then moving the head in the direction of the turn, and finally turning the body. As the patient progresses, head and eye movements may occur simultaneously with increased speed of turning.

Clinical Note: Scores from reliable tests and measures lend themselves to utilization as short-term goals. For example, if the stated outcome for the episode of care reads "The patient will score a 23/30 on the *Functional Gait Assessment* indicating that she is no longer at risk for falls," then an appropriate short-term goal might be "The patient will walk 20 feet with head turns to the left and right without stepping outside a 12-inch path."

Treadmill training provides practice walking under advanced conditions due to alterations in somatosensory inputs. Initially, light finger-touch support may be used in conjunction with slower gait speeds. As the patient progresses, upper extremity support should be discontinued and gait speeds increased to the patient's normal preferred walking pace. Superimposing head turning or dual-tasking activities further enhance difficulty.

Factors That Limit Recovery

Evidence supporting vestibular rehabilitation continues to accumulate, but certain factors limit the prognosis after vestibular insult.[2,5,7] Central nervous system involvement such as multiple sclerosis, stroke (including the anterior-inferior and posterior-inferior cerebellar arteries), and brain injuries respond more slowly to rehabilitation and are more likely to leave residual deficits. The therapist must consider this when establishing a prognosis and developing a POC. Similarly, the potential for recovery after bilateral vestibular loss is limited when compared with unilateral loss. Because bilateral involvement does not imply that both sides sustained equal damage, recovery depends on the extent of remaining function of the system, and restoration of activities relies heavily on compensation from the visual and somatosensory systems. Ménière's disease responds to vestibular rehabilitation strategies early in the disease process, but not with chronic Ménière's disease, and medical management may be indicated (e.g., surgical or chemical ablation of the remaining neurons to alleviate ongoing episodes and decrease disparity between sides). Preexisting conditions and comorbidities that limit the postural control system (such as blindness or diabetes mellitus) reduce the potential for recovery as compensation and adaptation strategies are constrained. The training and experience of the therapist play a critical role in the outcomes achieved with vestibular rehabilitation. As stated earlier in this chapter, skillful management of vestibular disorders requires extensive study to achieve advanced competency in this area of clinical practice. Specifically, the conditions of atypical BPPV, cervicogenic dizziness, concussion involving conjugate gaze abnormalities, including tropia and phoria, and pediatric vestibular disorders deserve the attention of advanced practitioners.

For more in-depth information on the treatment of vestibular disorders, the reader is directed to the published works of Susan Herdman,[5] Janet Helminski,[8] and Susan Whitney.[9] Information regarding continuing education in vestibular rehabilitation is available at the American Physical Therapy Association's website www.apta.org, Careers and Education tab. Specific information regarding appropriate tests and measures is available at the American Physical Therapy Association Neurology Section website at www.neuropt.org/professional-resources/neurology-section-outcome-measures-recommendations and at the Rehabilitation Measures Database at www.rehabmeasures.org.

Student Practice Activities

Student practice activities in Box 13.4 focus on interventions to examine, evaluate, and treat patients with vestibular disorders. Activities in Box 13.5 provide opportunities for clinical decision making by having the student determine appropriate interventions for selected clinical problems. In Box 13.6 students are directed to analyze Case Study 9: Peripheral Vestibular Dysfunction and provide answers to the guiding questions. Reviewing the case history, evaluative data, and videotaped segments provides additional opportunities for clinical decision making and promotes integration of the principles of vestibular rehabilitation.

(text continues on page 321)

BOX 13.4 STUDENT PRACTICE ACTIVITY: INTERVENTIONS TO EXAMINE, EVALUATE, AND TREAT VESTIBULAR DISORDERS

OBJECTIVE: Practice administering and assessing vestibular tests and interventions

EQUIPMENT NEEDS: Mat table, ETDRS chart

DIRECTIONS: Working in groups of three to four students, perform the vestibular activities presented below. Members of the group will assume different roles (described below) and will rotate roles each time the group progresses to a new item on the outline.

▲ One person assumes the role of therapist and participates in discussion.
▲ One person serves as the patient and participates in discussion.
▲ The remaining members participate in discussion and provide supportive feedback during demonstrations. One member of this group should be designated as a "fact checker" to return to the text content to confirm elements of the discussion (if needed) or if agreement cannot be reached.

Thinking aloud, brainstorming, and sharing thoughts should be continuous throughout this activity! Carry out the following activities for activity listed below.

1. Discuss the *activity,* including patient and therapist positioning, indications for use, and appropriate verbal cues and manual contacts.
2. Discuss the *performance* of the activity and assessment of the technique by the designated therapist and patient, including proper safety precautions, recommendations and suggestions for improvement, and strategies to make the activity either *more* or *less* challenging for the patient.
3. Discuss the *answers to the guiding questions* presented after each activity.

If any member of the group feels he or she requires practice with the activity and technique, the group should allocate time to accommodate the request. All group members providing input (recommendations, suggestions, and supportive feedback) should also accompany this practice.

Perform the Following Examination Techniques:
▲ Spontaneous gaze
▲ Gaze-evoked nystagmus

Guiding Questions

1. If eye beats purely up and down, what type of vestibular impairment is implicated?
2. If eye beats to left in all three positions in the orbit (center, looking right, looking left), what type of vestibular impairment is implicated?
3. If eye beats to right in the center of the orbit and when looking right, what type of vestibular impairment is implicated?
4. If eye beats to right when looking right, and left when looking left, what type of vestibular impairment is implicated?

Perform the Following Examination Techniques:
▲ Smooth pursuits—track a moving target across the visual field
▲ Saccades—ability to locate and alternate between two targets

The therapist notes the patient's ability to complete the movement smoothly.

Guiding Questions

1. What might an abnormal finding look like to the therapist?
2. If the patient is unable to perform one or both of these tests, what type of vestibular impairment is implicated?

Perform the Following Examination Techniques:
▲ Head Impulse Test
▲ Dynamic visual acuity using ETDRS chart

The therapist determines the presence or absence of gaze stability.

Guiding Questions

1. If the patient is unable to maintain gaze on the clinician's nose to both the right and left, what type of vestibular impairment is implicated?

Perform the Following Examination Techniques for Positional Nystagmus/BPPV:
▲ Dix-Hallpike test
▲ Roll test

The therapist directs patient to keep eyes open and (if able) determines direction of nystagmus.

Guiding Questions

1. If the patient does not demonstrate nystagmus but complains of dizziness, what type of impairment is implicated?
2. If patient demonstrates nystagmus that begins 5 to 10 seconds after being in the test position and lasts for less than 1 minute, what type of vestibular impairment is implicated?
3. If during the Dix-Hallpike test the patient demonstrates a clockwise, up-beating nystagmus, what type of vestibular impairment is implicated? What intervention is required to remediate the problem?
4. If during the roll test, the patient demonstrates a right-beating nystagmus with the head rotated to the right and a left-beating nystagmus with the head rotated to the left, what type of vestibular impairment is implicated? What intervention is required to remediate the problem?

Demonstrate the Following Interventions for BPPV:
▲ Practice the repositioning maneuvers selected above.
▲ Practice the modified Epley maneuver to the opposite side.
▲ Practice the bar-b-que maneuver to the opposite side.

(box continues on page 320)

BOX 13.4 STUDENT PRACTICE ACTIVITY: INTERVENTIONS TO EXAMINE, EVALUATE, AND TREAT VESTIBULAR DISORDERS (continued)

Guiding Question

1. What directions are important for the patient to understand prior to beginning these interventions?

Demonstrate the Following Interventions for Gaze Stability:

▲ Practice instructing the patient in gaze-shifting exercises as part of the home exercise program.

▲ Practice instructing the patient in ×1 viewing exercises as part of a home exercise program.

Guiding Question

1. Under what conditions would you chose one technique over the other?

BOX 13.5 STUDENT PRACTICE ACTIVITY: PRACTICE SELECTING APPROPRIATE INTERVENTIONS FOR SELECTED CLINICAL PROBLEMS

OBJECTIVE: Based on selected clinical problems and patient data, identify factors contributing to complaints of "dizziness" and choose appropriate therapeutic interventions to remediate them. The significant findings from a physical therapy evaluation of a patient diagnosed with vestibular disorder are presented for each clinical case.

DIRECTIONS: Based on the clinical information provided, determine a working diagnosis and list three appropriate therapeutic interventions for that patient. Interventions chosen should be those that would be employed during the first three therapy sessions.

Case 1

Subjective Complaints: feels as if being pushed to left when walking; feels unsteady when getting into and out of bed

History: sudden onset of dizziness began 3 weeks ago; imbalance with vomiting that lasted 3 days with gradual improvement; moderate hearing loss in L ear

Tests and Measures

Oculomotor Examination: Right-beating nystagmus with gaze in middle, L and R positions

Gaze Stability Tests: (+) HIT to left; (–) HIT to right; two-line difference on ETDRS for DVA, but test reproduces symptoms

Postural Control and Gait: DGI = 18/24; unsteady when walking with head turns right/left and up/down; >3 secs to turn around and stop with stepping strategies to prevent LOB

Positional Tests: (–) Dix-Hallpike; (–) roll test

Activity Limitations and Participation Restrictions: DHI = 32/100; unable to return to work as letter carrier for U.S .Postal Service

Working Diagnosis:_____

INTERVENTIONS:

1.

2.

3.

Case 2

Subjective Complaints: feels unsteady and reports blurred vision, difficulty reading at night; denies vertigo

History: vision and hearing intact

Tests and Measures

Oculomotor Examination: Direction-changing gaze-end nystagmus with looking to right and left; poor control with saccades and smooth pursuits

Gaze Stability Tests: (–) HIT to right and left

Postural Control and Gait: FGA= 21/30; ↓ stability with changing gait speed; steps over one shoe box; takes five steps in tandem; deviates 13 inches outside walking path when walking with eyes closed; unable to walk backward without losing balance

Positional Tests: (–) Dix-Hallpike; (–) roll test

Activity Limitations and Participation Restrictions: Trips frequently when walking outdoors and while shopping; difficulty completing work on the computer

Working Diagnosis:_____

INTERVENTIONS:

1.

2.

3.

Case 3

Subjective Complaints: reports spinning dizziness/vertigo when washing hair in shower, lying down in bed, and reclining in arm chair; reports symptoms last for seconds

History: sudden onset of symptoms that began 6 weeks ago; denies hearing loss but reports "pressure" in right ear

Tests and Measures

Oculomotor Examination: WNL

Gaze Stability Tests: (+) HIT to R; (–) HIT to L

BOX 13.5 STUDENT PRACTICE ACTIVITY: PRACTICE SELECTING APPROPRIATE INTERVENTIONS FOR SELECTED CLINICAL PROBLEMS (continued)

Postural Control and Gait: mCTSIB; WNL; no LOB with Romberg; LOB with Sharpened Romberg

Positional Tests: (–) Dix-Hallpike on L; (+) Dix-Hallpike on R; (–) roll test L and R

Activity Limitations and Participation Restrictions: DHI = 14/100; difficulty sleeping; must use three pillows and cannot lie flat.

INTERVENTIONS:

1.

2.

3.

Working Diagnosis:_____

Key: R, right; L, left; HIT, head impulse test; ETDRS, Early Treatment Diabetic Retinopathy Study; DHI, Dizziness Handicap Inventory; DGI, Dynamic Gait Index; LOB, loss of balance; mCTSIB: modified Clinical Test for Sensory Interaction in Balance; WNL, within normal limits

BOX 13.6 STUDENT PRACTICE ACTIVITY: CASE STUDY ANALYSIS—PUTTING IT ALL TOGETHER

OBJECTIVE: **To integrate the principles of vestibular evaluation and interventions in patient case format**

DIRECTIONS: **Read Case Study 9: Peripheral Vestibular Dysfunction (p. 387), view the video segments of the case online and answer the guiding questions.**

SUMMARY

This chapter presented an overview of the anatomy, physiology, and basic functions of the vestibular system to provide the entry-level therapist with foundational information needed to provide effective interventions to a person with a vestibular disorder. Common central and peripheral vestibular disorders were introduced together with fundamental differences in clinical presentation. Evidence-based examination tools were provided as well as a basic framework for the selection of appropriate interventions. Because of their versatility, the modified Epley and bar-b-que maneuvers were presented as tools to treat BPPV, and the concepts of habituation, adaptation, and compensation were explained.

REFERENCES

1. Kandel, ER, et al. Principles of Neural Science, ed 5. New York, McGraw-Hill, 2013.
2. Shubert, MC. Vestibular disorders. In O'Sullivan, SB, Schmitz, TJ, and Fulk, GD (eds): Physical Rehabilitation, ed 6. Philadelphia, F.A. Davis, 2014.
3. Lundy-Ekman, L. Neuroscience Fundamentals for Rehabilitation, ed 4. St. Louis, Elsevier Saunders, 2013.
4. Baloh, RW, and Kerber, KA. Clinical Neurophysiology of the Vestibular System, ed 4. New York, Oxford University Press, 2011.
5. Herdman, SJ. Vestibular Rehabilitation, ed 3. Philadelphia, F.A. Davis, 2007.
6. Shumway-Cook, A, and Horak, B. Assessing the influence of sensory interaction on balance: suggestions from the field. Phys Ther, 1986; 66:1548–1550.
7. VEDGE Task Force. Application of the Vestibular EDGE Task Force Recommendations. Presented at: American Physical Therapy Association Combined Sections Meeting. February 3–6, 2014; Las Vegas, Nevada.
8. Helminski, JO, Holmberg, J, and Rabbitt, R. Translating the biomechanics of benign paroxysmal positional vertigo to the differential diagnosis and treatment. Presented at: American Physical Therapy Association Combined Sections Meeting. February 3–6, 2014; Las Vegas, Nevada.
9. Furman, JM, Cass, SP, and Whitney, SL. Vestibular Disorders: A Case-Study Approach to Diagnosis and Treatment, ed 3. New York, Oxford University Press, 2010.
10. Shumway-Cook, A, and Woollacott, M. Motor Control—Theory and Practical Applications, ed 4. Baltimore, Williams & Wilkins, 2012.
11. Jacobson, GP, and Newman, CW. The development of the Dizziness Handicap Inventory. Arch Otolaryngol Head Neck Surg, 1990; 116:424.

Case Studies

In Part 2, we are privileged to bring together a group of outstanding clinicians from across the country to contribute case studies in both written (Part 2) and visual (videos online at Davis*Plus*) format. The contributing therapists demonstrate an exceptional commitment to student learning. Their collective expertise is reflected in the presentation of the cases, the guiding questions posed, and critical decisions required as students progress through the cases.

The overriding goals of Part 2 are to provide the student an opportunity to interact with the content and to promote clinical decision-making skills by evaluating the examination data to determine *diagnosis, prognosis,* and *plan of care.* These case studies present diagnoses familiar to the rehabilitation setting, with an overriding emphasis on improving activities and skills that are meaningful to the patient and typically contribute to improved functional outcomes and quality of life. The cases are guided by the conceptual framework and practice patterns presented in the *Guide to Physical Therapist Practice.*

We present 15 unique case studies in both written and video formats. The written case content is further divided into (1) *examination* and (2) *evaluation, diagnosis and prognosis, and plan of care* categories. Student evaluation of the physical therapy examination data (history, systems review, and specific tests and measures) provides the needed information on which to base decisions in determining the diagnosis, predicting the optimal levels of recovery and the time frame in which this will occur, and developing the plan of care. Challenges to student decision-making are introduced through guiding questions addressing specific considerations of the case example.

The videos presented online (www.fadavis.com) consist of a 6-minute visual segment distributed among sample components of the initial *examination,* sample *interventions,* and functional *outcomes.* The three segments include a planned time-lapse between episodes of filming to depict patient progress toward, or achievement of, functional outcomes. Most of the case

(text continues on page 324)

P A R T

II

studies were filmed over a 4- to 6-week period. Following is a brief description of each visual segment.

- **Examination** (Video Clip 1): The first video segment focuses on elements of the physical therapy examination. Content varies based on patient presentation. The intention is to provide a more complete understanding of the patient's impairments and activity limitations as well as how they affect function.
- **Intervention** (Video Clip 2): Based on the contributing therapists' intervention strategies selected to improve functional outcomes, the second video segment presents elements of a physical therapy treatment session.
- **Outcomes** (Video Clip 3): The third video segment depicts functional outcomes toward the end of the episode of care (i.e., the efficacy of interventions on the resolution of impairments and activity limitations). Some case studies depict activities similar to those presented in the first video clip (examination) to provide a *before* and *after* comparison of the impact of intervention.

During each visual segment, the accompanying narration directs the viewer to the specific elements depicted or calls attention to unique aspects of the case. A text version of each narration is presented online at Davis*Plus* (www.fadavis.com).

The following is a recommended sequence for students' use of the case studies. However, based on desired learning strategies, goals, and objectives, the sequence may vary.

1. **Consider the text case content.** Begin with the written case content. Assume you are the physical therapist managing the case, and you have just completed the initial examination. Analyze and organize data from the history, systems review, and tests and measures.
2. **View examination.** View the clip several times while observing the impairments or activity limitations (examination data) presented.
3. **Answer the text guiding questions.** With information gained from the examination data and from observing the patient's motor performance, progress to the case study guiding questions. These questions are designed to promote clinical decision-making skills through evaluating the examination data, determining the physical therapy diagnosis, establishing the prognosis, and developing the plan of care.
4. **View intervention.** The second video clip presents segments of a patient/therapist treatment session. It provides a unique opportunity to observe a sample intervention selected by the contributing therapist to improve functional outcomes. While viewing this segment, compare and contrast the interventions presented with those you selected.
5. **View outcomes.** Finally, the third video clip depicts functional outcomes at the end of the episode of care as well as the impact of training on the resolution of impairments and functional limitations. While viewing this segment,

compare and contrast the goals and expected outcomes you identified with
the functional outcomes achieved.

6. **View answers to the case study questions.** (This activity should be completed in student groups.) The therapists presenting the cases have shared
their perspectives by providing answers to the guiding questions. Answers
to the guiding questions for Case Studies 1 to 10 are available online at
Davis*Plus* (www.fadavis.com). While reviewing the answers provided:

• Compare and contrast your responses with those presented.

• Develop a rationale for the answers provided. Does the rationale match
the one on which you based your response?

• Be aware that your answers will not concisely match those provided.
Remember that this *does not necessarily mean your answers are incorrect.*
Often, there is more than one acceptable response to the questions. Determining the efficacy of your response requires careful reflection about the
rationale for your clinical decisions. It may also require one or more of
the following: discussion with peers, a return to text content (or other
resources) to confirm or refute your response, and/or consultation with a
physical therapy faculty member or colleague.

Note to Students

A collaborative learning environment with small groups of students working
on a single case can optimize learning. Each component of the sequence can
be discussed among group members. Discussion provides an opportunity to
compare your thoughts and ideas with those of classmates, instructors, or
colleagues.

Note to Instructors

Feedback from our readers has suggested that a portion of the case studies
(11–15) be presented with answers to the guiding questions made available
only to instructors. The intention is to provide faculty greater flexibility when
integrating these cases into specific course assignments designed to promote
clinical decision-making skills and/or into classroom discussions. Answers
to these guiding questions are available for faculty online at Davis*Plus*
(www.fadavis.com). The answers to the guiding questions can then be made
available to students after the assignments and discussions are completed.

Outcome Measures

A variety of outcome measures are incorporated into the case studies. Some
are general measures of function applicable to a broad spectrum of patients,
and others are diagnosis specific. These standardized instruments provide

important information about a patient's activity limitations and participation restrictions. In clinical practice, outcome measures have a range of applications, including providing baseline patient data on which to base function-oriented goals and outcomes at the start of an episode of care, as a measure of patient progress toward goals and outcomes, as indicators of patient safety, and as evidence to support the effectiveness of a specific intervention.

The clinical reasoning process that leads to sound clinical decision-making is a course of action involving a range of cognitive skills that physical therapists use to process information, reach decisions, and determine actions. In a health-care environment that demands efficiency and cost-effectiveness, physical therapists are required to make complex decisions under significant practice restraints. Owing to the importance of this critical phase of physical therapy intervention, clinical decision making requires continual practice and feedback throughout professional preparation. The intent of the case studies is to offer an opportunity to guide and facilitate development of this important process.

CASE STUDY

1

Patient With Traumatic Brain Injury

TEMPLE T. COWDEN, PT, MPT

Examination

History

- **Demographic Information:**

Patient is a 41-year-old, Filipino-Caucasian man. He is English speaking and right-hand dominant. He was admitted to the adult brain injury service for inpatient rehabilitation following a motorcycle accident.

- **Social History:**

Patient is an ex-Marine; he has one son and is divorced from his wife. He lives with his fiancée in a single-story home. His fiancée has three children who live with them, ages 12, 13, and 15. The patient's fiancée does not work outside of the home but is responsible for the cooking, laundry, cleaning, and upkeep of the home, as well as taking care of the children.

- **Employment:**

Patient worked as an inspector for a fire safety company. His job involved driving to various locations where he inspected and tested various fire safety equipment (such as fire alarms, fire extinguishers, and so forth), which involved a moderate amount of physical activity.

- **Living Environment:**

Patient resides in a single-story home, which is split level, with one step to enter the home's main living room area. There are three steps to enter the home, with no handrails or ramp in place.

- **General Health Status:**

Patient is medically stable and able to participate in a rehabilitation program. Prior to this injury, patient was believed to be in good general health.

- **Social and Health Habits:**

Patient enjoys playing basketball and softball with his friends. Prior to injury, he was not involved in a formal exercise program but remained active playing sports, spending time with the children and through work activities. Patient states his favorite activities are riding motorcycles and "hanging out at the bars." While it is unclear how much, the patient has a history of alcohol use; his use of other drugs is unknown.

- **Medical/Surgical History:**

Medical history is unknown due to incomplete medical records from previous facility. Patient is agitated and unable to consistently and appropriately answer questions. Surgical history prior to this injury is unknown.

- **History of Present Illness:**

This is a 41-year-old male, status post motorcycle accident while intoxicated on June 28. The patient was reportedly found approximately 70 feet (21 m) from the site of impact. He was brought in by ambulance to an acute hospital with a Glasgow Coma Scale (GCS) score of 1-1-1; blood pressure was 90 systolic (diastolic not documented), with a heart rate of 160 beats per minute and an oxygen saturation measurement (SpO_2) of 80% using pulse oximetry. Owing to the low GCS score and decreased oxygenation, the patient was immediately intubated and ventilated. He was noted to have 2-mm pupils bilaterally and was nonreactive with motor function evident on only the left side. There were multiple skin abrasions on the right shoulder, chest, and hip. Upon admission to the acute facility, the patient underwent computed tomography (CT) scan and was diagnosed with the following: flailed chest with multiple rib fractures, lung contusions, pneumothorax, contusion and laceration of the right lobe of the liver with hemoperitoneum (presence of blood in the peritoneal cavity), fracture subluxation of the right acromioclavicular joint, and fractures of the bases of the right fourth and fifth metacarpals. A CT of the brain showed blood in the fourth ventricle, brain stem, upper cervical spinal cord, and subarachnoid space (subarachnoid hemorrhage and intracranial hemorrhage). The patient was transferred to the intensive care unit (ICU), where consultations were done by neurosurgery, infectious disease, and orthopedics. A triple lumen catheter and gastrostomy tube were inserted. No further operative intervention was planned at that time. The patient remained in critical condition in the ICU with full ventilatory support for approximately 2 weeks. On July 3, the patient had a tracheotomy. The patient underwent drainage and débridement of the right hip wound and a vacuum-assisted closure (VAC) device placement on July 23. On July 24, due to deteriorating renal function, the patient was diagnosed with acute renal failure caused by sepsis and contrast toxicity. On July 31, the patient underwent irrigation, drainage and open reduction, and internal fixation of the carpometacarpal joint of the right fourth and fifth metacarpals, with plans for immobilization for 6 weeks. On August 4, the patient experienced an episode of asystole after the removal of a triple lumen catheter, which required cardiopulmonary resuscitation (CPR) and atropine to resolve. Due to closure of the right hip wound and suspicion of necrotizing fasciitis, he underwent further wound débridement and irrigation of the subcutaneous tissue and muscle on August 13. It was then discovered that the patient had bilateral common femoral popliteal and left peroneal deep venous thromboses (DVTs), and an inferior vena cava filter was placed. By early September, the patient was considered medically stable. He was able to tolerate a tracheostomy collar; he was more alert and able to respond to questions and communicate his basic wants and needs at times. However, he frequently became agitated. Patient was decannulated (removal of tracheostomy) prior to transfer to the rehabilitation facility, but the exact date was not indicated.

Admission to Rehabilitation Facility

- **Chief Complaints:**
  At the time of the initial examination (September 10), patient appears to be very agitated, restless, and impulsive. He complains of stomach and back pain. He also repeatedly yells out for his girlfriend and "Doc" (doctor). Patient appears to have hypersensitivity to touch and pain throughout right upper extremity (UE). Patient appears to be diaphoretic, with blood pressure of 150/110 mm Hg and a heart rate of 132 beats per minute.
- **Functional Status:**
  Before the injury, patient was independent with all basic activities of daily living (BADL) and instrumental activities of daily living (IADL).
- **Medications:**
  Upon admission, patient was taking the following medications: Colace, Dulcolax, buspirone, clothiapine, metoprolol, omeprazole, ranitidine (changed to Prevacid upon admission), Lovenox, sertraline, and olanzapine. The patient was also taking Vicodin and levetiracetarn for prophylactic use (patient has no history of seizures). Upon admission, this was changed to Neurontin because levetiracetarn has been found to increase agitation in some patients.

Systems Review

- **Cardiovascular/Pulmonary System:**
  - Heart rate: 132 beats per minute seated at edge of bed with regular rhythm
  - Respiratory rate: 18 breaths per minute
  - Blood pressure: 150/110 mm Hg
  - Oxygen saturation: 98% on room air

- Temperature: 98.2°F (36.8°C)
- Edema: mild bilateral pitting edema of legs and feet; right foot 2+, left foot 1+
- **Integumentary System:**
  - Scar(s): right hip with well-healed scar. Upper abdominal midline scar (from gastrostomy tube placement). Right hand has sutures in place on fourth and fifth fingers.
  - Skin color: black, necrotic tissue of left second and third toes. Face is pale, sweaty, and warm to the touch.
  - Skin integrity: healing tracheostomy scar. Excessive dryness and flaking of both feet. Excessively thick and long toenails bilaterally. Left UE excoriation.
- **Musculoskeletal System:**
  - Gross symmetry: obvious right shoulder deformity due to separation. Patient maintains right elbow flexed at about 90 degrees. Patient does not have normal midline orientation. He requires some assistance to maintain upright sitting balance without back support.
  - Gross range of motion (ROM): right UE limitations noted at shoulder (flexion, abduction, and external rotation), elbow, and wrist. Left UE ROM within functional limits (WFL). Decreased ROM evident at both knees (Fig. CS1.1).
  - Gross strength of right extremities: right UE demonstrates significant weakness and is typically maintained in a flexed position (Fig. CS1.2). The patient is able to actively move the right lower extremity (LE) against gravity (Fig. CS1.3).
  - Height: 6 ft, 4 in. (2.9 m)
  - Weight: 198 lb (89.9 kg)
- **Neuromuscular System:**
  - Gross coordinated movement: patient is able to move from supine to sitting at the edge of the bed without assistance. However, he requires supervision when sitting

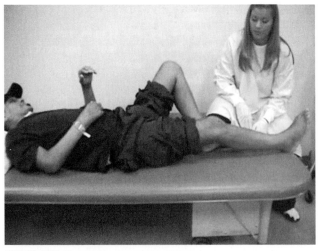

FIGURE CS1.1 Range of motion limitations are evident in the right knee (lacks full extension). *Not shown:* Limitations also exist in the left knee.

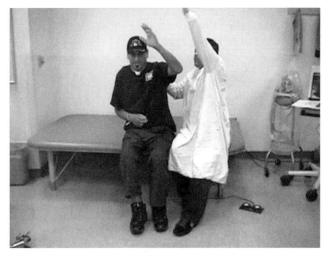

FIGURE CS1.2 In sitting, significant weakness is evident in the right UE (unable to move against gravity). The right UE is flexed and adducted with the hand tightly fisted. The left UE is able to move against gravity (shoulder abducts, externally rotates with elbow flexion).

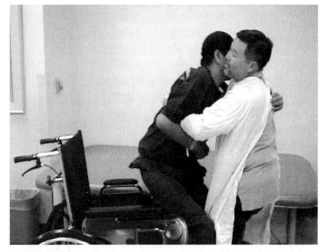

FIGURE CS1.4 Patient requires maximal assistance to transfer from wheelchair-to-platform mat. The patient lacks extension control at both hips and knees. Right UE remains flexed and adducted with hand tightly fisted.

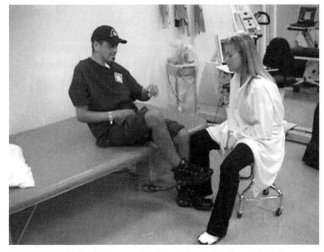

FIGURE CS1.3 In sitting, patient is able to lift the right LE against gravity (hip flexes with knee flexion). Note posterior shift of the trunk that accompanies the lift; patient moves into a sacral sitting position.

without a back support for prolonged periods, owing to poor balance and forwardly flexed posture with decreased trunk control. When sitting, he is unable to reach outside of his base of support (BOS) without loss of balance. He is unable to perform sit-to-stand transfers, even with the bed elevated, without maximal assistance from the therapist due to difficulty with task planning and diminished LE strength (Fig. CS1.4). Patient requires maximal assistance to move from bed to wheelchair owing to impulsivity, decreased strength, and impaired balance. Ambulation ability could not be examined initially because of safety concerns as well as patient agitation.
- Motor function (motor control and motor learning): Patient is able to voluntarily move all four extremities.

Weakness of right UE is greater distally than proximally. He is able to follow simple commands for movement, but with poor consistency, which appears to be a result of restless, agitated behavior. No ankle clonus is present.
- Communication and cognition: The patient is alert and oriented to person and place. Voice is slightly dysarthric, but patient is generally understandable. At previous facility, patient had participated minimally in a speech-language program; he had not received any previous physical therapy services. Patient is very restless, demonstrating continual writhing and movement from supine to sitting up in bed. Patient demonstrates impulsive behavior; he attempts to climb over bedrails and lies down without regard to his position in bed or the presence of bedrails. He answers simple personal questions appropriately but is highly distractible and has only about 60% accuracy for known personal information.

Tests and Measures

- **Sensory Integrity:**
  - Light touch and superficial pain sensations appear grossly intact for both LEs and the left UE.
  - The therapist is unable to perform even a general light touch examination on the right UE secondary to patient guarding. Unable to formally test light touch and superficial pain sensations because of patient's inability to follow testing instructions (secondary to cognitive impairments and decreased attention).
- **Strength:**
  - Unable to accurately examine strength, secondary to difficulty following testing instructions. (*Note:* Approximately 2 days after the initial consult, the therapist

was able to complete the manual muscle test [MMT].) Right LE is weak; patient is unable to move all joints through complete range against gravity. See Table CS1.1. Patient is unwilling to even attempt movement of right UE due to complaints of pain and weakness. Atrophy of right deltoid is noted. Left UE demonstrates functional strength throughout.

- **Range of Motion:**
  See Table CS1.2.
- **Cranial Nerve Function:**
  - Visual fields are grossly intact (CN II). Pupils are equal, round, and reactive to light and accommodation; extraocular muscles are intact (CN III, IV, V); face is symmetrical (CN VII).
  - Hearing is grossly intact (CN VIII). Palate is symmetrical in elevation; phonation is clear (CN IX, X). Tongue is midline with protrusion and limited ROM (CN XII).
- **Deep Tendon Reflexes:**
  Left UE 1+, right LE 2+, bilateral patellar reflex 2+, bilateral Achilles tendon reflex 1+. Key to grading:
  - 0, no response
  - 1+, present but depressed, low normal
  - 2+, average, normal
  - 3+, increased, brisker than average possibly but not necessarily abnormal
  - 4+, very brisk, hyperactive with clonus, abnormal
- **Balance:**
  - Patient demonstrates poor seated balance, although he is able to sit upright independently using a back support. He is unable to reach outside of his BOS for functional activities without loss of balance or fall. He typically demonstrates a kyphotic posture.
  - Patient has poor standing balance, as he is unable to achieve or maintain full standing without maximal assistance from the therapist. He is unable to perform

TABLE CS1.1 Lower Extremity Manual Muscle Test

Joint	Motion	Left	Right
Hip	Flexion	3/5	3/5
	Extension	2/5	2/5
	Abduction	2/5	2/5
Knee	Flexion	3/5	3/5
	Extension	3/5	3/5
Ankle	Dorsiflexion	3/5	2/5
	Plantarflexion (tested supine)	2/5	2/5

All scores are based on a 0 to 5 scale: 5, normal; 4, good; 3, fair; 2, poor; 1, trace; 0, no contraction.

TABLE CS1.2 Passive Range of Motion Examination (in Degrees)

Joint	Motion	Left	Right
Shoulder	Flexion	WFL	0–90*
	Extension	WFL	WFL
	Abduction	WFL	0–80*
	Internal rotation	WFL	WFL
	External rotation	WFL	0–30*
Elbow	Flexion	WFL	15–150
Wrist	Flexion	WFL	0–60
	Extension	WFL	0–30
Hip	Flexion	WFL	WFL
	Extension	WFL	WFL
	Abduction	WFL	WFL
Knee	Flexion	5–110	3–110
	Extension	Unable to achieve full knee extension	
Ankle	Dorsiflexion	WFL*	WFL*
	Plantar flexion	WFL	WFL

*Indicates movement was accompanied by pain.
WFL, within functional limits.

dynamic movements during standing without loss of balance.
- **Gait:**
  Unable to examine
- **Activities of Daily Living (ADL):**
  - BADL: Requires moderate to maximal assistance or total dependence for execution of all BADL
  - IADL: Dependent

Evaluation, Diagnosis and Prognosis, and Plan of Care

Note: Before considering the guiding questions below, view the Case Study 1 Examination video segment to enhance your understanding of the patient's impairments and activity limitations. *After completing the guiding questions,* view the Case Study 1 Intervention video segment to compare and contrast the interventions presented with those you selected. Last, view the Case Study 1 Outcomes video segment to compare and contrast the goals and expected outcomes you identified with the functional outcomes achieved.

Guiding Questions

1. Describe this patient's clinical presentation in terms of:
   a. Impairments
   b. Activity limitations
   c. Participation restrictions
2. Identify three impairments you would address initially to improve this patient's activity limitations and participation restrictions.
3. Identify three goals to address the impairments you identified above and the expected outcomes to improve the patient's activity limitations and participation restrictions.
4. Describe three treatment interventions focused on functional outcomes that could be used during the first 2 weeks of therapy. Indicate how you could progress each intervention, and include a brief rationale that justifies your choices.
5. What important safety precautions should be observed during treatment of this patient?
6. Identify factors, both positive (assets) and negative, that play a part in determining the patient's prognosis for recovery.
7. Describe strategies that can be used to develop self-management skills and promote self-efficacy in achieving goals and outcomes.
8. How can the physical therapist facilitate interdisciplinary teamwork to assist in reaching identified goals and functional outcomes?

Reminder: Answers to the case study guiding questions are available online at Davis*Plus* (www.fadavis.com).

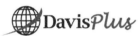 VIEWING THE CASE: Patient With Traumatic Brain Injury

As students learn in different ways, the video case presentation (examination, intervention, and outcomes) is designed to promote engagement with the content, allow progression at an individual (or group) pace, and use of the medium or combination of media (written, visual, and auditory) best suited to the learner(s). The video, presented online at Davis*Plus* (www.fadavis.com), includes both visual and auditory modes.

Video Summary

Patient is a 41-year-old man with traumatic brain injury undergoing active rehabilitation. The video shows examination and intervention segments for both inpatient and outpatient rehabilitation episodes of care. Outcomes are filmed at 3 weeks and 7 weeks after the initial examination.

DavisPlus For additional resources and to view the accompanying video associated with this case, please visit **www.davisplus.com.**

Patient With Traumatic Brain Injury: Balance and Locomotor Training

Heidi Roth, PT, MSPT, NCS, and Jason Barbas, PT, MPT, NCS

Examination

History

- **Demographic Information:**
  Patient is a 47-year-old, right-handed Caucasian man.
- **Social History:**
  Patient is single; patient's mother lives in the area.
- **Employment:**
  Patient has not been employed since his injury 2 years ago, but he previously worked for a garage manufacturing company.
- **Education:**
  Patient has a college degree.
- **Living Environment:**
  Patient currently resides in an assisted living apartment.
- **General Health Status:**
  Patient is in generally good health, mildly overweight, with decreased activity tolerance.
- **Social and Health Habits:**
  Patient leads a primarily sedentary lifestyle, is a cigarette smoker, and reports drinking five to six alcoholic beverages per week. His social network is limited to visiting his mother and other residents at the assisted living facility. He reports using a local gym occasionally.
- **Family History:**
  Patient does not report any significant family history of major medical conditions.
- **Medical/Surgical History:**
  Patient suffered a traumatic brain injury approximately 2 years ago during a motor vehicle collision.
- **Current Condition/Chief Complaint:**
  The patient presents for outpatient physical therapy services. He reports a decline in endurance and difficulty moving his left leg. He also reports a worsening of balance with falls at home (two falls in the past 2 months).
- **Activity Level:**
  Patient is independent in the home environment in all basic activities of daily living (BADL) and requires assistance in the community and for instrumental activities of daily living (IADL) (e.g., managing his finances and medications). He reports walking with a cane at times, but he also uses a rolling walker. He recently purchased a motorized scooter and reports a decrease

in activity level since buying the scooter. Prior to his injury, patient was independent with all BADL and IADL.
- **Medications:**
  Upon admission to outpatient services, the patient was taking the following medications: Metformin, 500 mg twice a day; Metoprolol, 50 mg twice a day; trazodone, 50 mg once a day; Zanaflex, 2 mg four times a day; hydrochlorothiazide, 25 mg once a day; vitamin B$_1$, 100 mg once a day; Prilosec, 20 mg once a day; Reglan, 10 mg three times a day; dicyclomine, 20 mg twice a day; amantadine HCl, 100 mg once a day; Tramadol, 50 mg every 6 hours as needed; folic acid, 1 mg once a day; ibuprofen, 800 mg three times a day as needed; multivitamin, once a day; BuSpar HCl 5 mg twice a day.

Systems Review

- **Communication/Cognition:**
  - Rancho Los Amigos Levels of Cognitive Functioning scale: level 7.
  - Although the patient is independent with verbal communication, he demonstrates concrete thinking, decreased short-term memory, increased time for new learning, and decreased safety awareness.
  - Learning: The patient requires multiple demonstrations of new activities, with both written and verbal reinforcement.
- **Cardiovascular/Pulmonary System:**
  - Resting heart rate (HR) = 72; Exercise HR = 90; 5 minutes post exercise HR = 82
  - Resting blood pressure (BP) = 130/76; exercise BP = 146/92; 5 minutes post exercise BP = 138/80
  - 6-Minute walk test = 418 feet with straight cane
  - Edema = absent
- **Integumentary System:**
  - No skin abnormalities are noted.
- **Musculoskeletal System:**
  - Height: 5 ft, 10 in. (1.77 m)
  - Weight: 220 lb (99.8 kg)
  - Gross strength: Bilateral upper extremities (UEs) within functional limits (WFL); decreased strength noted in bilateral lower extremities (LEs), with left lower extremity (LE) weaker than right LE (Table CS2.1).

TABLE CS2.1 Manual Muscle Test: Lower Extremities

Lower Extremity Motions Tested	Initial Examination		Discharge*	
	Left	Right	Left	Right
Hip extension	2/5	3/5	3–/5	4/5
Hip flexion	4/5	5/5	5/5	5/5
Hip adduction	3/5	3/5	4/5	5/5
Hip abduction	2/5	3/5	4/5	5/5
Knee flexion	4/5	4/5	4/5	5/5
Knee extension	4/5	5/5	5/5	5/5
Ankle DF	3/5	4/5	3/5	4/5
Ankle PF	3/5	3/5	3/5	3/5

*Discharge occurred 8 weeks after initial examination.

All scores are based on a 0 to 5 scale: 5, normal; 4, good; 3, fair; 2, poor; 1, trace; 0, no contraction.

Abbreviations: DF, dorsiflexion; PF, plantarflexion.

TABLE CS2.2 Modified Ashworth Scale for Grading Spasticity

LE Muscle Groups	Left LE	Right LE
Hip extensors	1+	0
Hip flexors	1+	0
Hip adductors	1+	0
Hip abductors	0	0
Knee extensors	2	0
Knee flexors	3	0
Ankle dorsiflexors	1	0
Ankle plantarflexors	1+	0

Key: 0, no increase in tone; 1, slight increase in tone, manifested by a catch and release or by minimal resistance at the end of the ROM when the affected part(s) is (are) moved into flexion or extension; 1+, slight increase in muscle tone manifested by a catch, followed by minimal resistance throughout the remainder (less than half) of the ROM; 2, more marked increase in muscle tone through most of the ROM, but the affected part(s) is (are) easily moved; 3, considerable increase in muscle tone; passive movement is difficult; 4, affected part(s) is (are) rigid in flexion or extension.

- Gross range of motion (ROM): WFL throughout bilateral UEs and LEs.
- **Neuromuscular System:**
  - Gross coordinated movement: decreased coordination and speed of movement bilaterally, more exaggerated in left UE and left LE
  - Spasticity: increased spasticity noted throughout left LE (Table CS2.2)
  - Sitting balance: independent, with static and dynamic sitting balance with eyes open (EO) and eyes closed (EC); able to reach outside base of support (BOS) without compensatory movements of opposite UE or LEs
  - Standing static balance: able to maintain static standing balance on level surface without UE support; demonstrates increased postural sway and loss of balance with EC, with decreased BOS, and when standing on soft (compliant) surfaces; delayed balance reactions noted in all planes
  - Standing dynamic balance: demonstrates loss of balance during all dual-task activities, such as turning the head during forward walking (up/down/right/left), changing speed and direction, and stepping over and around obstacles
- **Functional Status:**
  - Transfers: He is able to perform all transfers and bed mobility with modified independence (requires assistive device); however, extra time is needed to accomplish the transfers. He has difficulty transitioning from sit-to-stand from low or soft surfaces.

- **Gait:**
  - Patient ambulates with a straight cane in the home and community. He demonstrates significantly decreased gait speed. He ambulates with a decreased step length (right > left), decreased left weight shift, decreased left knee extension during stance, and decreased left terminal knee extension (Fig. CS2.1). He also exhibits a wide BOS, decreased left push-off at terminal stance, decreased left heel strike (initial contact), and diminished arm swing bilaterally. During swing phase of the left LE, spasticity is increased and inadequate dorsiflexion is noted. Decreased left hip extension is evident during terminal stance. Although the patient typically demonstrated a wide walking BOS, when asked to negotiate an obstacle course placed on the floor (requiring heightened cognitive monitoring), his BOS tended to decrease (Fig. CS2.2).
  - Community mobility: Before purchasing a motorized scooter, the patient ambulated with a cane and reports experiencing frequent loss of balance with curbs, ramps, uneven surfaces, and busy environments. Primary means of community mobility is now the scooter (past 5 months).

Tests and Measures

- **Sensation:**
  - Diminished light touch distal to left knee
  - Proprioception: intact at right ankle, knee, and hip; left hip and knee intact, left ankle decreased joint position sense (4/10 accuracy)

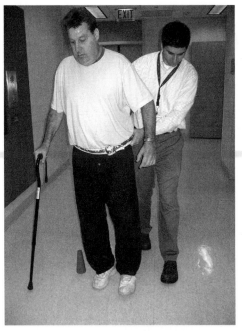

FIGURE CS2.1 Patient ambulates with a straight cane with decreased step length, decreased left weight shift, and decreased left knee extension. He also exhibits decreased arm swing on the left.

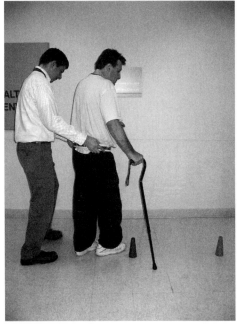

FIGURE CS2.2 Patient ambulates with a decreased BOS while walking through an obstacle course.

- **Strength:**
  - *Manual muscle test (MMT)* scores at initial examination and at discharge (8 weeks later) are reported for both LEs in Table CS2.1.
- **Spasticity:**
  - *Modified Ashworth Scale* scores for both LEs are reported in Table CS2.2. Scores were unchanged

from initial examination to discharge (8 weeks later).

- **Endurance, Balance, and Gait:**
  - The results of standardized tests for endurance, balance, and gait are reported at the initial examination, at 4 weeks, and at 8 weeks (discharge) in Table CS2.3.
  - Among the data reported in Table CS2.3 are scores from the Functional Reach Test. This is a practical, easily administered screen for balance problems originally developed for use with older adults. It is the maximal distance one can reach forward beyond arm's length as measured by a yardstick attached to a wall. The patient stands sideward next to a wall with the shoulder flexed to 90 degrees, the elbow extended, and the hand fisted (Fig. CS2.3). Using the yardstick,

TABLE CS2.3 Standardized Tests for Endurance, Balance, and Gait

Test Performed	Initial Examination	4 Weeks	8 Weeks
6-Minute Walk (ft)	413 (126 m)	518 (158 m)	602 (183 m)
10-Meter Walk (sec)	22	20	15
Gait Speed (m/sec)	0.45 (1.5 ft/sec)	0.50 (1.6 ft/sec)	0.67 (2.1 ft/sec)
Timed Up and Go (sec)	24	21	20
Dynamic Gait Index	7/24	11/24	17/24
Berg Balance Test	30/56	30/56	40/56
Romberg (EO) (sec)	5	10	30
Romberg (EC) (sec)	0	3	10
Tandem Stance (right or left LE front) (sec)	0	0	0
Semitandem Stance (sec)	7	10	30
Functional Reach (in.)	4 (10 cm)	6 (15 cm)	>10 (25 cm)
Assistive Device	Straight cane	Straight cane	Straight cane

Abbreviations: EO, eyes open; EC, eyes closed.

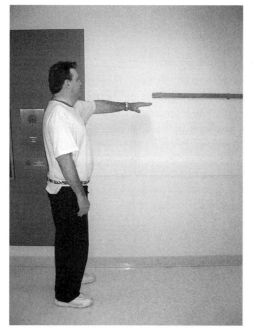

FIGURE CS2.3 Patient is standing sideward next to a wall with the left shoulder flexed to 90 degrees and the elbow extended (start of the Functional Reach Test). Note the relatively wide stance. Typically, this test is performed with a fisted hand. Owing to the patient's decreased short-term memory and increased time required for new learning, difficulty was experienced understanding the directions for keeping the hand in a fisted position. Based on this limitation, the test was modified and measures taken from the tip of the middle phalanx.

an initial measurement is taken of the position of the third metacarpal. The patient is then asked to lean as far forward as possible without losing balance or taking a step (Fig. CS2.4). A second measure is then taken and subtracted from the first to obtain a final measure in inches.

Evaluation, Diagnosis and Prognosis, and Plan of Care

Note: Before considering the guiding questions below, view the Case Study 2 Examination segment of the video to enhance understanding of the patient's impairments and activity limitations. After completing the guiding questions, view the Case Study 2 Intervention segment of the video to compare and contrast the interventions presented with those you selected. Last, progress to the Case Study 2 Outcomes segment of the video to compare and contrast the goals and expected outcomes you identified with the functional outcomes achieved.

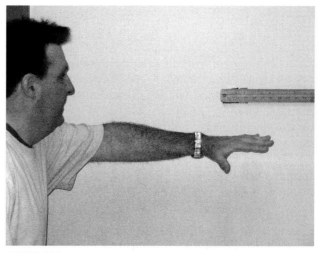

FIGURE CS2.4 Patient is instructed to reach forward as far as possible without raising the heels from the floor (end of the Functional Reach Test).

Guiding Questions

1. Describe this patient's clinical presentation in terms of:
   a. Impairments
   b. Activity limitations
   c. Participation restrictions
2. Identify five patient assets from the history and examination that would positively influence his physical therapy outcomes.
3. Identify five factors from the patient's history and examination that might negatively influence his physical therapy outcomes.
4. What impairments would you focus on during the physical therapy episode of care to address the patient's activity limitations and participation restrictions?
5. Identify anticipated goals (8 weeks) for balance and gait and the expected functional outcomes.
6. Describe three interventions focused on improving balance and gait that you would implement during the first 1 or 2 weeks of therapy. Indicate how you could progress each intervention, and include a brief rationale for your choice.
7. What strategies would you utilize to optimize motor learning within a therapy session as well as for carryover (retention) of learned activities?
8. Identify appropriate goals for the home exercise program (HEP).
9. Describe the elements and activities of a HEP.
10. What strategies can you include in your plan of care regarding fall prevention in the home?

Reminder: Answers to the case study guiding questions are available online at Davis*Plus* (www.fadavis.com).

VIEWING THE CASE: Patient With Traumatic Brain Injury: Balance and Locomotor Training

As students learn in different ways, the video case presentation (examination, intervention, and outcomes) is designed to promote engagement with the content, allow progression at an individual (or group) pace, and use of the medium or combination of media (written, visual, and auditory) best suited to the learner(s). The video, presented online at Davis*Plus* (www.fadavis.com), includes both visual and auditory modes.

Video Summary
Patient is a 47-year-old man with traumatic brain injury undergoing active rehabilitation. The video shows examination and intervention segments during outpatient rehabilitation, with an emphasis on balance and locomotor training. Outcomes are filmed 8 weeks after the initial examination.

Davis*Plus* For additional resources and to view the accompanying video associated with this case, please visit **www.davisplus.com.**

Patient With Incomplete Spinal Cord Injury, T4: Locomotor Training

ELIZABETH ARDOLINO, PT, MS; ELIZABETH WATSON, PT, DPT, NCS; ANDREA L. BEHRMAN, PT, PhD; SUSAN HARKEMA, PhD; AND MARY SCHMIDT-READ, PT, DPT, MS

Examination

History

The patient presents with incomplete paraplegia, secondary to an anterior spinal cord infarction that occurred while he was snowboarding. The patient was admitted to a pediatric acute trauma center and then completed a 4-week stay in an acute rehabilitation facility. He was referred to a locomotor training clinic for outpatient therapy and initiated this therapy 4 months after his injury.

- **Demographic Information:**
  The patient is a 17-year-old Caucasian boy.
- **Medical History:**
  Patient history is unremarkable except for occasional migraine headaches and delayed sleep phase syndrome (dissociation between the patient's circadian rhythm and the external environment).
- **Social History:**
  The patient is a junior in high school. Prior to his injury, he ran cross-country and played lacrosse. He is an honors student and is active in his church youth group. At the time of the initial outpatient locomotor training evaluation, the patient was being home-schooled.
- **Living Environment:**
  The patient lives with his parents and three older siblings in a two-story house with a stair glide to the second floor. There is a ramp at the main entrance to the house. The patient has a Quickie TNT ("Takes No Tools") manual wheelchair, as well as a tub bench and a commode at home.
- **Current Medications:**
  Baclofen, 10 mg twice a day; gabapentin/Neurontin, 600 mg twice a day; aspirin, 80 mg daily; and Detrol LA twice a day
- **Patient Goals:**
  Patient has identified the following goals for the physical therapy episode of care:
  - Ambulate independently with or without an assistive device
  - Return to high school at an ambulatory level

Systems Review

- **Cardiovascular/Pulmonary System:**
  Heart rate (HR): sitting at rest in manual wheelchair, HR = 82 beats per minute; supine on flat mat, HR = 71 beats per minute
  Blood pressure (BP): sitting at rest in manual wheelchair, BP = 108/65
  Orthostatic Testing:
  - BP resting in supine = 105/61
  - Immediately upon passive return to upright supported sitting, BP = 66/42
  - After 2 minutes of upright supported sitting, BP = 90/60
  - After 5 minutes of upright supported sitting, BP = 99/58
  - After 10 minutes of upright supported sitting, BP = 101/63
- **Musculoskeletal System:**
  - Gross range of motion (ROM): within normal limits (WNL) in both upper extremities (UEs) and lower extremities (LEs).
  - Gross strength testing: both UEs are symmetrical and strength is WNL. The left LE has good to fair voluntary movement, and the right LE has trace to absent voluntary movement.
  - Height: 5.75 ft (1.75 m)
  - Weight: 138 lb (62.6 kg)
- **Integumentary System:**
  Skin is intact with no open lacerations, abrasions, or pressure ulcers. There is no history of pressure ulcers.
- **Neuromuscular System:**
  Balance: The patient is able to sit unsupported in a chair but is unable to stand without support.
  - Sitting posture: In a relaxed seated position with UEs resting on thighs, the patient demonstrates increased thoracic and lumbar kyphosis (Fig. CS3.1). When asked to sit fully upright, the patient presents with an increased lumbar lordosis. He uses minimal UE support with his hands on his thighs to attain an upright sitting posture (Fig. CS3.2).

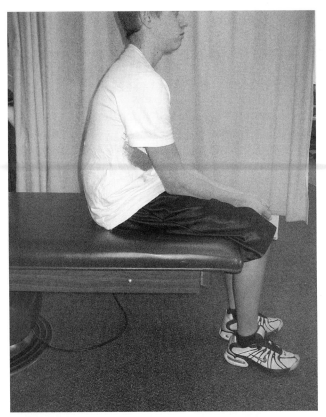

FIGURE CS3.1 Initial relaxed sitting posture with UEs resting on thighs. Note the increased thoracic and lumbar kyphosis.

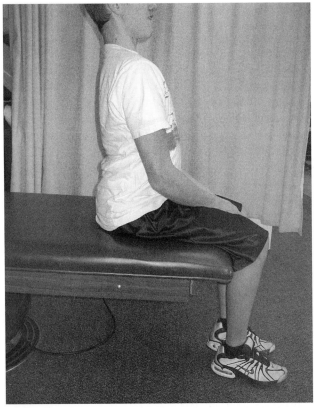

FIGURE CS3.2 Initial upright sitting posture achieved using UE support from hands placed on thighs. Note the increased lumbar lordosis.

- Standing posture: In supported standing, the patient presents with a severely increased lumbar lordosis, hyperextension of the thoracic spine, and genu recurvatum of the right knee (Fig. CS3.3).

Tests and Measures

- **Functional Status:**
  - Transfers: The patient is independent, with squat pivot transfers to even and uneven surfaces.
  - Locomotion: The patient is primarily a manual wheelchair user; he requires maximum assistance from two therapists to ambulate 5 ft (1.52 m) with a rolling walker.
- **Communication/Cognition:**
  The patient is alert and oriented to person, place, and time. He is able to answer questions appropriately regarding his needs and goals for therapy. He prefers to learn through demonstration.
- **Sensory/Motor Function:**
  The American Spinal Injury Association's (ASIA) *Standard Neurological Classification of Spinal Cord Injury*

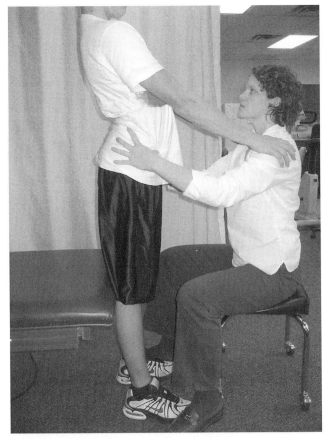

FIGURE CS3.3 Initial standing posture with UE support from hands placed on therapist's shoulders. Note the increased lumbar lordosis and hyperextension of the thoracic spine. Although obscured in the image, genu recurvatum of the right knee is also present.

form was used to document sensory and motor function (Fig. CS3.4)

- **Muscle Tone:**
  The *Modified Ashworth Scale* was used to grade spasticity (Table CS3.1).
- **Balance:**
  - The *Modified Functional Reach Test* was used to examine sitting balance (Table CS3.2).
  - The purpose of the Modified Functional Reach Test is to determine how far the patient can reach outside of his base of support (BOS) while positioned in short-sitting. The patient begins with his back resting against the chair backrest and then raises one UE to 90 degrees of shoulder flexion, parallel to a yardstick positioned on the wall next to him. The examiner notes the patient's starting point; the patient reaches forward with a fisted hand as far as possible without losing his balance. The examiner notes the farthest point that the patient reaches (measure taken at third metacarpal), and then the patient returns to the starting position. The test is performed three times, and the results are averaged.
  - *The Berg Balance Scale* was used to examine standing balance (Table CS3.3). The patient scored a 9/56, with difficulty performing any standing tasks that required standing without UE support, indicating a 100 percent risk of falls at an ambulatory level.
  - The patient's fall risk was determined using the *Performance-Oriented Mobility Assessment (POMA)* (Table CS3.4). The patient scored a total of 6/28, with difficulty performing any standing tasks that required standing without an assistive device, indicating 100 percent risk of falls at an ambulatory level.
- **Ambulation:**
  - The 10-meter walk test: The patient was unable to complete this test without physical assistance.
  - The 6-minute walk test: The patient was unable to complete this test without physical assistance.

Patient Name_____ Date of Exam_____

Examiner Name_____ Comments_____

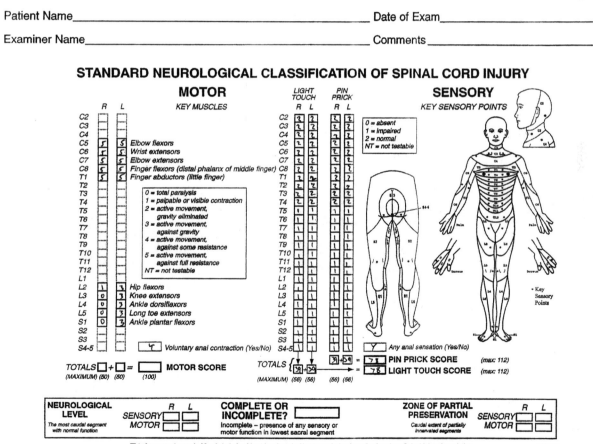

FIGURE CS3.4 The patient's sensory and motor scores using the American Spinal Injury Association (ASIA) Examination Form: *Standard Neurological Classification of Spinal Cord Injury.* American Spinal Injury Association: International Standards for Neurological Classification of Spinal Cord Injury, 2006; Atlanta, GA, with permission. (Note: An overview of changes with the new ISNCSCI worksheet is available at http://www.asia-spinalinjury.org/elearning/ISNCSCI.php (retrieved April 6, 2015).)

TABLE CS3.1 Modified Ashworth Scale for Grading Spasticity[a]

Muscle Group	Right LE	Left LE
Hip Flexors	0	0
Hip Extensors	1+	1+
Hip Adductors	1	1
Knee Flexors	0	1
Knee Extensors	1	1
Plantarflexors	1	1+
Invertors	0	0
Evertors	0	1

Key: 0, no increase in tone; 1, slight increase in tone, manifested by a catch and release or by minimal resistance at the end of the ROM when the affected part(s) is(are) moved into flexion or extension; 1+, slight increase in muscle tone manifested by a catch, followed by minimal resistance throughout the remainder (less than half) of the ROM; 2, more marked increase in muscle tone through most of the ROM, but the affected part(s) is (are) easily moved; 3, considerable increase in muscle tone; passive movement is difficult; 4, affected part(s) is (are) rigid in flexion or extension.

[a]Bohannon, R, and Smith, M. Interrater reliability of a modified Ashworth scale of muscle spasticity. Phys Ther 67:206, 1987.

TABLE CS3.2 Modified Functional Reach Test[a]

Forward Reaches	Length, in. (cm)
Reach 1	21.0 (53.34)
Reach 2	20.5 (52.07)
Reach 3	22.5 (57.15)
Mean	21.3 (54.10)

[a]Lynch, SM, Leahy, P, and Barker, SP. Reliability of measurements obtained with a modified functional reach test in subjects with spinal cord injury. Phys Ther 78(2):128, 1998.

Step Training With Body Weight Support System and a Treadmill

Four main elements comprise the examination in the step training environment: *stand retraining, stand adaptability, step retraining,* and *step adaptability.*

1. **Stand retraining:**
   The test begins with the patient standing on the treadmill (TM) with 75 percent of body weight supported. The amount of body weight supported is then lowered until the patient can no longer maintain an upright standing posture, even with maximal assistance from the trainers. Each trainer (physical therapist or physical therapist

assistant) then states the amount of assistance being provided at each body segment (e.g., foot/ankle, knee, and hip/pelvis) (Table CS3.5).

2. **Stand adaptability:**
   The purpose of this test is to examine the body weight parameters needed to maintain independence at different body segments. Stand adaptability includes: *static standing, lateral weight shifts,* and *step weight shifts.*
   - Static standing: The therapist examines the amount of body weight support (BWS) necessary for each body segment to attain independence. The test begins at the lowest BWS achieved during the stand retraining portion. The BWS is then slowly raised. As the amount of BWS increases, the trainers are able to decrease the amount of assistance provided/required at each segment. Each trainer verbally identifies when assistance is no longer needed and the body segment becomes independent (Table CS3.6).
   - Lateral weight shifts: Starting with the patient in a stance position, the therapist determines the amount of BWS and assistance necessary for the patient to perform lateral weight shifts in both directions. The trainers verbally identify the amount of assistance required at each body segment (Table CS3.7). The body weight supported is the amount that allows the majority of the body segments to be independent during the weight shifts.
   - Step weight shifts: The trainers determine the amount of BWS and assistance necessary for the patient to perform an anterior weight shift when one LE is in a forward step position. The test begins at the same amount of BWS used during the lateral weight shifts, starting with the right LE forward. The test is repeated with the left LE in a forward step position. Each trainer identifies the amount of assistance required at each segment (Tables CS3.8 and CS3.9).

3. **Step retraining:**
   The purpose of this test is to determine the optimal BWS and TM speed parameters to establish a kinematically correct stepping pattern. The test begins using the amount of BWS established during the stand adaptability weight shifting. The speed on the TM is gradually increased until a normal walking speed is reached (~2.4 mph [3.9 km/hr]). The amount of trainer assistance necessary to achieve an optimal stepping pattern is reported and documented (Table CS3.10).

4. **Step adaptability:**
   The purpose of this test is to determine the amount of BWS and TM speed parameters necessary to maintain independence (no trainer assistance) at each body segment. The test begins at the parameters established during step retraining. The amount of BWS is slowly increased and the speed is slowly decreased until independence is reached at each segment of the body. If independence is not reached with 75 percent of the patient's body weight supported at a speed of 0.6 mph,

(text continues on page 344)

TABLE CS3.3 Berg Balance Scale[a,b,c]

Item	Score
1. Sitting to standing	1—needs minimal aid to stand or stabilize
2. Standing unsupported	0—unable to stand 30 seconds without support
3. Sitting with back unsupported but feet supported on floor or on a stool	4—able to sit safely and securely for 2 minutes
4. Standing to sit	1—sits independently but has uncontrolled descent
5. Transfers	3—able to transfer safely with definite need of hands
6. Standing unsupported with eyes closed	0—needs help to keep from falling
7. Standing unsupported with feet together	0—needs help to assume position and unable to stand for 15 seconds
8. Reaching forward with outstretched arm while standing	0—loses balance while trying, requires external support
9. Picking up object from the floor from a standing position	0—is unable to try/needs assistance to keep from losing balance/falling
10. Turning to look behind over the left and right shoulders while standing	0—needs assistance while turning
11. Turn 360 degrees	0—needs assistance while turning
12. Place alternate foot on step or stool while standing unsupported	0—needs assistance to keep from falling/unable to try
13. Standing unsupported one foot in front	0—loses balance while stepping or standing
14. Standing on one leg	0—is unable to try or needs assist to prevent falls
	Total Score: 9/56

[a]Berg, K, et al. Measuring balance in the elderly: Preliminary development of an instrument. Physiotherapy Canada, 41:304, 1989.

[b]Berg, K, et al. A comparison of clinical and laboratory measures of postural balance in an elderly population. Arch Phys Med Rehabil, 73:1073, 1992.

[c]Berg, K, et al. Measuring balance in the elderly: Validation of an instrument. Can J Public Health, 83 (suppl 2):S7, 1992.

TABLE CS3.4 Performance-Oriented Mobility Assessment (POMA)[a]

	Balance Portion		
Task	**Description of Balance**	**Possible**	**Score**
Sitting Balance	Leans or slides in chair Steady, safe	= 0 = 1	1
Arises	Unable without help	= 0	1
	Able, uses arms to help	= 1	
	Able without using arms	= 2	

(table continues on page 342)

TABLE CS3.4 Performance-Oriented Mobility Assessment (POMA)[a] *(continued)*

Balance Portion

Task	Description of Balance	Possible	Score
Attempts to Arise	Unable without help	= 0	1
	Able requires more than one attempt	= 1	
	Able to rise on one attempt	= 2	
Immediate Standing Balance (first 5 seconds)	Unsteady (swaggers, moves feet, trunk sway)	= 0	1
	Steady but uses walker or other support	= 1	
	Steady without walker or other support	= 2	
Standing Balance	Unsteady	= 0	1
	Steady but wide stance (medial heels more than 4 inches apart) and uses cane or other support	= 1	
	Narrow stance without support	= 2	
Nudged	Begins to fall	= 0	0
	Staggers, grabs, catches self	= 1	
	Steady	= 2	
Eyes Closed	Unsteady	= 0	0
	Steady	= 1	
Turning 360 Degrees	Discontinuous steps	= 0	0
	Continuous steps	= 1	
	Unsteady	= 0	0
	Steady	= 1	
Sitting Down	Unsafe (falls into chair)	= 0	1
	Uses arms or not a smooth motion	= 1	
	Safe, smooth motion	= 2	
Balance Score			**6/16**

Gait Portion

Task	Description of Balance	Possible	Score
Initiation of Gait	Any hesitancy	= 0	0
	No hesitancy	= 1	
Step Length and Height	a. Right swing foot does not pass left stance foot	= 0	0
	b. Right foot passes left stance foot with step	= 1	
	c. Right foot does not clear floor completely with step	= 0	0
	d. Right foot completely clears floor	= 1	

TABLE CS3.4 Performance-Oriented Mobility Assessment (POMA)[a] (continued)

Gait Portion

Task	Description of Balance	Possible	Score
	e. Left swing foot does not pass right stance foot with step	= 0	0
	f. Left foot passes right stance foot	= 1	
	g. Left foot does not clear floor completely with step	= 0	0
	h. Left foot completely clears floor	= 1	
Step Symmetry	Right and left step length not equal	= 0	0
	Right and left step appear equal	= 1	
Step Continuity	Stopping or discontinuing between steps	= 0	0
	Steps appear continuous	= 1	
Path	Marked deviation	= 0	0
	Mild/moderate deviation or uses walking aid	= 1	
	Straight without walking aid	= 2	
Trunk	Marked sway or uses walking aid	= 0	0
	No sway but flexion of knees or back, or spreads arms out while walking	= 1	
	No sway, no flexion, no use of arms, and no use of walking aid	= 2	
Step Width	Heels apart	= 0	0
	Heels almost touching while walking	= 1	
Gait Score			**0/12**
Balance + Gait Score			**6/28**

[a]Tinetti, ME. Performance-oriented assessment of mobility problems in elderly patients. J Am Geriatr Soc, 34:119–126, 1986.

TABLE CS3.5 Stand Retraining

Body Segment	Level of Assistance	Percent of BWS
Right Knee	Minimal	10
Right Ankle	Independent	10
Left Knee	Independent	10
Left Ankle	Independent	10
Trunk	Moderate	10
Hips/Pelvis	Moderate	10

TABLE CS3.6 Stand Adaptability: Static Standing

Body Segment	Level of Assistance	Percent of BWS
Right Knee	Minimal	75
Right Ankle	Independent	10
Left Knee	Independent	10
Left Ankle	Independent	10
Trunk	Independent	25
Hips/Pelvis	Minimal	75

Abbreviation: BWS, body weight support.

TABLE CS3.7 Stand Adaptability: Lateral Weight Shifting

Body Segment	Level of Assistance	Percent of BWS
Right Knee	Minimal	50
Right Ankle	Independent	50
Left Knee	Minimal	50
Left Ankle	Independent	50
Trunk	Independent	50
Hips/Pelvis	Minimal	50

TABLE CS3.8 Stand Adaptability: Step Weight Shifting (Right Foot Forward)

Body Segment	Level of Assistance	Percent of BWS
Right Knee	Moderate	50
Right Ankle	Independent	50
Left Knee	Minimal	50
Left Ankle	Independent	50
Trunk	Independent	50
Hips/Pelvis	Maximal	50

TABLE CS3.9 Stand Adaptability: Step Weight Shifting (Left Foot Forward)

Body Segment	Level of Assistance	Percent of BWS
Right Knee	Moderate	50
Right Ankle	Independent	50
Left Knee	Minimal	50
Left Ankle	Independent	50
Trunk	Independent	50
Hips/Pelvis	Moderate	50

then the level of assistance required at the given body segment is reported and documented (Table CS3.11).

Evaluation, Diagnosis and Prognosis, and Plan of Care

Note: Before considering the guiding questions below, view the Case Study 3 Examination segment of the video to enhance understanding of the patient's impairments and activity limitations. After completing the guiding questions, view the Case Study 3 Intervention segment of the video to compare and contrast the interventions presented with those you selected. Last, progress to the Case Study 3 Outcomes segment of the video to compare and contrast the goals and expected outcomes you identified with the functional outcomes achieved.

Guiding Questions

1. Based on the ASIA examination data presented in Figure CS3.4, what is the patient's LE motor score?
2. Based on the ASIA examination data presented in Figure CS3.4, what is the patient's neurological level? Using Box CS3.1 below, what is the patient's impairment classification?
3. Using the *Guide to Physical Therapist Practice,* identify the patient's physical therapy diagnosis.
4. Formulate a physical therapy problem list for the patient. For each problem identified, indicate whether it is a *direct impairment, indirect impairment, composite impairment,* or *activity limitation.*
5. For patients with spinal cord injury (SCI), the LE motor score (LEMS) from the ASIA examination as well as the ASIA Impairment Scale classification has been used to predict ambulation ability. Based on the patient's LEMS and Impairment Scale classification, what is your prediction for this patient's ambulatory potential? Consider whether the patient has the potential to be either a household or community ambulator or whether he will be primarily a wheelchair user. What assistive or orthotic devices might be used to improve this patient's function?
6. *Activity-based therapy,* including the use of locomotor training (LT), offers another perspective on predicting ambulation ability. Activity-based therapy focuses on the use of task-specific training to provide appropriate sensory and kinematic cues to the nervous system in order to foster neurological recovery. Again, consider the patient's ambulatory potential. Before making a decision about ambulatory potential, consider (a) the patient's performance during the step retraining portion of the initial examination (see Table CS3.10), and (b) the principles of LT (weight-bearing is maximized, kinematics and sensory cues are optimized with emphasis placed on motor recovery while

TABLE CS3.10 Step Retraining

Body Segment	Level of Assistance	Percent of BWS	TM Speed, mph (km/hr)
Right Knee	Maximal	35	2.4 (3.9)
Right Ankle	Maximal	35	2.4 (3.9)
Left Knee	Moderate	35	2.4 (3.9)
Left Ankle	Moderate	35	2.4 (3.9)
Trunk	Independent	35	2.4 (3.9)
Hips/Pelvis	Moderate	35	2.4 (3.9)

TABLE CS3.11 Step Adaptability

Body Segment	Level of Assistance	Percent of BWS[a]	TM Speed, mph (km/hr)
Right Knee	Maximal	55	0.6 (1)
Right Ankle	Maximal	55	0.6 (1)
Left Knee	Moderate	55	0.6 (1)
Left Ankle	Moderate	55	0.6 (1)
Trunk	Independent	35	2.4 (3.9)
Hips/Pelvis	Moderate	55	0.6 (1)

[a]Unable to raise BWS to greater than 55% because patient no longer able to achieve foot flat (loading response) during stepping at greater BWS.

Abbreviations: BWS, body weight support; TM, treadmill.

BOX CS3.1 ASIA Impairment Scale (AIS)[a]

A = Complete: No motor or sensory function is preserved in the sacral segments S4 to S5.
B = Incomplete: Sensory but not motor function is preserved below the neurological level and includes the sacral segments S4 to S5.
C = Incomplete: Motor function is preserved below the neurological level, and more than half of key muscles below the neurological level have a muscle grade less than 3.
D = Incomplete: Motor function is preserved below the neurological level, and at least half of key muscles below the neurological level have a muscle grade of 3 or more.
E = Normal: motor and sensory function is normal.

[a]American Spinal Injury Association. International Standards for Neurological Classification of Spinal Cord Injury. American Spinal Injury Association, Atlanta, GA, 2006.

minimizing compensatory strategies). Consider also the patient's LEMS identified in question 1 and the patient's impairment scale classification identified in question 2.

7. Identify the duration of the episode of care needed to achieve the level of ambulation identified in question 5 (e.g., household or community ambulator or primarily a wheelchair user).

8. Identify the duration of the episode of care needed to achieve the level of ambulatory potential identified in question 6 using activity-based therapy, including the use of LT.

9. Table CS3.12 identifies a series of assistive devices and one entry labeled orthotic intervention. In the spaces provided in the table, state how these devices are, and are not, consistent with the following LT principles.

• *Maximize LE weightbearing:* Patients are encouraged to stand as often as possible, using the UEs as little as possible.

TABLE CS3.12 Assistive Device/Orthoses: Consistency/Inconsistency With Locomotor Training Principles

Assistive Device/Orthoses	Consistent Aspects	Inconsistent Aspects
Rolling Walker		
Bilateral Lofstrand Crutches		
Bilateral Single-Point Canes		
Unilateral Single-Point Cane		
Orthotic Intervention		

• *Provide appropriate sensory cues:* These cues include providing the correct tactile information during stepping on the treadmill and while walking at as close to normal walking speed (2.0 to 2.6 mph [3.2 to 4.2 km/hr]) as possible.

• *Provide appropriate kinematics:* Patients are encouraged to attain an upright trunk with a neutral pelvis throughout the entire gait cycle, hip extension during terminal stance, and heel strike at initial contact.

• *Maximize independence and minimize compensation:* Patients attempt to use the least restrictive assistive device possible and minimize the use of bracing.

10. Box CS3.2 identifies the *focus of progression for LT* using (A) BWS and a TM and (B) overground walking as well as (C) a sample progression of LT for the patient, using sessions 1 and 20 as examples. Examine the focus of progression for both BWS and TM training and the overground progression. Next, examine the sample progression of LT for the patient (sessions 1 and 20). Based on each example, list two goals for progression during the next treatment sessions (2 and 21) in each of the following areas:
    • Step training on the BWS system
    • Sit-to-stand transfers
    • Standing balance
    • Overground ambulation

Reminder: Answers to the case study guiding questions are available online at Davis*Plus* (www.fadavis.com).

BOX CS3.2 Focus of Progression for LT Using BWS and a TM, Focus of Progression for LT Overground, and Sample Progression of LT for the Case Study Patient

A. **Focus of Progression: LT Using BWS and a TM**
   • Decreasing the amount of body weight supported (i.e., increase LE weightbearing)
   • Achieving a normal walking speed (2.0–2.6 mph [3.2–4.2 km/hr])
   • Improving endurance (the goal is to maintain 60 minutes of weightbearing on a TM with at least 20 minutes of stepping)
   • Promoting independence of body segments (initial focus on the trunk and pelvis)

B. **Focus of Progression: LT Overground**
   • Achieving proper kinematics during functional mobility (e.g., sit-to-stand transfers, standing, and ambulation)
   • Minimizing the use of compensatory strategies
   • Minimizing the use of assistive devices

C. **Sample Progression of LT for the Case Study Patient**
   Session 1 Example: During session 1 using the BWS system and a TM, the patient completed a total of 49 minutes of weightbearing, with 22 minutes of stepping at a TM speed of 2.4 mph (3.9 km/hr) with an average of 37% BWS. He required moderate assistance at his pelvis, maximal assistance at his right knee and ankle, and moderate assistance at his left knee and ankle. In the overground environment, he performed sit-to-stand transfers from a standard-height mat table with UE support from a rolling walker; he required minimal assistance at pelvis and right knee. Once standing, he required increased

UE support to maintain standing balance and minimal assistance at the right LE to prevent knee buckling. He ambulated 10 ft (3 m) with a rolling walker, with minimal assistance of one physical therapist at his pelvis and minimal assistance of two physical therapists (one at each LE) to advance the limb during swing and to maintain hip and knee extension during stance. Increased lumbar lordosis was noted during all standing and ambulation activities.

   Session 20 Example: During session 20 using the BWS system and a TM, the patient completed a total of 60 minutes of weightbearing, with 30 minutes of step retraining at a TM speed of 2.6 mph (4.2 km/hr), with an average of 33% BWS. He required minimal assistance at the pelvis to attain proper alignment, moderate assistance at the right knee and ankle, and minimal assistance at the left knee and ankle. In the overground environment, he performed sit-to-stand transfers from a standard-height mat, with minimal assistance at the pelvis without UE support. Using a wide BOS, he was able to maintain standing balance with supervision without UE support for 30 seconds. He ambulated 250 ft (76.2 m) using bilateral Lofstrand crutches with contact guard at pelvis for balance and alignment. The patient was independent in advancing each LE. He continued to present with increased lumbar lordosis, although it is slightly diminished compared to session 1.

VIEWING THE CASE: Patient With Incomplete Spinal Cord Injury, T4: Locomotor Training

As students learn in different ways, the video case presentation (examination, intervention, and outcomes) is designed to promote engagement with the content, allow progression at an individual (or group) pace, and use of the medium or combination of media (*written, visual,* and *auditory*) best suited to the learner(s). The video, presented online at Davis*Plus* (www.fadavis.com), includes both *visual* and *auditory* modes.

Video Summary

Patient is a 17-year-old male with an incomplete SCI (T4, ASIA C) referred to an LT clinic for outpatient rehabilitation, initiated 4 months post injury. The video shows examination and intervention segments with an emphasis on balance and locomotor training. Outcomes are filmed after 75 treatment sessions.

DavisPlus For additional resources and to view the accompanying video associated with this case, please visit **www.davisplus.com.**

Patient With Stroke: Home Care Rehabilitation

LYNN WONG, PT, MS, DPT, GCS

Examination

History

- **Demographic Information:**
  The patient is an 86-year-old widowed woman, status post mild ischemic cerebrovascular accident (CVA) with left hemiparesis. She is receiving skilled nursing care, physical therapy (PT), occupational therapy (OT), and home health aide services through a home health agency. The patient was born in Austria and is a Holocaust survivor.

- **Living Environment/General Health Status:**
  The patient is currently living with her son and daughter-in-law in their small two-story home. The family room is used as her bedroom, which is one step down from the main level of the home (the guest bedroom is up 10 steep steps from the main level). She is using a hospital bed. The patient previously lived alone in a one-level condominium and was independent and active in the community, although she did not drive. She previously ambulated without an assistive device and enjoyed reading, crocheting, cooking, and baking. She also enjoyed playing Scrabble (a word game in which words are formed from individual lettered tiles on a game board) and participated in exercise classes through the local recreation department 2 or 3 days per week (tai chi, water walking in season, and general exercise classes). Her son, daughter-in-law, and the patient state that their collective goal is for her to return to her own home, with added services if necessary.

- **Medical History:**
  CVA sustained 3 weeks ago, hypertension, depression after her husband's death, urinary incontinence, and bilateral tibia/fibula fracture secondary to a motor vehicle accident approximately 15 years ago.

- **Medications:**
  Sertraline, 25 mg daily; metoprolol, 50 mg daily; Aggrenox, 1 tablet twice a day; hydrochlorothiazide, 12.5 mg twice a day; valsartan, 160 mg twice a day; Acidophilus, 2 tablets three times a day; Zofran, 4 mg as needed; milk of magnesia, as needed; bisacodyl, as needed; acetaminophen, 650 mg as needed; Pepcid, 20 mg twice a day; Ambien, 5 mg at bedtime; Detrol LA, 2 mg twice a day; Colace, 100 mg twice a day.

- **History of Present Illness:**
  Patient presented to her local hospital with left-sided weakness and inability to ambulate. Initial computed tomography (CT) scan was negative. She was seen by a physical therapist and a speech and language pathologist. She was placed on nectar thick liquids secondary to dysphagia. After 5 days, she was transferred to an acute rehab hospital. She received PT, OT, and speech therapy there for approximately 2 weeks, with steady improvements in left-sided return and function. Patient experienced an episode of near syncope and was transferred back to an acute care hospital. She was diagnosed with near syncope, dehydration, and a urinary tract infection (UTI). Her UTI was treated with ciprofloxacin, 250 mg twice a day for 7 days, and her dehydration was treated with intravenous hydration. Physical therapy was resumed, and a swallowing evaluation was requested. The evaluation noted adequate improvement in swallowing to discontinue the thickened liquids. After 7 days in the acute care hospital, the patient was discharged to her son and daughter-in-law's home with 24-hour supervision and assistance from family and companions as well as home care as mentioned above (skilled nursing, PT, OT, and home health aide services).

Systems Review

- **Mental Status:**
  - Alert, oriented to person, place, and time, and cooperative and motivated
- **Neuromuscular System:**
  - Mild left hemiparesis
  - No synergy influence noted
  - Tone normal
- **Cardiopulmonary System:**
  - Resting heart rate: 80 beats per minute; heart rate after ambulation: 80 beats per minute
  - Resting blood pressure: 168/62 mm Hg; blood pressure after ambulation: 200/82 mm Hg
  - Resting respiratory rate: 18 breaths per minute; 26 breaths per minute after ambulation
  - SpO_2: 99% on room air at rest
  - Edema: none present

- **Integumentary System:**
  - Skin integrity is intact.
  - Skin color is slightly pale.
  - No scars are noted, and her skin is normally mobile.
- **Musculoskeletal System:**
  - Height: 5 ft, 2 in. (1.6 m)
  - Weight: 132 lb (60 kg)
  - No complaints of pain
  - Range of motion (ROM): All joints are within normal limits (WNL) except the left lower extremity (LE) presents with 0 degrees of dorsiflexion.
  - Strength: Manual muscle test (MMT) grades are presented in Table CS4.1.

Tests and Measures

- **Sensation:**
  - Light touch: intact
  - Proprioception: decreased in left upper extremity (UE)
- **Functional Status:**
  - Bed mobility
    - Rolling: modified independence; pulls on rail of hospital bed with right UE to assist
    - Scooting: supervision (minimal verbal cues required for technique and foot placement)
    - Sit-to-supine: supervision for LE placement
    - Supine-to-sit: independent; requires increased time and effort

TABLE CS4.1 Manual Muscle Test[a]

Motion Tested	Left	Right
Shoulder Flexion	4+/5	4+/5
Shoulder Abduction	4+/5	4+/5
Elbow Flexion	4–/5	4+/5
Elbow Extension	4–/5	4+/5
Mass Grasp	4/5	4+/5
Hip Flexion	4/5	4/5
Hip Extension	3/5	4–/5
Hip Abduction	3/5	4–/5
Knee Extension	4+/5	4+/5
Knee Flexion	4+/5	4+/5
Dorsiflexion	4/5	5/5
Plantarflexion	4/5	5/5

[a]All scores are based on a 0 to 5 scale: 5, normal; 4, good; 3, fair; 2, poor; 1, trace; 0, no contraction.

- Transfers
  - Sit-to-stand: modified independence; once standing, requires standard straight cane to maintain initial balance
  - Stand-to-sit: supervision; lowers self using right UE to control descent
  - Symmetry: asymmetrical, with increased weightbearing on the right
- **Gait/locomotion:**
  - Ambulated 75 ft (23.6 m) with standard straight cane and supervision
  - Gait deviations include decreased step length bilaterally, decreased left stance time and weightbearing, and minimally decreased left toe clearance during swing.
- **Balance:**
  - Static sitting: able to withstand minimal challenges (perturbations) in all directions
  - Dynamic sitting: able to reach minimal distances outside her base of support (BOS) in all directions
  - Static standing: able to maintain static standing without an assistive device or assistance; unable to withstand any challenges (perturbations)
  - Dynamic standing: requires supervision and use of a standard straight cane at all times for balance and safety
- **Activities of daily living:**
  - Able to dress self while sitting in a chair once clothing is laid out on an adjoining table
  - Requires increased time to don and doff socks and tie and untie shoes secondary to decreased fine motor coordination of left distal UE
  - Requires minimum assist for sponge bathing (for back and feet)
  - Requires minimum to moderate assist to shower using a handheld shower nozzle and a tub seat without a back

Evaluation, Diagnosis and Prognosis, and Plan of Care

Note: Before considering the guiding questions below, view the Case Study 4 Examination segment of the video to enhance understanding of the patient's impairments and activity limitations. After completing the guiding questions, view the Case Study 4 Intervention/Outcomes segment of the video to compare and contrast the interventions and functional outcomes presented with those you identified.

Guiding Questions

1. Develop a problem list for this patient, including:
   a. Impairments
   b. Activity limitations
   c. Participation restrictions
2. Using the *Guide to Physical Therapist Practice*, determine the PT diagnosis for this patient. Provide justification for your decision.

3. Identify five goals and outcomes for this patient that could be accomplished within the next 4 weeks.

4. Using three goals and outcomes identified in question 3, describe the interventions you would use to achieve each. If appropriate, indicate a progression for each intervention. Provide a brief rationale for the interventions you selected.

5. What activities should be included in the patient's home exercise program (HEP)? Provide a brief rationale for each activity selected.

6. What motor learning strategies would enhance this patient's ability to achieve the stated goals and outcomes?

7. The patient and her family express a desire for her to return to her one-level condominium and live alone. How realistic is this goal? Provide a rationale for your decision.

8. What do you think is an appropriate discharge plan for this patient? Provide justification for your response.

Reminder: Answers to the case study guiding questions are available online at Davis*Plus* (www.fadavis.com).

VIEWING THE CASE: Patient With Stroke

As students learn in different ways, the video case presentation (examination, intervention, and outcomes) is designed to promote engagement with the content, allow progression at an individual (or group) pace, and use of the medium or combination of media (written, visual, and auditory) best suited to the learner(s). The video, presented online at Davis*Plus* (www.fadavis.com), includes both visual and auditory modes.

Video Summary

Patient is an 86-year-old woman with stroke and left hemiparesis. The video shows examination and intervention/outcomes segments during two sessions of home care PT following inpatient rehabilitation (2 weeks). Emphasis is on balance and locomotor training. The intervention/outcomes segment was filmed after eight visits over 4 weeks.

DavisPlus For additional resources and to view the accompanying video associated with this case, please visit **www.davisplus.com**.

Patient With Stroke: Constraint-Induced Movement Therapy

David M. Morris, PT, PhD; Sonya L. Pearson, PT, DPT; and Edward Taub, PhD

Examination

History

- **Demographic Information:**
  The patient is a 63-year-old African American man who sustained an ischemic cerebrovascular accident (CVA) 6 months previously, resulting in right-side hemiparesis.
- **Social History:**
  The patient is married and lives in a single-level home with his wife and daughter. He reports a history of smoking (quit more than 40 years ago) and drinks alcohol socially on occasion. He enjoyed carpentry, fishing, and hunting prior to his stroke.
- **Employment:**
  Patient is a retired steel mill worker.
- **Medical History:**
  The patient reports no previous surgeries or significant medical problems except for hypertension and type II diabetes; both are currently under control with lifestyle changes and medications.
- **History of Present Illness:**
  Patient sustained an ischemic CVA, resulting in right-side hemiparesis. Magnetic resonance imaging revealed a left pontine infarction. Cerebral angiography revealed severe stenosis of the right vertebral artery and proximal basilar artery. Prior to the stroke, the patient was right-handed.
- **Chief Complaint:**
  Patient complains he is unable to use his right arm and hand effectively. His goals are to use his right arm and hand well enough to perform household chores and return to his hobbies.
- **Medications:**
  Current medications include aspirin, Glucotrol, glucophage, Coumadin, and warfarin.

Systems Review

- **Communication/Language:**
  - Patient exhibits mild dysarthria.
- **Cognition/Affect:**
  - There is no cognitive impairment as evidenced by his mini–mental state examination[1] score of 30.
  - No abnormalities in affect are noted.

- **Cardiovascular/Pulmonary System:**
  - Heart rate: 72 beats per minute and strong
  - Blood pressure: 110/80 mm Hg (sitting)
  - Respiratory rate: 16 breaths per minute, regular and unlabored
- **Integumentary System:**
  - No abnormalities are noted.
- **Musculoskeletal System:**
  - Height: 6 ft, 1 in. (1.9 m)
  - Weight: 205 lb (93 kg)
  - Passive range of motion is within normal limits (WNL) in all extremities, except for shoulder flexion, abduction, and external rotation in the right upper extremity (UE).
  - Gross strength is WNL in the left upper and lower extremities (LEs); patient demonstrates weak, active movement in the right UE and LEs.
- **Neuromuscular System:**
  - There is mild right facial droop (lower quadrant).
  - Hemiparesis is present in the right extremities.
  - Patient is able to actively extend his right wrist to 10 degrees past neutral and able to extend his second, third, and fourth digits (i.e., index, middle, and ring fingers, respectively) beyond 10 degrees at each finger joint. He is unable to extend his fifth digit.
- **Learning Style:**
  Patient reports that he likes to observe prior to learning a new movement skill.

Tests and Measures

- **Tone:**
  The examination results of tone in elbow flexors, forearm pronators, and wrist flexors from the *Modified Ashworth Scale*[2] for grading spasticity are presented in Table CS5.1.
- **Range of Motion:**
  UE range of motion (ROM) results are presented in Tables CS5.2 (passive ROM) and CS5.3 (active ROM).
- **Balance:**
  Balance was examined using the following:
  - *The Established Populations for Epidemiologic Studies of the Elderly (EPESE)*[3,4] short performance battery (Table CS5.4)

TABLE CS5.1 Modified Ashworth Scale for Grading Spasticity[a]

Muscle Group	Left	Right
Elbow Flexors	0	2
Forearm Pronators	0	1+
Wrist Flexors	0	1+

[a]All movements measured in sitting position.

Key: 0, no increase in tone; 1, slight increase in tone, manifested by a catch and release, or by minimal resistance at the end of the ROM when the affected part(s) is (are) moved into flexion or extension; 1+, slight increase in muscle tone manifested by a catch, followed by minimal resistance throughout the remainder (less than half) of the ROM; 2, more marked increase in muscle tone through most of the ROM, but the affected part(s) is (are) easily moved; 3, considerable increase in muscle tone; passive movement is difficult; 4, affected part(s) is (are) rigid in flexion or extension.

TABLE CS5.2 Upper Extremity Passive Range of Motion (in degrees)

Motion	Left	Right
Shoulder Flexion	0–135	0–100
Shoulder Abduction	0–130	0–80
Shoulder Internal Rotation	0–15	0–15
Shoulder External Rotation	0–85	0–75
Elbow Flexion	0–155	0–155
Forearm Supination	0–90	0–60
Forearm Pronation	0–90	0–90
Wrist Elexion	0–90	0–70
Wrist Extension	0–85	0–50

TABLE CS5.3 Upper Extremity Active Range of Motion (in degrees)[a]

Joint	Left	Right
Thumb CMC Abduction	0–37	0–28
Second Finger MCP Extension	0–5	0–40
Fifth Finger MCP extension	0–5	0–37
Wrist Flexion	0–80	0–50
Wrist Extension	0–65	0–10
Elbow Flexion	0–145	0–140
Elbow Extension	90–0	90–64
Forearm Supination	0–90	0–30
Shoulder Flexion	0–115	0–50
Shoulder Abduction	0–110	0–55

CMC, carpometacarpal; MCP, metacarpophalangeal.

[a]All movements measured in sitting position.

- The 360-degree turn test, a brief examination of dynamic balance that is scored on qualitative characteristics in the Physical Performance Test[5] and as a timed quantitative item on the Berg Balance Scale.[6–8] Results are displayed in Table CS5.5.
- Motor Function:
  Detailed examination of motor function was conducted using the following:
  - *The Fugl-Meyer Assessment of Physical Performance (FMA)*[9] is an impairment-based test of motor ability that examines sensation, ROM, pain, and quality of movement during a series of increasingly more difficult motor tasks. The pretreatment FMA recording sheet is displayed in CS5 Appendix A (located at the end of this case study).

- *The Wolf Motor Function Test (WMFT)*[10–12] is a laboratory performance test that employs 17 motor tasks; 15 are timed and 2 involve measures of strength. The testing administration is standardized and ordered sequentially from simple to complex. The 15 timed tasks are filmed and later rated by masked scorers for functional ability using a six-point rating scale (0 to 5) (Box CS5.1). The two strength tasks are (1) forward flexion of the shoulder in a seated position to the top of a 10-inch box on a facing table using weights up to 20 lb (9 kg) strapped to the forearm and (2) dynamometer grip strength for 3 seconds with the elbow flexed to 90 degrees. The pretreatment WMFT score sheet is displayed in Table CS5.6.
- *The Motor Activity Log (MAL)* is a structured interview that includes the MAL Amount of Use Scale and the MAL How Well Scale (see Chapter 12, Tables 12.5 and 12.6, respectively). Respondents are asked to rate how much and how well they use their more affected UE for 30 activities of daily living tasks outside the clinical setting. (See Chapter 12, Table 12.7 for the activities included in the MAL and Table 12.1 for grading criteria [minimum active ROM and MAL scores]). The pretreatment MAL scores are presented in CS5 Appendix B.
- *The Stroke Impact Scale (SIS)*[13–15] is a full-spectrum health status interview that measures changes in eight impairment, function, and quality-of-life subdomains following stroke. The pretreatment SIS score sheets

TABLE CS5.4 Performance in Tests of Standing Balance (EPESE Protocol)[a]

Test	Scoring	Patient Time (sec)
Side-by-Side Stand	0 = Unable to hold position for more than 9 seconds (inability to complete test) 1 = Able to stand with feet side by side for 10 seconds, unable to hold in semi-tandem for 10 seconds. If able to hold for 10 seconds, go to next posture.	10
Semitandem Stand	2 = Able to stand in semi-tandem position for 10 seconds, unable to hold a full tandem position for more than 2 seconds. If able to hold for 10 seconds, go to next posture.	10
Full Tandem Stand	3 = Able to stand in full tandem position for 3 to 9 seconds 4 = Able to stand in full tandem position for 10 seconds, highest possible score	10
		Total Score: 4

[a]The patient was asked to stand using three foot positions: side-by-side, semi-tandem (heel of one foot next to the great toe of the other foot), and full tandem (heel of one foot directly in front of other foot) for 10 seconds each.

TABLE CS5.5 Performance in Test of Dynamic Balance: 360-Degree Turn

Trial/ Average	Turn to Right	Turn to Left
Trial 1	11.15 sec; 13 steps	13 sec; 13 steps
Trial 2	9.84 sec; 10 steps	12.56 sec; 12 steps
Average	10.5 sec; 12 steps	12.78 sec; 12.5 steps

Scoring: Total time and steps per turn.

BOX CS5.1 Wolf Motor Function Test Functional Ability Rating Scale

0 = Does not attempt with UE being tested
1 = UE being tested does not participate functionally; however, an attempt is made to use the UE. In unilateral tasks, the UE not being tested may be used to move the UE being tested.
2 = Does, but requires assistance of the UE not being tested for minor readjustments or change of position, or requires more than two attempts to complete, or accomplishes very slowly. In bilateral tasks, the UE being tested may serve only as a helper.
3 = Does, but movement is influenced to some degree by synergy or is performed slowly or with effort.
4 = Does, movement is close to normal* but slightly slower; it may lack precision, fine coordination, or fluidity.
5 = Does, movements appear to be normal.*

UE, upper extremity.

*For the determination of normal, the less involved UE can be utilized as an available index for comparison, with premorbid UE dominance taken into consideration.

are presented in CS5 Appendix C. Although not included for this patient, a ninth question (titled Stroke Recovery) asks the patient for an estimate of the amount of recovery of function he or she has experienced. The directions for this question read: On a scale of 0 to 100, with 100 representing full recovery and 0 representing no recovery, how much have you recovered from your stroke? The patient responds by selecting one of the following options: 100, 90, 80, 70, 60, 50, 40, 30, 20, 10, 0. The patient completes a daily activity log as presented in CS5 Appendix D.

Evaluation, Diagnosis and Prognosis, and Plan of Care

Note: Before considering the guiding questions below, view the Case Study 5 Examination segment of the video to enhance understanding of the patient's impairments and activity limitations. After completing the guiding questions, view the Case Study 5 Intervention segment of the video to compare and contrast the interventions presented with those you selected. Last, progress to the Case Study 5 Outcomes segment of the video to compare and contrast the goals and expected outcomes you identified with the functional outcomes achieved.

Note: The reader is referred to Chapter 12: Constraint-Induced Movement Therapy, for a detailed discussion of constraint-induced movement (CI) therapy.

Note: See CS5 Appendix E for a list of additional materials available at Davis*Plus* (www. fadavis.com).

TABLE CS5.6 Pretreatment Wolf Motor Function Scores

Task	Performance Time (sec)	Functional Ability Rating[a]
1. Forearm to table (side)	2.40	3
2. Forearm to box (side)	11.87	2
3. Extend elbow (side)	2.59	2
4. Extend elbow (weight)	3.50	3
5. Hand to table (front)	1.40	3
6. Hand to box (front)	3.21	2
7. Reach and retrieve	0.93	3
8. Lift can	120+	1
9. Lift pencil	4.18	3
10. Lift paper clip	120+	1
11. Stack checkers	120+	1
12. Flip cards	21.56	2
13. Turn key in lock	12.34	3
14. Fold towel	50.59	2
15. Lift basket	16.34	2
Median Score	11.87	NA
Mean Score	32.73	2.2
Log Squared Mean	2.29	NA
Strength Measures		
Weight to box	0 lb (0 kg)	
Grip strength	5.14 lb (2.33 kg)	

[a]See Box CS5.1.

Guiding Questions

1. Using the *Guide to Physical Therapist Practice,* identify the preferred practice pattern that best describes this patient's diagnosis.
2. Using the University of Alabama grading system (see Chapter 12, Table 12.1) for UE function, which category would be assigned to this patient?
3. Identify UE movement impairments that should be considered as targets for designing shaping and task practice activities.
4. Discuss factors that will likely negatively influence this patient's participation in the CI therapy protocol.
5. Discuss factors that will likely positively influence this patient's participation in the CI therapy protocol.
6. Using the patient's typical routine (see CS5 Appendix D), identify activities that could be listed in the *"mitt on, more affected UE only"* category of the behavioral contract. (***Note:*** Activities can be modified to allow for inclusion in this category.)
7. Using the patient's typical routine (see CS5 Appendix D), identify activities that for safety reasons should be placed in the *"mitt off, both hands"* and *"mitt off, less affected UE only"* categories.
8. Using MAL change scores, what are the expected outcomes of application of the CI therapy protocol?
9. Describe two shaping and two task practice activities that would be appropriate for this patient.
10. Describe the appropriate delivery schedule of the CI therapy protocol for this patient.

Reminder: Answers to the Case Study Guiding Questions are available online at Davis*Plus* (www.fadavis.com).

REFERENCES

1. Folstein, MF, Folstein, SE, and McHugh, PR. "Mini-mental state." A practical method for grading the cognitive state of patients for the clinician. J Psychiatr Res, 1975; 12:189.
2. Bohannon, R, and Smith, M. Interrater reliability of a modified Ashworth scale of muscle spasticity. Phys Ther, 1987; 67:206.
3. Guralnik, J, et al. Lower-extremity function in persons over the age of 70 years as a predictor of subsequent disability. N Engl J Med, 1995; 332:556.
4. Guralnik, J, et al. A short physical performance battery assessing lower extremity function: Association with self-reported disability and prediction of mortality and nursing home admission. J Gerontol, 1994; 49:M85–M94.
5. Reuben, DB, and Siu, AL. An objective measure of physical function of elderly outpatients: The Physical Performance Test. J Am Geriatr Soc, 1990; 38:1105.
6. Berg, K, et al. Measuring balance in the elderly: Preliminary development of an instrument. Physiother Can, 1989; 41:304.
7. Berg, K, et al. A comparison of clinical and laboratory measures of postural balance in an elderly population. Arch Phys Med Rehabil, 1992; 73:1073.
8. Berg, K, et al. Measuring balance in the elderly: Validation of an instrument. Can J Public Health, 1992; 83(suppl. 2):S7.
9. Fugl-Meyer, A, Jaasko, L, Leyman, I, et al: The post stroke hemiplegic patient, 1. A method for evaluation of physical performance. Scand J Rehabil Med, 1975; 7:13.
10. Wolf, SL, et al. Forced use of hemiplegic upper extremities to reverse the effect of learned nonuse among chronic stroke and head injured patients. Exp Neurol, 1989; 104:125.

11. Wolf, SL, et al. Assessing Wolf Motor Function Test as outcome measure for research in patients after stroke. Stroke, 2001; 32:1635.
12. Morris, DM, et al. The reliability of the Wolf Motor Function Test for assessing upper extremity function after stroke. Arch Phys Med Rehabil, 2001; 82:750.
13. Duncan, PW, et al. Stroke Impact Scale-16: A brief assessment of physical function. Neurology, 2003; 60(2):291.
14. Lai, SM, et al. Physical and social functioning after stroke: Comparison of the Stroke Impact Scale and Short Form-36. Stroke, 2003; 34:488.
15. Duncan, PW, et al. Rasch analysis of a new stroke-specific outcome scale: The Stroke Impact Scale. Arch Phys Med Rehabil, 2003; 84:950.

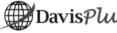

VIEWING THE CASE: Patient With Stroke: Constraint-Induced Movement Therapy

As students learn in different ways, the video case presentation (examination, intervention, and outcomes) is designed to promote engagement with the content, allow progression at an individual (or group) pace, and use of the medium or combination of media (written, visual, and auditory) best suited to the learner(s). The video, presented online at Davis*Plus* (www.fadavis.com), includes both visual and auditory modes.

Video Summary

Patient is a 63-year-old man with stroke and right hemiparesis (6 months post stroke). The video shows examination and interventions segments during outpatient rehabilitation receiving CI movement therapy. Outcomes are filmed at 2 weeks and 1 year posttreatment.

DavisPlus For additional resources and to view the accompanying video associated with this case, please visit **www.davisplus.com**.

CASE STUDY 5 APPENDIX

A Components of the Fugl-Meyer Evaluation of Physical Performance Used to Examine Patient

Components of the Meyer Evaluation of Physical Performance Used to Examine Patient

Range of Motion

Joint	Movement	Score	Scoring Criteria
Shoulder	Flexion	1	0 = Only a few degrees of motion
	Abduction to 90 degrees	1	1 = Decreased passive range of motion
	External rotation	1	2 = Normal passive range of motion
	Internal rotation	1	
Elbow	Flexion	2	
	Extension	2	
Wrist	Flexion	1	
	Extension	1	
Fingers	Flexion	1	
	Extension	2	
Forearm	Pronation	2	
	Supination	1	
	Total ROM Score:	**16**	

Pain

Joint	Movement	Pain Score	Scoring Criteria
Shoulder	Flexion	1	0 = Marked pain at end of range or pain through range
	Abduction to 90 degrees	1	
	External rotation	1	1 = Some pain
	Internal rotation	1	
Elbow	Flexion	2	2 = No pain
	Extension	2	

Components of the Meyer Evaluation of Physical Performance Used to Examine Patient (continued)

Pain (continued)

Joint	Movement	Pain Score	Scoring Criteria
Wrist	Flexion	2	
	Extension	2	
Fingers	Flexion	2	
	Extension	2	
Forearm	Pronation	2	
	Supination	2	
	Total Pain Score:	**20**	

Sensation Center Sensation

Type of Sensation	Area	Score	Scoring Criteria
Light touch	Upper arm	1	0 = Anesthesia
	Palm of hand	1	1 = Hyperesthesia/dysesthesia
Proprioception	Shoulder	2	2 = Normal
	Elbow	2	0 = No sensation
	Wrist	2	1 = Three-quarters of answers are correct, but considerable difference in sensation compared with unaffected side
	Thumb	2	
			2 = All answers correct, little or no difference
	Total Sensation Score:	**10**	

Motor Function (in sitting)

	Item	Score	Scoring Criteria
Reflexes	Biceps	2	0 = No reflex activity can be elicited.
	Triceps	2	2 = Reflex activity can be elicited.
Flexor Synergy	Elevation	1	0 = Cannot be performed at all
	Shoulder retraction	1	1 = Performed partly
	Abduction (at least 90 degrees)	1	2 = Performed faultlessly
	External rotation	1	
	Elbow flexion	1	
	Forearm supination	1	

(continues on page 358)

Components of the Meyer Evaluation of Physical Performance Used to Examine Patient *(continued)*

Motor Function (in sitting) (continued)

Joint	Movement	Pain Score	Scoring Criteria
Extensor Synergy	Shoulder adduction/internal rotation	1	0 = Cannot be performed at all
	Elbow extension	1	1 = Performed partly
	Forearm pronation	1	2 = Performed faultlessly
Movement Combining Synergies	Hand to lumbar spine	1	0 = No specific action performed 1 = Hand must pass anterior superior iliac spine 2 = Performed faultlessly
	Shoulder flexion to 90 degrees; elbow at 0 degrees	0	0 = Arm is immediately abducted, or elbow flexes at start of motion. 1 = Abduction or elbow flexion occurs in later phase of motion. 2 = Performed faultlessly
	Pronation/supination of forearm with elbow at 90 degrees and shoulder at 0 degrees	1	0 = Correct position of shoulder and elbow cannot be attained and/or pronation or supination cannot be performed at all. 1 = Active pronation or supination can be performed even within a limited range of motion, and at the same time the shoulder and elbow are correctly positioned. 2 = Complete pronation and supination with correct positions at elbow and shoulder
Movement Out of Synergy	Shoulder abduction to 90 degrees, elbow at 0, and forearm pronated	0	0 = Initial elbow flexion occurs or any deviation from pronated forearm occurs. 1 = Motion can be performed partly, or, if during motion, elbow is flexed or forearm cannot be kept in pronation. 2 = Faultless motion
	Shoulder flexion 90 degrees –180 degrees, elbow at 0 degrees, and forearm in midposition	0	0 = Initial flexion of elbow or shoulder abduction occurs. 1 = Elbow flexion or shoulder abduction occurs during shoulder flexion. 2 = Faultless motion

Components of the Meyer Evaluation of Physical Performance Used to Examine Patient *(continued)*

Motor Function (in sitting) (continued)

Joint	Movement	Pain Score	Scoring Criteria
	Pronation/supination of forearm, elbow at 0 degrees, and shoulder between 30 degrees and 90 degrees of flexion	0	0 = Supination and pronation cannot be performed at all or elbow and shoulder positions cannot be attained. 1 = Elbow and shoulder properly positioned, and pronation and supination performed in a limited range 2 = Faultless motion
Normal Reflex Activity (This stage is included only if the patient attains a score of 6 in stage above: *Movement out of synergy.*)	Biceps and/or finger flexors and triceps	0	0 = At least two of the three phasic reflexes are markedly hyperactive. 1 = One reflex is markedly hyperactive, or at least two reflexes are lively. 2 = No more than one reflex is lively, and none are hyperactive.
Wrist	Stability, elbow at 90 degrees and shoulder at 0 degrees	0	0 = Patient cannot dorsiflex (extend) wrist to required 15 degrees. 1 = Dorsiflexion (extension) is accomplished, but no resistance is taken. 2 = Position can be maintained with some (slight) resistance.
	Flexion/extension, elbow at 90 degrees and shoulder at 0 degrees	1	0 = Volitional movement does not occur. 1 = Patient cannot actively move the wrist joint throughout the total range of motion. 2 = Faultless, smooth movement
	Stability, elbow at 0 degrees and shoulder at 30 degrees	0	0 = Patient cannot dorsiflex (extend) wrist to required 15 degrees. 1 = Dorsiflexion (extension) is accomplished, but no resistance is taken. 2 = Position can be maintained with some (slight) resistance.
	Flexion/extension, elbow at 0 degrees and shoulder at 30 degrees	1	0 = Volitional movement does not occur. 1 = Patient cannot actively move the wrist joint throughout the total range of motion. 2 = Faultless, smooth movement

(continues on page 360)

Components of the Meyer Evaluation of Physical Performance Used to Examine Patient *(continued)*

Motor Function (in sitting) (continued)

Joint	Movement	Pain Score	Scoring Criteria
	Circumduction	1	0 = Cannot be performed
			1 = Jerky motion or incomplete circumduction
			2 = Complete motion with smoothness
Hand	Finger mass flexion	1	0 = No flexion occurs.
			1 = Some flexion, but not full motion
			2 = Complete active flexion (compared with unaffected hand)
	Finger mass extension	1	0 = No extension occurs.
			1 = Patient can release an active mass flexion grasp.
			2 = Full active extension
	Grasp #1: MCP joints are extended and proximal and distal IP joints are flexed; grasp is tested against resistance.	0	0 = Required position cannot be acquired.
			1 = Grasp is weak.
			2 = Grasp can be maintained against relatively great resistance.
	Grasp #2: Patient is instructed to adduct thumb with a scrap of paper interposed; all other joints are at 0 degrees.	0	0 = Function cannot be performed.
			1 = Scrap of paper interposed between the thumb and index finger can be kept in place, but not against a slight tug.
			2 = Paper is held firmly against a tug.
	Grasp #3: Patient opposes thumb pad against the pad of index finger, with a pencil interposed.	1	0 = Function cannot be performed.
			1 = Pencil interposed between the thumb and index finger can be kept in place, but not against a slight tug.
			2 = Pencil is held firmly against a tug.
	Grasp #4: The patient should grasp a small can by opposing the volar surfaces of the first and second fingers against each other.	1	0 = Function cannot be performed.
			1 = A can interposed between the thumb and index finger can be kept in place, but not against a slight tug.
			2 = A can is held firmly against a tug.

Components of the Meyer Evaluation of Physical Performance Used to Examine Patient *(continued)*

Motor Function (in sitting) (continued)

Joint	Movement	Pain Score	Scoring Criteria
	Grasp #5: The patient grasps a tennis ball with a spherical grip or is instructed to place his/her hand in a position of thumb abduction with abduction and flexion of the second, third, fourth, and fifth fingers.	1	0 = Function cannot be performed. 1 = A tennis ball can be kept in place with a spherical grasp, but not against a slight tug. 2 = A tennis ball is held firmly against a tug.
Coordination/Speed: Finger to nose (five repetitions in rapid succession while patient is blindfolded)	Tremor	2	0 = Marked tremor 1 = Slight tremor 2 = No tremor
Dysmetrial	1		0 = Pronounced or unsystematic dysmetria 1 = Slight or systematic dysmetria 2 = No dysmetria
Speed	1		0 = Activity is more than 6 seconds longer than unaffected hand. 1 = Activity is 2 to 5 seconds longer than unaffected hand. 2 = Less than 2 seconds difference
	Total Motor Score:	**27**	

MCP, metacarpophalangeal; IP, interphalangeal.

Pretreatment Motor Activity Log (MAL) Scores

Task Number	Task	Amount of Use[a]	How Well[b]
1	Turn on a light with a light switch	1	1
2	Open a drawer	1	2
3	Remove an item of clothing from a drawer	1	2.5
4	Pick up the phone	0	0
5	Wipe off a kitchen counter or other surface	0	0
6	Get out of a car (includes only the movement needed to get the body from sitting to standing outside of the car, once the door is open)	2	2
7	Open the refrigerator	1	3
8	Open a door by turning a doorknob	1	1
9	Use a TV remote control	1	1
10	Wash hands (includes lathering and rinsing; does not include turning water on and off with a faucet handle)	5	1
11	Turn water on and off with knob or lever on the faucet	0	0
12	Dry hands	5	1
13	Put on socks	2	1.5
14	Take off socks	0	0
15	Put on shoes (includes tying shoestrings and fastening straps)	1	1.5
16	Take off shoes (includes untying shoestrings and unfastening straps)	0	0
17	Get up from a chair with armrests	0	0
18	Pull a chair away from the table before sitting down	0	0
19	Pull chair toward the table after sitting down	0	0
20	Pick up a glass, bottle, drinking cup, or can (does not need to include drinking)	1	1.5
21	Brush teeth (does not include preparing toothbrush or brushing dentures)	0	0
22	Put makeup, lotion, or shaving cream on face	0	0

Task Number	Task	Amount of Use[a]	How Well[b]
23	Use a key to unlock a door	0	0
24	Write on paper (if dominant arm was most affected, "Do you see it to write?"; if nondominant arm was most affected, drop the item and assign "NA")	1	0.5
25	Carry an object in hand (draping an item over the arm is not acceptable)	1	2
26	Use a fork or spoon for eating (refers to the action of bringing food to the mouth with a fork or spoon)	0	0
27	Comb hair	0	0
28	Pick up a cup by a handle	0	0
29	Button a shirt	4	2
30	Eat half a sandwich or finger foods	0	0
	Mean Score:	**0.7**	**0.8**

[a]Amount of Use Scale: 0 = did not use my weaker arm (not used); 1 = occasionally tried to use my weaker arm (very rarely); 2 = sometimes used my weaker arm but did most of the activity with my stronger arm (rarely); 3 = used my weaker arm about half as much as before the stroke (half prestroke); 4 = used my weaker arm almost as much as before the stroke (3/4 prestroke); 5 = used my weaker arm as normal as before the stroke (same as prestroke).

[b]How Well Scale: 0 = the weaker arm was not used at all for that activity (never); 1 = the weaker arm was moved during that activity but was not helpful (very poor); 2 = the weaker arm was of some use during that activity but needed some help from the stronger arm or moved very slowly or with difficulty (poor); 3 = the weaker arm was used for the purpose indicated but movements were slow or were made with only some effort (fair); 4 = the movements made by the weaker arm were almost normal but not quite as fast or accurate as normal (almost normal); 5 = the ability to use the weaker arm for that activity was as well as before the injury (normal).

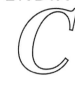

C Stroke Impact Scale (SIS): Pretreatment Scores

1. In the past week, how would you rate the strength of your . . .	A Lot of Strength	Quite a Bit of Strength	Some Strength	A Little Strength	No Strength at All
a. arm that was most affected by your stroke?	5	4	3	**2**	1
b. grip of your hand that was most affected by your stroke?	5	4	3	**2**	1
c. leg that was most affected by your stroke?	5	4	**3**	2	1
d. foot/ankle that was most affected by your stroke?	5	4	**3**	2	1

2. In the past week, how difficult was it for you to . . .	Not Difficult at All	A Little Difficult	Somewhat Difficult	Very Difficult	Extremely Difficult
a. remember things that people just told you?	**5**	4	3	2	1
b. remember things that happened the day before?	**5**	4	3	2	1
c. remember to do things (e.g., keep scheduled appointments or take medication)?	**5**	4	3	2	1
d. remember the day of the week?	**5**	4	3	2	1
e. concentrate?	**5**	4	3	2	1
f. think quickly?	**5**	4	3	2	1
g. solve problems?	**5**	4	3	2	1

3. In the past week, how often did you . . .	None of the Time	A Little of the Time	Some of the Time	Most of the Time	All of the Time
a. feel sad?	**5**	4	3	2	1
b. feel that there is nobody you are close to?	**5**	4	3	2	1
c. feel that you are a burden to others?	**5**	4	3	2	1
d. feel that you have nothing to look forward to?	**5**	4	3	2	1

3. In the past week, how often did you . . .	None of the Time	A Little of the Time	Some of the Time	Most of the Time	All of the Time
e. blame yourself for mistakes that you made?	**5**	4	3	2	1
f. enjoy things as much as ever?	5	4	3	2	**1**
g. feel quite nervous?	**5**	4	3	2	1
h. feel that life is worth living?	5	4	3	**2**	1
i. smile and laugh at least once a day?	5	4	3	2	**1**

4. In the past week, how difficult was it to . . .	Not Difficult at All	A Little Difficult	Somewhat Difficult	Very Difficult	Extremely Difficult
a. say the name of someone who was in front of you?	**5**	4	3	2	1
b. understand what was being said to you in a conversation?	**5**	4	3	2	1
c. reply to questions?	**5**	4	3	2	1
d. correctly name objects?	**5**	4	3	2	1
e. participate in a conversation with a group of people?	**5**	4	3	2	1
f. have a conversation on the telephone?	**5**	4	3	2	1
g. call another person on the telephone, including selecting the correct phone number and dialing?	**5**	4	3	2	1

5. In the past 2 weeks, how difficult was it to . . .	Not Difficult at All	A Little Difficult	Somewhat Difficult	Very Difficult	Could Not Do at All
a. cut your food with a knife and fork?	5	4	3	**2**	1
b. dress the top part of your body?	5	4	**3**	2	1
c. bathe yourself?	5	4	3	**2**	1
d. clip your toenails?	5	4	3	**2**	1
e. get to the toilet on time?	**5**	4	3	2	1
f. control your bladder (not have an accident)?	5	**4**	3	2	1
g. control your bowels (not have an accident)?	**5**	4	3	2	1

(continues on page 366)

5. In the past 2 weeks, how difficult was it to . . .	Not Difficult at All	A Little Difficult	Somewhat Difficult	Very Difficult	Could Not Do at All
h. do light household tasks/chores (e.g., dust, make a bed, take out garbage, do the dishes)?	5	4	**3**	2	1
i. go shopping?	5	4	3	2	**1**
j. do heavy household chores (e.g., vacuum, laundry, or yard work)?	5	4	**3**	2	1

6. In the past 2 weeks, how difficult was it to . . .	Not Difficult at All	A Little Difficult	Somewhat Difficult	Very Difficult	Could Not Do at All
a. stay sitting without losing your balance?	**5**	4	3	2	1
b. stay standing without losing your balance?	**5**	4	3	2	1
c. walk without losing your balance?	5	**4**	3	2	1
d. move from a bed to a chair?	5	**4**	3	2	1
e. walk one block?	5	4	**3**	2	1
f. walk fast?	5	4	**3**	2	1
g. climb one flight of stairs?	5	4	**3**	2	1
h. climb several flights of stairs?	5	4	3	**2**	1
i. get in and out of a car?	5	4	**3**	2	1

7. In the past 2 weeks, how difficult was it to use your hand that was most affected by your stroke to . . .	Not Difficult at All	A Little Difficult	Somewhat Difficult	Very Difficult	Could Not Do at All
a. carry heavy objects (e.g., bag of groceries)?	5	4	3	2	**1**
b. turn a doorknob?	5	4	3	2	**1**
c. open a can or jar?	5	4	3	2	**1**
d. tie a shoelace?	5	4	3	2	**1**
e. pick up a dime?	5	4	3	2	**1**

8. During the past 4 weeks, how much of the time have you been limited in . . .	None of the Time	A Little of the Time	Some of the Time	Most of the Time	All of the Time
a. your work (paid, voluntary, or other)?	5	**4**	3	2	1
b. your social activities?	5	**4**	3	2	1
c. quiet recreation (crafts, reading)?	5	4	3	**2**	1
d. active recreation (sports, outings, travel)?	5	**4**	3	2	1
e. your role as a family member and/or friend?	5	4	**3**	2	1
f. your participation in spiritual or religious activities?	5	4	3	**2**	1
g. your ability to control?	5	**4**	3	2	1
h. your ability to help others?	5	**4**	3	2	1

D The Patient's Typical Daily Activity Log

Daily Activity Schedule

Weekdays:

Time	Activity	Details (if needed)
6:00 a.m.	Wake up	
6:05 a.m.	Make coffee	Automatic coffeemaker
6:15 a.m.	Let dogs out/feed dogs	Dry dog food
6:30 a.m.	Drink coffee/watch news on TV	
6:45 a.m.	Eat breakfast	Cereal, toast, juice
7:00 a.m.	Shower	
7:15 a.m.	Shave	Disposable safety razor
7:20 a.m.	Brush teeth	Electric toothbrush
7:30 a.m.	Get dressed	
8:00 a.m.	Leave home for clinic	
12 noon	Leave clinic for home	
12:30 p.m.	Eat lunch	Sandwich, chips, fruit, iced tea
1:30 p.m.	Walk dogs	Two small dogs on sidewalk
2:30 p.m.	Read mail/newspaper; check e-mails	
4:00 p.m.	Yard work/housework	
5:00 p.m.	Watch news on TV	
6:00 p.m.	Eat dinner	Meat, veg., salad, bread, iced tea
7:00 p.m.	Watch TV	
9:30 p.m.	Wash face/brush teeth	
9:45 p.m.	Put on pajamas	
10:00 p.m.	Go to bed	

Daily Activity Schedule

Saturdays:

Time	Activity	Details (if needed)
8:00 a.m.	Wake up	
8:05 a.m.	Make coffee	Automatic coffeemaker
8:15 a.m.	Let dogs out/feed dogs	Dry dog food
8:30 a.m.	Drink coffee/watch news on TV	
8:45 a.m.	Eat breakfast	Waffles, bacon, juice
9:00 a.m.	Shower	
9:15 a.m.	Shave	Disposable safety razor
9:20 a.m.	Brush teeth	Electric toothbrush
9:30 a.m.	Get dressed	
10:00 a.m.	Grocery shopping with wife	
12 noon	Lunch out with wife	
1:00 p.m.	Movies, park, or mall with wife	
3:30 p.m.	Laundry	
4:30 p.m.	Read mail/newspaper; check e-mails	
6:00 p.m.	Eat dinner	Meat, veg., salad, bread, iced tea
7:00 p.m.	Play cards/board games with neighbors	
9:30 p.m.	Wash face/brush teeth	
9:45 p.m.	Put on pajamas	
10:00 p.m.	Go to bed	

Daily Activity Schedule

Sundays:

Time	Activity	Details (if needed)
8:00 a.m.	Wake up	
8:05 a.m.	Make coffee	Automatic coffeemaker
8:15 a.m.	Let dogs out/feed dogs	Dry dog food
8:30 a.m.	Drink coffee/watch news on TV	
8:45 a.m.	Eat breakfast	Omelet, sausage, juice

Daily Activity Schedule

Sundays:

Time	Activity	Details (if needed)
9:00 a.m.	Shower	
9:15 a.m.	Shave	Disposable safety razor
9:20 a.m.	Brush teeth	Electric toothbrush
9:30 a.m.	Get dressed	
10:00 a.m.	Church with wife	
12:00 noon	Lunch out with family at brother's home	Meat, veg., salad, bread, iced tea
2:30 p.m.	Watch sports on TV with brother	
4:30 p.m.	Read mail/newspaper; check e-mails	
6:00 p.m.	Eat light dinner	Sandwiches, chips, iced tea
7:00 p.m.	Watch TV	
9:30 p.m.	Wash face/brush teeth	
9:45 p.m.	Put on pajamas	
10:00 p.m.	Go to bed	

E Additional Materials Available at Davis*Plus*

The following additional Case Study 5 materials are available for review online at Davis*Plus* (www.fadavis.com).

Note: The additional Case Study 5 materials are ordered based on their relevance to the case and the progression the materials would be used with or by the patient.

Examination

History

- **Demographic Information:**
  The patient is an 84-year-old man with a 9-year history of Parkinson's disease.
- **History of Present Illness:**
  The patient has experienced a recent deterioration of balance, gait, endurance, and strength. He was hospitalized for 12 days to monitor the deterioration and adjust medications accordingly. The patient was then transferred to an inpatient rehabilitation facility for 2 weeks, has received home physical therapy for 4 weeks, and now has been referred for outpatient physical therapy.
- **Medical History:**
  Patient reports prostate cancer, left upper extremity (UE) adhesive capsulitis (status post trauma from a motor vehicle accident), and depression.
- **Surgical History:**
  Patient reports right total knee arthroplasty (status post 8 years), left total knee arthroplasty (status post 4 years), and left total hip arthroplasty (status post 3 years).
- **Medications:**
  Sinemet, Mirapex, Lexapro, iron, and Zocor.
- **Social History:**
  The patient is retired and lives with his wife. She is also retired and able to provide limited assistance during the day secondary to her history of cardiac disease. A recently hired aide provides 4 hours of assistance per day.
- **Living Environment:**
  The patient lives in an apartment with no steps. He has the following durable medical equipment: straight cane, tripod rollator, shower chair, commode, and two grab bars installed in the bathroom.
- **General Health Status:**
  Fair
- **Prior Level of Function:**
  Prior to last hospitalization, the patient ambulated independently with a straight cane.
- **Current Level of Function:**
  The patient ambulates using a straight cane at home for short distances and ambulates outside with a rollator

*Filmed at Rusk Institute of Rehabilitation Medicine, New York.

and contact guard assistance secondary to imbalance and fall risk. The patient reports an average of three falls per month. He uses a motorized scooter when traveling farther than four blocks. He reports difficulty with rolling in bed in both directions, transferring from supine-to-sit and sit-to-stand, donning and doffing clothes, and eating.

Systems Review

- **Cardiovascular/Pulmonary System:**
  - Heart rate: 70 beats per minute
  - Respiratory rate: 24 breaths per minute
  - Blood pressure: 128/76 mm Hg
- **Musculoskeletal System:**
  - Height: 5 ft, 8 in. (1.7 m)
  - Weight: 185 lb (84 kg)
  - Gross symmetry: The patient presents with decreased lumbar lordosis, rounded shoulders, increased thoracic kyphosis, and forward head posture.
  - Gross range of motion (ROM): The patient presents with gross limitations in active ROM in both UEs and both lower extremities (LEs), with greater limitations in the left UE and LE.
  - Gross strength: The patient presents with gross limitations in the strength of both UEs and both LEs, with greater limitations in the left UE and LE.
- **Neuromuscular System:**
  - Motor function (motor control, motor learning): The patient's impaired motor control is apparent; increased difficulty is noted during initiation of bed mobility, transfers, and ambulation. The patient presents with daily freezing episodes (inability to continue an activity). When he is asked to perform functional activities, including transfers, ambulation, and fine motor tasks with increased speed or with additional task demands, the quality and safety of movement deteriorate.
  - Tone: Moderate cogwheel rigidity is present in both UEs and LEs and is particularly apparent during elbow and knee extension. The left UE and LE are more impaired than the right.
  - Balance: The patient presents with good static sitting balance and fair dynamic sitting balance. He presents with poor static and dynamic standing balance.
  - Gait: The patient ambulates 400 ft (122 m) with a rollator and contact guard assistance secondary to imbalance

and fall risk. He ambulates up and down four steps with bilateral handrails and minimal assistance to maintain balance and encourage weight shift. The patient uses a step-to gait pattern on stairs.

- **Functional Status:**
  - Functional mobility: The patient performs bed mobility with contact guard assistance for rolling in both directions and minimal assistance for scooting in bed. He transfers supine-to-sit with contact guard assistance. Transfers from sit-to-stand require minimal assistance to initiate motion and encourage anterior progression of the torso.
  - Self-care and home management: The patient requires minimal assistance when donning and doffing clothes. He requires supervision to minimal assistance when eating secondary to tremors and decreased fine motor control.

Tests and Measures

- **Posture:**
  Reedco Posture Score Sheet: 40/100. The patient presents with deficits in all planes, with the most pronounced postural abnormalities being increased thoracic kyphosis, rounded shoulders, forward head, and anteriorly inclined torso.
- **Aerobic Capacity/Endurance:**
  Results of the *6-Minute Walk Test*[1] are presented in Table CS6.1. Patient ambulates with a rollator and minimal assistance.
- **Sensory Integrity:**
  - Impaired response to light touch on bilateral plantar surfaces (no response to light touch during 4 of 10 trials on right foot and during 6 of 10 trials on left foot).
  - Impaired ability to discriminate between sharp and dull sensations on bilateral plantar surfaces (inability to discriminate during 5 of 10 trials on feet bilaterally).
  - Impaired proprioceptive awareness on great toe bilaterally (incorrect response 4 of 10 trials on right foot and 6 of 10 trials on left foot). Intact proprioceptive awareness at ankles bilaterally.
- **Strength:**
  Results of the *manual muscle test* and grip strength values (dynamometer) are presented in Table CS6.2.

TABLE CS6.1 6-Minute Walk Test Results

Test	HR	BP	RR	SaO$_2$
Pretest	63	128/76	24	90
Posttest	66	138/79	24	96

Note: Lowest O$_2$ saturation during walking: 86; total distance covered: 528 ft (177 m).

Patient required two rest intervals during the test.

BP, blood pressure; HR, heart rate; RR, respiratory rate; SaO$_2$, oxygen saturation.

TABLE CS6.2 Manual Muscle Test and Grip Strength Values[a]

Joint	Motion	Right	Left
Hip	Flexion	4/5	4/5
	Extension	3/5	3/5
	Abduction	4–/5	4–/5
	Adduction	4–/5	4–/5
Knee	Flexion	4+/5	4+/5
	Extension	5/5	5/5
Ankle	Plantarflexion	3+/5	4+/5
	Dorsiflexion	3+/5	4+/5
Shoulder	Flexion	4–/5	3/5
	Extension	4/5	3/5
	Abduction	3+/5	3–/5
	Internal rotation	4/5	3/5
	External rotation	4/5	3/5
Hand	Grip strength	55 lb (25 kg)	20 lb (9 kg)

[a]With the exception of grip strength, all scores are based on a 0 to 5 scale: 5, normal; 4, good; 3, fair; 2, poor; 1, trace; 0, no contraction. Strength tested within available ROM

- **Range of Motion:**
  - Results of the active ROM (AROM) examination for the cervical and lumbar spine are presented in Table CS6.3.
  - AROM values for the hips, ankles, and shoulders are presented in Table CS6.4.
  - Passive ROM (PROM) values for the hips, ankles, and shoulders are presented in Table CS6.5.
- **Deep Tendon Reflexes:**
  Patient presents with bilateral 1+ (present but depressed, low normal) triceps response and 0 (no response) for bilateral bicep, hamstring, patellar, and ankle responses.
- **Tone:**
  - On the *Modified Ashworth Scale*[2] bilateral hamstrings present with minimal resistance through range and moderate resistance at end range (3/4)
  - Bilateral quadriceps present with minimal resistance through the entire range (2/4).
- **Coordination:**
  Results of coordination tests are presented in Table CS6.6.
- **Pain:**
  Patient reports 3/10 left shoulder pain at rest and 9/10 left shoulder pain with activity (0 = no pain and 10 = worst possible pain).

TABLE CS6.3 Active Range of Motion: Cervical and Lumbar Spine

Body Segment	Motion	Range (degrees)
Cervical Spine	Flexion	0–30
	Extension	0–18
	Rotation right	0–52
	Rotation left	0–38
	Side bend right	0–10
	Side bend left	0–30
Lumbar Spine	Flexion	0–15
	Extension	0–5
	Rotation right	0–6
	Rotation left	0–4
	Side bend right	0–10
	Side bend left	0–20

TABLE CS6.4 Active Range of Motion: Hips, Ankles, and Shoulders

Joint	Motion	Right (degrees)	Left (degrees)
Hip	Straight leg raise	0–35	0–25
	Flexion	0–100	5–90
	Extension	0–0	Lacks 5 degrees to full extension
	Abduction	0–20	0–10
Ankle	Plantarflexion	0–10	0–10
	Dorsiflexion	0–5	0–5
Shoulder	Flexion	0–110	0–70 (painful)
	Extension	0–20	0–20
	Abduction	0–120	0–60 (painful)
	Internal rotation	0–18	0–10 (painful)
	External rotation	0–40	0–36 (painful)

TABLE CS6.5 Passive Range of Motion: Hips, Ankles, and Shoulders

Joint	Motion	Right (degrees)	Left (degrees)
Hip	Straight leg raise	0–40	0–30
	Flexion	0–110	5–90
	Extension	0–0	Lacks 5° to full extension
	Abduction	0–25	0–10
Ankle	Plantarflexion	0–10	0–10
	Dorsiflexion	0–5	0–5
Shoulder	Flexion	0–120	0–100 (painful)
	Extension	0–20	0–20
	Abduction	0–120	0–80 (painful)
	Internal rotation	0–20	0–10 (painful)
	External rotation	0–45	0–45 (painful)

TABLE CS6.6 Coordination Tests

Coordination Test	Grade Right	Grade Left
Finger-to-nose	4	3
Finger-to-therapist's finger	3	3
Pronation/supination	4	4
Heel-on-shin	4	3
Tapping (foot)	4	4

Scoring: 5, normal performance; 4, minimal impairment; 3, moderate impairment; 2, severe impairment; 1, activity impossible.

- **Balance:**
  - *Berg Balance Scale*[3–5] (with use of rollator): score of 26/56, indicating a 100% risk for falls
  - *Functional Reach Test*[6–8]: result of 4 in. (10 cm), indicating a high risk for falls
  - *Dynamic Gait Index*[9] (with use of rollator): score of 10/24, indicating an increased risk of falls with dynamic activities

- *EquiTest Balance Analysis* (NeuroCom International, Inc., Clackamas, Oregon)
  - *Sensory Organization Test* (SOT) composite score = 39. The patient presents with below-normal balance for his age group in conditions 3, 4, 5, and 6. The patient fell on every trial in conditions 5 and 6. Sensory analysis indicates moderate deficits in the visual system and maximal deficits in the vestibular system.
  - Strategy analysis: Results show a reliance on ankle strategies and decreased hip strategies.
  - Center of gravity analysis: Results indicate decreased weightbearing on the right LE in neutral and in squat positions at different angles of knee flexion. Most significant was a 13% decrease in weightbearing on the right LE with a 60-degree squat.
  - Adaptation test: Patient presents with minimal reflexive response to rotary toe up/down perturbations.
  - Rhythmic weight shift: Directional control composite scores were 79% in the frontal plane and 64% in the sagittal plane. The patient demonstrated deficits in directional control that were most apparent in the sagittal plane at faster speeds.
- **Gait:**
  Timed Up and Go Test[10] (patient performed test with rollator and contact guard assist): 26 seconds, indicating high risk for falls.
- **Functional Status**
  Functional Independence Measure (FIM)[11]: Results of the FIM are presented in Table CS6.7.
- **Disease-Specific Measures:**
  - *The Parkinson's Disease Quality of Life* (PDQL)[12] questionnaire:
    - Parkinsonian symptoms: 37
    - Systemic symptoms: 23
    - Social functioning: 22

- Emotional functioning: 28
- Total: 110/185

Note: The PDQL is a self-administered measure that contains 37 items in four subscales: *Parkinsonian symptoms*, *systemic symptoms*, *social functioning*, and *emotional functioning*. An overall score can be derived, with a higher score indicating better perceived quality of life.

- *The Unified Parkinson's Disease Rating Scale* (UPDRS)[13]:
  - Mentation, behavior, and mood: 4
  - Activities of Daily Living: 19
  - Motor: 23
  - *Total: 46/199*

Note: The UPDRS is a rating tool designed to follow the longitudinal course of Parkinson's disease. It is made up of several sections, including *Mentation, Behavior, and Mood*; *Activities of Daily Living;* and *Motor Examination*. Items are evaluated by interview. Some sections require multiple grades assigned to each extremity. A total of 199 points are possible; 199 points represent the worst (total) disability, and 0 represents no disability. The UPDRS also includes the *Modified Hoehn and Yahr Staging* (disease severity is divided over five stages into unilateral or bilateral signs; higher numbered stages represent progressively more difficulty with mobility and balance) and the *Schwab and England Activities of Daily Living Scale* (estimates are made of the percentage of impairment ranging from 0% = vegetative functions [bedridden] to 100% = completely independent).

- The *Modified Hoehn and Yahr Staging:* The results place the patient in stage 3 and indicate significant slowing of body movements, early impairment of equilibrium while walking or standing, and generalized dysfunction that is moderately severe.
- The *Schwab and England Activities of Daily Living Scale:* Score is 70%, which indicates that the patient is not completely independent, has greater difficulty with some chores, takes twice as long to accomplish tasks, and is conscious of difficulty and slowness.

Evaluation, Diagnosis and Prognosis, and Plan of Care

Note: Before considering the guiding questions below, view the Case Study 6 Examination segment of the video to enhance understanding of the patient's impairments and activity limitations. After completing the guiding questions, view the Case Study 6 Intervention segment of the video to compare and contrast the interventions presented with those you selected. Last, progress to the Case Study 6 Outcomes segment of the video to compare and contrast the goals and expected outcomes you identified with the functional outcomes achieved.

TABLE CS6.7 Components of Functional Independence Measure (FIM): Transfers and Locomotion

Activity	FIM Score[a]
Transfers: Bed/Chair/Wheelchair	4
Transfers: Toilet	6
Locomotion: Walk	4
Locomotion: Wheelchair	7
Locomotion: Stairs	2

[a]Scoring: 7 = Complete independence (timely, safety); 6 = Modified independence (device); 5 = Supervision (subject = 100%); 4 = Minimal assistance (subject = 75% or more); 3 = Moderate assistance (subject = 50% or more); 2 = Maximal assistance (subject = 25% or more); 1 = Total assistance or not testable (subject less than 25%).

Guiding Questions

1. Identify or categorize this patient's clinical presentation in terms of the following:
   a. Direct impairments
   b. Indirect impairments
   c. Composite impairments
   d. Activity limitations and participation restrictions
2. Identify anticipated goals (remediation of impairments) and expected outcomes (remediation of activity limitations/participation restrictions) that address the attainment of functional outcomes.
3. Formulate three treatment interventions focused on functional outcomes that could be used during the first 2 or 3 weeks of therapy. Indicate a progression for each selected intervention. Provide a brief rationale for your choices.
4. For each of the three phases of motor learning (cognitive, associated, and autonomous), describe what strategies can be used to enhance achievement of the stated goals and outcomes.
5. What strategies can be used to develop self-management skills and promote self-efficacy to enhance the achievement of stated goals and outcomes?

Reminder: Answers to the Case Study Guiding Questions are available online at Davis*Plus* (www.fadavis.com).

REFERENCES

1. Schenkman, M, et al. Reliability of impairment and physical performance measures for persons with Parkinson's disease. Phys Ther, 1997; 77:19.
2. Bohannon, R, and Smith, M. Interrater reliability of a modified Ashworth scale of muscle spasticity. Phys Ther, 1987; 67:206.
3. Berg, K, et al. Measuring balance in the elderly: Preliminary development of an instrument. Physiother Can, 1989; 41:304.
4. Berg, K, et al. A comparison of clinical and laboratory measures of postural balance in an elderly population. Arch Phys Med Rehabil, 1992; 73:1073.
5. Berg, K, et al. Measuring balance in the elderly: Validation of an instrument. Can J Public Health, 1992; 83(suppl 2):S7.
6. Duncan, P, et al. Functional reach: A new clinical measure of balance. J Gerontol, 1990; 45:M192.
7. Duncan, P, et al. Functional reach: Predictive validity in a sample of elderly male veterans. J Gerontol, 1992; 47:M93.
8. Weiner, D, et al. Functional reach: A marker of physical frailty. J Am Geriatr Soc, 1992; 40:203.
9. Shumway-Cook, A, and Woollacott, M. Motor Control Translating Research into Clinical Practice. Baltimore: Lippincott Williams & Wilkins, 2007.
10. Podsiadlo, D, and Richardson, S. The timed "up and go": A test of basic functional mobility for frail elderly patients. J Am Geriatr Soc, 1991; 39:142.
11. Guide for the Uniform Data Set for Medical Rehabilitation (including the FIM instrument), Version 5.0. Buffalo, NY, State University of New York, 1996.
12. Hobson, P, Holden, A, and Meara, J. Measuring the impact of Parkinson's disease with the Parkinson's Disease Quality of Life questionnaire. Age Ageing, 1999; 28:341.
13. Fahn, S, and Elton, R. Unified Parkinson's Disease Rating Scale. In Fahn, S, et al (eds): Recent Developments in Parkinson's Disease, vol 2. Florham Park, NJ, Macmillan Health Care Information, 1987, 153–163.

VIEWING THE CASE: Patient With Parkinson's Disease

As students learn in different ways, the video case presentation (examination, intervention, and outcomes) is designed to promote engagement with the content, allow progression at an individual (or group) pace, and use of the medium or combination of media (written, visual, and auditory) best suited to the learner(s). The video, presented online at Davis*Plus* (www.fadavis.com), includes both visual and auditory modes.

Video Summary

Patient is an 84-year-old man with a 9-year history of Parkinson's disease. The video shows examination and intervention segments during outpatient rehabilitation following episodes of inpatient rehabilitation (2 weeks) and home physical therapy (4 weeks). Outcomes are filmed after 6 weeks of intervention.

Davis*Plus* For additional resources and to view the accompanying video associated with this case, please visit **www.davisplus.com**.

CASE STUDY 7

Patient With Complete Spinal Cord Injury, T9

Paula Ackerman, MS, OTR/L; Myrtice Atrice, PT, BS; Teresa Foy, BS, OTR/L; Sarah Morrison, PT, BS; Polly Hopkins, MOTR/L; and Shari McDowell, PT, BS

Examination

History

The patient is a 21-year-old woman involved in a motor vehicle accident on January 4. She was a restrained passenger in a reclined position when the car hydroplaned head-on into a guard rail. The patient denied loss of consciousness (Glasgow Coma Scale = 15). She was taken to a local medical center, where she presented with immediate loss of movement and sensation in her lower extremities (LEs).

Imaging revealed a burst fracture of the L1 vertebral body and lamina, an L2–3 right transverse process fracture, and bony fragments were noted to have extended into the spinal canal. There was a 40% lateral displacement of the spinal cord in relation to the vertebral bodies. In addition to the spinal cord injury (SCI), she sustained a right pneumothorax, right pulmonary contusion, and multiple rib fractures on the right. The methylprednisolone (a high-dose steroid aimed at reducing the swelling) protocol was initiated in the emergency room. A T11–L3 posterior spinal stabilization was performed on January 5. Postoperatively she remained paraplegic and had sensation to her abdominal area. A computed tomography (CT) scan of the head was negative. A prophylactic vena cava filter was placed during the surgery on January 5.

- Demographic Information:
  - Height: 5 ft, 5 in. (1.7 m)
  - Weight: 114 lb (52 kg); previously 125 lb (57 kg) at the time of her accident
- **Social History:**
  Patient lives with her mother and grandmother. Her parents are divorced. She denies tobacco or alcohol use.
- **Employment:**
  Patient is a full-time student at a local community college and is interested in obtaining her degree in early childhood education. She also worked part-time as a dance instructor at a local dance studio.
- **Living Environment:**
  The family lives in a one-story rental home. There are two steps leading up to the front door. They do not have plans to move or the financial means to purchase a home at this time.

- **General Health Status:**
  Prior to her injury, the patient was in very good health. She is an accomplished dancer, having won multiple state and national dance competitions. She had asthma as a child; however, she has had no difficulties with asthma in adulthood.
- **History of Present Illness:**
  The patient was admitted to a SCI Model System of Care for rehabilitation on January 16. The initial examination indicated a T9 SCI with an American Spinal Injury Association (ASIA) Impairment Scale designation of A: complete injury (no motor or sensory function is preserved in the sacral segments S4 to S5).[1] Initial radiological films revealed a stable T11 to L3 fusion (Fig. CS7.1). She arrived in a thoracolumbosacral orthosis (TLSO), which was replaced with a less-restrictive Jewett brace to decrease the risk of skin breakdown in areas of no sensation and to allow greater ease of forward flexion at the hips during transfers. The brace was discontinued on February 11. The admission motor and sensory screening examinations revealed right upper extremity (UE) paresthesias and weakness, which were monitored and eventually resolved without specific intervention. The patient presented with a chest tube for a residual pneumothorax. The pneumothorax resolved over the course of 10 days, at which time the chest tube was removed without complications.

  The patient presented with a neurogenic bladder and bowel upon admission. A Foley catheter had been placed to manage her bladder at the previous medical center. This was discontinued, and intermittent catheterizations were initiated, which she eventually learned to manage independently. Manual evacuation of the rectal vault and suppositories were initiated to establish a program to manage her neurogenic bowel. Her hospital course was complicated by a urinary tract infection (UTI), multiple episodes of insufficient rectal vault evacuation, and intermittent abdominal discomfort. The clinical examination of the lower abdomen was negative. A kidney ureter and bladder (KUB) x-ray revealed constipation, which remained unresolved despite adherence to a routine bowel program. Results of an abdominal and pelvic CT scan revealed moderate to marked stool in the colon. This resolved prior to discharge. However, the patient

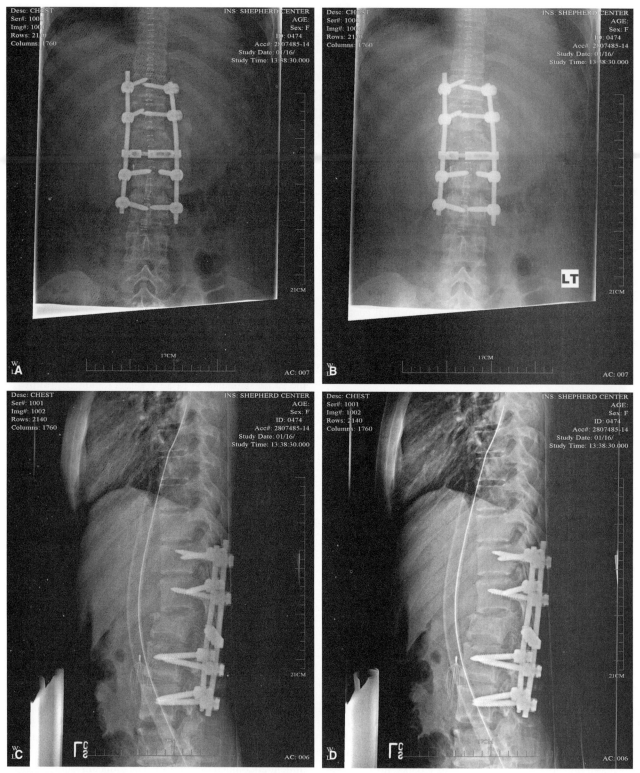

FIGURE CS7.1 Thoracolumbar x-rays of T11–L3 posterior spinal stabilization using cross-linking devices (A and B: posterior views; C and D: lateral views).

had a poor appetite throughout her stay, and supplemental nutritional support was provided. Her prealbumin level (indicator of visceral protein status) was within normal limits (24.6 mg/dL).

- **Medications:**
Macrobid, Fragmin, and Pepcid

Systems Review

- **Cardiovascular/Pulmonary System:**
Lungs were clear to auscultation with a chest tube in place on the right. The patient denied chest pain (other than the chest tube site), shortness of breath, nausea, or

vomiting. She had pneumonia and asthma as a small child but has had no problems as an adult.

- Heart rate: normal (regular) heart rate and rhythm without murmurs
- Respiratory rate: 15 breaths per minute (deep breaths were painful)
- Vital capacity: 1 L
- Blood pressure: 110/68 mm Hg

Tests and Measures

- ASIA Impairment Scale:[1]
  - The patient is classified as a complete SCI (ASIA designation: A [Box CS7.1]).
  - Sensory and motor neurological level is T9 bilaterally (Fig. CS7.2).
- **Function:**
  Functional Independence Measure (FIM)[2]: Results from the FIM are presented in Table CS7.1.
- **Strength:**
  Results from the *Manual Muscle Test* (admission data) are presented in Table CS7.2.
- **Range of Motion (ROM):**
  - Left UE ROM was within normal limits (WNL).
  - At admission, right shoulder ROM was limited to 90 degrees of flexion and 90 degrees of abduction. Pain noted as 9/10 on numeric pain scale (10 = worst pain; 0 = no pain); described as a sharp pain. An empty end-feel was noted.
- **Balance:**
  - On admission *Modified Functional Reach Test*[3] = 10.5 in. (26.67 cm)

- At discharge Modified Functional Reach Test = 27.5 in. (70 cm)
- Tone and Reflexes:
  - Deep tendon reflexes (DTR) for bilateral quadriceps tendons: 0/4 (no response)
  - Babinski sign: Positive
  - Hypotonic
- **Pain:**
  - The patient reported 8/10 pain in the area of the chest tube and rib fractures (10 = worst pain; 0 = no pain).
  - A Fentanyl patch and Dilaudid (as needed) were initiated to manage pain.
  - All pain medication was discontinued by the time of discharge.
  - See the ROM section above for shoulder pain information.

Evaluation, Diagnosis and Prognosis, and Plan of Care

Note: Before considering the guiding questions below, view the Case Study 7 Examination segment of the video to enhance understanding of the patient's impairments and activity limitations. After completing the guiding questions, view the Case Study 7 Intervention segment of the video to compare and contrast the interventions presented with those you selected. Last, progress to the Case Study 7 Outcomes segment of the video to compare and contrast the goals and expected outcomes you identified with the functional outcomes achieved.

BOX CS7.1 ASIA Impairment Scale (AIS)[a]

A = Complete. No sensory or motor function is preserved in the sacral segments S4–5.

B = Sensory Incomplete. Sensory but not motor function is preserved below the neurological level and includes the sacral segments S4–5 (light touch or pin prick at S4–5 or deep anal pressure) AND no motor function is preserved more than three levels below the motor level on either side of the body.

C = Motor Incomplete. Motor function is preserved below the neurological level**, and more than half of key muscle functions below the neurological level of injury (NLI) have a muscle grade less than 3 (Grades 0–2).

D = Motor Incomplete. Motor function is preserved below the neurological level**, and at least half

(half or more) of key muscle functions below the NLI have a muscle grade ≥3.

E = Normal. If sensation and motor function as tested with the ISNCSCI are graded as normal in all segments, and the patient had prior deficits, then the AIS grade is E. Someone without an initial SCI does not receive an AIS grade.

Note: When assessing the extent of motor sparing below the level for distinguishing between AIS B and C, the ***motor level*** on each side is used; whereas to differentiate between AIS C and D (based on proportion of key muscle functions with strength grade 3 or greater) the ***neurological level of injury*** is used.

---

[a]From: American Spinal Injury Association. International Standards for Neurological Classification of Spinal Cord Injury. Atlanta, GA, American Spinal Injury Association, 2006. Used with permission. (*Note:* An overview of changes with the new ISNCSCI worksheet is available at http://www.asia-spinalinjury.org/elearning/ISNCSCI.php [retrieved April 6, 2015]).

**For an individual to receive a grade of C or D, i.e. motor incomplete status, they must have either (1) voluntary anal sphincter contraction or (2) sacral sensory sparing <u>with</u> sparing of motor funtion more than three levels below the motor level for that side of the body. The International Standards at this time allows even non-key muscle function more than 3 levels below the motor level to be used in determining motor incomplete status (AIS B versus C).

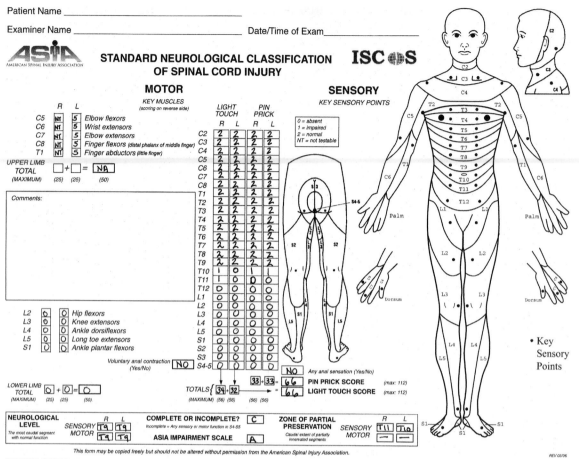

FIGURE CS7.2 The patient's sensory and motor scores using the ASIA *Standard Neurological Classification of Spinal Cord Injury*. From: American Spinal Injury Association. International Standards for Neurological Classification of Spinal Cord Injury. Atlanta, GA, American Spinal Injury Association, 2006. Used with permission. (*Note:* An overview of changes with the new ISNCSCI worksheet is available at http://www.asia-spinalinjury.org/elearning/ISNCSCI.php (retrieved April 6, 2015)).

Guiding Questions

1. In addition to those mentioned in the case, what other examination tools could you perform to measure the patient's activity level?
2. Organize and analyze the available data to develop a problem list. Identify:
   a. Impairments, direct
   b. Impairments, indirect
   c. Activity limitations
   d. Participation restrictions
3. What are the concerns with the patient losing 11 pounds since the injury?
4. This patient presents with T9 paraplegia with an ASIA Impairment Scale (AIS) designation of A. What classification is this (see Box CS7.1)?
5. Describe components of transfer training for this patient. What modifications are necessary? Progression?

What additional wheelchair skills should be included in her POC?
6. How might your treatment plan for mobility skills and transfers differ if the patient had presented with an AIS designation of B, C, or D (as described in Box CS7.1)?
7. Based on her history of being a dancer and dance teacher, what are the patient assets that can be used to her advantage during rehabilitation?
8. What additional goals would you develop for the patient's postacute rehabilitation? What functional outcomes would you identify?
9. Considering that the patient lives in a rental property, what basic recommendations would you have for home modifications?
10. What durable medical equipment needs do you anticipate?

TABLE CS7.1 Functional Independence Measure (FIM)[a]

	FIM Scores:[b] Admission	FIM Scores:[b] Discharge (6 weeks later)
Self-Care		
Eating	7	7
Grooming	7	7
Bathing	1	7
Dressing, upper	2	7
Dressing, lower	1	7
Toileting	1	6
Sphincter Control		
Bladder	1	6
Bowel	1	5
Transfers		
Transfer, bed	1	5
Transfer, toilet	1	5
Transfer, tub	1	5
Locomotion		
Wheelchair	3	6
Stairs	1	1
Communication		
Comprehension	7	7
Expression	7	7
Social Cognition		
Social interaction	7	7
Problem-solving	7	7
Memory	7	7

[a]From Guide for the Uniform Data Set for Medical Rehabilitation.

[b]Scoring is as follows: 7 = complete independence (timely, safety); 6 = modified independence (device); 5 = supervision (subject = 100%); 4 = minimal assistance (subject = 75% or more); 3 = moderate assistance (subject = 50% or more); 2 = maximal assistance (subject = 25% or more); 1 = total assistance or not testable (subject less than 25%).

TABLE CS7.2 Manual Muscle Test Scores (admission)[a]

Joint	Muscle	Right	Left
Shoulder	Medial rotators	3/5	5/5
	Lateral rotators	3/5	5/5
	Flexion	3/5	5/5
	Abduction	3/5	5/5
	Extension	3/5	5/5
Elbow	Flexion	3/5	5/5
	Extension	4/5	5/5
Wrist	Flexion	3/5	5/5
	Extension	3/5	5/5
Fingers	Flexion	4/5	5/5
	Extension	4/5	5/5
Hip	Flexion	0/5	0/5
	Extension	0/5	0/5
Knee	Flexion	0/5	0/5
	Extension	0/5	0/5
Ankle	Dorsiflexion	0/5	0/5
	Plantarflexion	0/5	0/5
Toes	Flexion	0/5	0/5
	Extension	0/5	0/5

[a]All scores are based on a 0–5 scale: 5, normal; 4, good; 3, fair; 2, poor; 1, trace; 0, no contraction.

Note: At the time of discharge, strength in the right UE improved to 5 out of 5 throughout.

Reminder: Answers to the Case Study Guiding Questions are available online at DavisPlus (www.fadavis.com).

REFERENCES

1. American Spinal Injury Association (ASIA). Examination form. Standard neurological classification of spinal cord injury. In International Standards for Neurological Classification of Spinal Cord Injury. Chicago, IL, American Spinal Injury Association, 2006.
2. Guide for the Uniform Data Set for Medical Rehabilitation (including the FIM instrument), Version 5.0. Buffalo, NY, State University of New York, 1996.
3. Lynch, SM, Leahy, P, and Barker, SP. Reliability of measurements obtained with a modified functional reach test in subjects with spinal cord injury. Phys Ther, 1998; 78(2):128.

VIEWING THE CASE: Patient With Complete Spinal Cord Injury, T9

As students learn in different ways, the video case presentation (examination, intervention, and outcomes) is designed to promote engagement with the content, allow progression at an individual (or group) pace, and use of the medium or combination of media (written, visual, and auditory) best suited to the learner(s). The video, presented online at Davis*Plus* (www.fadavis.com), includes both visual and auditory modes.

Video Summary

Patient is a 21-year-old woman with a complete SCI (T9, ASIA A) undergoing active rehabilitation. The video shows examination and intervention segments during inpatient rehabilitation, with an emphasis on transfer and wheelchair mobility skills training. Outcomes are filmed 4 weeks after the initial examination.

Davis*Plus* For additional resources and to view the accompanying video associated with this case, please visit **www.davisplus.com.**

8

Patient With Incomplete Spinal Cord Injury, C7

MARIA STELMACH, PT, DPT, NCS,
AND SOPHIE BENOIST, PT, DPT

Examination

History

- **Demographic Information:**
  The patient is a 49-year-old woman who was referred to outpatient physical therapy with a diagnosis of incomplete spinal cord injury.
- **History of Present Illness:**
  About 1.5 years ago, the patient was working as a train conductor and suffered a whiplash injury to her neck while dodging a spitball in a moving train. She went to the emergency room for further evaluation and was discharged home. A few weeks later, the patient experienced pain in her arms, shoulders, and back. Pain persisted, and approximately 2 months later the patient went to the emergency room again. An x-ray was performed with inconclusive findings, and the patient was discharged with pain medication. Over the next couple months, patient began to experience tremor in her hand, bladder incontinence, and difficulty balancing while walking. A neurologist examined her and magnetic resonance imaging (MRI) of the spine was performed. The MRI revealed multiple disc herniations in the cervical spine with spinal cord impingement. The patient underwent C6-C7 decompression and fusion surgery 1 week later. She was unable to move her lower extremities (LEs) after the surgery. The patient remained in the hospital for 4 months and was discharged home with a power tilt-in-space wheelchair and attendant care. She was then frequently readmitted to the hospital for the next year owing to development of urinary tract infections, stage 4 sacral pressure ulcer, and methicillin-resistant staphylococcus aureus (MRSA) in her eye. She was admitted to inpatient rehabilitation approximately 1.5 years after the decompression surgery. She received 1 month of inpatient rehabilitation and then was discharged home. She now presents to outpatient therapy to continue to improve her functional mobility status.

- **Medical/Surgical History:**
  Unremarkable
- **Current Medications:**
  Baclofen, gabapentin, lorazepam, temazepam, folic acid, docusate sodium, protein liquid for wound

- **Living Environment:**
  Patient lives alone in an apartment with one step to enter. She has a ramp to enter building. She utilizes a tilt-in-space power wheelchair, commode, Hoyer lift, and hospital bed with air mattress, leg lifter, and a reacher. She has a home health aide 10 hours per day for 7 days a week. She uses an indwelling catheter. She currently sponge bathes.
- **Social Support:**
  Patient has a supportive daughter.
- **Employment:**
  Patient is currently on disability. She previously worked as a subway train conductor.
- **Prior Level of Function:**
  Patient was independent with all aspects of functional mobility skills, leisure activities, activities of daily living (ADL) and instrumental activities of daily living (IADL), and worked full time as a subway train conductor.

Systems Review

- **Cardiovascular/Pulmonary System:**
  - Within normal limits
  - Patient has a history of orthostatic hypotension that is now managed with bilateral compression stockings and abdominal binder.
- **Musculoskeletal System:**
  - Gross range of motion (ROM): The patient's bilateral upper extremities (UEs) are within normal limits (WNL). Bilateral LEs are WNL throughout except for moderate tightness of hamstrings, hip flexors, and hip internal/external rotators bilaterally.
  - Gross strength (manual muscle test [MMT]): The patient's bilateral UE strength is 5/5 except for right long finger flexion 4/5; right fifth digit abduction 1/5; and left fifth digit abduction 3/5 (Fig. CS8.1). No active movement in bilateral LEs. No anal contraction present.
- **Neuromuscular System:**
  - Reflexes: absent in both LEs throughout; WNL for bilateral biceps, triceps, and brachioradialis (2+ = normal response)

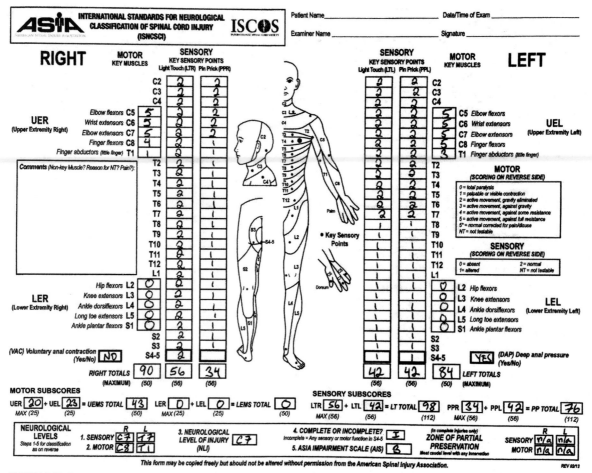

FIGURE CS8.1 Sensory and motor scores. From American Spinal Injury Association. International Standards for Neurological Classification of Spinal Cord Injury, rev 2013. Atlanta, GA, American Spinal Injury Association, 2013. Reprinted 2013, with permission.

- Sensation: impaired sensation in both LEs and right UE; anal sensation present
- Sitting balance: impaired static and dynamic sitting balance in both short and long sitting
- **Integumentary System:**
  - Stage 2 sacral pressure ulcer

Tests and Measures

- **Cognition:**
  - Alert and oriented ×3
- **Pain:**
  - Bilateral shoulder pain 5/10
- **International Standards for Classification of Spinal Cord Injury** (see Fig. CS8.1):
  - Sensory: Right C7, left T7
  - Motor: Right C8, left T1
  - Neurological level: C7
  - American Spinal Injury Association Impairment Scale (Box CS8.1): Category B: Incomplete

- **Bed Mobility:**
  - Rolling from supine to right sidelying: minimal assistance (Fig CS8.2)
  - Rolling from supine to left sidelying: minimal assistance
  - Supine to long-sit position: moderate assistance
  - Short sit to supine: moderate assistance for leg management and balance
- **Transfers:**
  - Sliding board transfer wheelchair to and from mat (level height): maximal assistance for board placement and removal
  - Maximal assistance for LE positioning during transfer
  - Moderate assistance for balance during transfer
- **Balance:**
  - Static sitting: (Fair) Patient able to maintain static short sitting balance without loss of balance and without UE support
  - Dynamic sitting balance: (Poor) Patient able to minimally weight shift ipsilaterally (toward one side), able to weight shift in anterior/posterior direction but experiences difficulty crossing midline

BOX CS8.1 ASIA Impairment Scale (AIS)ᵃ

A = Complete. No sensory or motor function is preserved in the sacral segments S4–5.

B = Sensory Incomplete. Sensory but not motor function is preserved below the neurological level and includes the sacral segments S4–5 (light touch or pin prick at S4–5 or deep anal pressure) AND no motor function is preserved more than three levels below the motor level on either side of the body.

C = Motor Incomplete. Motor function is preserved below the neurological level**, and more than half of key muscle functions below the neurological level of injury (NLI) have a muscle grade less than 3 (Grades 0–2).

D = Motor Incomplete. Motor function is preserved below the neurological level**, and <u>at least half</u> (half or more) of key muscle functions below the NLI have a muscle grade ≥3.

E = Normal. If sensation and motor function as tested with the ISNCSCI are graded as normal in all segments, and the patient had prior deficits, then the AIS grade is E. Someone without an initial SCI does not receive an AIS grade.

Note: When assessing the extent of motor sparing below the level for distinguishing between AIS B and C, the *motor level* on each side is used; whereas to differentiate between AIS C and D (based on proportion of key muscle functions with strength grade 3 or greater) the *neurologic level of injury* is used.

ᵃFrom American Spinal Injury Association. International Standards for Neurological Classification of Spinal Cord Injury. Atlanta, GA, American Spinal Injury Association, 2006. Used with permission. (*Note:* An overview of changes with the new ISNCSCI worksheet is available at www.asia-spinalinjury.org/elearning/ISNCSCI.php [retrieved April 6, 2015].)

**For an individual to receive a grade of C or D, that is, motor incomplete status, they must have either (1) voluntary anal sphincter contraction or (2) sacral sensory sparing <u>with</u> sparing of motor function more than three levels below the motor level for that side of the body. The International Standards at this time allows even non–key muscle function more than three levels below the motor level to be used in determining motor incomplete status (AIS B versus C).

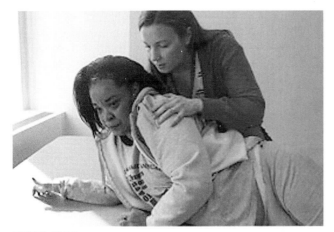

FIGURE CS8.2 Movement transition from supine to right sidelying.

Evaluation, Diagnosis and Prognosis, and Plan of Care

Note: Before considering the guiding questions below, view the Case Study 8 Examination segment of the video to enhance understanding of the patient's impairments and activity limitations. After completing the guiding questions, view the Case Study 8 Intervention segment of the video to compare and contrast the interventions presented with those you selected. Last, progress to the Case Study 8 Outcomes segment of the video to compare and contrast the goals and expected outcomes you identified with the functional outcomes achieved.

Guiding Questions

1. Describe the patient's clinical presentation in terms of impairments, activity limitations, and participation restrictions.
2. What should be included in a home exercise program for this patient?
3. Describe interventions that could be used to improve the patient's bed mobility and transfer skills.
4. In terms of patient education, what key components should be addressed with the patient to assure safety at home and prevention of recurrent issues?
5. If the patient demonstrated active movement of her right ankle dorsiflexors, would her ASIA Impairment Scale classification change, and if so how?

Reminder: Answers to the Case Study Guiding Questions are available online at Davis*Plus* (www.fadavis.com).

VIEWING THE CASE: Patient With Incomplete Spinal Cord Injury, C7

As students learn in different ways, the video case presentation (examination, intervention, and outcomes) is designed to promote engagement with the content, allow progression at an individual (or group) pace, and use of the medium or combination of media (written, visual, and auditory) best suited to the learner(s). The video, presented online at Davis*Plus* (www.fadavis.com), includes both visual and auditory modes.

Video Summary
The patient is a 49-year-old woman who was referred to outpatient physical therapy with a diagnosis of incomplete spinal cord injury. The video shows examination and intervention segments for rehabilitation episodes of care. Outcomes are filmed at 12 weeks after the initial examination.

Davis*Plus* For additional resources and to view the accompanying video associated with this case, please visit **www.davisplus.com.**

Examination

History

- **Demographic Information:**
  Patient is a 65-year-old woman who presents for evaluation and treatment owing to complaints of dizziness that began 4 to 6 weeks ago. She is ambidextrous and wears glasses and contact lenses.
- **Employment, Living Environment, and Social History:**
  Patient is a retired high school guidance counselor but works as part-time summer help in a perennial garden nursery. She lives alone but has a busy social life and travels frequently.
- **Medical History:**
  She states she is in excellent health but has a history of cervical and lumbar arthritis, thyroid disease, high blood pressure, and elevated cholesterol levels. She also reveals that she had a lumpectomy more than 30 years ago for a benign tumor and underwent surgery for trigger finger (stenosing tenosynovitis) 3 years ago. She reports a "bout of viral meningitis" over 20 years ago and experienced an isolated episode of atrial fibrillation approximately 1 year ago. She is scheduled for left foot neuroma removal surgery in 2 weeks. She exercises four or five times per week for 20 to 60 minutes and enjoys walking and going to the gym.
- **Current Condition/Chief Complaints:**
  Patient reports that when she awoke dizzy one morning 4 to 6 weeks ago, she experienced nausea and difficulty walking that lasted for a few days. She went to her primary care physician, who put her on meclizine for 10 days. She notes gradual improvement in her symptoms and describes her current condition as "stable." She denies falling. She states that, at this time, looking up and turning to the right continues to cause increased symptoms. She experiences occasional spinning dizziness with quick head movements and states that sometimes she does not spin but also does not feel normal. She states she frequently feels off balance. She denies tinnitus, hearing loss, or fullness or pressure in her ears.

Systems Review

Musculoskeletal System

No formal examination was performed given the nature of the patient's complaints and lack of observable physical impairments.

Tests and Measures

- **Rating of Symptom Severity:**
  - At the start of today's examination, the patient rated her symptoms as a "1 to 2" on a scale of 0 to 10.
- **Dizziness Handicap Index:**
  - Her score on the Dizziness Handicap Index (DHI)[1] is a 26 on a scale of 0 to 100.
- **Balance and Visual Testing:**
  - Modified Clinical Test for Sensory Integration in Balance (mCTSIB)[2]: Results from the mCTSIB are presented in Table CS9.1.
  - Walking with quick head turns to left and right: When performing this activity, the patient demonstrates minor disruption in gait.
  - Oculomotor testing in room light: The patient's gaze and nystagmus are normal in room light. She was able to perform smooth pursuits in horizontal, vertical, and diagonal planes without interruption. Tests for saccadic control in the horizontal and vertical planes were also normal but more difficult to perform to the right.
  - Head Thrust test: The patient's head thrust test was positive to the right. The patient performed a saccadic eye movement to return her gaze to the target following a quick head movement to the right.
  - Dynamic Visual Acuity test (DVA): This test was performed in the standing position using a *Lighthouse ETDRS* (Early Treatment Diabetic Retinopathy Study) wall chart. It was negative, as there was a one-line discrepancy between what the patient could read with her head still (no movement) compared to when her head was moving at a rate of approximately two repetitions per second (2 Hz). However, she reported an increase

TABLE CS9.1 Modified Clinical Test for Sensory Integration and Balance (mCTSIB)

Standing Position	Time (sec)	Postural Sway	Loss of Balance
EO, FT, SS	30	WNL	No
EO, FT, CS	30	Min increased sway	No
EO, FT, on foam	30	WNL	No
EC, FT, on foam	25	Min-mod increased sway	No
EO, tandem, SS sharpened Romberg	5	Increased sway to right	To the right
EC, tandem, SS sharpened Romberg	Immediate fall	N/A	To the left

CS, compliant surface; EO, eyes open; EC, eyes closed; FT, feet together; min, minimal; min-mod, minimal to moderate; N/A, not applicable; SS, solid surface; WNL, within normal limits.

in symptoms from "1 to 2" to "3 to 4" on a 0 to 10 scale with this activity.

- Observation for nystagmus using the infrared video goggles without a visual reference: Under observation in the video goggles, the patient demonstrated a consistent, left-beating nystagmus with forward, left, and right gaze.
- The Head Shaking Induced Nystagmus test[3] (HSN) using the infrared video goggles: This test provoked a slightly left-beating nystagmus. The patient reported feeling "woozy" with a symptom intensity of "2 to 3" on a 0 to 10 scale.
- The Dix-Hallpike test[4] using the infrared video goggles:
  - The right Dix-Hallpike test: Positive for an up-beating, counterclockwise nystagmus of short duration. The patient complained of feeling dizzy while in the test position and reported that she was "slightly" dizzy upon returning to the sitting position.
  - The left Dix-Hallpike test: The patient denied symptoms with the left Hallpike-Dix test but demonstrated a consistent left-beating nystagmus.
- The Roll test using the infrared video goggles:
  - Right Roll test: This test revealed a left-beating nystagmus.
  - Left Roll test: This test also revealed a left-beating nystagmus.

Evaluation, Diagnosis and Prognosis, and Plan of Care

Note: Before considering the guiding questions, view the Case Study 9 Examination segment of the video to enhance understanding of the patient's clinical presentation. After completing the guiding questions, view the Case Study 9 Intervention segment of the video to compare and contrast the interventions presented with those you selected. Last, progress to the Case Study 9 Outcomes segment of the video to compare and contrast the goals and expected outcomes you identified with the functional outcomes achieved.

Guiding Questions

1. Given this patient's report at the initial examination, identify the most likely cause(s) of her complaints of dizziness, disequilibrium, and motion sensitivity.
2. Which clinical examination findings reveal abnormality in the vestibular system? Analyze and interpret these results.
3. Determine a working diagnosis (diagnostic hypothesis) for this patient.
4. Describe this patient's clinical presentation in terms of:
   a. Impairments
   b. Activity limitations
   c. Participation restrictions
5. Using the *Guide to Physical Therapist Practice,* identify the appropriate practice pattern for the patient.
6. Describe the plan of care (therapeutic interventions) you will use to address the impairments.
7. What are your anticipated goals and expected outcomes for the patient? State the time frame in which you expect to meet these expectations.
8. Explain how your working diagnosis would change if a positive Dix-Hallpike test was your only abnormal finding.
9. Describe the therapeutic intervention you will employ to address impairments associated with a positive Dix-Hallpike test.

Reminder: Answers to the Case Study Guiding Questions are available online at Davis*Plus* (www.fadavis.com).

REFERENCES

1. Jacobsen, GP, and Newman, CW. The development of the dizziness handicap inventory. Arch Otolaryngol Head Neck Surg, 1990; 116:424.
2. Rose, DJ. Fallproof!: A Comprehensive Balance and Mobility Training Program. Champaign, IL, Human Kinetics, 2003.
3. Hain, TC, Fetter, M, and Zee, D. Head-shaking nystagmus in patients with unilateral peripheral vestibular lesions. Am J Otolaryngol, 1987; 8:36.
4. Dix, R, and Hallpike, CS. The pathology, symptomatology and diagnosis of certain common disorders of the vestibular system. Ann Otol Rhinol Laryngol, 1952; 6:987.

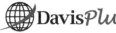

VIEWING THE CASE: Patient With Peripheral Vestibular Dysfunction

As students learn in different ways, the video case presentation (examination, intervention, and outcomes) is designed to promote engagement with the content, allow progression at an individual (or group) pace, and use of the medium or combination of media (written, visual, and auditory) best suited to the learner(s). The video, presented online at Davis*Plus* (www.fadavis.com), includes both visual and auditory modes.

Video Summary

Patient is a 65-year-old woman referred to a vestibular clinic with peripheral vestibular dysfunction. The video shows examination and intervention segments during outpatient rehabilitation, with an emphasis on oculomotor, balance, and locomotor training. Outcomes are filmed after seven treatment sessions within 10 weeks.

DavisPlus For additional resources and to view the accompanying video associated with this case, please visit **www.davisplus.com.**

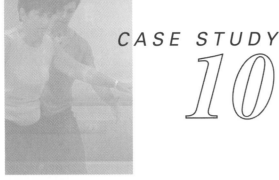

Patient With Complete Spinal Cord Injury, T10

DARRELL MUSICK, PT, AND LAURA S. WEHRLI, PT, DPT, ATP

Examination

History

- **Demographic Information:**
  The patient is a 43-year-old Caucasian, English-speaking man with a postgraduate education.
- **Social History:**
  The patient is married with two teenage children. He recently moved to the state of Washington with the military and participates in social athletics, including baseball, basketball, and ice hockey.
- **Employment:**
  Patient is a member of the executive staff in a military medical group as a nurse practitioner and chief of nursing.
- **Living Environment:**
  Patient lives in a one-story private home with one 6-in. (15 cm) step to enter.
- **General Health Status:**
  Patient is an active, healthy individual.
- **Medical History:**
  Hypertension (controlled with lisinopril), bradycardia, basal cell carcinoma (removed without complication), kidney stone several years ago, hyperlipidemia (controlled with Zocor), allergic rhinitis (controlled with Singulair); no known drug allergies.
- **Current Condition/Chief Complaints:**
  On November 21, patient was driving a borrowed all-terrain vehicle (ATV) when he lost control. He was thrown from the vehicle and hit his head/helmet on a pipe in a gully. He felt immediate pain in his back. He reports that he had difficulty breathing owing to rib pain and immediately had no feeling in his legs ("I couldn't feel or move my legs"). He was transported by helicopter to a hospital in Reno, Nevada. The patient also reported he was able to contract his quadriceps slightly until just prior to reaching the hospital. He was found to have:
  - L1 burst fracture
  - Left 1st through 10th rib fractures with left pulmonary contusion
  - Left hemopneumothorax requiring chest tube placement

- Left T1 transverse process fracture
- T2 to T7 spinous process fractures
- T10 to T12 right posterior medial rib fractures
- Left scapular body fracture

On November 24, the patient underwent surgery for a T11–L3 laminectomy and posterior lateral fixation. He was immobilized in a custom thoracolumbosacral orthosis (TLSO); weightbearing as tolerated (WBAT) on left upper extremity (UE).

Systems Review

- **Cardiovascular/Pulmonary System:**
  - Heart rate: 79 beats per minute
  - Blood pressure: 104/67 mm Hg
  - Respiratory rate: 16 breaths per minute
- **Musculoskeletal System:**
  - Gross symmetry: visible rib deformities on left thorax; left lower extremity (LE) swelling
  - Gross range of motion (ROM): LE ROM generally within functional limits (WFL), with the exception of moderately tight hamstrings and hip rotation bilaterally; contracted left plantarflexors. UE ROM is also generally WFL, with the exception of tightness in bilateral shoulder flexion, abduction, and rotation (greater on left).
  - Gross strength: Grossly normal strength throughout UEs; 0/5 strength in bilateral LEs
  - Height: 6 ft 2 in (1.9 m)
  - Weight: 170 lb (77 kg)
- **Integumentary System:**
  - Multiple ecchymoses on all four extremities
  - Prominent ecchymoses on left chest wall and right lateral chest wall
  - Small open wounds on right posterior upper arm and anterior forearm
  - No pressure ulcers
- **Neuromuscular System:**
  - Normal reflexes on bilateral UEs
  - Diminished reflexes on bilateral LEs
  - Impaired sensation of lower trunk and LEs bilaterally

- Diminished rectal tone and no voluntary anal contraction
- Balance impaired in short- and long-sitting

Tests and Measures

- **Arousal, Attention, and Cognition**
  - No signs or symptoms of traumatic brain injury (TBI) noted
  - Oriented to time, place, and person
  - Arousal, attention, cognition, and recall appear to be within normal limits (WNL)

  Note: The following sensory and muscle performance examination data is based on the *International Standards for Neurological Classification of Spinal Cord Injury (ISNCSCI)* (Fig. CS10.1)

- **Sensation** (Fig. CS10.1):
  - Pinprick sensation normal C2–T12 bilaterally
  - Light touch sensation normal C2–T10 left; C2–L1 right
  - No sensation at S4–5 or deep anal sensation
- **Muscle Performance** (Fig. CS10.1):
  - 5/5 strength: C5–T1 bilaterally
  - 0/5 strength: L2–S1 bilaterally
  - No voluntary anal contraction
  - Trunk and upper abdominal muscles present but unable to test owing to TLSO
- **Pain:**
  - Left shoulder pain at rest without pain medication 2/10
  - Left shoulder pain with activity without pain medication 6/10
- **Posture** (*Examined in short-sitting with UE support*):
  - Forward head posture
  - Trunk stabilized in TLSO

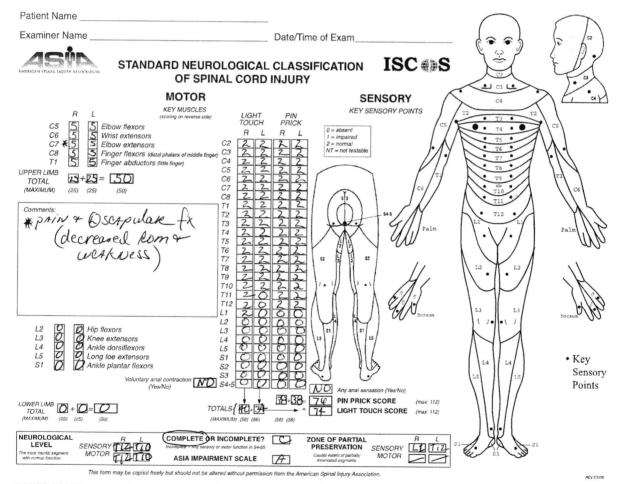

FIGURE CS10.1 The patient's sensory and motor scores using the American Spinal Injury Association (ASIA) Examination Form: *Standard Neurological Classification of Spinal Cord Injury.* (American Spinal Injury Association. International Standards for Neurological Classification of Spinal Cord Injury. Atlanta, GA, American Spinal Injury Association, 2006.) (*Note:* An overview of changes with the 2013 revision of the ISNCSCI worksheet is available at http://www.asia-spinalinjury.org/elearning/ISNCSCI.php (retrieved March 31, 2015).)

- Neutral pelvic tilt
- LEs in neutral alignment
- **Range of Motion (ROM):**
  - Goniometric measures of the LEs indicated bilateral tightness in hip flexion, hip internal and external rotation, straight leg raises, ankle dorsiflexion; contracted left plantarflexors (right plantarflexion WNL) (Table CS10.1).
  - UE ROM limitations include shoulder flexion, abduction, and internal and external rotation. Greater limitations noted at left shoulder secondary to left scapular body fracture and associated pain.
- **Functional Status:**
  - Functional mobility skills require dependent assistance at this time.
- **Home/Work Environment:**
  Review of house floor plans and discussion with patient and family provided the following information:
  - The one-story private home has one 6-in. (15-cm) step to enter. The bedroom, kitchen, and living areas are wheelchair accessible from the main entrance. The master bathroom doorway is 30 inches (76 cm) wide. The toilet is in a separated area of the bathroom with a 28-inch (71-cm) wide entry and privacy wall. The

shower stall is 60 × 60 in. (1.5 × 1.5 m) with a 1.5-in. (3.8-cm) lip at the entrance.
  - At work, administrative areas, office, and desk are accessible. The patient must give presentations and speeches frequently and would like to stand at a lectern in bilateral knee-ankle-foot orthoses (KAFO).

Evaluation, Diagnosis and Prognosis, and Plan of Care

Note: Before considering the guiding questions below, view the Case Study 10 Examination segment of the video to enhance understanding of the patient's impairments and activity limitations. After completing the guiding questions, view the Case Study 10 Intervention segment of the video to compare and contrast the interventions presented with those you selected. Last, progress to the Case Study 10 Outcomes segment of the video to compare and contrast the goals and expected outcomes you identified with the functional outcomes achieved.

Guiding Questions

1. Review Figure CS10.1. What is the patient's physical therapy diagnosis? More specifically, what is the neurological level of injury and where does the patient place on the ASIA Impairment Scale (Box CS10.1)?
2. What Preferred Practice Pattern from the *Guide to Physical Therapist Practice* should be used?
3. How many weeks of treatment would you anticipate will be needed for inpatient rehabilitation?
4. Identify the patient's impairments and the resulting activity limitations.
5. From the information gathered during the examination, what impairments do you anticipate will affect the patient's prognosis?
6. List the interventions that you would include in the plan of care.
7. What will the patient need to consider to ensure home accessibility?
8. Identify three pieces of equipment the patient will require at discharge.
9. What is the patient's prognosis with respect to functional outcomes at the end of his rehabilitation stay? How would you describe his anticipated activity limitations and participation restrictions at 1 year after discharge?

Reminder: Answers to the Case Study Guiding Questions are available online at Davis*Plus* (www.fadavis.com).

TABLE CS10.1 Range of Motion Values (in degrees) Indicating Areas of Joint Motion Limitations[a]

Joint	Motion	Right	Left
Shoulder	Flexion	0–160	0–150
	Abduction	0–130	0–105
	Internal Rotation	0–65	0–50
	External Rotation	0–70	0–65
Hip	Flexion	0–112	0–110
	Internal Rotation	0–23	0–30
	External Rotation	0–35	0–30
	Straight Leg Raise	0–70	0–70
Ankle	Dorsiflexion	0–3	None[b]
	Plantarflexion	0–55	13–50

[a]All other ROM values WNL.
[b]Unable to achieve neutral starting position for measurement.

BOX CS10.1 ASIA Impairment Scale (AIS)ᵃ

A = Complete. No sensory or motor function is preserved in the sacral segments S4-5.

B = Sensory Incomplete. Sensory but not motor function is preserved below the neurological level and includes the sacral segments S4-5 (light touch or pin prick at S4-5 or deep anal pressure) AND no motor function is preserved more than three levels below the motor level on either side of the body.

C = Motor Incomplete. Motor function is preserved below the neurological level**, and more than half of key muscle functions below the neurological level of injury (NLI) have a muscle grade less than 3 (grades 0-2).

D = Motor Incomplete. Motor function is preserved below the neurological level**, and at least half (half

or more) of key muscle functions below the NLI have a muscle grade ≥3.

E = Normal. If sensation and motor function as tested with the ISNCSCI are graded as normal in all segments, and the patient had prior deficits, then the AIS grade is E. Someone without an initial SCI does not receive an AIS grade.

Note: When assessing the extent of motor sparing below the level for distinguishing between AIS B and C, the ***motor level*** on each side is used; whereas to differentiate between AIS C and D (based on proportion of key muscle functions with strength grade 3 or greater) the ***neurologic level of injury*** is used.

ᵃFrom American Spinal Injury Association. International Standards for Neurological Classification of Spinal Cord Injury. Atlanta, GA, American Spinal Injury Association, 2006. Used with permission. (***Note:*** An overview of changes with the new ISNCSCI worksheet is available at http://www.asia-spinalinjury.org/elearning/ISNCSCI. php [retrieved April 6, 2015].)

**For an individual to receive a grade of C or D, that is, motor incomplete status, they must have either (1) voluntary anal sphincter contraction or (2) sacral sensory sparing with sparing of motor function more than three levels below the motor level for that side of the body. The International Standards at this time allows even non–key muscle function more than three levels below the motor level to be used in determining motor incomplete status (AIS B versus C).

 VIEWING THE CASE: Patient With Spinal Cord Injury, T10

As students learn in different ways, the video case presentation (examination, intervention, and outcomes) is designed to promote engagement with the content, allow progression at an individual (or group) pace, and use of the medium or combination of media (written, visual, and auditory) best suited to the learner(s). The video, presented online at Davis*Plus* (www.fadavis.com), includes both visual and auditory modes.

Video Summary

Patient is a 43-year-old man with a complete spinal cord injury (T10, AIS A) and multiple fractures undergoing active rehabilitation. The video shows examination and intervention segments during inpatient rehabilitation. Outcomes are filmed 9 weeks after initial examination.

DavisPlus For additional resources and to view the accompanying video associated with this case, please visit **www.davisplus.com**.

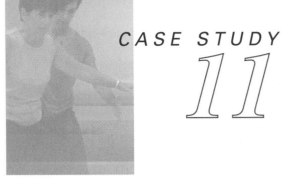

CASE STUDY

11

Patient With Cerebellar Glioblastoma

Catherine Printz, PT, DPT, NCS;
Melissa S. Doyle, PT, DPT, NCS;
and Carter McElroy, PT, MP

Examination

History

- **Demographic Information:**
  The patient is a 71-year-old right-handed man with a large, right-sided cerebellar brain tumor status post-resection and ongoing chemotherapy.

- **History of Present Illness:**
  Two years ago the patient developed an insidious onset of headache, nausea, vomiting, and progressive gait instability. A visit to the emergency department and subsequent magnetic resonance imaging revealed a large right cerebellar mass measuring 4 cm (1.6 in.). He underwent tumor resection 5 days later. The pathology report revealed Stage 4 glioblastoma multiforme. At that time, he required a wheelchair as his primary mode of locomotion. He was then sent to inpatient rehabilitation for 3 weeks and chemotherapy and radiation was initiated, which was completed 6 months ago. The patient is now taking an experimental study drug to prevent tumor regrowth and was referred to outpatient physical therapy to address incoordination and impaired balance and gait. He failed a driving test 1 month ago owing to coordination impairments. In the last 6 months, he has not required an assistive device and has not experienced any falls.

- **Medical History:**
  Patient has a history of hypertension. Current medications include methylphenidate, atenolol, and levetiracetam.

- **Social History:**
  The patient is married, lives with spouse, and is a retired mechanical engineer. Wife is very supportive. Patient is active in church activities and enjoyed bicycling.

- **Living Environment:**
  Patient lives in a multiple-level home with three flights of stairs. He has the following durable medical equipment: wheelchair, front-wheeled walker, cane, and gait belt.

- **General Health Status:**
  Good. His prior level of functioning was fully independent and active. Before brain tumor diagnosis, the patient rode his bicycle from California to Florida.

The authors extend their thanks to Elizabeth Trawinski, Idaho State University, for her assistance in preparing this case study.

Systems Review

- **Cardiovascular/Pulmonary System:**
- Blood pressure: 132/77
- Pulse: 63 beats per minute
- Respiratory rate: 17 breaths per minute
- **Musculoskeletal System:**
- Height: 5 ft, 9 in.
- Weight: 147 lbs
- Gross symmetry: normal anatomical symmetry; with movement, right hemibody ataxia greater than left (Fig. CS11.1)
- Gross range of motion (ROM): within normal limits (WNL) bilaterally
- Gross strength: generally 5/5 throughout both upper extremities (UEs) and lower extremities (LEs), except mild impairment in right grip strength

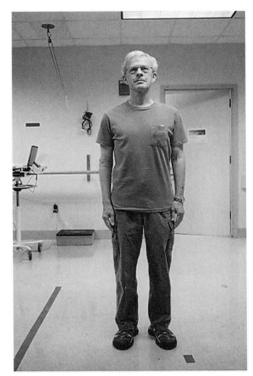

FIGURE CS11.1 Postural examination The patient demonstrates normal postural alignment during static standing.

- **Neuromuscular System:**
  - Sensation: intact for light touch, pressure, and joint position sense of hallux and ankles
  - Coordination: impaired
  - Tone: normal
  - Postural control: impaired in both sitting and standing
  - Balance: impaired static and dynamic balance
  - Gait: ataxic gait; requires close supervision without an assistive device
  - Cognition: mild impairments in short-term recall (able to recall two of three items after 10-minute period). Patient reports difficulty with complex thought processes.
- **Integumentary System:**
  - Surgical site on scalp healed well
  - Otherwise intact

Tests and Measures (initial examination)

Note: This case begins during the 8th week of outpatient physical therapy. The initial examination data are included to provide information about progress made since initiation of treatment.

- **Vision:**
  - Oculomotor exam: see Table CS11.1 and Fig. CS11.2
  - Gaze stability testing: impaired vestibulo-ocular reflex (VOR); see Table CS11.1
- **Strength:**
  - Strength testing (manual muscle test [MMT]): 5/5 throughout bilateral UEs and LEs
- **Range of Motion:**
  - WNL throughout bilateral UEs and LEs
- **Gait Assessment:**
  - Wide-based ataxic gait

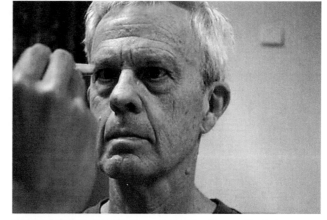

FIGURE CS11.2 Oculomotor examination The patient demonstrates difficulty with smooth pursuit, dysmetric saccades, and impaired VOR during oculomotor and gaze stability examinations.

- Impaired foot placement, right greater than left
- Diminished trunk rotation and arm swing throughout gait cycle
- Utilizes excess anterior trunk lean to compensate for inadequate anticipatory postural adjustments when preparing to ambulate (Fig. CS11.3)
- Rapid forward progression into weight acceptance following initial contact
- Instability in single limb support (stance); excess hip flexion noted throughout stance phase
- Inadequate knee flexion during swing phase limits limb advancement

- **Balance:**
  - Sitting
    - Static: independent (feet flat on floor, no UE support; patient holds himself upright)

TABLE CS11.1 Oculomotor and Gaze Stability Exam

	Initial Examination	8 Weeks
Vestibulo-ocular Reflex (VOR)	Abnormal VOR 1 with retinal slip.	Mildly abnormal VOR 1, no retinal slip noted.
VOR Cancellation	Abnormal. Patient reports moderate subjective dizziness, imbalance.	Abnormal. Patient reports mild subjective dizziness, imbalance.
Smooth Pursuits	Full ocular ROM, abnormal saccades especially in horizontal plane. No gaze-evoked nystagmus provoked at end range of motion.	Lower amplitude dysmetric saccades in horizontal plane.
Saccadic Eye Movement Testing	Abnormal. Overshooting in horizontal and vertical directions.	Abnormal. Less overshooting noted in horizontal and vertical directions. Improved velocity of saccadic movement.
Convergence Testing	Moderate oscillopsia present with convergence.	Mild oscillopsia present with convergence.

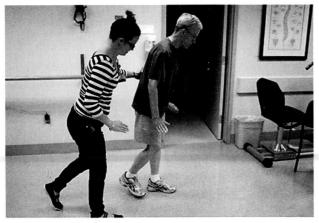

FIGURE CS11.3 Pregait anticipatory postural adjustments The patient demonstrates a forward lean to initiate the anticipatory postural adjustments required for gait.

- Dynamic: responds to perturbations with hypermetric postural responses. Limits of stability (LOS) testing with eyes closed (EC), in lateral and posterior directions, shows decreased excursion. Upon returning to midline, hypermetric responses and overcorrections evident.
- Standing
  - Tandem standing: Left LE posterior: 1.25 seconds; right LE posterior: unable to complete without loss of balance (LOB)
- *Modified Clinical Test for Sensory Interaction in Balance (mCTSIB):*
  - Eyes open (EO)/firm: 30 standing seconds
  - EC/firm: 30 seconds: (slight sway anterior/posterior)
  - EO/foam: 30 seconds (more sway in anterior/posterior direction)
  - EC/foam: 4.46 seconds, with posterior LOB
- **Single Limb Stance:**
  - Unable bilaterally; greater difficulty with attempted balance on right LE (Fig. CS11.4)
- *Mini BESTest* (9/28 points [32%]):
  - Anticipatory control: 0/6 points
  - Reactive postural control: 1/6 points
  - Sensory orientation: 3/6 points
  - Dynamic gait: 5/10 points
- *Activities-Specific Balance Confidence Scale*: See Table CS11.2.
  Scale for the Assessment and Rating of Ataxia: See Table CS11.3.
  Reactive Postural Control Standing:
  - Anterior: unable to elicit a step, resulting in LOB
  - Posterior: three steps to recover equilibrium
  - Left lateral: three steps to recover equilibrium
  - Right lateral: unable to elicit a step, resulting in LOB
- *5 Time Sit-To-Stand (5× STS):* 7.65 seconds (without UE support)
  Timed Up and Go: 10.2 seconds without an assistive device

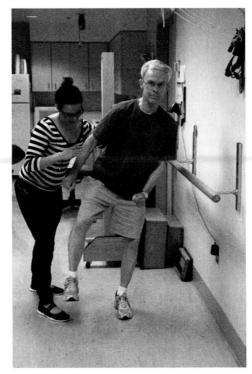

FIGURE CS11.4 Single limb balance The patient demonstrates an excessive lateral weight shift outside his base of support to attempt single limb balance. He is unable to maintain single limb balance bilaterally.

TABLE CS11.2 Activities-Specific Balance Confidence Scale		
	Initial Exam	**8 Weeks**
Patient Self-assessment	54%	90%
Spouse Assessment	61%	91%

- **Coordination:**
  - Finger-to-nose-to-finger: severely dysmetric right UE, mildly dysmetric left UE; (Fig. CS11.5)
  - Rapid alternating movements: right hand accuracy impaired. Wrist/hand contact with the knee is maintained during pronation/supination to decrease the multijoint control of this movement (dyssynergia).

Tests and Measurements (after 8 weeks of intervention)

- **Vision:**
  - Oculomotor exam: See Table CS1.1.
  - Gaze stability exam: See Table CS1.1.
- **Strength:**
  - Grossly 5/5 throughout bilateral UEs/LEs
- **Range of Motion:**
  - WNL throughout bilateral UEs/LEs

TABLE CS11.3 Scale for the Assessment and Rating of Ataxia

	Initial Examination	8 Weeks
1. Gait	5–Severe staggering, permanent support of one stick or light support by one arm required	4–Marked staggering, intermittent support of the wall required
2. Stance	3–Able to stand for >10 sec without support in natural position, but not with feet together	3–Able to stand for >10 sec without support in natural position, but not with feet together
3. Sitting	2–Constant sway, but able to sit >10 sec without support	1–Slight difficulties, intermittent sway
4. Speech disturbance	3–Occasional words difficult to understand	2–Impaired speech, but easy to understand
5. Finger chase	3–Dysmetria, under/overshooting target >15 cm	2–Dysmetria, under/overshooting target <15 cm
6. Nose-finger test	1–Tremor with an amplitude <2 cm	1–Tremor with an amplitude <2 cm
7. Fast alternating hand movements	1.5–Right =2: Clearly irregular, single movements difficult to distinguish but performs <10s; Left =1: Slightly irregular (performs <10s)	1–Slightly irregular (performs <10s)
8. Heel-shin slide	1.5–Right =2: Clearly abnormal, goes off shin up to three times during three cycles Left =1: Slightly abnormal, contact to shin maintained	1–Slightly abnormal, contact to shin maintained
TOTAL SCORE	**20/42**	**15/42**

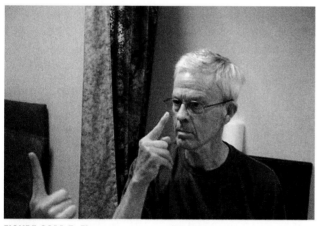

FIGURE CS11.5 Finger-to-nose coordination test The patient demonstrates difficulty with multiple joint control (dyssynergia) and hypermetric responses to finger-nose-finger testing.

- **Gait Assessment:**
  - Improved base of support (BOS) with periods of wide-base gait required in times of instability (for example, turning)
  - Decrease in compensatory forward trunk lean to initiate postural adjustments for gait
  - Increased trunk rotation and arm swing with improved coordination between upper and LE movements
  - Impaired foot placement, right greater than left
  - Increased stance time with improved static stability in single limb support
- **Balance:**
  - Sitting
    - Static: independent (feet flat on floor, no UE support). Patient holds himself upright.
    - Dynamic: increased LOS noted; faster and more precise return to midline
  - Standing
    - Tandem standing: left LE posterior: 7.65 seconds; right LE posterior: 19.95 seconds
- **Modified CTSIB:**
  - EO/firm: 30 seconds
  - EC/firm: 30 seconds (slight sway anterior/posterior)
  - EO/foam: 30 seconds (more sway in anterior/posterior direction)
  - EC/foam: 2.38 seconds, with posterior/ left lateral LOB
- **Single Leg Balance**: right LE 2.32 seconds; left LE unable

- **Mini BESTest:** (16/28 points [57%])
  - Anticipatory control: 2/6 points
  - Reactive postural control: 4/6 points
  - Sensory orientation: 4/6 points
  - Dynamic gait: 6/10 points
- **Activities-Specific Balance Confidence Scale:** See Table CS11.2
- **Scale for the Assessment and Rating of Ataxia:** See Table CS11.3
  Reactive Postural Control Standing:
  - Anterior: 1 step to recover equilibrium
  - Posterior: 2 steps to recover equilibrium
  - Left lateral: 2 steps to recover equilibrium
  - Right lateral: 1 step to recover equilibrium
  - 5 Timed Sit-to-Stand (5× STS): 6.36 seconds (without UE support)
  - Timed Up and Go: 8.50 seconds without an assistive device
- **Coordination:**
  - Finger-to-nose-to-finger: dysmetric right UE, but improved accuracy/coordination compared to the initial evaluation; left UE normal.
  - Rapid alternating movements: right hand accuracy mildly impaired; able to increase excursion of wrist and hand without excess dyssynergia.

Evaluation, Prognosis and Diagnosis, and Plan of Care

Note: Before considering the guiding questions below, view the Case Study 11 Examination segment of the video to enhance understanding of the patient's impairments and activity limitations. After completing the guiding questions, view the Case Study 11 Intervention segment of the video to compare and contrast the interventions presented with those you selected. Last, progress to the Case Study 11 Outcomes segment of the video to compare and contrast the goals and expected outcomes you identified with the functional outcomes achieved.

Guiding Questions

1. Using the *International Classification of Functioning, Disability and Health (ICF)* framework, describe key features of the patient's clinical presentation in terms of body structures and functions, activities, and participation.
2. Considering the anatomy and functional divisions of the cerebellum, how is the patient's clinical presentation consistent with the diagnosis of right cerebellar glioblastoma?
3. Identify three key impairments that should be addressed to improve this patient's activity limitations and participation restrictions.
4. Formulate one treatment intervention for each of the three key impairments you identified earlier. Indicate a progression for each selected intervention.
5. What would be appropriate to include in a home exercise program for this patient?
6. What motor learning considerations are specific to designing intervention programs for individuals with cerebellar dysfunction?
7. Establish anticipated short-term goals (4 weeks) and long-term goals (8 weeks) for this patient.
8. This patient might benefit from referral to which other disciplines?
9. What special considerations are indicated when working with patients with cancer?

Note: To allow instructors greater opportunity to integrate selected cases into assignments, laboratory activities, and/or class discussions, answers to the Guiding Questions for Case Studies 11 to 15 are available only to instructors online at Davis*Plus* (www.fadavis.com). Student feedback to guiding questions based on the answers developed by the case study contributors can be obtained from the course instructors(s).

🌐 VIEWING THE CASE: Patient With Cerebellar Glioblastoma

As students learn in different ways, the video case presentation (examination, intervention, and outcomes) is designed to promote engagement with the content, allow progression at an individual (or group) pace, and use of the medium or combination of media (written, visual, and auditory) best suited to the learner(s). The video, presented online at Davis*Plus* (www.fadavis.com), includes both visual and auditory modes.

Video Summary
The patient is a 71-year-old man with a large, right-sided cerebellar brain tumor status postresection and ongoing chemotherapy. The video shows examination and intervention segments for active rehabilitation episodes of care. Outcomes are filmed at 8 weeks after the initial examination.

🌐 **DavisPlus** For additional resources and to view the accompanying video associated with this case, please visit **www.davisplus.com.**

CASE STUDY

12

Patient With Guillain Barré Syndrome and Tetraplegia

KATE ROUGH, PT, DPT, NCS; VICTORIA STEVENS PT, NCS; STACIA LEE, PT, NCS; AND KATIE R. SWEET, PT, DPT

Examination

History

- **Demographic Information:**
  The patient is a 38-year-old man diagnosed with Guillain Barré syndrome (GBS).
- **History of Present Illness:**
  Approximately 4 weeks before his admission the patient began to notice sensory changes and distal weakness in his hands and feet following an upper respiratory infection. He also reported weakness of his arms and midline neck pain that radiated into both arms. During the acute care phase of his hospitalization, the patient was treated with two rounds of intravenous immunoglobulin (IVIG) infusions. Over a period of 3 weeks, his weakness progressed proximally through both legs and arms to his trunk and facial muscles. He was transferred to an inpatient rehabilitation facility for intensive speech, occupational, and physical therapy to maximize his communication skills, functional mobility, and ability to perform activities of daily living (ADL) before returning home with his family. At time of admission to inpatient rehabilitation, complications included atrial fibrillation, autonomic dysfunction, aspiration pneumonia, hyponatremia, panic attacks, dysphasia (requiring placement of a percutaneous endoscopic gastrostomy [PEG] tube and continuous feedings), and a 20-pound weight loss.
- **Medications:**
  - Enoxaparin 40 mg to prevent blood clots
  - Ocular lubricant one drop each eye every 12 hours to prevent dry eyes
  - Lansoprazole 30 mg for acid reflux
  - Lisinopril 10 mg for autonomic dysfunction
  - Metoprolol 50 mg for autonomic dysfunction
  - Pregabalin 25 mg for neuropathic pain
  - Promethazine 25 mg for nausea/vomiting
  - Acetaminophen-oxycodone 325 mg for pain as needed (PRN)
  - Bisacodyl 10 mg for constipation PRN
  - Hydromorphone 1 to 2 mg for pain PRN
  - Lorazepam 0.5 to 1 mg for anxiety PRN
  - Metoclopramide 5 mg for nausea PRN

- **Diagnostic Tests**
  - Lumbar puncture: elevated protein level consistent with GBS
  - Magnetic resonance imaging (MRI) of cervical spine: C7 neural foraminal narrowing indicating radiculopathy (right greater than left); mild canal narrowing at C6–C7 without cord impingement
  - Computerized tomography (CT) scan: atelectasis of lower lobe of the left lung
  - Modified barium swallow: good swallowing and control of yogurt and pudding (i.e., thick semisolid material); less than optimal handling of nectar thick and thick liquids with anterior penetration and significant tracheal aspiration
  - Electrocardiogram (EKG): atrial fibrillation
- **Medical History:**
  - Before the onset of GBS, the patient's medical history was unremarkable.
- **Social History:**
  The patient lives with his wife and two children, age six and three. They live in a one-story ranch style home with one stair to enter. The bathroom has a walk-in shower with grab bars. His wife is able to provide intermittent physical assistance and supervision. The patient is self-employed doing home remodeling and landscaping. He enjoys yard work and going out to dinner with his wife and friends.

Systems Review

- **Cardiovascular/Pulmonary:**
  - Temperature: 97.88°F (36.6°C)
  - Pulse: 100 beats per minute
  - Blood pressure: 129/88 mmHg
  - Respirations: 16 breaths/minute
  - Oxygen saturation: 91% (room air)
- **Integumentary:**
  - Skin is intact; however, patient has very little adipose tissue over bony prominences and is at high risk for skin breakdown.
- **Musculoskeletal:**
  - Height: 5 ft, 9 in.
  - Weight: 124.5 pounds
  - Body mass index (BMI): 18.2 kg/m^2

- Gross symmetry: Patient has a slight build with evidence of atrophy-based weight loss. He has a flat thoracic spine and slight forward head posture.
- Strength: bilateral impairments in upper and lower extremities
- Gross range of motion (ROM): tightness and pain bilaterally in shoulder flexion and abduction; decreased hamstring length
- Sensation: impaired light touch and proprioception
- Coordination: not tested secondary to weakness
- Postural control: Impaired
- **Language and Communication:**
The patient demonstrated dysarthric speech and was unable to produce facial expressions. Communication was also impaired by weak facial musculature. Owing to these deficits, it was difficult for him to communicate with his family and the rehabilitation staff.

Note: The patient experienced a panic attack during his acute care hospitalization. He also demonstrated some ongoing anxiety during his course of rehabilitation. He was very independent before developing GBS and was initially reluctant to seek assistance from family or staff.

Tests and Measures

- **Sensation:**
  - Light touch diminished bilaterally from elbow to hand and bilaterally from knees through the great toe and digits.
  - Proprioception absent at bilateral great toes; patient reports 3/6 trials correctly but admits to guessing on all trials.
- **Cranial Nerve (CN) Examination**
  - CN I: not tested
  - CN II: normal acuity in all visual fields
  - CN III/IV/VI: right eye difficulty adducting past midline leading to diplopia
  - CN V: intact sensation all three divisions, motor function intact
  - CN VII: impaired in all divisions of the facial nerve; unable to close eyes or open mouth
  - CV VIII: intact hearing
  - CN IX/X: autonomic dysfunction, no hoarseness, uvula midline
  - CN XI: symmetric weakness during shoulder shrug, graded 2/5
  - CN XII: tongue protrudes to midline without fasciculations or deviation
- **Coordination:**
  - Unable to perform coordination tests secondary to weakness
- **Postural Control:**
  - Unable to maintain static sitting without assistance; unable to support himself with upper extremities owing to weakness

- **Range of Motion:**
  - Upper extremity (UE) passive range of motion (PROM): within normal limits (WNL), except for shoulder flexion and shoulder abduction (See Table CS12.1.)
  - Lower extremity (LE) PROM: WNL, except for hip flexion with knee extension and ankle dorsiflexion (DF) (See Table CS12.2.)
- **Strength:**
  - Manual muscle test (MMT) scores: See Tables CS12.3 and CS12.4.
- **Gait and Wheelchair Mobility:**
  - Unable to ambulate owing to significant trunk and LE weakness
  - A tilt-in-space wheelchair required owing to poor sitting balance and trunk weakness
  - Dependent for wheelchair mobility and pressure relief

TABLE CS12.1 Upper Extremity PROM Measurements

Motion	Right	Left
Shoulder flexion	0–90°	0–150°
Shoulder abduction	0–70°	0–110°

TABLE CS12.2 Lower Extremity PROM Measurements

Motion	Right	Left
Hip flexion with knee extension	0–20°	0–20°
Ankle dorsiflexion	0–0°	0–0°

TABLE CS12.3 UE Manual Muscle Testing

Motion	Right	Left
Shoulder abduction	1	1
Shoulder flexion	1	1
Shoulder internal rotation	2+	2+
Shoulder external rotation	2+	2+
Elbow flexion	2	2+
Elbow extension	2–	2–
Wrist extension	1	1
Finger flexion	1	1
Finger abduction	1	1

TABLE CS12.4 Lower Extremity Manual Muscle Testing

Motion	Right	Left
Hip flexor	2–	2–
Hip abduction	2+	2+
Hip adduction	2+	2+
Knee extension	3+	3+
Dorsiflexion	2+	2+
Plantarflexion	2+	2+
Great toe extension	1	1

- **Pain:**
  - *Visual Analogue Scale (VAS):* 5/10 in both calves, as well as his PEG tube site.
- **Fatigue:**
  - *Modified Fatigue Impact Scale (MFI):* Total score: 40/84
    - Physical subscale: 25/36
    - Cognitive subscale: 10/40
    - Psychosocial subscale: 5/8
- **Balance:**
  - Timed sitting balance test: trial 1= 3 sec; trial 2 = 5 sec
  - *Modified Functional Reach Test* (measured from the acromion because the patient could not hold his arm at 90 degrees of flexion):
    - Forward average: 9.25 inches

- Right average: 6 inches
- Left average: 5.25 inches
- **Tone:**
  - Bilateral UEs: flaccid
  - Bilateral LEs: hypotonic
  - Modified Ashworth Scale: 0 for all major muscle groups in both upper and LEs
  - Clonus: absent in both LEs
  - Reflexes: diminished bilaterally at knee, biceps, and Achilles tendon
- **Mobility:**
  - *Boston University Activity Measure for Post Acute Care (AM-PAC)* "6-Click" Inpatient Short Form (Basic Mobility and Daily Activity domains): raw score 7/24, indicating maximal assistance required to perform functional mobility. (See Table CS12.5.)
  - *Functional Independence Measure* (FIM): total score: 52/126. (See Table CS12.6.)
    - Motor subscale: 18/91
    - Cognitive subscale: 34/35
- **Gait:**
  - Unable to perform examination of gait owing to weakness

Evaluation, Diagnosis and Prognosis, and Plan of Care

Note: Before considering the guiding questions below, view the Case Study 12 Examination segment of the video to enhance understanding of the patient's impairments and activity limitations. After completing the guiding questions, view the Case Study 12 Intervention segment of the video to

TABLE CS12.5 Boston University Activity Measure for Post Acute Care (AM-PAC) "6-Click" Inpatient Short Form (Basic Mobility and Daily Activity Domains)

How much difficulty does the patient currently have . . . ?	Unable/1	A Lot/2	A Little/3	None/4
Turning over in bed (including adjusting bedclothes, sheets, and blankets)		X		
Sitting down on and standing up from a chair with arms (e.g., wheelchair, bedside commode, etc.)	X			
Moving from lying on back to sitting on the edge of the bed	X			
How much help from another person does the patient currently need . . . ?	Unable/1	A Lot/2	A Little/3	None/4
Moving to and from a bed to a chair (including a wheelchair)	X			
Need to walk in hospital room	X			
Climbing steps with a railing	X			
Raw Score:	7			

TABLE CS12.6 Functional Independence Measure	
Self-Care	**Scoring**[a]
A. Eating	1
B. Grooming	1
C. Bathing	1
D. Dressing - Upper	1
E. Dressing - Lower	1
F. Toileting	1
Sphincter Control	
G. Bladder	1
H. Bowel	7
Transfers	
I. Bed, Chair, Wheelchair	1
J. Toilet	1
K. Tub, Shower	1
Locomotion	
L. Walk/Wheelchair	1
M. Stairs	1
Communication	
N. Comprehension (auditory)	7
O. Expression (vocal)	6
Social Cognition	
P. Social Interaction	7
Q. Problem Solving	7
R. Memory	7

[a]Scoring is as follows: 7 = complete independence (timely, safety); 6 = modified independence (device); 5 = supervision (subject = 100%); 4 = minimal assistance (subject = 75% or more); 3 = moderate assistance (subject = 50% or more); 2 = maximal assistance (subject = 25% or more); 1 = total assistance or not testable (subject less than 25%).

compare and contrast the interventions presented with those you selected. Last, progress to the Case Study 12 Outcomes segment of the video to compare and contrast the goals and expected outcomes you identified with the functional outcomes achieved.

Guiding Questions

1. Identify the physical therapy diagnosis.
   - Identify the impairments, activity limitations, and participation restrictions you will address in determining the prognosis and the plan of care.
   - Identify the practice pattern(s) consistent with the examination findings (physical therapy diagnosis) using the *Guide to Physical Therapy Practice.*
2. Establish anticipated goals (short term) and expected outcomes (long term). Include with each goal/outcome, the area of intended impact (using the list below).
   - Impact on impairments
   - Impact on activity limitations
   - Impact on participation restrictions
   - Impact on risk reduction/prevention
   - Impact on health, wellness, and fitness
   - Impact on patient/client satisfaction
3. Determine prognosis: Prognosis refers to *"the predicted optimal level of improvement in function and the amount of time needed to reach that level"* (*Guide to Physical Therapist Practice*).
   - Set a time frame for the episode of care.
   - Identify the number of visits per week needed to achieve the goals/outcomes.
4. Develop a plan of care. The plan of care should address each of the following components:
   - Interventions (in order of application with rationale)
   - Patient/client-related instruction
   - Required coordination, communication, and/or documentation
5. Describe the discharge plan. Your plan should include each of the following components of an effective discharge plan:
   - Patient, family, or caregiver education
   - Plans for appropriate follow-up care or referral to another agency
   - Instruction in a home exercise program (HEP)
   - Evaluation and modification of the home environment to assist the patient's return to home
6. What important safety precautions should be observed during treatment of this patient?

   Note: To allow instructors greater opportunity to integrate selected cases into assignments, laboratory activities, and/or class discussions, answers to the guiding questions for Case Studies 11 to 15 are available only to instructors online at Davis*Plus* (www.fadavis.com). Student feedback to guiding questions based on the answers developed by the case study contributors can be obtained from the course instructors(s).

As students learn in different ways, the video case presentation (examination, intervention, and outcomes) is designed to promote engagement with the content, allow progression at an individual (or group) pace, and use of the medium or combination of media (written, visual, and auditory) best suited to the learner(s). The video, presented online at Davis*Plus* (www.fadavis.com), includes both visual and auditory modes.

Video Summary

The patient is a 38-year-old man diagnosed with Guillain Barré syndrome. The video shows examination and intervention segments for active rehabilitation episodes of care. Outcomes are filmed at 6 weeks after the initial examination.

DavisPlus For additional resources and to view the accompanying video associated with this case, please visit **www.davisplus.com.**

Patient With Stroke

LAUREN SNOWDON, PT, DPT, ATP

Examination

History

- **Demographic Information:**
  The patient is a 55-year-old African American man presenting to inpatient rehabilitation status post left basal ganglia hemorrhage with right hemiparesis.
- **Medical History:**
  The patient has a medical history significant for hypertension, hyperlipidemia, and chronic renal insufficiency.
- **History of Present Illness:**
  The patient presented to the emergency room 1 week ago with a complaint of right-sided weakness and was noted to be hypertensive. During his acute hospital stay, he was found to be positive for right posterior tibial deep vein thrombosis (DVT), with resultant inferior vena cava (IVC) filter placement. His acute hospital course was otherwise uncomplicated, and he was transferred to inpatient rehabilitation to address the chief complaints of gait and balance deficits and difficulties with activities of daily living (ADL).
- **Diagnostic and Laboratory Findings:**
  - A computed axial tomography (CAT) scan of the brain revealed left basal ganglia hemorrhage with minimal mass effect (midline displacement) and no intraventricular hemorrhage. Magnetic resonance imaging (MRI) showed a 0.59-in. (1.5-cm) intracranial hemorrhage in the left basal ganglia region, left lateral thalamus, and left internal capsule. No neurosurgical intervention was recommended (the IVC filter was placed, as anticoagulation was contraindicated).
  - White blood cell count = 5.2, hemoglobin = 11.4, hematocrit = 34.7, platelets = 221.
- **Medications:**
  - Prior to admission: Zocor, Coreg, Lopressor
  - Admission medications: Labetalol, hydrochlorothiazide, Lotrel, Nexium, Singulair, Ambien
- **Social History:**
  Prior to admission, the patient was independent in ambulation without an assistive device and independent in all ADL. He lived alone in a two-level house with three steps to enter with one right-side railing. Inside the home, 12 steps lead to the second floor with a right-side railing, where the bedroom and bathroom are located. Both of his parents are alive and healthy, and the patient denies a family history of diabetes, hypertension, or stroke. The patient denies tobacco use and notes minimal use of alcohol for social occasions.
- **Employment:**
  Patient was employed full time as a registered nurse in a rehabilitation hospital, working a 12-hour overnight shift 3 or 4 days per week.

Systems Review

- **Cardiovascular/Respiratory:**
  - Heart rate: 68 beats per minute
  - Blood pressure: 108/76 mm Hg
  - Respiratory rate: 18 breaths per minute
- **Cognition and Communication:**
  - Alert and oriented times three and able to follow multistep commands.
  - Independent for basic and social communication; speech is fluent, with biographical naming intact.
  - Pleasant and cooperative throughout the examination process, with a mildly flat affect noted.
  - Mild difficulty with short- and long-term recall, number skills, concentration, and auditory comprehension/processing time.
- **Vision:**
  - Slight ptosis of right eye noted.
  - Extraocular motions intact, with pupils equally round and reactive to light and accommodation.
  - Reports no loss of vision, blurred vision, or double vision; wears glasses for distance.
- **Musculoskeletal System:**
  - Gross range of motion (ROM): Right lower extremity (LE) shows mild limitations, with greatest limitations in hip extension and ankle dorsiflexion (Table CS13.1).
  - Gross strength: Right LE shows mild losses in hip and knee strength, with greatest loss in ankle dorsiflexion (Table CS13.2).
  - Height: 6 ft, 5 in. (196 cm)
  - Weight: 230 lb (104 kg)
- **Neuromuscular System:**
  - Patient presents with decreased initiation of movement, decreased smooth coordinated movements, and diminished speed (velocity) of movement.

TABLE CS13.1 Lower Extremity Range of Motion (in degrees)

Joint	Motion	Right	Left
Hip	Flexion	0–100	0–110
	Extension	0–5	0–10
	Internal rotation	0–20	0–30
	External rotation	0–50	0–40
	Abduction	0–45	0–45
	Adduction	0–20	0–20
	Straight leg raise	0–70	0–85
Knee	Flexion	0–125	0–125
	Extension	0–0	0–0
Ankle	Dorsiflexion	0–2	0–8
	Plantarflexion	0–45	0–45

TABLE CS13.2 Muscle Test[a]

Joint	Motion	Right	Left
Hip	Flexion	3–/5	4+/5
	Extension	3+/5	5/5
	Internal rotation	4/5	4+/5
	External rotation	4/5	5/5
	Abduction	3+/5	5/5
	Adduction	4/5	5/5
Knee	Flexion	3/5	5/5
	Extension	3–/5	5/5
Ankle	Dorsiflexion	1/5	4+/5
	Plantarflexion	3/5	5/5

[a]All scores are based on a 0 to 5 scale: 5, normal; 4, good; 3, fair; 2, poor; 1, trace; 0, no contraction.

- Tone: Patient presents with hypotonia of right LE; tone within normal limits (WNL) in left LE.
- Patient is left-hand dominant.
- **Other Systems:**
  - No significant findings noted for integumentary, gastrointestinal, and genitourinary systems.

- Patient presents with no significant complaints of depression or change in mood and has no psychiatric history.

Tests and Measures

- **Edema (Circumferential Measurements):**
  - Right LE: 18.7 in. (47.5 cm) at midcalf, 13.2 in. (33.5 cm) at ankle, inferior to malleoli
  - Left LE: 17.9 in. (45.5 cm) at midcalf, 13.2 in. (33.5 cm) at ankle, inferior to malleoli
- **Sensory Integrity:**
  - Intact to light touch and pinprick in left LE
  - Decreased to light touch and pinprick throughout distal right LE, with inconsistent responses noted for L3–L5 dermatomes
- **Pain:**
  - Pain of 2/10 noted in distal right LE at rest (10 = worst pain; 0 = no pain).
  - Pain of 5/10 in right hamstring with standing or elongation (10 = worst pain; 0 = no pain).
- **Coordination:**
  - Demonstrates a positive response for finger-to-nose test (dysmetria) using right upper extremity (UE).
  - Positive right pronator drift evident (indicative of spasticity). Note: To test for pronator drift, the patient is asked to hold the position of 90 degrees of shoulder flexion, with the elbows extended, forearms supinated, and eyes closed. Forearm pronation indicates the patient has a pronator drift.
  - Difficulty noted with rapid alternating movements (dysdiadochokinesia) bilaterally, including forearm pronation/supination and foot tapping.
- **Posture**
  - Sitting: The patient sits with a forward head, rounded shoulders, increased thoracic kyphosis, reduced lumbar lordosis, and excessive posterior pelvic tilt (Fig. CS13.1); he also demonstrates a sloped right shoulder position with shortening of right-side trunk musculature (Fig. CS13.2). In sitting, the patient typically demonstrates excessive left lateral lean and increased weightbearing on the left ischial tuberosity.
  - Standing: The patient demonstrates decreased right knee (Fig. CS13.3) and hip extension in stance. When standing without an assistive device, the patient maintains a forwardly flexed posture (Fig. CS13.4) and requires minimal assistance.
- **Functional Status**
  - Wheelchair mobility: Moderate assistance is required to propel a wheelchair 10 ft (3 m).
  - Rolling: Supervision is required for rolling toward both left and right. Decreased initiation of movement is noted when rolling toward left side. Movement transitions for supine-to/from-prone require supervision.

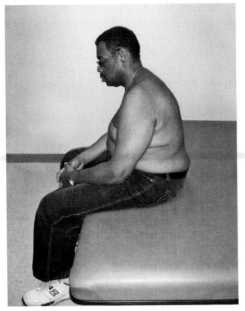

FIGURE CS13.1 Lateral view of seated posture Note the forward head, rounded shoulders, increased thoracic kyphosis, and reduced lumbar lordosis.

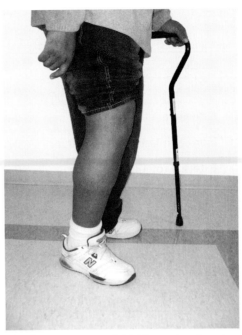

FIGURE CS13.3 Lateral view of right knee showing decreased knee extension in stance position. Although not visible here, diminished hip extension is also noted. Note swelling of right calf.

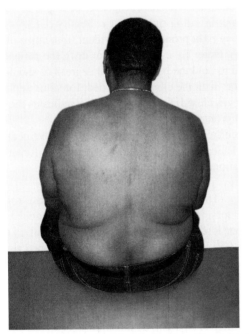

FIGURE CS13.2 Posterior view of seated posture The right shoulder is slightly lower than the left with shortening of right-side trunk musculature.

- Supine-to-sidelying-to-sitting: Close supervision is required from supine-to-sidelying on left. Minimal assistance is required from supine-to-sidelying on right, with use of bilateral UEs to assist in right LE management. Minimal assistance is required for moving from sidelying-to-sitting.
- Sit-to-supine: Close supervision is required. The patient uses both UEs and left LE to assist with right LE placement onto mat.

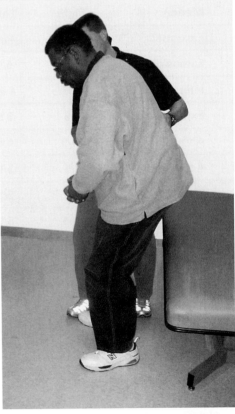

FIGURE CS13.4 Lateral view of standing posture without use of an assistive device. The patient assumes a forwardly flexed posture of head, neck, and trunk with increased hip and knee flexion. Minimal assistance from the therapist is required.

- Sit-to-stand: requires minimal assistance (Fig. CS13.5).
- Stand-to-sit: requires minimal assistance to control descent
- Sit-pivot transfer from wheelchair to mat: requires minimal assistance
- Sit-pivot transfer from mat to wheelchair: requires minimal assistance
- **Balance**
  - Static sitting balance: supervision
  - Dynamic sitting balance: supervision
  - Static standing balance: minimal assistance
  - Dynamic standing balance: minimal assistance
- **Ambulation**
  - Walks 5 ft (1.5 m) on level surfaces with minimal to moderate assistance using a narrow-base quadruped (quad) cane held in left hand
  - Demonstrates decreased thoracic trunk extension, excessive left lateral lean, and greater weightbearing through the less-involved left LE. During swing, there is insufficient right hip and knee flexion and ankle dorsiflexion (decreased foot clearance). During stance, there is

decreased right hip and knee extension. Decreased step length is noted bilaterally.
- Decreased endurance for upright standing and ambulation
- Stairs: unable to examine secondary to impairments in strength, balance, and tolerance for upright position
- **Patient's Goal**
  - "To walk and do things by myself at home and work."

Evaluation, Diagnosis and Prognosis, and Plan of Care

Note: Before considering the guiding questions below, view the Case Study 13 Examination segment of the video to enhance understanding of the patient's impairments and activity limitations. After completing the guiding questions, view the Case Study 13 Intervention segment of the video to compare and contrast the interventions presented with those you

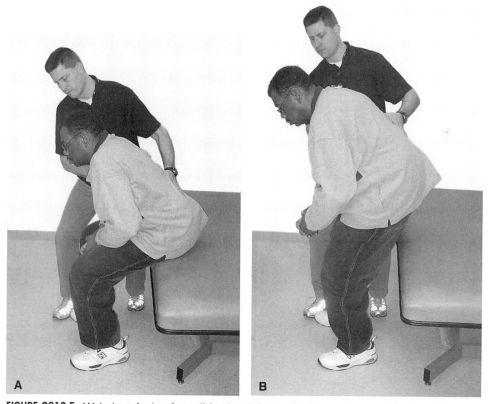

FIGURE CS13.5 (A) In transferring from sit-to-stand, the patient experiences difficulty with forward translation of the upper body over the feet. As the patient typically sits with a posterior pelvic tilt and increased thoracic kyphosis, he attempted to bring body weight forward by increasing thoracic kyphosis as he flexed the hips (body weight too far posterior). This brings the head forward but does not effectively translate the body mass horizontally. In addition, limitations in ankle ROM reduced the ability to position the feet behind the knees to allow the lower leg to rotate effectively over the foot. (B) Attempts to achieve upright standing posture and balance following sit-to-stand transfer. Note that the patient maintains a downward gaze toward the floor and keeps the upper trunk flexed (instead of extended) when weight is shifted forward. This posturing impairs his sense of postural alignment and vertical orientation.

selected. Last, progress to the Case Study 13 Outcomes segment of the video to compare and contrast the goals and expected outcomes you identified with the functional outcomes achieved.

Guiding Questions

1. Develop a clinical problem list for this patient, including the following:
   a. Impairments
   b. Activity limitations
   c. Participation restrictions
2. How might the patient's impairments in right ankle ROM and strength affect his gait?
   a. What phases of gait will be affected?
   b. Describe three interventions to address the impairments at the right ankle.
   c. If therapeutic interventions do not improve right ankle function, what compensatory strategies/devices might you consider?
3. In the inpatient rehabilitation setting, the patient receives 3 hours of therapy per day, 5 days a week. Establish one goal and a logical time frame for goal achievement for the following activity limitations:
   a. Sit-to/from-stand transfers
   b. Sit-pivot (lateral) transfers
   c. Ambulation
   d. Stair climbing

4. Based on the patient's clinical presentation, develop a plan of care (POC) for motor learning and describe appropriate strategies, including the following:
   a. Schedule of practice
   b. Types of feedback
   c. One other motor learning strategy to enhance achievement of this patient's outcomes
5. Based on the patient's goal of returning to home and work:
   a. Describe two task-specific treatments that will address the goal of *returning to work* as a nurse.
   b. Describe two task-specific treatments that will address the goal of *returning to home*.
6. The patient is unable to perform stair climbing.
   a. From a therapeutic exercise perspective, identify three muscle groups critical to the patient's ability to climb stairs and one exercise for each group identified.
   b. Describe one *part-task* and one *whole-task* practice strategy with a progression of each that could be used to improve the patient's ability to climb stairs.

   Note: To allow instructors greater opportunity to integrate selected cases into assignments, laboratory activities, and/or class discussions, answers to the guiding questions for Case Studies 11–15 are available only to instructors online at Davis*Plus* (www.fadavis.com). Student feedback to guiding questions based on the answers developed by the case study contributors can be obtained from the course instructors(s).

⊕ VIEWING THE CASE: Patient With Stroke

As students learn in different ways, the video case presentation (examination, intervention, and outcomes) is designed to promote engagement with the content, allow progression at an individual (or group) pace, and use of the medium or combination of media (written, visual, and auditory) best suited to the learner(s). The video, presented online at Davis*Plus* (www.fadavis.com), includes both visual and auditory modes.

Video Summary
Patient is a 55-year-old man with stroke and right hemiparesis. The video shows examination and intervention segments during inpatient rehabilitation. Outcomes are filmed after 4 weeks.

⊕ **Davis*Plus***   For additional resources and to view the accompanying video associated with this case, please visit **www.davisplus.com**.

14 Patient With Motor Incomplete Spinal Cord Injury, C4

Sally Taylor, PT, DPT, NCS

Examination

History

- **Demographic Information:**
  The patient is a 50-year-old, married, Caucasian, English-speaking man.
- **History of Present Illness:**
  The patient slipped and fell backward while walking his dog outside the home. He did not lose consciousness, but was immediately unable to move his arms or legs and experienced altered sensation below the neck. Magnetic resonance imaging (MRI) revealed a spinal cord contusion, cord stenosis, and cord compression between C2 and C4. He underwent spinal fusion of C2-C4 with posterior cervical laminectomy and lateral plating.
- **Admitting Diagnosis:**
  The admitting diagnosis was C4 spinal cord injury (SCI). Based on the American Spinal Injury Association Impairment Scale (AIS), the lesion was designated as a Category C: Incomplete. Sensory and motor function is preserved below the neurological level and includes the sacral segments S4-S5. The patient was admitted wearing a cervical orthosis (Fig. CS14.1).
- **Medical History:**
  Hypertension and hyperlipidemia (no medications prior to admission)
- **Surgical History:**
  None prior to admission
- **Social History:**
  The patient enjoys his work, family, grandchildren, and attending college athletic events. He works at a nuclear power plant full time as the director of maintenance.
- **Living Environment:**
  He lives in a ranch-style home with one step to enter with a tub/shower combination in the bathroom.
- **Prior Level of Function:**
  He was fully independent prior to the accident and stayed active by walking his dog daily.

Systems Review

- **Cardiovascular/Pulmonary System:**
  - Heart rate: 49 beats per minute (BPM)
  - Respiratory rate: 18 BPM
  - Blood pressure: 128/69
- **Musculoskeletal System:**
  - Gross range of motion (ROM):
    - Bilateral upper extremities (UEs): within normal limits (WNL)
    - Bilateral lower extremities (LEs): WNL except for straight-leg raise bilaterally owing to hamstring tightness; tightness also noted in hip rotation
  - Gross strength: Significant weakness noted in bilateral UE and LE (Fig. CS14.2).
- **Neuromuscular System:**
  - Sensation: light touch intact bilateral UEs and right LE; reduced light touch noted in left LE
  - Normal reflexes (2+) on bilateral UE and LE
  - Rectal tone present with voluntary anal contraction

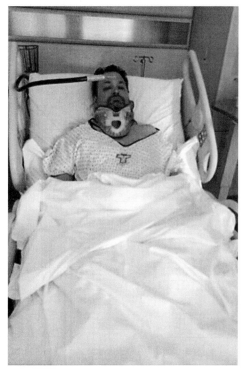

FIGURE CS14.1 The patient was admitted to the inpatient rehabilitation unit wearing a cervical orthosis. He was provided with a sip-and-puff call light in his room.

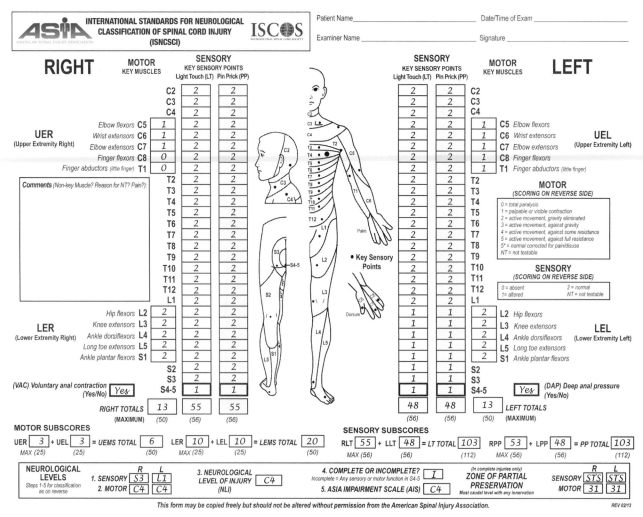

FIGURE CS14.2 Sensory and motor scores American Spinal Injury Association. International Standards for Neurological Classification of Spinal Cord Injury, rev 2013. Atlanta, GA, American Spinal Injury Association, 2013, with permission.

- Coordination: unable to perform owing to decreased strength
- Postural control: requires maximal assistance
- Balance: requires maximal assistance
- Gait: nonambulatory
- **Integumentary System:**
  - No abrasions noted
  - No pressure ulcers noted

Test and Measures

- **Sitting Balance:**
  - Maximal assistance for short-sitting balance on mat without UE support
  - Minimal assistance for short-sitting balance on mat with bilateral UE support for 30 seconds
  - *Modified Functional Reach Test:* unable to complete secondary to loss of balance

- **Transfers, Locomotion, and Upright Tolerance:**
  - Functional Independence Measure (FIM)
    - Transfers bed = 1 (Fig. CS14.3)
    - Transfers toilet = 1
    - Transfers tub/shower = 1
    - Locomotion wheelchair = 1
    - Locomotion stairs = 1
  - Upright tolerance: impaired tolerance on tilt table (Fig. CS14.4)

  Note: The following examination data is based on the *International Standards for Neurological Classification of Spinal Cord Injury (ISNCSCI)* (see Fig. CS14.2).

- **Sensation:**
  - Pinprick
    - Right: normal for C2-S3 segments; impaired for S4-5
    - Left: normal for C2-L1 segments; impaired for L2-S4-5

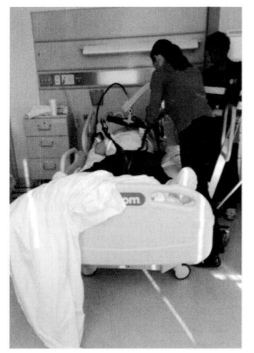

FIGURE CS14.3 The patient is initially transferred from hospital bed to wheelchair using a hydraulic lift and two-person assist to ensure safety.

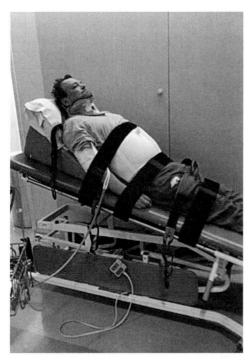

FIGURE CS14.4 Upright tolerance is initiated with a tilt table. Vital signs are closely monitored.

- Light touch
  - Right: normal for C2-S3 segments; impaired for S4-5
  - Left: normal for C2-L1 segments, impaired for L2-S4-5
- Deep anal sensation present

- **Muscle Performance:**
  - ASIA motor test (see Fig. CS14.2)
  - Strength C5 1/5 bilaterally; C6 1/5 bilaterally; C7 1/5 bilaterally; C8 0/5 bilaterally; T1 0/5 bilaterally
  - Strength L2-S1 2/5 bilaterally
  - Voluntary anal contraction
- **ASIA Impairment Scale:**
  - Based on the ASIA Impairment Scale (Box CS14.1), the patient is classified as a sensory and motor incomplete SCI (Category C = Incomplete: motor function is present below the neurological level and has a muscle grade of 2).

Evaluation, Diagnosis and Prognosis, and Plan of Care

Note: Before considering the guiding questions below, view the Case Study 14 Examination segment of the video to enhance understanding of the patient's impairments and activity limitations. After completing the guiding questions, view the Case Study 14 Intervention segment of the video to compare and contrast the interventions presented with those you selected. Last, progress to the Case Study 14 Outcomes segment of the video to compare and contrast the goals and expected outcomes you identified with the functional outcomes achieved.

Guiding Questions

1. Using the *Guide to Physical Therapy Practice*, identify the primary practice pattern consistent with examination findings.
2. Describe the patient's presentation using the domains (i.e., body function and structure, activity limitations, and participation restrictions) included in the International Classification of Functioning, Disability, and Health (ICF) adopted by the World Health Organization (WHO).
3. At what point during the course of his recovery should you initiate upright positioning in standing to prepare for progression of gait training?
4. What is the neurological level of injury? What features of the clinical presentation place the patient in a classification of C of the American Spinal Injury Association Impairment Scale (ASI)?
5. What interventions would you include in the plan of care (POC) for this patient?
6. What devices or adaptive equipment are required for safe return to the home environment?
7. What outcomes (long-term goals) would you establish for this patient?
8. What duration of inpatient rehabilitation would you anticipate for this patient?
9. As the patient presents with an incomplete injury, what tests and measures would be indicated on a regular basis?

BOX CS14.1 ASIA Impairment Scale (AIS)[a]

A = Complete. No sensory or motor function is preserved in the sacral segments S4-5.

B = Sensory Incomplete. Sensory but not motor function is preserved below the neurological level and includes the sacral segments S4-5 (light touch or pin prick at S4-5 or deep anal pressure) AND no motor function is preserved more than three levels below the motor level on either side of the body.

C = Motor Incomplete. Motor function is preserved below the neurological level**, and more than half of key muscle functions below the neurological level of injury (NLI) have a muscle grade less than 3 (Grades 0–2).

D = Motor Incomplete. Motor function is preserved below the neurological level**, and at least half (half or more) of key muscle functions below the NLI have a muscle grade ≥ 3.

E = Normal. If sensation and motor function as tested with the ISNCSCI are graded as normal in all segments, and the patient had prior deficits, then the AIS grade is E. Someone without an initial SCI does not receive an AIS grade.

Note: When assessing the extent of motor sparing below the level for distinguishing between AIS B and C, the ***motor level*** on each side is used; whereas to differentiate between AIS C and D (based on proportion of key muscle functions with strength grade 3 or greater) the ***neurological level of injury*** is used.

[a]From American Spinal Injury Association. International Standards for Neurological Classification of Spinal Cord Injury. Atlanta, GA, American Spinal Injury Association, 2006. Used with permission. (*Note:* An overview of changes with the new ISNCSCI worksheet is available at www.asia-spinalinjury.org/elearning/ISNCSCI.php [retrieved April 6, 2015]).

**For an individual to receive a grade of C or D, that is, motor incomplete status, they must have either (1) voluntary anal sphincter contraction or (2) sacral sensory sparing <u>with</u> sparing of motor function more than three levels below the motor level for that side of the body. The International Standards at this time allows even non–key muscle function more than three levels below the motor level to be used in determining motor incomplete status (AIS B versus C).

10. Is there any type of clinical predication rule that can be utilized to predict the patient's ability to return to an ambulatory level? If yes, what score would you anticipate the patient to achieve?

Note: To allow instructors greater opportunity to integrate selected cases into assignments, laboratory activities, and/or class discussions, answers to the guiding questions for Case Studies 11–15 are available only to instructors online at Davis*Plus* (www.fadavis.com). Student feedback to guiding questions based on the answers developed by the case study contributors can be obtained from the course instructors(s).

VIEWING THE CASE: Patient With Motor Incomplete Spinal Cord Injury, C4

As students learn in different ways, the video case presentation (examination, intervention, and outcomes) is designed to promote engagement with the content, allow progression at an individual (or group) pace, and use of the medium or combination of media (written, visual, and auditory) best suited to the learner(s). The video, presented online at Davis*Plus* (www.fadavis.com), includes both visual and auditory modes.

Video Summary
Patient is a 50-year-old man with a motor incomplete SCI, C4 undergoing active rehabilitation. The video shows examination and intervention segments during inpatient rehabilitation. Outcomes are filmed 7 weeks after initial examination.

Davis*Plus* For additional resources and to view the accompanying video associated with this case, please visit **www.davisplus.com.**

REFERENCES

1. American Spinal Injury Association (ASIS). International Standards for Neurological Classification of Spinal Cord Injury Clinical Summary. Atlanta, GA, American Spinal Injury Association, 2013 Retrieved March 26, 2015, from www.scireproject.com/outcome-measures-new/american-spinal-injury-association-impairment-scale-ais-international-standards.

2. Kirshblum S, and Waring W. Updates for the International Standards for Neurological Classification of Spinal Cord Injury. Phys Med Rehabil Clin N Am, 2014; 25:505–517.

3. Kirshblum S, et al. International Standards for Neurological Classification of Spinal Cord Injury. J Spinal Cord Med, 2011; 34: 535–46.

CASE STUDY
15
Patient With Transfemoral Amputation

Kyla L. Dunlavey, PT, MPT, OCS, and Barri L. Schnall, PT, MPT

Examination

History

- **Demographic Information:**
The patient is a 23-year-old man, status posttraumatic left transfemoral amputation secondary to military trauma. In addition to the amputation, he sustained bilateral femoral fractures, comminuted right fibular and medial malleolar fractures, and trauma to internal organs. He is status post-open reduction internal fixation of the distal fibula with side plate and screw fixation.

- **History of Present Illness:**
Owing to his age and excellent premorbid fitness level, the patient progressed rapidly through an initial intensive (5 day per week) rehabilitation program. Within 4 months of injury, he achieved modified independence in ambulation (single point cane) on level surfaces, uneven terrain and elevations (community distances). At 6 months, the patient was cleared to pursue college classes. Although pain was not an issue, efficiency of gait was impaired, and the patient was having difficulty negotiating on campus.

- **Medical History:**
Unremarkable

- **Social History/Prior Level of Function:**
Patient was an active-duty service member in peak physical condition. He lives with his girlfriend on the lower floor of an elevator building. He has recently obtained a service dog. The dog's role is to provide physical support and assistance to his owner. An additional benefit is the emotional calming that comes from the bond established. This emotional support is especially important when the service member is walking in a new or busy environment.

He returns to outpatient physical therapy to achieve his long-term goal of being able to run. In the short term, he would like to improve the quality and efficiency of walking without using a cane in the community. At initial examination, he is wearing his prosthesis 10 hours per day without excess pressure or compromised skin integrity. He has a definitive carbon fiber socket with flexible inner liner, suction suspension, four-ply socks, microprocessor knee, and a K4 level energy storage and return foot. Dual x-ray absorptiometry (DEXA) scan results are acceptable, indicating that bone density is sufficient to progress to higher impact activities without increased risk of fracture.

Systems Review

- **Cardiovascular System:**
  - Vital signs: within normal limits (WNL)
  - Patient reports ongoing use of rowing machine and hand crank bike for 30 minutes, three times per week.
- **Integumentary System:**
  - Skin on residual limb is intact without evidence of focal pressure points, callous, blisters, or adhesions. (See Fig. CS15.1.)
  - Intact limb presents mild adhesions at scared area (anteriorly at level of midtibia and malleoli). Femoral scars from external fixation hardware are mobile.
- **Neuromuscular System:**
  - Denies phantom sensation or pain
  - Right foot intact for light touch with paresthesia at scars sites
  - Proprioception intact
  - Balance impaired
- **Musculoskeletal System:**
  - Well-developed upper body and core musculature
  - Posture in standing: Center of mass (COM) is shifted over the intact limb. Although subtle, it results in relative adduction of the right lower extremity (LE). In addition, the pelvis is slightly retracted on the left as determined by palpation of the iliac crests. Palpation helps to differentiate between potential leg length discrepancy versus

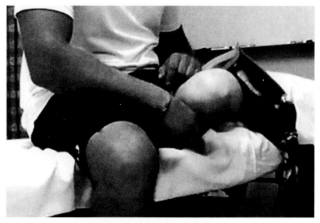

FIGURE CS15.1 Residual limb skin inspection reveals a well-shaped limb free of abrasions, cuts, and other skin problems.

compensatory postural adaptations. There is an anterior pelvic tilt and resultant increase in trunk extension.
• Left hip range of motion (ROM) is limited.

Tests and Measures

• **Cognition:**
  • No barriers to learning were identified.
  • Patient denies symptoms of posttraumatic stress disorder (PTSD).
• **Range of Motion:**
  • Upper extremities (UEs): WNL
  • LEs: Left hip lacks 10 degrees to full extension with springy end-feel; right LE WNL except for limited ankle eversion.
• **Strength:**
  • UEs and LEs: 5/5 (available musculature) on manual muscle test (MMT)
  • Impaired functional strength demonstrated by inability to perform single-leg squat with his prosthetic limb on the Power Tower (resistive exercise unit) at maximum height. Prior to physical therapy intervention, the patient achieved 34% body weight (65% after 24 treatment sessions) (see Fig. CS 15.2).
• **Balance:**
  • Standing balance impaired: unable to perform single limb stance (SLS) on left LE without UE support
  • Right LE SLS is mildly impaired owing to ankle trauma with a duration of 25 seconds before physical therapy with progression to 60 seconds after 24 treatment sessions.
• **Pain:**
  • Denied, no medications
• **Functional Status:**
  • Bed mobility: The patient is independent with and without prosthesis.

• Transfers: Sit-to-stand is at the level of modified independence from standard height surface. Quality of movement is compromised; the patient minimizes weightbearing on the prosthetic limb. Floor-to-stand transfer is also at the modified independence level.
• Gait: Patient is able to ambulate without an assistive device, but gait deviations become magnified. The most obvious deviations are increased lateral trunk flexion, rotation, and pelvic obliquity and left LE abduction.
• Stairs/ramps: Patient demonstrates modified independence using a step-to gait.
• **Functional Outcome Measures:**
  • *Timed Up and Go* (TUG): 19 seconds with cane
  • *Six Minute Walk Test* (6 MWT): 265 meters with cane
  • *Four Square Step Test* (4 SST): 27 seconds with assistive device
  • *Stair Assessment Index* (SAI): 2/13
  • *Hill Assessment Index* (HAI): 0/11
  • *Comprehensive High-Level Activity Mobility Predictor* (CHAMP)[1]
    • Single limb stance: unable to perform on left LE without UE support; 25 seconds on right LE
    • Edgren side step: 6 cones
    • T-Test: 1:20 seconds
    • Illinois Agility Test: 1:55 seconds (Fig. CS15.3)

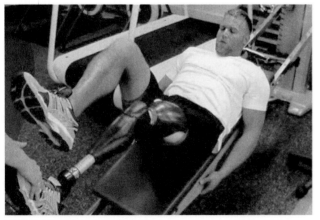

FIGURE CS15.2 Patient performing single-leg squat.

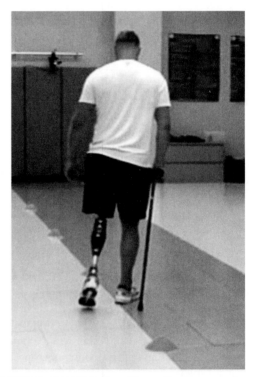

FIGURE CS15.3 CHAMP Testing: The patient weaves through cones as he negotiates the Illinois Agility Test component of the CHAMP.

Evaluation, Diagnosis and Prognosis, and Plan of Care

Note: Before considering the guiding questions below, view the Case Study 15 Examination segment of the video to enhance understanding of the patient's impairments and activity limitations. After completing the guiding questions, view the Case Study 15 Intervention segment of the video to compare and contrast the interventions presented with those you selected. Last, progress to the Case Study 15 Outcomes segment of the video to compare and contrast the goals and expected outcomes you identified with the functional outcomes achieved.

Guiding Questions

1. What possible implications or impact could data from the patient history and systems review have on patient performance during the initial examination?
2. Identify the patient's impairments.
3. Develop anticipated short-term goals to be achieved in 4 to 6 weeks. Provide an example of the intended impact on function for each goal.
4. Consider the following primary impairments: (a) decreased hip extension ROM in residual limb, (b) impaired motor planning and balance, and (c) diminished endurance. Discuss the functional implication of addressing these impairments early in the plan of care.
5. Describe treatment interventions to address balance, strength, and motor control that could be used during the first weeks of therapy. Indicate how you would progress each.
6. What information should the physical therapist provide the patient, family, and/or the interdisciplinary team to promote desired outcomes?
7. What limiting factor might affect the patient's return to high-level activities? What are the patient's assets? What discharge recommendations will you make?
8. How many weeks of treatment do you anticipate being needed before discharge?

   Note: To allow instructors greater opportunity to integrate selected cases into assignments, laboratory activities, and/or class discussions, answers to the guiding questions for Case Studies 11 to 15 are available only to instructors online at Davis*Plus* (www.fadavis.com). Student feedback to guiding questions based on the answers developed by the case study contributors can be obtained from the course instructors(s).

 VIEWING THE CASE: Patient With Transfemoral Amputation

As students learn in different ways, the video case presentation (examination, intervention, and outcomes) is designed to promote engagement with the content, allow progression at an individual (or group) pace, and use of the medium or combination of media (written, visual, and auditory) best suited to the learner(s). The video, presented online at Davis*Plus* (www.fadavis.com), includes both visual and auditory modes.

Video Summary

The patient is a 23-year-old man, status posttraumatic left transfemoral amputation secondary to military trauma. The video shows examination and intervention segments for outpatient rehabilitation episodes of care. Outcomes are filmed at 12 weeks after the initial examination.

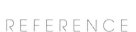 For additional resources and to view the accompanying video associated with this case, please visit **www.davisplus.com.**

REFERENCE

1. Gailey, RS, et al. Construct validity of Comprehensive High-Level Activity Mobility Predictor (CHAMP) for male service members with traumatic lower-limb loss. J Rehabil Res Dev, 2013; 50:919.

INDEX

Note: Page numbers followed by *b* indicates boxes; *f*, figures; *t*, tables.